MILD TRAUMATIC BRAIN INJURY
IN CHILDREN AND ADOLESCENTS

Also from Keith Owen Yeates

Pediatric Neuropsychology, Second Edition:
Research, Theory, and Practice
*Edited by Keith Owen Yeates, M. Douglas Ris,
H. Gerry Taylor, and Bruce F. Pennington*

MILD TRAUMATIC BRAIN INJURY IN CHILDREN AND ADOLESCENTS

From Basic Science to Clinical Management

EDITED BY

Michael W. Kirkwood
Keith Owen Yeates

THE GUILFORD PRESS
New York   London

Last digit is print number: 9   8   7   6   5   4   3   2   1

The authors have checked with sources believed to be reliable in their efforts to provide information that is complete and generally in accord with the standards of practice that are accepted at the time of publication. However, in view of the possibility of human error or changes in behavioral, mental health, or medical sciences, neither the authors, nor the editors and publisher, nor any other party who has been involved in the preparation or publication of this work warrants that the information contained herein is in every respect accurate or complete, and they are not responsible for any errors or omissions or the results obtained from the use of such information. Readers are encouraged to confirm the information contained in this book with other sources.

Library of Congress Cataloging-in-Publication Data

Mild traumatic brain injury in children and adolescents: from basic science to clinical management / edited by Michael W. Kirkwood, Keith Owen Yeates.
    p. cm.
  Includes bibliographical references and index.
  ISBN 978-1-4625-0513-5 (hardback)
  1. Brain-damaged children—Rehabilitation. 2. Brain—Wounds and injuries—Patients—Rehabilitation. I. Kirkwood, Michael W. II. Yeates, Keith Owen.
  RJ496.B7M53 2012
  617.4′81044—dc23

                                                2012007610

To Jen and Finn, who frame my life's most important work,
and to my parents, who taught me early
the value of both knowledge and diligence
—M. W. K.

To Kiernan and Taylor, my amazing daughters,
who help me keep life in perspective
—K. O. Y.

About the Editors

Michael W. Kirkwood, PhD, ABPP, is Associate Clinical Professor in the Department of Physical Medicine and Rehabilitation at the University of Colorado School of Medicine and codirects the Children's Hospital Colorado Concussion Program in Aurora. He holds a Diplomate in Clinical Neuropsychology from the American Board of Professional Psychology. Dr. Kirkwood is a board member of the American Academy of Clinical Neuropsychology and has served as president of the Colorado Neuropsychological Society. He is an investigator or co-investigator for several state- and federally funded studies aimed at characterizing and treating the effects of pediatric traumatic brain injury, with a number of current projects focused on understanding persistent problems following concussion. Dr. Kirkwood is on the editorial board of *Child Neuropsychology* and serves as a reviewer for many neuropsychological and medical journals. A lecturer both nationally and internationally on traumatic brain injury in children and teens, Dr. Kirkwood is the author of more than 25 journal articles and book chapters and coauthor of the book *Board Certification in Clinical Neuropsychology: A Guide to Becoming ABPP/ABCN Certified without Sacrificing Your Sanity* (2008).

Keith Owen Yeates, PhD, ABPP, is Professor in the Departments of Pediatrics, Psychology, and Psychiatry at The Ohio State University College of Medicine. He is Director of the Center for Biobehavioral Health at The Research Institute and Chief of the Section of Pediatric Psychology and Neuropsychology, both at Nationwide Children's Hospital in Columbus. Dr. Yeates holds a Diplomate in Clinical Neuropsychology from the American Board of Professional Psychology and is a Fellow of the American Psychological Association. He has served as president of the Division of Clinical Neuropsychology of the American Psychological Association and of the Association of Postdoctoral Programs in Clinical Neuropsychology. Dr. Yeates was named the Canadian Association of Child Neurology John Tibbles Lecturer by the Royal College of Physicians and Surgeons of Canada in 2004, was a Visiting Fellow of the Australian Psychological Society in 2006, and was the recipient of the Arthur Benton Award from the International Neuropsychological Society in 2011 and the Independent Scientist Career Development Award from the National Institutes of

Health from 2003 to 2008. He has received extensive external grant funding for research that focuses on the neurobehavioral outcomes of childhood brain injuries and disorders. Dr. Yeates is Associate Editor of the *Journal of the International Neuropsychological Society*, serves on the editorial boards of several other neuropsychology journals, and has been a regular member of three federal grant review panels. He is the author of over 115 peer-reviewed journal articles and 35 book chapters and coeditor of *Pediatric Neuropsychology: Research, Theory, and Practice* (2nd edition; 2010).

Contributors

Stephen Ashwal, MD, Department of Pediatrics, Loma Linda University, Loma Linda, California

Gunes Avci, PhD, Cognitive Neuroscience Laboratory, Department of Physical Medicine and Rehabilitation, Baylor College of Medicine, Houston, Texas

Talin Babikian, PhD, ABPP, Department of Psychiatry and Biobehavioral Sciences, David Geffen School of Medicine, University of California, Los Angeles, Los Angeles, California

Jerome Badaut, PhD, Departments of Pediatrics and Physiology, Loma Linda University, Loma Linda, California

Brenda Bartnik-Olson, PhD, Department of Radiology, Loma Linda University, Loma Linda, California

Rachel P. Berger, MD, MPH, Safar Center for Resuscitation Research, Department of Pediatrics, Children's Hospital of Pittsburgh of UPMC, Pittsburgh, Pennsylvania

Doug Bodin, PhD, ABPP, Department of Psychology, Nationwide Children's Hospital, Columbus, Ohio

Gerald H. Clayton, PhD, Department of Physical Medicine and Rehabilitation, University of Colorado School of Medicine, and Children's Hospital Colorado, Aurora, Colorado

Jacqueline S. Coats, BA, Department of Biophysics and Bioengineering, Loma Linda University, Loma Linda, California

R. Dawn Comstock, PhD, Center for Injury Research and Policy, The Research Institute at Nationwide Children's Hospital; Department of Pediatrics, The Ohio State University College of Medicine; and Division of Epidemiology, The Ohio State University, College of Public Health, Columbus, Ohio

Gavin A. Davis, MBBS, FRACS, Department of Neurosurgery, Cabrini Hospital, Malvern, Victoria, Australia

John DiFiori, MD, Division of Sports Medicine, David Geffen School of Medicine, University of California, Los Angeles, Los Angeles, California

Jeanne E. Dise-Lewis, PhD, Department of Physical Medicine and Rehabilitation, University of Colorado School of Medicine, and Children's Hospital Colorado, Aurora, Colorado

Jacobus Donders, PhD, ABPP, Psychology Service, Mary Free Bed Hospital, Grand Rapids, Michigan

Isabelle Gagnon, PT, PhD, School of Physical and Occupational Therapy, McGill University, and Trauma Programs, The Montreal Children's Hospital, McGill University Health Center, Montreal, Quebec, Canada

Gerard A. Gioia, PhD, Division of Pediatric Neuropsychology, Children's National Medical Center, Rockville, Maryland

Christopher C. Giza, MD, Department of Neurosurgery, David Geffen School of Medicine, University of California, Los Angeles, Los Angeles, California

Grace S. Griesbach, PhD, Department of Neurosurgery, David Geffen School of Medicine, University of California, Los Angeles, Los Angeles, California

Joseph A. Grubenhoff, MD, Section of Emergency Medicine, Department of Pediatrics, University of Colorado School of Medicine, and Children's Hospital Colorado, Aurora, Colorado

Kevin M. Guskiewicz, PhD, Department of Exercise and Sport Science, University of North Carolina at Chapel Hill, Chapel Hill, North Carolina

Gerri Hanten, PhD, Cognitive Neuroscience Laboratory, Department of Physical Medicine and Rehabilitation, Baylor College of Medicine, Houston, Texas

Richard Hartman, PhD, Department of Psychology, Loma Linda University, Loma Linda, California

Barbara A. Holshouser, PhD, Department of Radiology, Loma Linda University, Loma Linda, California

Lei Huang, MD, Department of Biophysics and Bioengineering, Loma Linda University, Loma Linda, California

Alyssa P. Ibarra, BS, Cognitive Neuroscience Laboratory, Department of Physical Medicine and Rehabilitation, Baylor College of Medicine, Houston, Texas

Grant L. Iverson, PhD, Faculty of Medicine, Department of Psychiatry, University of British Columbia, Vancouver, British Columbia, Canada

Jennifer A. Janusz, PsyD, ABPP, Department of Pediatrics, University of Colorado School of Medicine, Aurora, Colorado

James P. Kelly, MD, FAAN, Department of Neurosurgery, University of Colorado School of Medicine, Aurora, Colorado

John W. Kirk, PsyD, ABPP, Department of Physical Medicine and Rehabilitation, University of Colorado School of Medicine, and Children's Hospital Colorado, Aurora, Colorado

Michael W. Kirkwood, PhD, ABPP, Department of Physical Medicine and Rehabilitation, University of Colorado School of Medicine, and Children's Hospital Colorado, Aurora, Colorado

Harvey S. Levin, PhD, ABPP, Cognitive Neuroscience Laboratory, Departments of Physical Medicine and Rehabilitation, Neurology, and Neurosurgery, Baylor College of Medicine, Houston, Texas

Kelsey Logan, MD, MPH, Departments of Internal Medicine and Pediatrics, The Ohio State University College of Medicine, and Department of Athletics, The Ohio State University, Columbus, Ohio

Stephen R. McCauley, PhD, Cognitive Neuroscience Laboratory, Departments of Physical Medicine and Rehabilitation, Neurology, and Pediatrics, Baylor College of Medicine, Houston, Texas

Michael McCrea, PhD, ABPP, Department of Neurosurgery, Medical College of Wisconsin, Milwaukee, Wisconsin

Audrey McKinlay, PhD, Department of Psychology, University of Canterbury, Christchurch, New Zealand; School of Psychology and Psychiatry, Monash University, Melbourne, Australia

Tamara C. Valovich McLeod, PhD, ATC, Athletic Training Program, A. T. Still University, Mesa, Arizona

Jason P. Mihalik, PhD, ATC, Matthew Gfeller Sport-Related Traumatic Brain Injury and Research Center, Department of Exercise and Sport Science, University of North Carolina at Chapel Hill, Chapel Hill, North Carolina

Andre Obenaus, PhD, Department of Pediatrics, Loma Linda University, Loma Linda, California

Aaron Provance, MD, Department of Orthopaedics, University of Colorado School of Medicine, and Children's Hospital Colorado, Aurora, Colorado

Christopher Randolph, PhD, ABPP, Department of Neurology, Loyola University Medical Center, Chicago, Illinois

Maegan D. Sady, PhD, Division of Pediatric Neuropsychology, Children's National Medical Center, Rockville, Maryland

Nicole Shay, PhD, Outpatient Services, Emma Pendleton Bradley Hospital, East Providence, Rhode Island

Beth Slomine, PhD, ABPP, Department of Neuropsychology, Kennedy Krieger Institute, Johns Hopkins University, Baltimore, Maryland

H. Gerry Taylor, PhD, ABPP, Department of Pediatrics, Case Western Reserve University, Rainbow Babies and Children's Hospital, University Hospitals Case Medical Center, Cleveland, Ohio

Karen A. Tong, MD, Department of Radiology, Loma Linda University, Loma Linda, California

Elisabeth A. Wilde, PhD, Cognitive Neuroscience Laboratory, Departments of Physical Medicine and Rehabilitation, Neurology, and Radiology, Baylor College of Medicine, Houston, Texas

Pamela E. Wilson, MD, Department of Physical Medicine and Rehabilitation, University of Colorado School of Medicine, and Children's Hospital Colorado, Aurora, Colorado

Keith Owen Yeates, PhD, ABPP, Departments of Pediatrics, Psychology, and Psychiatry, The Ohio State University College of Medicine, and Center for Biobehavioral Health, The Research Institute at Nationwide Children's Hospital, Columbus, Ohio

Noel Zuckerbraun, MD, Safar Center for Resuscitation Research, Department of Pediatrics, Children's Hospital of Pittsburgh of UPMC, Pittsburgh, Pennsylvania

Preface

Mild traumatic brain injury (mTBI) has been recognized as a distinct form of head injury for centuries but has been largely neglected historically as a topic of scientific interest. Since the early 1990s, however, the attention devoted to concussion and other types of mTBI has grown exponentially. Indeed, over the last few years, one would be hard pressed to identify another medical condition that has received as much scientific or popular scrutiny. Even so, pediatric mTBI remains a frequent source of misunderstanding, confusion, and controversy.

With these issues in mind, we thought the time was right to assemble an authoritative book focused on mTBI in children and teens. In our initial discussions, we agreed that the book's ultimate utility would depend on finding a diverse collection of authors who could provide a cutting-edge, comprehensive synthesis of the most important advances and findings in the field. Fortunately, a multidisciplinary group of preeminent pediatric clinicians and researchers agreed to contribute, and the resulting book thoroughly covers mTBI from the disciplines of neuroscience, medicine, neuropsychology, and athletics.

This book is intended to serve as a primary resource or general reference for professionals who work with children and teens who have suffered mTBI. The intended audience is diverse and includes health care providers and researchers; students in neuropsychology, psychology, neurology, sports medicine, rehabilitation, primary care, emergency medicine, and the basic neurosciences; and school nurses, school psychologists, special educators, athletic trainers, and coaches. Policymakers and attorneys may also find the book useful because mTBI is of major public health importance and is not an uncommon cause of legal disputation.

Collectively, the chapters provide a summary and critique of the existing research and delineate the implications of this knowledge base for those in health care and community settings. Because excellent resources that focus on mTBI in adults (e.g., McCrea, 2008) and pediatric TBI more broadly already exist (e.g., Anderson & Yeates, 2010), the current book covers pediatric mTBI exclusively. At the same time, the book is meant to be a wide-ranging resource, reviewing mTBI throughout childhood and the teenage years, from evidence-based outcomes to clinical evaluation tools and management strategies, and from straightforward sport-related concussions to more severe or "complicated" mTBIs.

Since an edited book is only as valuable as the individual chapters, we first and foremost want to extend our heartfelt thanks to our chapter authors, who generously found time amid hectic academic and clinical schedules to skillfully summarize the current literature and add an impressive amount of new scholarship to the field, while remaining receptive and responsive to our editorial suggestions. We also want to thank Rochelle Serwator, Senior Editor at The Guilford Press, who was fully behind the project from day one and helped to bring it to fruition through her gentle but consistent direction and timely encouragement. We additionally want to extend our appreciation to the many colleagues, students, and families with whom we have had the privilege to work, as their stories, perspectives, and critical questions about mTBI have shaped our thinking for the better. Last, but definitely not least, we want to thank our families and friends, who have supported us with enthusiasm and a generous dose of patience and understanding.

REFERENCES

Anderson, V., & Yeates, K. O. (2010). *Pediatric traumatic brain injury: New frontiers in clinical and translational research.* Cambridge, UK: Cambridge University Press.

McCrea, M. A. (2008). *Mild traumatic brain injury and postconcussion syndrome.* New York: Oxford University Press.

Contents

PART I

INTRODUCTION

CHAPTER 1

History, Diagnostic Considerations, and Controversies

Elisabeth A. Wilde, Stephen R. McCauley, Gerri Hanten, Gunes Avci, Alyssa P. Ibarra, and Harvey S. Levin

M ild traumatic brain injury (mTBI)—which also traditionally incorporates terms such as *concussion, minor head injury, minor brain injury,* or *minor head trauma*— occurs when a forceful motion of the head (with or without impact) results in a transient alteration of mental status, such as confusion or disorientation, loss of memory for events immediately before or after the injury, or brief loss of consciousness. Traumatic brain injury (TBI) in children has garnered increasing attention among clinicians, researchers, parents, educators, communities, and sports- and recreation-related professionals working with children in recent years, as data indicate that the rates of hospital admissions and emergency department visits for head injuries are indeed higher among children than the general adult population, particularly among children under 5 years and in adolescents ages 15–19 (Faul, Xu, Wald, & Coronado, 2010). In addition to mechanisms such as motor vehicle crashes and falls, each year an estimated 135,000 cases of TBI, treated in emergency departments, occur due to sports and recreation injuries in children ages 5–18 years (Centers for Disease Control and Prevention, 2007). mTBI accounts for the overwhelming majority (at least 75%) of all TBI in the United States (Sosin, Sniezek, & Thurman, 1996)—though, due to lack of data on individuals who do not seek immediate medical attention, this is a probably an underestimate of the true incidence of mTBI. Despite growing acknowledgment of the potential for long-term disability in at least a subset of children and adolescents with mTBI, the long-term consequences of pediatric mTBI have been difficult to estimate.

This chapter provides a brief introduction to early research findings that have influenced current methodology in pediatric mTBI research, and we review general trends in current literature in contrast to literature from approximately two to three decades ago. Diagnostic considerations and commonly used criteria are introduced in the context of developmental considerations in children. Finally, a series of remaining controversies in the field of pediatric mTBI are briefly introduced.

TRENDS IN mTBI RESEARCH IN CHILDREN

Historically, mTBI has not received a great deal of scholarly attention because it was generally accepted as clinically benign (Echemendia & Julian, 2001; Segalowitz & Brown, 1991). Until more recently, lukewarm interest, a lack of controlled studies, and underestimation of the sequelae of mTBI all presented significant obstacles to developing a solid understanding of its long-term consequences. However, highly publicized sports-related mTBI and media focus upon military-related mTBI in the adult literature have aroused an interest in the consequences of this condition at all ages, including in children and adolescents, as demonstrated by a dramatic increase in published studies in pediatric mTBI in recent years (see Figure 1.1). Nevertheless, some aspects of early methodological design continue to exert a notable influence on current studies in this area.

Early History

Modern research on mTBI in children was pioneered by child psychiatrist Michael Rutter and his associates. Following earlier investigation of outcomes of depressed skull fracture with dural tears, using a retrospective design (Shaffer, Chadwick, & Rutter, 1975), these investigators shifted their focus to prospective investigation of children who sustained closed-head trauma (Brown, Chadwick, Shaffer, Rutter, & Traub, 1981; Chadwick, Rutter, Brown, Shaffer, & Traub, 1981a; Chadwick, Rutter, Shaffer, & Shrout, 1981b; Rutter, Chadwick, Shaffer, & Brown, 1980). This seminal series of studies was distinguished by longitudinal designs that involved serial assessments of children at 4 months, 1 year, and 2.5 years postinjury. Secondly, these investigators used a "dose–response" strategy of comparing outcomes of children

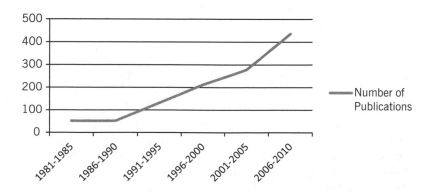

FIGURE 1.1. Results of a PubMed search for articles related to mTBI in children between the years 1981 and 2010 by 5-year increments, indicating a steady increase in publications in the last 20 years. The most dramatic increase occurs in the last 5 years.

who sustained mild head injury with children who sustained severe head injury. In addition, a group of children who experienced orthopedic injury without trauma to the head were also studied to control for more general injury-related risk factors. Standard interviews with the parents shortly after the injury were conducted to obtain information about preinjury medical history and psychiatric disorder in addition to characterizing the family environment. Serial Performance IQ scores showed a recovery curve after severe head injury, whereas repeated assessment of children in the mTBI group revealed little change in performance over time. Rutter inferred that a threshold for brain injury was exceeded in the severe head injury group, but not in the patients with mild head injury. Although the rate of preinjury psychiatric disorder was highest in the mTBI group (31%) relative to the severe TBI (14%) and control (11%) groups, the rate of novel psychiatric disorder in the postinjury assessments was markedly increased only in the children who sustained severe TBI. These studies also called attention to the contribution of preinjury comorbidities to psychiatric sequelae of the injuries and the effects of disadvantageous environment, which were controlled through this study design. The legacy of Rutter's research is seen in contemporary studies on mTBI in children that have incorporated aspects of the earlier work.

One focus of studies in the early 1990s was related to the epidemiology and incidence of mTBI. The 1991 National Health Survey revealed that motor vehicle accidents were responsible for 28% of brain injuries, sports and physical activities were responsible for 20%, and assaults were responsible for 9%. The study highlighted the fact that the risk of sustaining brain injury was highest among teens, young adults, males, and people with low income who lived alone (Sosin et al., 1996). Although the national survey did not separately categorize mTBI and moderate brain injury, the study did begin to highlight the magnitude of the issue. In another study from this era, Segalowitz and Brown (1991) reported that 2–3% of high-school-age adolescents (14–18 years) were hospitalized for mTBI. However, when the authors conducted a survey in a high school with a sample size of 616, they found that reports of mTBI (including nonhospitalized cases) in the same age group were almost 10 times higher than hospital-reported incidence.

In addition to incidence and prevalence, assessment of the cognitive sequelae (e.g., Levin, Eisenberg, Wigg, & Kobayashi, 1982; Winogron, Knights, & Bawden, 1984) and behavioral outcome (e.g., Boll & Barth, 1983; Stern, Melamed, Silberg, Rahmani, & Groswasser, 1985) in children was a focus of mTBI research from early on. Segalowitz and Brown (1991) reported that adolescents with mTBI between 14 and 18 years of age displayed problems with hyperactivity, stuttering, mixed handedness, and dislike of mathematics. On the other hand, Knights et al. (1991) reported few behavioral changes in children ages 5–17 years with mTBI. Interestingly, and consistent with the general trend at the time, this study did not utilize a control group, reflecting the notion that children with mTBI were appropriate controls for children with moderate and severe brain injury.

Advances in technology, especially in regard to brain imaging and measures of the brain injury associated with abnormal neuropsychological outcomes, have also played a role in bolstering interest in mTBI. For example, between 1981 and 1990, electroencephalograghy (EEG) was used to demonstrate abnormalities not visualized by clinical computer tomography (CT) scans (Sugiura et al., 1981). EEG was also used to distinguish minor and mild concussions, with a reported potential value of determining the risk of later posttraumatic epilepsy (Geets & Zegher, 1985). The reliance on EEG to assess brain abnormalities postinjury lessened somewhat thereafter, as routine clinical use of EEG post head trauma was shown to be unrevealing in some instances and initiated concern related to the burden of unnecessary diagnostic procedures (Oster, Shamdeen, Gottschling, Gortner, & Meyer, 2010). Near the late 1980s, mTBI research shifted to the use of magnetic resonance imaging (MRI) as a measure to assess structural alterations of the brain postinjury (Levin et al., 1987, 1989). In one study, MRI scans revealed 44 more intracranial lesions than did concurrent CT scans in 85% of patients (Levin et al., 1987). In comparison to EEG, the higher density of prognostic information obtained from MRI proved it superior to electrophysiological testing (Wedekind, Fischbach, Pakos, Terhaag, & Klug, 1999). In addition, the use of MRI seemed to more accurately detect specific types of brain injury, namely, diffuse axonal injury found in the cerebral white matter (Yokota, Kobayashi, Nakazawa, Tsuji, & Taniguti, 1989). This finding, among others, revealed the presence of injuries possibly associated with neuropsychological outcomes that required more sensitive measures.

Recent Trends in Research

In contrast to the paucity of research on pediatric mTBI 30 years ago, recent research on mTBI has flourished and covers a more diverse range of topics, including epidemiology, research methodology, diagnostic techniques such as behavioral assessment and brain imaging, neurocognitive and social outcomes, and consequences of brain imaging techniques on children's health.

Advances in technology continue to facilitate the advancement of research in mTBI, especially the development of more sensitive, noninvasive, advanced MRI techniques such as diffusion tensor imaging (DTI). This MRI technique reveals potential alteration in white matter microstructure, and has been cited as a promising prognostic tool (Inglese et al., 2005). The use of DTI in adult mTBI has grown particularly rapidly in recent years, but has also been used in children and adolescents. In addition to advanced structural MRI techniques, Keightley et al. (2011) investigated the effect of sports-related mTBI using functional MRI and the Head Impact Telemetry (HIT) System to localize and assess the changes in neural activity in the brain as a result of mild injury. Moreover, HIT allowed the detection and recording of the magnitude and location of head impacts during sport activities. With the aid of technology, the head impact location can now be assessed, as well as the possible neural networks affected by mTBI. Other forms of advanced structural and functional neuroimaging are also being used in the study of pediatric mTBI and are the focus of a later chapter.

Technological developments have paved the way not only for improvement in brain imaging techniques, but also for the analysis of mTBI at a molecular level (Menascu, Brezner, Tshechmer, & Rumeny, 2010). For example, Filippidis, Papadopoulos, Kapsalaki, and Fountas (2010) reviewed studies examining the role of the S100B serum biomarker in the treatment of children who sustained mTBI. Although the specificity of that particular marker has yet to be demonstrated in mTBI in children (see Geyer, Ulrich, Grafe, Stach, & Til, 2009; Piazza et al., 2007), such studies suggest that serum protein biomarkers may be eventually identified that could facilitate diagnosis and avoid unnecessary head CT scans to alleviate the risks of radiation exposure in children (Klig & Kaplan, 2010).

Another topic of recent research is the emphasis on long-term outcome from childhood mTBI in terms of neurocognitive and sociocognitive functioning, as well as later neuroimaging. For example, Beauchamp et al. (2011) investigated the changes in hippocampal, amygdalar, and global brain volume 10 years after childhood TBI in patients with a range of severity that included mTBI. This group of investigators has also examined persistent changes in the corpus callosum in relation to social skills (Beauchamp et al., 2009) and predictors of educational skills in long-term outcome following injury during childhood (Catroppa et al., 2009). Anderson, Brown, Newitt, and Hoile (2011) have investigated consequences of head injury in the domains of intellectual ability, personality, and quality of life.

Another appealing feature in recent research has been the increased acknowledgment of children's phenomenological experience following mTBI. For example, Woodrome et al. (2011) investigated children's coping strategies after mTBI and reported that coping strategies collectively account for 10–15% of the variance in children's posttraumatic symptoms over time.

As noted above, research on pediatric mTBI has undergone a noticeable proliferation. Technological developments and acknowledgment of mTBI as a more serious health concern have ignited interest in the topic and helped shape the direction of research. New techniques to measure brain injury, although progressively more advanced than the methods used 30 years ago, still aim to answer some of the fundamental questions sought from the start: that is, to examine the scope of the problem, accurately assess outcome, identify any persistent sequelae, understand the mechanism underlying any persistent deficits, and reveal factors that influence recovery.

DIAGNOSTIC CONSIDERATIONS IN mTBI

This section is included to inform clinical investigators and clinicians who retrospectively obtain information about the acute phase of injury based on medical record review and/or parent interview. However, readers are referred to pediatric neurosurgical sources for more detailed information on the clinical guidelines for assessment and management of acute TBI in children (see Luerssen, 1994).

Definition of mTBI

Definitions of mTBI used by clinicians and investigators vary significantly (Culotta, Sementilli, Gerold, & Watts, 1996). As noted by Yeates and Taylor (2005), various definitions and terminologies, published by professional organizations representing different medical specialties, and have contributed to a lack of consensus about what is referred to here as *mild traumatic brain injury* (mTBI). The American Academy of Pediatrics (1999) published treatment guidelines for "minor closed head injury," which are described in Table 1.1. Although symptoms are presented, no mention is made of altered brain function. In contrast to the AAP definition, which includes "normal mental status on initial examination," the Mild Traumatic Brain Injury Committee of the Head Injury Interdisciplinary Special Interest Group of the American Congress of Rehabilitation Medicine (1993) refers to this clinical condition as mTBI and includes alteration of consciousness in the definition (see Table 1.2) with the presumption of a "physiological disruption of brain function." The World Health

TABLE 1.1. American Academy of Pediatrics Definition of "Minor Closed Head Injury"

Inclusion criteria

- Normal mental status on initial examination
- No abnormal or focal neurological findings
- No physical evidence of skull fracture
- Loss of consciousness < 1 minute
- May have had a seizure immediately after injury
- May have vomited after injury
- May exhibit other signs and symptoms (e.g., headaches, lethargy)

Exclusion criteria

- Multiple trauma
- Unobserved loss of consciousness
- Known of suspected cervical spine injury
- Suspected intentional head trauma

Note. Reprinted from Yeates and Taylor (2005). Copyright 2005 by Taylor & Francis Ltd. Reprinted by permission.

Organization (WHO) specifies several *International Classification of Diseases*, 10th revision (ICD-10) codes as mild closed-head injury, including a concussion (code 850), which is referred to as a "transient impairment of function as a result of a blow to the brain." The ICD-10 also has diagnostic codes to specify whether a mild closed-head injury is associated with loss of consciousness, skull fracture, or brain lesions.

Age and Developmental Issues in Assessments during the Acute Phase of mTBI

Assessment of Impaired Consciousness

Historically, clinicians and investigators have classified TBI as mild, moderate, and severe using the Glasgow Coma Scale (GCS), a widely used scoring system to assess impaired consciousness and coma (Teasdale & Jennett, 1974). Patients with scores of 8 or less are classified as "severe," scores of 9–12 are "moderate," and scores of 13–15 are "mild." Alteration of consciousness is a key diagnostic feature of mTBI, but administering the verbal component of the GCS assumes that comprehension

TABLE 1.2. American Congress of Rehabilitation Medicine Definition of "Mild Traumatic Brain Injury"

Inclusion criteria (at least one must be present)

- Any loss of consciousness
- Any loss of memory for events immediately before or after the accident
- Any alteration in mental state at the time of the accident
- Focal neurological deficits that may be transient

Exclusion criteria

- Loss of consciousness > 30 minutes
- Glasgow Coma Scale score < 13 after 30 minutes
- Posttraumatic amnesia > 24 hours

Note. Reprinted from Yeates and Taylor (2005). Copyright 2005 by Taylor & Francis Ltd. Reprinted by permission.

of language is sufficiently developed to reliably assess the ability to follow simple commands. Consequently, modifications of the GCS and use of pediatric scales to measure impaired consciousness have been proposed for use with infants. For example, among children under 36 months, a pediatric coma scale that is intended to approximate the GCS can be used (Simpson, Cockington, Hanieh, Raftos, & Reiley, 1991). Assessment of "confusion," the level of verbal response immediately below "oriented" on the verbal component of the GCS, is also age-dependent. Although an experienced pediatric clinician might be capable of evaluating confused speech in a young child, reliance on temporal orientation could be problematic because this ability is not reliably developed until approximately age 8 years. Despite these caveats, the GCS continues to be widely used in emergency centers that treat children with mTBI (Kapapa, Konig, Pfister, Sasse, & Woischneck, 2010).

Assessment of Posttraumatic Amnesia

Postraumatic amnesia (PTA) refers to the interval following injury for which the child has no recall of events. mTBI may be diagnosed based on PTA and confirmation of trauma to the head even without loss of consciousness. Evaluated in real time, PTA could extend to the circumstances of injury, the immediate postinjury period, arrival of first responders, and transport to hospital. Later evaluations rely on the child's recall of the aforementioned events surrounding the injury and the events immediately before the injury (e.g., climbing a tree, prior play preceding injury in a football game), which may be vulnerable to retrograde amnesia. With dependence on orientation to person, place, and time, developmental status must be considered in the clinical assessment of PTA. Consequently, Ewing-Cobbs, Levin, Fletcher, Miner, and Eisenberg (1990) designed the Children's Orientation and Amnesia Test (COAT) to evaluate PTA during the acute and subacute phases of TBI in children ages 3–15 years. Measures of PTA developed for use with adults (e.g., Galveston Orientation and Amnesia Test) could be given to adolescents 16 years and older. The COAT evaluates general orientation (e.g., person and place), temporal orientation, and short term memory. Scoring of the COAT is referenced to control data obtained in typically developing children. Items pertaining to temporal orientation are not included in the assessment of children younger than 8 years because this capacity is not well developed in young children. A total score falling two standard deviations or more below the mean for the child's age is interpreted as evidence for residual PTA. Repeated administration of the COAT could show resolution of PTA over time, which corresponds to 24 hours or less in mTBI. During the resolution of PTA, cognitive performance is typically variable and often limited by fatigue and poor attention. Deferring more comprehensive neuropsychological assessment until after PTA resolves, postconcussion symptoms diminish, and the child returns home from the emergency center is advisable to obtain reliable data.

CONSIDERATIONS AND CONTROVERSIES

Despite significant advances in the field of pediatric mTBI, several important considerations and controversies remain, including a number related to clinical assessment and research methodology.

Complicated versus Uncomplicated mTBI in Children

As noted earlier, the results of CT are not typically considered in most definitions of mTBI, and variation exists across emergency centers in the clinical guidelines for obtaining CT in mTBI. However, estimates are that 14% of children with GCS scores of 13–15 show evidence of pathology on CT scans acquired within 24 hours after sustaining TBI associated with mild impairment of consciousness (Simon, Letourneau, Vitorino, & McCall, 2001). In a longitudinal study of cognitive recovery in 80 children ages 5–15 years who underwent CT within 24 hours of sustaining a TBI associated with mild impairment of consciousness, the data obtained on four occasions over the first 12 months were compared to 32 children with pathology on CT scan and 48 children with normal CT (Levin, Hanten, Roberson, Li, & Ewing-Cobbs, 2008). Evidence of slower or reduced recovery of episodic memory, resistance to cognitive interference, visual–motor speed, and academic achievement was apparent in the group of children whose mTBI was complicated by pathology on the CT scan. These authors proposed that presence of early CT abnormalities may indicate the need for follow-up examination and increase the risk for neurobehavioral sequelae of an otherwise mTBI.

Influence of Multiple or Repeat mTBI

Although multiple mTBI has not been a very popular research area among scholars, the prevalence and outcome of the condition beg for further interest and research. For example, Zemper (2005), in a large prospective cohort study that included a total of 15,304 football players age 18 years or less, reported that individuals with a concussion history were almost 6 times more likely to have another concussion and almost twice as likely to include loss of consciousness. In another study of collegiate football players, repeated head injuries were also associated with slower recovery (Guskiewicz, McCrea, Marshall, Cantu, & Randolph, 2003). For example, in this study, 30.3% of the participants with one previous concussion recovered in less than a day, whereas none of the patients with three or more previous concussion displayed such rapid recovery. Moreover, the recovery was prolonged (i.e., more than 7 days) for 30% of the patients with three or more previous concussions, whereas only 9% of patients with one previous concussion showed prolonged recovery. Whether children and adolescents demonstrate an increased vulnerability to subsequent injury, the degree to which this vulnerability changes over the developmental spectrum throughout childhood and adolescence, and alteration of the expected trajectory of recovery with repeat injury remain topics of controversy.

Some researchers investigating high school and collegiate athletes have reported that the level of cognitive impairment as a result of repeated mTBI is no different than cognitive impairment caused by a single mTBI (e.g., Broglio, Ferrara, Piland, Anderson, & Collie, 2006; Iverson, Brooks, Lovell, & Collins, 2006; Macciocchi, Barth, Littlefield, & Cantu, 2001). On the other hand, other studies report that a history of multiple previous concussions results not only in lingering consequences, as demonstrated in inferior performance on baseline preseason testing on a neuropsychological battery (e.g., Collins et al., 1999), but also in differences in on-field signs/symptoms, such as greater likelihood of loss of consciousness and confusion in high school athletes (Collins et al., 2002).

A recent meta-analysis by Belanger, Spiegel, and Vanderploeg (2009) aimed to measure the magnitude of cognitive impairment caused by multiple mTBI in athletes. They analyzed eight studies, all conducted with athletes, which involved 614 cases of multiple mTBI and 926 control cases of a single mTBI with no previous history. These two groups were evaluated across seven cognitive domains: attention, executive functioning, fluency, memory acquisition, delayed memory, motor abilities, and postconcussion symptom reporting. Although the overall effect on neuropsychological functioning was not significant, exploratory follow-up analyses showed that multiple mTBI was associated with deficits on measures of executive functioning and delayed memory, although the effect sizes were small (0.24 and 0.16, respectively). In general, this meta-analysis revealed that in studies to date, sustaining two or more mTBI has modest association with cognitive performance in only a few domains that may last several months after the most recent TBI.

Although it is intuitive that multiple mTBI should have greater adverse effect on cognitive functioning than a single mTBI, as reviewed above, the literature presents conflicting results. This discrepancy might be caused by the methodological variability among the studies (Macciocchi, Barth, & Littlefield, 1998), especially regarding age and postinjury time variables. Age at injury is important because age seems to have an effect on the recovery from mTBI (Field, Collins, Lovell, & Maroon, 2003). Additionally, *second-impact syndrome* is a commonly discussed postconcussion clinical sequela that is reported to occur when an athlete sustains a second head injury before fully recovering from the first head injury (Cantu, 1998), presumably from diffuse cerebral swelling that does not resolve prior to a second concussion. To date, this phenomenon has been observed mostly in children and teenagers. However, the existence of a second-impact syndrome has been a source of some controversy because of its rarity and the lack of closely spaced concussions in most observed cases (McCrory & Berkovic, 1998; Randolph, 2011). Diffuse cerebral swelling is also a well-documented phenomenon in the neurosurgical literature following a single minor brain trauma (Mandera, Wencel, Bazowski, & Krauze, 2000; Snoek, Minderhoud, & Wilmink, 1984).

Finally, potential methodological variability concerning the interval between recurrent concussions may affect results. For example, there plausibly may be a difference between sustaining consecutive traumas within a short time frame (i.e., within a single game) as opposed to over a longer time frame (i.e., months or years apart). However, the outcome of recurrent concussions with longer intervals and in children at specific developmental stages remains incompletely understood.

As noted, studies with human subjects cannot provide a clear picture of the outcome of repeated mTBI due to methodological constraints. Animal models, on the other hand, can shed light on this topic because animal studies lack some confounding variables that are associated with human subjects (see Obenaus et al., Chapter 4, and Babikian, DiFiori, & Giza, Chapter 5, this volume). For example, studies on adult animal models for repeated head traumas suggest that multiple concussions, compared to single concussion, result in impaired cognitive performance (e.g., Kanayama et al., 1996; Laurer et al., 2001). Taken together, the animal and human literature suggests that the effect of multiple mTBI, both in cognition and pathophysiology, appears more pronounced in patients with three or more concussions.

However, the literature review above indicates that conclusions regarding the effect of multiple mTBI on cognitive functioning are premature. Several reasons can be cited to direct scholarly attention to this topic. Distinct populations from different backgrounds sustain multiple mTBI regularly; it is of value to determine the consequences of repeated head trauma in each of these populations for implementation of intervention, which may lead to more effective rehabilitation. As noted above, the current literature on multiple head injuries is currently limited to sports-related injuries. Underprivileged populations, such as children with a history of abuse and prison inmates, are also subject to repeated head trauma. For example, a study by Diamond, Harzke, Magaletta, Cummins, and Frankowski (2007) reported that of the 998 prison inmates who were interviewed for the study, 82.8% reported having had one or more head injuries during their lifetime. Recurrent mTBI incidents have not yet been shown definitively to have an additive effect that can lead to cognitive deficits comparable to sequelae of more severe TBI. Although knowledge on repeated sports-related head injuries is increasing, we cannot safely argue that other sources of repeated head trauma (e.g., blast exposure, abuse) result in the same pathophysiology and related neurobehavioral phenotype. Given that the existing literature on the effects of multiple mTBI has yielded equivocal findings, it is important to identify the source of this variation for proper diagnosis, prognosis, and rehabilitation, particularly as it relates to infants, children, and adolescents.

Importance of Time Postinjury in Cognitive Symptom and Imaging Resolution in Acute mTBI

Despite widespread agreement that mTBI may be associated with initial neuropsychological problems and changes detectable on some forms of advanced imaging in *some* patients, disagreement continues about the frequency and relevance of these findings, even in the acute phase of recovery, as well as their persistence. Knowledge surrounding the time course underlying recovery also remains incomplete, as do the factors that may influence this pattern in any given child. The inconsistency in reported findings likely results from several factors, including the absence of a standard definition of mTBI and differences in selection criteria, sample characteristics, and methodology. Impaired attention, concentration, information-processing speed, and memory continue to be cited as the most common initial and persistent complaints following mTBI, with other common symptoms including headaches, dizziness, nausea, fatigue, and emotional problems such as impulsiveness and mood swings. We note that considerable variability exists in the frequency with which individuals with mTBI report postinjury complaints, and clearly further study is warranted.

Imaging studies of acute mTBI in children have also struggled to identify the direction, time course, and persistence of parenchymal, or brain tissue, changes associated with mTBI. For example, some researchers utilizing advanced modalities such as DTI with children and adolescents have reported initial increases in metrics such as fractional anisotropy and decreases in measures of mean diffusivity or apparent diffusion coefficient, which have been ascribed to cytotoxic edema or inflammation in the acute or subacute stage (Wilde et al., 2008; Wu et al., 2010). In contrast, others have reported an opposite pattern in DTI-related metrics in a subacute stage in adults with poor outcome (e.g., Messe et al., 2011). In addition to the direction of change, the persistence of these changes remains unknown, particularly in pediatric populations, and additional understanding of the pattern and time course of these changes is needed.

Outcome Measures

The question as to whether pediatric mTBI results in long-term deficits has been controversial, and study results have been mixed. Perhaps not surprisingly, comprehensive review articles on this topic have failed to conclusively resolve the issue (Beers, 1992; Boll & Barth, 1983; Carroll et al., 2004; Satz, 2001; Satz, Zaucha, McCleary, & Light, 1997), but they have served to highlight many of the shortcomings of work in this area. In addition to persistent problems, including the lack of a consistent definition of mTBI and the lack of agreement on appropriate groups to be used for comparison, numerous other factors that limit progress have been cited, such as wide age ranges of study samples, relatively short follow-up duration, narrow age ranges of instruments hampering longitudinal follow-up, fundamental differences in constructs of cognitive abilities over the developmental spectrum (e.g., executive function in a toddler vs. an adolescent), demonstrated validity of an instrument's use in TBI, and the sensitivity of some instruments (although standardized) in detecting impairment following mTBI in particular. Additionally, the sources of information regarding emotional/psychiatric features, cognition, and behavioral disturbance can greatly influence the quality and veridicality of the data. For example, how well can a very young child estimate and report his or her own level of fatigue or thinking more slowly, and so forth? Conversely, a parent may have difficulty accurately estimating the severity of his or her child's somatic and emotional symptoms, as these are purely subjective experiences that cannot be precisely assessed by an informant. Clinical lore suggests that parent and child reports often result in contradictory symptom pictures. Although it is beyond the scope of this chapter to address these issues, it is obvious that if persisting deficits indeed do occur following mTBI in some children and adolescents, the selection of the most appropriate outcome measures is paramount.

In an effort to advance the field of TBI more quickly, an interagency Common Data Elements (CDE) initiative was recently formed (Thurmond et al., 2010), and the TBI Outcomes Workgroup was charged with the task of selecting a set of instruments recommended for use in TBI (Wilde et al., 2010). However, the original CDE workgroup did not include measures appropriate for infants, children, and adolescents with TBI, so an additional set of measures was later selected to specifically address this gap (McCauley et al., 2012). The intent of the pediatric CDE is to present a starting point to stimulate further research and also to highlight the limitations of existing measures in certain domains, in order to lead to further test development. Newly developed measures may help to clarify the presence or absence of long-term deficits in infants, children, and adolescents with mTBI. At present, the CDE acknowledges the need for specific recommendations for mTBI, and additional work is planned. Further information on specific measures for the assessment of mTBI in children and adolescents is contained in chapters that follow.

Suboptimal Effort and Negative Impression Management

In mTBI literature in adults, consideration is often given to suboptimal effort and symptom exaggeration in the context of secondary gain, often related to litigation and financial compensation. However, in children, this issue has received much less attention, presumably due to the assumptions that youth are less capable of deception than adults and that examiners can readily detect suboptimal effort in youth.

Additionally, the role that external and psychological incentives may play in symptom report and performance on testing in youth has been assumed to be different than that of adults. Consequently, few studies in mTBI in children have specifically examined the role of effort validity.

Two recent studies have suggested that suboptimal effort may indeed require further consideration in both clinical practice and research, at least in children older than 8 years. Kirkwood and Kirk (2010) examined performance on the Medical Symptom Validity Test (MSVT) in 193 consecutively referred patients with mTBI, ages 8–17 years, and reported a base rate of suboptimal effort of 17%, based upon failure of at least one of the three primary effort indices of the MSVT. A comparison of the groups that passed versus failed the MSVT revealed no difference in gender, ethnicity/race, maternal education, history of premorbid learning disability, attention-deficit/hyperactivity disorder or reading problems, litigation status, time since injury, or whether the injury was associated with loss of consciousness or neuroimaging pathology. In a subsequent report that utilized a larger sample of approximately the same age range, 18.5% of the sample failed at least one of the three primary effort indices of the MSVT (Kirkwood, Yeates, Randolph, & Kirk, 2011). Again, the samples of children that failed versus passed symptom validity measures did not differ in terms of demographic variables, history of premorbid conditions, litigation status, or injury severity. The underlying reasons for suboptimal effort in children with mTBI may not be readily apparent, but the authors of the above studies indicate that factors may include both conscious and unconscious processes and attempts to obtain external gains (e.g., additional support at school) or to fulfill internal psychological needs (e.g., somatization). It is also possible that failure on symptom validity tests in children simply reflects noncompliance or other factors that increase performance variability.

Appropriate Comparison Groups in Pediatric mTBI Research

The question of the appropriate control group is important in the study of mTBI, and premorbid conditions and factors not directly related to injury must be carefully considered to gain a clear understanding of the consequences of mTBI (Asarnow et al., 1995; Bijur, Haslum, & Golding, 1990). Many recent studies of pediatric TBI have used children with orthopedic injuries as a comparison group. This approach derives from the impetus to control for confounds on measures of outcome by factors ancillary to brain injury, such as risk factors that predispose to injury (Stancin et al., 1998) or the psychological impact of trauma (Basson et al., 1991).

Risk factors for TBI can be broadly divided into personal and demographic characteristics of the injured person and general effects of the trauma experience. Among personal and demographic factors, socioeconomic status (SES), psychiatric status, race, gender, and family environment have been identified as relevant to TBI. For example, lower SES is associated with greater propensity for injury of any type (Collins, 1990), including TBI (Selassie, Pickelsimer, Frazier, & Ferguson, 2004; Yates, Williams, Harris, Round, & Jenkins, 2006), a pattern that has been ascribed to greater exposure to more physically demanding occupations, neighborhood violence, and less safe residences or vehicles (Hoofien, Vackil, Gilboa, & Donovick, 2003). In children with TBI, lower SES is associated with poorer psychosocial outcome (e.g., Taylor et al., 1999) and worse performance on tests of cognition (e.g., Hanten et al.,

2009). Stancin et al. (1998) found that even among children with orthopedic injuries alone, preinjury family status predicted later parental and family distress. Thus, SES is an important variable to consider, both in studies of incidence and outcome of children with TBI and in the effect of injury on the family. Other demographic factors shown to influence incidence and outcome of TBI include gender and age, with older children having an advantage over younger children (depending on injury severity), and race, with African American or American Indian populations being more affected than European American (Bazarian et al., 2005; Rutland-Brown, Langlois, Thomas, & Xi, 2006).

Controlling for demographic variables, however, may not be sufficient to account for non-injury-related effects, especially on outcome research. Babikian et al. (2011) studied the outcome of three groups of children well matched on age, gender, race, and socioeconomic status: those with mild TBI (n = 124), other injuries not involving the head (n = 115), and a demographically comparable group of children without injuries (n = 145). On measures of memory, verbal learning, and executive function, the authors found that for five of the six variables on which there were differences between the mTBI group and the noninjury control group, the other-injury group also showed deficits, suggesting that the impairment observed in the TBI group could be due to the general effects of trauma, rather than to brain injury. Notably, however, the other-injury group had Abbreviated Injury Scale scores that were significantly higher than the mTBI group, and the mTBI was not verified or classified by neuroimaging data. Nonetheless, other studies of children who have experienced trauma and hospitalization have revealed effects of the experience that could potentially confound outcome measures of mTBI (Daviss et al., 2000).

Psychiatric status has been implicated as a factor in TBI research. For example, attention-deficit/hyperactivity disorder has been associated with the propensity to sustain injury (Bruce, Kirkland, & Waschbusch, 2007; Ozer, Gillani, Williams, & Hak, 2010; Schwebel & Gaines, 2007), including TBI (Gerring et al., 1998). On the other hand, studies have reported effects of depression (Han et al., 2011), anxiety (Max et al., 2011), and posttraumatic stress disorder (PTSD) on recovery after injury (Holbrook et al., 2005), which have been found to be related to quality of life. Daviss et al. (2000) reported that of 83 children hospitalized for trauma, 69% showed posttraumatic stress symptoms at baseline, and 59% at 6 months postinjury. In a study of children with mTBI, Hajek et al. (2010) found higher PTSD in orthopedically injured children at baseline, as compared to children with TBI, but did not find that symptoms persisted in either group. Literature linking PTSD to reading and academic achievement (Delaney-Black et al., 2002) highlights the importance of controlling for psychiatric variables when studying cognitive outcomes of TBI.

Although the consensus for a number of years has been that children with orthopedic injury are well matched to those with TBI on many of the above-mentioned factors, some evidence suggests that the risk factors may not equate between groups. Loder, Warschausky, Schwartz, Hensinger, and Greenfield (1995) investigated the relation of premorbid family environment and behavioral profiles of children who had sustained orthopedic trauma. They reported significantly higher rates of premorbid social problems and behavioral dysfunction in the orthopedically injured children than in the general population, although the direct comparison to children with TBI was not made.

Other studies also suggest that orthopedic injury groups may not be equitable (at least quantitatively) to children with TBI on some risk factors. For example, Basson et al. (1991) used a parent interview to assess behavior problems of children with TBI, children with general traumatic injuries (not involving the head), and children who had undergone emergency appendectomies. They found that the greatest behavioral change was experienced by the group of children with general trauma, which exceeded that of children with TBI. In contrast, none of the children with appendectomies met criteria for behavior change, suggesting that the experience of trauma itself may lead to behavior change, and that the propensity for behavior change may differ in children with orthopedic injuries (or general trauma) and children with TBI.

CONCLUSION

In many respects, the field of pediatric mTBI is still in its infancy, with less than a half century of research behind it. However, interest in this topic is rapidly increasing in both depth and breadth, and significant advances in understanding have emerged in the last 20 years. Nonetheless, significant unresolved issues remain regarding the classification and diagnostic criteria for mTBI, and these are particularly worthy of further consideration in infants and young children, where traditional assessment of signs and symptoms is difficult. Additionally, several existing and emerging controversies are apparent in current research related to the use of an appropriate control group; the impact of repeat mTBI in terms of increased vulnerability to subsequent injury; the existence and selection of appropriate outcome measures for use mTBI with infants and children who have sustained mTBI; the assessment of suboptimal effort in children; and the magnitude, direction, and persistence of change on imaging-related indices and measures of symptoms and cognitive performance, particularly in the acute or subacute period.

REFERENCES

American Academy of Pediatrics. (1999). The management of minor closed head injury in children. *Pediatrics*, *104*, 1407–1415.

Anderson, V., Brown, S., Newitt, H., & Hoile, H. (2011). Long-term outcome from childhood traumatic brain injury: Intellectual ability, personality, and quality of life. *Neuropsychology*, *25*(2), 176–184.

Asarnow, R. F., Satz, P., Light, R., Zaucha, K., Lewis, R., & McCleary, C. (1995). The UCLA study of mild closed head injury in children and adolescents. In S. Broman & M. E. Michel (Eds.), *Traumatic brain injury in children* (pp. 117–146). New York: Oxford University Press.

Babikian, T., Satz, P., Zaucha, K., Light, R., Lewis, R. S., & Asarnow, R. F. (2011). The UCLA Longitudinal Study of Neurocognitive Outcomes Following Mild Pediatric Traumatic Brain Injury. *Journal of the International Neuropsychological Society*, *4*, 1–10.

Basson, M. D., Guinn, J. E., McElligott, J., Vitale, R., Brown, W., & Fielding, L. P. (1991). Behavioral disturbances in children after trauma. *Journal of Trauma: Injury, Infection, and Critical Care*, *31*, 1363–1368.

Bazarian, J. J., McClung, J., Shah, M. N., Cheng, Y. T., Flesher, W., & Kraus, J. (2005). Mild traumatic brain injury in the United States, 1998–2000. *Brain Injury*, *19*, 85–91.

Beauchamp, M., Ditchfield, M., Maller, J., Catroppa, C., Godfrey, C., Rosenfeld, J., et al. (2011). Hippocampus, amygdala and global brain changes 10 years after childhood traumatic brain injury. *International Journal of Developmental Neuroscience, 29*(2), 137–143.

Beers, S. R. (1992). Cognitive effects of mild head injury in children and adolescents. *Neuropsychological Review, 3*, 281–320.

Belanger, H., Spiegel, E., & Vanderploeg, R. (2009). Neuropsychological performance following a history of multiple self-reported concussions: A meta-analysis. *Journal of the International Neuropsychological Society, 16*(2), 262–267.

Bijur, P. E., Haslum, M., & Golding, J. (1990). Cognitive and behavioral sequelae of mild head injury in children. *Pediatrics, 86*(3), 337–344.

Boll, T., & Barth, J. (1983). Mild head injury. *Psychiatric Developments, 1*(3), 263–275.

Broglio, S., Ferrara, M., Piland, S., Anderson, R., & Collie, A. (2006). Concussion history is not a predictor of computerised neurocognitive performance. *British Journal of Sports Medicine, 40*(9), 802–805.

Brown, G., Chadwick, O., Shaffer, D., Rutter, M., & Traub, M. (1981). A prospective study of children with head injuries: III. Psychiatric sequelae. *Psychological Medicine, 11*(1), 63–78.

Bruce, B., Kirkland, S., & Waschbusch, D. (2007). The relationship between childhood behaviour disorders and unintentional injury events. *Paediatric Child Health, 12*(9), 749–754.

Cantu, R. (1998). Second-impact syndrome. *Clinical Journal of Sports Medicine, 17*(1), 37–44.

Carroll, L. J., Cassidy, J. D., Peloso, P. M., Borg, J., von Holst, H., Holm, L., et al. (2004). Prognosis for mild traumatic brain injury: Results of the WHO Collaborating Centre Task Force on Mild Traumatic Brain Injury. *Journal of Rehabilitation Medicine*, (43, Suppl.), 84–105.

Catroppa, C., Anderson, V., Muscara, F., Morse, S., Haritou, F., Rosenfeld, J., et al. (2009). Educational skills: Long-term outcome and predictors following paediatric traumatic brain injury. *Neuropsychological Rehabilitation, 19*(5), 716–732.

Centers for Disease Control and Prevention. (2007, July 27). *Nonfatal traumatic brain injuries from sports and recreation activities: United States, 2001—2005.* Retrieved from *www.cdc.gov/mmwr/preview/mmwrhtml/mm5629a2.htm.*

Chadwick, O., Rutter, M., Brown, G., Shaffer, D., & Traub, M. (1981a). A prospective study of children with head injuries: II. Cognitive sequelae. *Psychological Medicine, 11*(1), 49–61.

Chadwick, O., Rutter, M., Shaffer, D., & Shrout, P. (1981b). A prospective study of children with head injuries: IV. Specific cognitive deficits. *Journal of Clinical Neuropsychology, 3*(2), 101–120.

Collins, M., Grindel, S., Lovell, M., Dede, D., Moser, D., Phalin, B., et al. (1999). Relationship between concussion and neuropsychological performance in college football players. *Journal of the American Medical Association, 282*(10), 964–970.

Collins, M., Lovell, M., Iverson, G., Cantu, R., Maroon, J., & Field, M. (2002). Cumulative effects of concussion in high school athletes. *Neurosurgery, 51*(5), 1175–1179.

Culotta, V., Sementilli, M., Gerold, K., & Watts, C. (1996). Clinicopathological heterogeneity in the classification of mild head injury. *Neurosurgery, 38*(2), 245–250.

Daviss, W. B., Mooney, D., Racusin, R., Ford, J. D., Fleischer, A., & McHugo, G. J. (2000). Predicting posttraumatic stress after hospitalization for pediatric injury. *Journal of the American Academy of Child and Adolescent Psychiatry, 39*, 576–583.

Delaney-Black, V., Covington, C., Ondersma, S. J., Nordstrom-Klee, B., Templin, T., Ager, J., et al. (2002). Violence exposure, trauma, and IQ and/or reading deficits among urban children. *Archives of Pediatric Adolescent Medicine, 156*(3), 280–285.

Diamond, P., Harzke, A., Magaletta, P., Cummins, A., & Frankowski, R. (2007). Screening for traumatic brain injury in an offender sample: A first look at the reliability and validity of the traumatic brain injury questionnaire. *Journal of Head Trauma Rehabilitation, 22*(6), 330–338.

Echemendia, R., & Julian, L. (2001). Mild traumatic brain injury in sports: Neuropsychology's contribution to a developing field. *Neuropsychology Review, 11*(2), 69–88.

Ewing-Cobbs, L., Levin, H., Fletcher, J., Miner, M., & Eisenberg, H. (1990). The Children's Orientation and Amnesia Test: Relationship to severity of acute head injury and to recovery of memory. *Neurosurgery, 27*(5), 683–691.

Faul, M., Xu, L., Wald, M. M., & Coronado, V. G. (2010). *Traumatic brain injury in the United States: Emergency department visits, hospitalizations, and deaths.* Atlanta, GA: Centers for Disease Control and Prevention, National Center for Injury Prevention and Control.

Field, M., Collins, M., Lovell, M., & Maroon, J. (2003). Does age play a role in recovery from sports-related concussion?: A comparison of high school and collegiate athletes. *Journal of Pediatrics, 142*(5), 546–553.

Filippidis, A., Papadopoulos, D., Kapsalaki, E., & Fountas, K. (2010). Role of the s100b serum biomarker in the treatment of children suffering from mild traumatic brain injury. *Neurosurgical Focus, 29*(5), E2.

Geets, W., & de Zegher, F. (1985). EEG and brainstem abnormalities after cerebral concussion: Short term observations. *Acta Neurologica Belgica, 85*(5), 277–283.

Gerring, J. P., Brady, K. D., Chen, A., Vasa, R., Grados, M., Bandeen-Roche, K. J., et al. (1998). Premorbid prevalence of ADHD and development of secondary ADHD after closed head injury. *Journal of the American Academy of Child and Adolescent Psychiatry, 37*(6), 647–654.

Geyer, C., Ulrich, A., Grafe, G., Stach, B., & Til, H. (2009). Diagnostic value of s100b and neuron-specific enolase in mild pediatric traumatic brain injury. *Journal of Neurosurgery: Pediatrics, 4*(4), 339–344.

Guskiewicz, K., McCrea, M., Marshall, S., Cantu, R., & Randolph, C. (2003). Cumulative effects associated with recurrent concussion in collegiate football players: The NCAA concussion study. *Journal of the American Medical Association, 290*(19), 2549–2555.

Hajek, C. A., Yeates, K. O., Taylor, H. G., Bangert, B., Dietrich, A., Nuss, K. E., et al. (2010). Relationships among post-concussive symptoms and symptoms of PTSD in children following mild traumatic brain injury. *Brain Injury, 24*(2), 100–109.

Han, P. P., Holbrook, T. L., Sise, M. J., Sack, D. I., Sise, C. B., Hoyt, D. B., et al. (2011). Postinjury depression is a serious complication in adolescents after major trauma: Injury severity and injury-event factors predict depression and long-term quality of life deficits. *Journal of Trauma: Injury, Infection, and Critical Care, 70*(4), 923–930.

Hanten, G., Li, X., Newsome, M. R., Swank, P., Chapman, S. B., Dennis, M., et al. (2009). Oral reading and expressive language after childhood traumatic brain injury: Trajectory and correlates of change over time. *Topics in Language Disorders, 29*, 236–248.

Holbrook, T. L., Hoyt, D. B., Coimbra, R., Potenza, B., Sise, M., & Anderson, J. P. (2005). Long-term posttraumatic stress disorder persists after major trauma in adolescents: New data on risk factors and functional outcome. *Journal of Trauma: Injury, Infection, and Critical Care, 58*(4), 764–769; discussion 769–771.

Hoofien, D. E., Vackil, E., Gilboa, A., & Donovick, P. (2003). Comparison of the predictive power of socioeconomic variables, severity of injury and age on long-term outcome of traumatic brain injury: Sample specific variables versus factors as predictors. *Brain Injury, 16*, 9–27.

Inglese, M., Makani, S., Johnson, G., Cohen, B., Silver, J., Gonen, O., et al. (2005). Diffuse axonal injury in mild traumatic brain injury: A diffusion tensor imaging study. *Journal of Neurosurgery, 103*(2), 298–303.

Iverson, G., Brooks, B., Lovell, M., & Collins, M. (2006). No cumulative effects for one or two previous concussions. *British Journal of Sports Medicine, 40*(1), 72–75.

Kanayama, G., Takeda, M., Niigawa, H., Ikura, Y., Tamii, H., Taniguchi, N., et al. (1996). The effects of repetitive mild brain injury on cytoskeletal protein and behavior. *Methods and Findings in Experimental and Clinical Pharmacology, 18*(2), 105–115.

Kapapa, T., Konig, K., Pfister, U., Sasse, M., & Woischneck, D. (2010). Head trauma in children: Part 1. Admission, diagnostics, and findings. *Journal of Child Neurology, 25*(2), 146–156.

Keightley, M., Green, S., Reed, N., Agnihotri, S., Wilkinson, A., & Lobaugh, N. (2011). An investigation of the effects of sports-related concussion in youth using functional magnetic resonance imaging and the head impact telemetry system. *Journal of Visualized Experiments, 47,* 2226.

Kirkwood, M. W., & Kirk, J. W. (2010). The base rate of suboptimal effort in a pediatric mild TBI sample: Performance on the Medical Symptom Validity Test. *The Clinical Neuropsychologist, 24*(5), 860–872.

Kirkwood, M. W., Yeates, K. O., Randolph, C., & Kirk, J. W. (2011). The implications of symptom validity test failure for ability-based test performance in a pediatric sample. *Psychological Assessment.* Advance online publication. doi:10.1037/a0024628.

Klig, J., & Kaplan, C. (2010). Minor head injury in children. *Current Opinion in Pediatrics, 22*(3), 257–261.

Knights, R., Ivan, L., Ventureyra, E., Bentivoglio, C., Stoddart, C., Winogron, W., et al. (1991). The effects of head injury in children on neuropsychological and behavioural functioning. *Brain Injury, 5*(4), 339–351.

Laurer, H., Bareyre, F., Lee, V., Trojanowski, J., Longhi, L., Hoover, R., et al. (2001). Mild head injury increasing the brain's vulnerability to a second concussive impact. *Journal of Neurosurgery, 95*(5), 859–870.

Levin, H., Amparo, E., Eisenberg, H., Miner, M., High, W., Jr., Ewing-Cobbs, L., et al. (1989). Magnetic resonance imaging after closed head injury in children. *Neurosurgery, 24*(2), 223–227.

Levin, H., Amparo, E., Eisenberg, H., Williams, D., High, W., McArdle C., et al. (1987). Magnetic resonance imaging and computerized tomography in relation to the neurobehavioral sequelae of mild and moderate head injuries. *Journal of Neurosurgery, 66*(5), 706–713.

Levin, H., Eisenberg, H., Wigg, N., & Kobayashi, K. (1982). Memory and intellectual ability after head injury in children and adolescents. *Neurosurgery, 11*(5), 668–673.

Levin, H., Hanten, G., Roberson, G., Li, X., & Ewing-Cobbs, L. (2008). Prediction of cognitive sequelae based on abnormal computed tomography findings in children following mild traumatic brain injury. *Journal of Neurosurgery: Pediatrics, 1*(6), 461–470.

Loder, R. T., Warschausky, S., Schwartz, E. M., Hensinger, R. N., & Greenfield, M. L. (1995). The psychosocial characteristics of children with fractures. *Journal of Pediatric Orthopedics, 15,* 41–46.

Luerssen, T. (1994). Acute traumatic cerebral injuries. In W. Cheek (Ed.), *Pediatric neurosurgery* (pp. 266–278). Philadelphia: Saunders.

Macciocchi, S., Barth, J., & Littlefield, L. (1998). Outcome after mild head injury. *Clinical Journal of Sports Medicine, 17*(1), 27–36.

Macciocchi, S., Barth, J., Littlefield, L., & Cantu, R. (2001). Multiple concussions and neuropsychological functioning in collegiate football players. *Journal of Athletic Training, 36*(3), 303–306.

Mandera, M., Wencel, T., Bazowski, P., & Krauze, J. (2000). How should we manage children after mild head injury? *Child's Nervous System, 16*(3), 156–160.

Max, J., Keatley, E., Wilde, E. A., Bigler, E. D., Levin, H. S., Schachar, R. J., et al. (2011). Anxiety disorder in children and adolescents in the first six months after traumatic brain injury. *Journal of Neuropsychiatry and Clinical Neuroscience, 23,* 29–39.

McCauley, S. R., Wilde, E. A., Anderson, V. A., Bedell, G., Beers, S. R., Chapman, S. B., et al. (2012). Recommendations for the use of common outcome measures in pediatric traumatic brain injury research. *Journal of Neurotrauma, 29*(4): 678–705.

McCrory, P., & Berkovic, S. (1998). Second impact syndrome. *Neurology, 50*(3), 677–683.

Menascu, S., Brezner, A., Tshechmer, S., & Rumeny, P. (2010). Serum biochemical markers for brain damage in children with emphasis on mild head injury. *Pediatric Neurosurgery, 46*(2), 82–88.

Messe, A., Caplain, S., Paradot, G., Garrigue, D., Mineo, J., Soto Ares, G., et al. (2011). Diffusion tensor imaging and white matter lesions at the subacute stage in mild traumatic brain injury with persistent neurobehavioral impairment. *Human Brain Mapping, 32*(6), 999–1011.

Mild Traumatic Brain Injury Committee of the Head Injury Interdisciplinary Special Interest Group of the American Congress of Rehabilitation Medicine. (1993). Definition of mild traumatic brain injury. *Journal of Head Trauma Rehabilitation, 8*, 86–87.

Oster, I., Shamdeen, G., Gottschling, S., Gortner, L., & Meyer, S. (2010). Electroencephalogram in children with minor traumatic brain injury. *Journal of Pediatrics and Child Health, 46*(7–8), 373–377.

Ozer, K., Gillani, S., Williams, A., & Hak, D. J. (2010). Psychiatric risk factors in pediatric hand fractures. *Journal of Pediatric Orthopedics, 30*, 324–327.

Piazza, O., Storti, M., Cotena, S., Stoppa, F., & Perrotta, D., Esposito, G., et al. (2007). S100b is not a reliable prognostic index in paediatric TBI. *Pediatric Neurosurgery, 43*(4), 258–264. PMID: 17627141

Randolph, C. (2011). Baseline neuropsychological testing in managing sport-related concussion: Does it modify risk? *Current Sports Medicine Reports, 10*(1), 21–26.

Rutland-Brown, W., Langlois, J. A., Thomas, K. E., & Xi, Y. L. (2006). Incidence of traumatic brain injury in the United States. *Journal of Head Trauma Rehabilitation, 21*(6), 544–548.

Rutter, M., Chadwick, O., Shaffer, D., & Brown, G. (1980). A prospective study of children with head injuries: I. Design and methods. *Psychological Medicine, 10*(4), 633–645.

Satz, P. (2001). Mild head injury in children and adolescents. *Current Directions in Psychological Science, 10*, 106–109.

Satz, P., Zaucha, K., McCleary, C., & Light, R. (1997). Mild head injury in children and adolescents: A review of studies (1970–1995). *Psychological Bulletin, 122*, 107–131.

Schwebel, D. C., & Gaines, J. (2007). Pediatric unintentional injury: Behavioral risk factors and implications for prevention. *Journal of Developmental and Behavioral Pediatrics, 28*(3), 245–254.

Segalowitz, S., & Brown, D. (1991). Mild head injury as a source of developmental disabilities. *Journal of Learning Disabilities, 24*(9), 551–559.

Selassie, A. W. E., Pickelsimer, E., Frazier, L., Jr., & Ferguson, P. L. (2004). The effect of insurance status, race, and gender on ED disposition of persons with traumatic brain injury. *American Journal of Emergency Medicine, 22*, 465–473.

Shaffer, D., Chadwick, O., & Rutter, M. (1975). Psychiatric outcome of localized head injury in children. *Ciba Foundation Symposium, 34*, 191–213.

Simon, B., Letourneau, P., Vitorino, E., & McCall, J. (2001). Pediatric minor head trauma: Indications for computed tomographic scanning revisited. *Journal of Trauma, 51*(2), 231–238.

Simpson, D., Cockington, R., Hanieh, A., Raftos, J., & Reiley, P. (1991). Head injuries in infants and young children: The value of the paediatric coma scale—review of literature and report on a study. *Child's Nervous System, 7*(4), 183–190.

Snoek, J., Minderhoud, J., & Wilmink, J. (1984). Delayed deterioration following mild head injury in children. *Brain, 101*(Pt. 1), 15–36.

Sosin, D., Sniezek, J., & Thurman, D. (1996). Incidence of mild and moderate brain injury in the United States, 1991. *Brain Injury, 10*(1), 47–54.

Stancin, T., Taylor, H. G., Thompson, G. H., Wade, S., Drotar, D., & Yeates, K. O. (1998). Acute psychosocial impact of pediatric orthopedic trauma with and without accompanying brain injuries. *Journal of Trauma: Injury, Infection, and Critical Care, 45*, 1031–1038.

Stern, J., Melamed, S., Silberg, S., Rahmani, L., & Groswasser, Z. (1985). Behavioral disturbances as an expression of severity of cerebral damage. *Scandinavian Journal of Rehabilitation Medicine, 12*(Suppl.), 36–41.

Sugiura, M., Mori, N., Yokosuka, R., Yamamoto, M., Imanaga, H., & Sugimori, T. (1981). [Head injury in children—with special reference to CT findings (author's transl).] *No Shinkei Geka, 9*(6), 697–704.

Taylor, H. G., Yeates, K. O., Wade, S. L., Drotar, D., Klein, S. K., & Stancin, T. (1999). Influences on first-year recovery from traumatic brain injury in children. *Neuropsychology, 13*(1), 76–89.

Teasdale, G., & Jennett, B. (1974). Assessment of coma and impaired consciousness: A practical scale. *Lancet, 2*(7872), 81–84.

Thurmond, V. A., Hicks, R., Gleason, T., Miller, A. C., Szuflita, N., Orman, J., et al. (2010). Advancing integrated research in psychological health and traumatic brain injury: Common data elements. *Archives of Physical Medicine and Rehabilitation, 91*, 1633–1636.

Wedekind, C., Fischbach, R., Pakos, P., Terhaag, D., & Klug, N. (1999). Comparative use of magnetic resonance imaging and electrophysiologic investigation for the prognosis of head injury. *Journal of Trauma: Injury, Infection, and Critical Care, 47*(1), 44–49.

Wilde, E. A., McCauley, S. R., Hunter, J. V., Bigler, E. D., Chu, Z., Wang, Z., et al. (2008). Diffusion tensor imaging of acute mild traumatic brain injury in adolescents. *Neurology, 70*(12), 948–955.

Wilde, E. A., Whiteneck, G., Bogner, J., Bushnik, T., Cifu, D. X., Dikmen, S., et al. (2010). Recommendations for the use of common outcome measures in traumatic brain injury research. *Archives of Physical Medicine and Rehabilitation, 91*, 1650–1660.

Winogron, H., Knights, R., & Bawden, H. (1984). Neuropsychological deficits following head injury in children. *Journal of Clinical Neuropsychology, 6*(3), 267–286.

Woodrome, S., Yeates, K., Taylor, H., Rusin, J., Bangert, B., Dietrich, A., et al. (2011). Coping strategies as a predictor of post-concussive symptoms in children with mild traumatic brain injury versus mild orthopedic injury. *Journal of the International Neuropsychological Society, 17*(2), 317–326.

Wu, T., Wilde, E., Bigler, E., Yallampalli, R., McCauley, S., Troyanskaya, M., et al. (2010). Evaluating the relationship between memory functioning and cingulum bundles in acute mild traumatic brain injury using diffusion tensor imaging. *Journal of Neurotrauma, 27*(2), 303–307.

Yates, P. J., Williams, W. H., Harris, A., Round, A., & Jenkins, R. (2006). An epidemiological study of head injuries in a UK population attending and emergency department. *Journal of Neurology, Neurosurgery, and Psychiatry, 77*, 699–701.

Yeates, K., & Taylor, H. (2005). Neurobehavioural outcomes of mild head injury in children and adolescents. *Pediatric Rehabilitation, 8*(1), 5–16.

Yokota, H., Kobayashi, S., Nakazawa, S., Tsuji, Y., & Taniguti, Y. (1989). [Significance of magnetic resonance imaging in diffuse axonal injury]. *No Shinkei Geka, 17*(12), 1133–1138.

Zemper, E. (2005). Track and field injuries. *Medicine and Sport Science, 48*, 138–151.

CHAPTER 2

Epidemiology and Prevention

R. Dawn Comstock and Kelsey Logan

Describing the epidemiology of mild traumatic brain injury (mTBI), including concussion, is challenging for several reasons. First, although the spectrum of mTBI ranges from milder concussions to complicated mTBI (i.e., Glasgow Coma Scale [GCS] 13–15 but with structural pathology on imaging), the term *concussion* is rapidly becoming ubiquitous for all mTBI. Many parents view the diagnostic terms *mild traumatic brain injury* and *concussion* as equivalent (Gordon, Dooley, Fitzpatrick, Wren, & Wood, 2010), and clinicians may use the term *concussion* to describe a broad range of mTBI diagnoses because it is less alarming to parents than the term *mild brain injury* (DeMatteo et al., 2010). The frequency of the use of the term *concussion* in the lay media also reflects this trend (see Figure 2.1). Second, despite recent efforts to provide a clear definition of concussion (Cantu, 2009) and mTBI (Carroll, Cassidy, Holm, Kraus, & Coronado, 2004), consensus on standard definitions has been difficult to reach (Meehan & Mannix, 2010). Finally, these injuries are diagnosed and managed in settings ranging from high school athletic training rooms to emergency departments (EDs) to neurosurgeons' offices by a wide range of clinicians. Currently no surveillance system or combination of systems captures a representative sample of these injuries from across these diverse settings. Despite these challenges, the recent sharp increase in the number of publications on both concussion and mTBI in the medical literature can be used to draw the most complete picture of these injuries to date.

EPIDEMIOLOGY OF mTBI/CONCUSSION

The most commonly cited statistics on TBI in the United States are those distributed by the Centers for Disease Control and Prevention (CDC), National Center for Injury Prevention and Control (*www.cdc.gov/TraumaticBrainInjury/statistics.html*), which

(A)

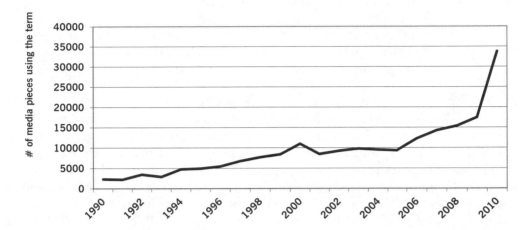

(B)

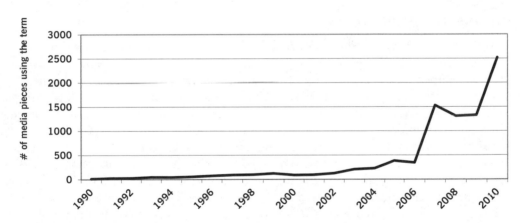

FIGURE 2.1. Trends in the use of the terms *concussion* (A) and *traumatic brain injury* (B) in the lay media. Google News keyword search using the terms "concussion" and "traumatic brain injury" conducted January 6, 2011.

include the following: (1) an estimated 1.7 million people sustain a TBI annually, with TBI a contributing factor to 30.5% of all injury-related deaths (Faul, Xu, Wald, & Coronado, 2010); (2) direct medical costs and indirect costs of TBI (lost productivity, etc.) totaled an estimated $60 billion in 2000 (Finkelstein, Corso, Miller, & Associates, 2006); and (3) about 75% of TBIs are concussions or other forms of mTBI (CDC, 2003). From this we can calculate that 1,275,000 people sustain an mTBI annually. We focus on the epidemiology of these mTBIs in the rest of this chapter.

Patterns of Injury by Age

Although the literature indicates that mTBI, including concussion, is more common among children from birth to 4 years and older youth ages 15–19 years (Faul et al.,

2010), age-related patterns of mTBI appear to be highly correlated with age differences in participation in sport and recreation activities commonly associated with these injuries. For example, a comparison of collegiate and high school athletes playing the same nine sports showed that although the overall rate of concussion was higher in the collegiate athletes than in their high school counterparts, concussions comprised a greater proportion of total injuries sustained by high school athletes than by collegiate athletes in seven of the nine sports studied (Gessel, Fields, Collins, Dick, & Comstock, 2007). Similarly, a study of ED visits for concussion from 2001 to 2005 among youth 8–19 found that the 14- to 19-year age group accounted for 65% of these injuries (Bakhos, Lockhart, Myers, & Linakis, 2010). More specifically, 4 in 1,000 youth ages 8–13 and 6 in 1,000 youth ages 14–19 had an ED visit for a sport- or recreation-activity-related concussion during the 5-year study period. Another study using a different source of ED data found that among children 0–19 presenting with concussions from 2002 to 2006, a greater proportion of the injuries was sustained by older children, with 15% of the visits by those 1–4 years, 14% by those 5–9, 28% by those 10–14, and 40% by those 15–19 (Meehan & Mannix, 2010).

Patterns of Injury by Sex

The literature consistently reports that males sustain more concussions and other mTBIs than females. In terms of incidence of injury, this is true. However, this strong disparity appears to be a function of the sex differences in participation in the various sport and recreation activities with the highest rates of injury (i.e., football and other full-contact, collision sports). Research indicates that females are at higher risk of injury than males when participating in gender-comparable sports. For example, a study of National Collegiate Athletic Association (NCAA) athletes reported female soccer and basketball players had significantly higher incidence of concussion than did men playing the same sport (Covassin, Swanik, & Sachs, 2003). Additionally, a recent critical literature review of sport concussion by gender found that 9 of 10 studies reviewed reported higher injury rates for females compared to males playing the same sport (Dick, 2009). More specifically, several studies have reported that in high school sports played by both sexes (basketball, soccer, and baseball/softball), girls sustained higher rates of concussions than boys (Gessel et al., 2007; Lincoln et al., 2011; Powell & Barber-Foss, 1999). However, it is unclear if the identified sex differences represent a true difference in risk of sustaining a concussion associated with biophysiological differences or if they represent sociocultural factors that lead to a higher likelihood of concussion diagnoses among females, whereas concussions sustained by males are more likely to go unreported and thus undiagnosed.

Patterns of Injury by Activity

Although estimated numbers of mTBI presenting to EDs have varied across studies, sport and recreation activities have consistently been most commonly associated with injury. For example, a study of concussions among those ages 0–19 treated in EDs from 2002 to 2006 reported the most common mechanism of injury was sport (30%), followed by motor vehicle crash (20%; Meehan & Mannix, 2010). Another study presenting data from 2001 to 2005 reported an estimated 502,784 ED visits for concussion by youth ages 8–19, 50% of which occurred during sport and recreation activities (Bakhos et al., 2010). The most common sport and recreation activities associated with injury were football (22.6%), bicycling (11.6%), basketball (9.2%), soccer (7.7%), and snow skiing (6.4%). Similarly, a third study found that from 2001 to 2005 there were an estimated 134,959 ED visits for sport- and recreation-related mTBIs among youth ages 5–18 (Gilchrist, Thomas, Wald, & Langlois, 2007). The activities most commonly associated with injury were bicycling (17.3%), football (15.0%), basketball (8.5%), playground activities (7.7%), soccer (5.7%), and baseball (5.5%). Patterns are also seen among high school athletes participating in team sports, with most studies reporting that generally, full-contact sports (football, boys' lacrosse, ice hockey, rugby, etc.) have the highest rates of concussion, sports in which athlete–athlete contact occurs frequently but is not the primary focus of the sport (basketball, soccer, etc.) have moderate rates of concussion, and sports where athlete–athlete contact is relatively rare (volleyball, baseball, softball, etc.) have the lowest rates of concussion (Gessel et al., 2007; Lincoln et al., 2011).

Patterns of Injury over Time

Evaluating patterns of mTBI over time is particularly challenging given (1) the wide variety of clinical settings in which these injuries are diagnosed and managed and (2) changes in the general population's access to health care over time (e.g., the recent proliferation of urgent care centers appears to have resulted in fewer sport-related injuries presenting to EDs). The rate of hospitalization for children with mTBI has decreased significantly over time, from 64.6 hospitalizations per 100,000 population in 1991–1993 to 23.8 per 100,000 in 2003–2005 (Bowman, Bird, Aitken, & Tilford, 2008). This apparent decrease likely reflects changes in clinical perspective regarding management of mTBI rather than a true decrease in incidence of these injuries. However, data from two large, comparable national surveillance studies of concussion among high school athletes indicate that although rates of concussion have remained relatively stable over the past decade, concussion represents a larger proportion of all injuries now compared to a decade ago (Table 2.1). Similarly, recent data from the National High School Sports-Related Injury Surveillance Study (High School Reporting Information Online [*http://injuryresearch.net/highschoolrio.aspx*]), a prospective study that captures data from athletes participating in nine sports in a nationally representative sample of 100 U.S. high schools, shows that whereas the overall rate of concussion has remained relatively stable (0.23 per 1,000 athlete exposures in 2005–2006 and 0.32 in 2009–2010) the proportion of all injuries represented by concussions has risen from 9.1% in 2005–2006 to 14.0% in 2009–2010. Conversely, a prospective 11-year study of concussion among athletes participating in 12 sports in one public high school system containing 25 schools found that concussion rates increased 4.2-fold between 1997–1998 and 2007–2008, with an annual increase of 15.5% (Lincoln et al., 2011). Even if rates of sport-related concussion have remained relatively stable over time, the actual numbers of concussions sustained annually has undoubtedly increased due to the continued increase in numbers of youth participating in sport and recreation activities. Any increase in injury rates more likely reflects a greater sensitivity to sports-related concussion, leading to diagnosis of a larger proportion of sustained concussions rather than to an actual increase in concussion rates.

TABLE 2.1. A Comparison of Sports-Related mTBI and Concussion Displayed as Rates per 1,000 Athlete Exposures and as a Percentage of All Injuries among High School Athletes over the Past Decade

Sport	1995/96–1997/98	2005/06–2009/10
Football		
Overall rate per 1,000 AE	0.59	0.54
Rate per 1,000 competition AE	2.82	1.99
% of all injuries	7.3%	13.3%
Girls' soccer		
Overall rate per 1,000 AE	0.23	0.30
Rate per 1,000 competition AE	0.71	0.86
% of all injuries	4.3%	13.3%
Boys' soccer		
Overall rate per 1,000 AE	0.18	0.20
Rate per 1,000 competition AE	0.57	0.55
% of all injuries	3.9%	10.2%
Girls' basketball		
Overall rate per 1,000 AE	0.16	0.20
Rate per 1,000 competition AE	0.42	0.52
% of all injuries	3.6%	11.3%
Boys' basketball		
Overall rate per 1,000 AE	0.11	0.10
Rate per 1,000 competition AE	0.28	0.23
% of all injuries	2.6%	6.4%
Wrestling		
Overall rate per 1,000 AE	0.25	0.18
Rate per 1,000 competition AE	0.51	0.37
% of all injuries	4.4%	7.8%
Baseball		
Overall rate per 1,000 AE	0.05	0.04
Rate per 1,000 competition AE	0.12	0.08
% of all injuries	1.7%	3.6%
Softball		
Overall rate per 1,000 AE	0.10	0.10
Rate per 1,000 competition AE	0.13	0.15
% of all injuries	2.7%	8.7%

Note. Data for mTBI, 1995/96–1997/98, from Powell and Barber-Foss (1999). Data for concussion, 2005/06–2009/10, from the National High School Sports-Related Injury Surveillance Study (High School RIO). AE, athlete exposure.

ECONOMIC AND PUBLIC HEALTH IMPACT

Economic Impact

Determining the economic impact of mTBI is difficult for the same reasons that describing the epidemiology of these injuries is difficult: These injuries are diagnosed and managed by a wide variety of clinicians in settings ranging from high school athletic training rooms to EDs to neurosurgeons' offices. For example, it is extremely difficult to evaluate the economic cost associated with sport-related concussions diagnosed and managed in the high school athletic training room as there is commonly no "out-of-pocket" expense to the concussed athlete's parents. However, some direct costs can be evaluated via insurance records (e.g., costs for hospitalization, ED visits, visits to physicians' offices, visits to concussion clinics) or survey of injured individuals' families (e.g., out-of-pocket expenses for co-pays/deductibles, medical supplies, etc., not covered by insurance). For example, one study reported that from 1997 to 2000 total annual health care expenditures for mTBI-related services for children ages 1–18 who were not hospitalized averaged $77.9 million, with an average per-capita health care expenditure of $1,044 (Brener, Harman, Kelleher, & Yeates, 2004). Nearly two-thirds of these expenditures were for acute care. Additionally, from 2000 to 2003, the total estimated hospital charges for sports-injury hospitalization among children ages 5–18 with possible or definite TBI (note this study did not differentiate between moderate–severe TBI and mTBI) was $66.4 million (Yang et al., 2007). These findings alone demonstrate the financial burden faced by families of injured children. However, the total cost associated with mTBI is undoubtedly underestimated in published studies due to the difficulty in evaluating additional costs (e.g., lost work days for parents providing care, lost lifetime income for injured individuals with diminished long-term work capabilities).

Broader Public Health Impact

Concussions and other forms of mTBI carry a large public health burden beyond simple economic cost because injured individuals can experience short-term physical, cognitive, behavioral, and emotional problems as well as potential long-term health and economic consequences. Such injuries can impact injured individuals' ability to return to school, work, and social and physical activities in the short term and can negatively impact their long-term work capabilities, physical activities, family dynamics, and social outlooks. For example, mTBI, including concussion, sustained by school-age children can affect their family functioning, causing significant increases in perceived burden (Ganesalingam et al., 2008).

INJURY RISK

The medical and lay communities have shown a booming interest in concussion in the past several years, largely driven by media coverage of high-profile athletes with the injury. This publicity and interest have resulted in some attitudinal change in concussion recognition and treatment and have led to sport-rule changes, in addition to state and federal legislation directed at improving concussion education, recognition, and management. Accordingly, interest in concussion risk reduction has grown. Research has been directed at protective equipment, age, gender, genetics, and preexisting conditions, among other factors. The epidemiology of mTBI, including concussion, discussed previously aims to determine where injury risk is greatest—a crucial first step toward development of effective concussion prevention programs.

Age Differences

Children are known to have the highest incidence of mTBI (Guerrero, Thurman, & Sniezek, 2000). In fact, at least one head injury warranting medical care is sustained in 16% of children by the time they are 10 years old (Barlow et al., 2010). Additionally, the majority of sport-related concussions occur in children ≤18 years of age (Halstead, 2010). The number of concussions sustained by youth has been found to be higher than previously estimated, and this number is likely to continue increasing. In sport, this is especially relevant, as the number of children participating in recreational and competitive athletics continues to grow.

Concussion risk in children is thought to be increased mainly by anatomical and physiological factors that make them both more susceptible to injury and more difficult to assess for injury. Larger head sizes in adults may account for the increased force needed to inflict the clinical symptoms typical of concussion (Ommaya, Goldsmith, & Thibault, 2002). Queen et al. theorize that smaller head mass in children increases head–neck linear and angular head acceleration in soccer heading (Queen, Weinhold, Kirkendall, & Yu, 2003). In addition, ongoing rapid brain development may make the young brain more susceptible to injury (McCrory, Collie, Anderson, & Davis, 2004). In addition, age-related differences in brain recovery mechanisms may contribute to longer recovery time in children. Lastly, concussion evaluation is more difficult in children, both because they have more trouble with symptom reporting and because it is more challenging to objectively assess cognitive function in a developing brain.

Sex Differences

Multiple studies have reported that female athletes have higher concussion rates than their male counterparts when competing in the same sport. Additionally, it appears that mechanisms of concussion also differ by sex. For example, concussions among females playing soccer and basketball have been reported to occur more often with ball or surface contact, whereas concussions in males more often occur with player–player contact (Dick, 2009). Even outside of sport, females seem to have higher incidence of concussion. Females had over 18 times higher concussion incidence than males in a study on work-related claims in a university system, even though the overall claims rate for females was only 1.36 times higher than for males (Saleh, Fuortes, Vaughn, & Bauer, 2001).

From current data, it appears that females at least trend toward higher concussion risk overall, and in some sports (i.e., soccer and basketball), it is clear that females are at higher risk. However, the reasons for this are not entirely clear, and it is important to gain an explanation so that appropriately targeted injury prevention efforts can be implemented. After all, the increased injury risk seen in these studies may be due in part to a reporting bias that would certainly affect reported incidence rates, symptom scores, etc. Culturally, females may be more likely to report injury. In a study of injured collegiate athletes (Granito, 2002), females were significantly more likely to recognize and discuss how an injury could impact health in the future. Similarly, among high school athletes, females appear to be more willing to delay return to play following concussion compared to males (Yard & Comstock, 2009). Additionally, a study of high school athletes found that the types of symptoms reported differed between sexes after sport-related concussion, with males reporting more cognitive symptoms and females reporting more neurobehavioral and somatic symptoms (Frommer et al., 2011). This difference may indicate that females are more willing to report symptoms less obvious to observers, or it could reflect anatomical and physiological sex differences. As we learn more about the potential long-term effects of concussion, the athlete's recognition of potentially more serious health risks from concussion may influence reporting. More research needs to be done in this area.

Assuming that reporting does not play a large role and that there is a real increase in concussion risk for females, anatomical and physiological differences may be contributors. Force transmitted to the brain through acceleration and deceleration of the skull is an important factor in concussion pathophysiology. Some thought has been given to differences between head mass and neck strength in males and females as a possible explanation for increased concussion risk in females, with females not having as much head and neck control as males do, perhaps increasing the force transmitted to the brain. Increased head mass has been shown to decrease linear and angular head acceleration in soccer heading (Queen et al., 2003). A 2005 comparison of sex differences in head–neck acceleration (Tierney et al., 2005) showed that physically active females had significantly less head–neck mass and neck girth, less neck muscle strength, higher angular acceleration, and higher overall muscle activity area than males. Another study by the same authors again showed less head–neck mass, neck girth, and neck muscular strength while studying the effect of headgear on head acceleration. When wearing headgear, female soccer players showed increases in head acceleration (32% and 44% with two types of headgear) during heading, compared to males wearing the same headgear (Tierney et al., 2008). This increased acceleration could contribute to females' inability to withstand a force transmitted to the head or neck with the same stability and strength as males do, which may affect concussion risk. Cross and Serenelli (2003) have suggested neck strengthening as a means of decreasing cervical injuries. However, there has been no definitive evidence that neck strengthening plays a role in concussion prevention. This is at least partly due to the lack of research in the area. A small prospective study of 19 collegiate women (Mansell, Tierney, Sitler, Swanik, & Stearne, 2005) reported that 8 weeks of cervical strength training did not affect force application, even though it increased neck girth and some strength measures.

Much more research must be done to determine exactly what accounts for the increased concussion incidence seen in females before effective injury prevention efforts can be developed.

Sport Differences

Obviously, the nature of the sport contributes to injury risk. Protective equipment, sport equipment (e.g., field hockey sticks), sport design (e.g., heading in soccer), and sport rules (e.g., checking in men's ice hockey) each play a role in the injuries likely to occur in a particular sport. In addition to the studies reported above describing the epidemiology of mTBI by activity and concussion by sport, other studies have attempted to define risk of concussion in specific sports. In collegiate sports, women's basketball and men's and women's lacrosse and soccer have shown higher concussion risk compared to other sports (Covassin et al., 2003). In a systematic review of concussion specific to male contact sports (Koh, Cassidy, & Watkinson, 2003), ice hockey and rugby had the highest concussion incidence in high school team sports, comparable to concussion incidence for professionals in those sports. Soccer had the lowest incidence. Understanding the specific risk factors associated with each sport is necessary before effective targeted, tailored prevention efforts can be developed.

Genetics

Although some researchers believe that genetic factors influence the risk of mTBI, research in this area is limited. The apolipoprotein E (ApoE) protein and ApoE promoter gene have been studied for association with concussion risk. Several years ago, the ApoE-E4 allele was proposed as a positive risk factor, but no association has been found in limited research. One retrospective study of collegiate male football and female soccer players (Terrell et al., 2008) did show a significant association between the ApoE-TT promoter genotype, increasing the odds of prior concussion nearly threefold. More research should be done in this area, as there is not enough data to provide clinical indication for genetic testing at this time.

Preexisting Conditions

Preexisting conditions, such as mood disorders and neurodevelopmental problems, have been hypothesized as a potential risk factor for prolonged recovery from mTBI, including concussion. Neuronal dysfunction is present in these disorders, as it is in concussion. However, it is not known if these conditions *predispose* an athlete to concussion in sport (Kutcher & Echner, 2010). Little to no research has been done in this area.

Development of depression, anxiety, learning disorders, or attention-deficit/ hyperactivity disorder following concussion or in postconcussion syndrome has been well established and should be treated when identified.

PREVENTION

Although a great deal of progress has been made in reducing the incidence of mTBI in workplace and daily settings (e.g., fall prevention programs, workplace safety regulations, automobile safety improvements, the introduction and promotion of helmet use in recreational activities ranging from bicycling to snow skiing), the current "hot topic" in the media and among clinicians and researchers is the prevention of sport-related concussion. Some prevention efforts have been implemented, with reports of at least limited success (e.g., improved protective equipment, coaching of proper sport technique, education regarding the importance of adherence to sports' rules); however, to date, nothing has been shown effective in preventing or significantly reducing the incidence of all sport-related concussion in even a single sport. Thus, as a recent clinical report noted, current recommendations focus on educating clinicians to recognize the signs and symptoms of concussion and the appropriate management of concussion to reduce the long-term symptoms and complications of this injury (Halstead, Walter, Council of Sports Medicine and Fitness, 2010).

Protective Equipment

Helmets have been introduced in various sport and recreational activities to attempt to reduce serious head injury, although for the most part they were not originally designed to decrease the risk of mTBI, including concussion (Delaney, Al-Kashmiri, Drummond, & Correa, 2008; Pettersen, 2002). Helmet design has changed, in some sports, with manufacturer attempts to focus on concussion prevention. Some sports, such as recreational skiing, snowboarding, and bicycling, do not require wearing a helmet for participation. However, data show helmet use in such sports is effective for head injury prevention. A case–control study of head injury (not specifically concussion) in skiers and snowboarders showed that those wearing a helmet had a 60% risk reduction (Sulheim, Holme, Ekeland, & Bahr, 2006). In skiers and snowboarders under the age of 13, helmet use significantly decreased the likelihood of head, face, and neck injury (Macnab, Smith, Gagnon, & Macnab, 2002). Similarly, studies in bicycling, including a Cochrane review in 1999, have shown decreased head injury risk with helmet use (Thompson, Rivara, & Thompson, 1999). Although no definitive research has been conducted on the association of concussion with head injury risk, these cited studies imply potential decreased concussion risk with helmet use.

American football is likely the most studied sport related to concussion. Helmets in football were originally designed to decrease risk of skull fracture and intracranial bleeding, which they do effectively (Halstead, 2010). Football is known to be associated with the highest absolute numbers of concussion, and much effort has been directed toward concussion prevention in football, mainly through helmet technology and playing techniques. At this time, no helmet is clearly shown to reduce concussion risk. A study of over 2,000 high school athletes in a prospective cohort (Collins, Lovell, Iverson, Ide, & Maroon, 2006) reported a 31% decreased relative concussion risk with a helmet designed to reduce force from contact to the side of the head or face; however, there are methodological problems with this study, and it will need to be replicated, with improved study design, before those results can be considered valid. The National Football League has shown mildly decreased force transmission in several newer helmet designs, when testing linear and rotational forces (Viano, Pellman, Withnall, & Shewchenko, 2006). Whether this improvement translates to actual decrease in injury rate is yet to be seen.

Soccer headgear has been introduced in the past several years, with the primary intention of reducing concussions in heading, and it has been marketed this way to the public. However, research has shown concussions in soccer most often occur not from heading the ball but from head-to-head, head-to-ground, or head-to-body-part contact. Several studies have investigated the potential of headgear to reduce force, with some promising results, but none has prospectively shown that this reduced force translates to decreased concussion risk. A large, nonrandomized study of youth soccer athletes (Delaney et al., 2008) showing fewer concussion symptoms in those wearing headgear, compared to those not wearing headgear, used a questionnaire with symptom self-report. The presence of any concussion symptom defined concussion in this study. These findings have not been replicated in a randomized controlled trial.

Similarly, rugby has investigated the use of headgear to decrease concussion. Two randomized controlled trials by the same author (one was a pilot study; McIntosh & McCrory, 2001; McIntosh et al., 2009) showed no protective effect of headgear. Marshall and colleagues (2005) also studied a cohort of over 300 rugby athletes to compare concussion incidence between those who wore headgear and those who did not and found no difference. Design changes in rugby headgear to reduce impact forces have been proposed, including increasing headgear thickness and density (McIntosh, McCrory, & Finch, 2004). Whether these changes would decrease concussion risk is not known.

Training Techniques

Unfortunately, no proven injury prevention strategies related to player-to-player or player-to-surface contact are available in sport-related concussion. These types of contact make up the large majority of concussions, and it makes sense to target this area for continued study. No fitness or other training program has been shown to decrease injury, although there certainly may be programs that will prove their merit in the future.

Continued study of the mechanism of concussion in various sports will lead to injury prevention specific to that sport. For example, in high school women's lacrosse, a recent study revealed concussions most often occurred from stick contact to the head or face (Lincoln, Hinton, Almquist, Lager, & Dick, 2007). The authors from that study proposed that injuries may be reduced with better stick and ball handling skills. Helmet use in sports such as women's lacrosse, in which no helmet is currently used, may well provide needed injury risk reduction.

TRENDS AND FUTURE RESEARCH DIRECTIONS

A dire need exists for the development of new or the combination of existing surveillance systems to provide researchers with access to a more comprehensive data set with which to evaluate the clinical, public health, economic, and epidemiological overviews of pediatric mTBI. Until such a data set can address the reality that these injuries are diagnosed and managed in a wide range of settings by a wide range of clinicians, the published literature will continue to provide only "snapshots" of these injuries rather than a comprehensive overview. Additional research efforts are needed in a broad array of areas, from diagnostic tools to prevention efforts, two of which are highlighted below.

Legislative Efforts

Recent efforts at local, state, and national levels have focused on implementing legislation regarding sport-related concussion (e.g., Washington's Zackery Lystedt Law). However, it is unknown how such efforts have changed knowledge, attitudes, beliefs, and behaviors of clinicians, coaches, parents, and student athletes. Research in this area is needed.

Helmet Technology

The fact that helmet and headgear manufacturers will continue to promote their products as "concussion-decreasing" gear is a given. What remains to be seen is whether specific helmets actually decrease concussion occurrence. As a large amount of pressure is placed on parents who want to keep their children safe by providing them with the "best" protective equipment, there is a strong need to fully research manufacturers' claims. Because helmets pad just the skull, with no way to actually pad the brain, helmet design has traditionally been targeted toward decreasing potentially catastrophic brain injuries, such as skull fracture and subdural and epidural hematomas. We are learning more about the forces that cause concussion and know that it is not just the "big hit" that inflicts injury. Smaller forces to the brain often cause the same problem, and repetitive small forces may pose a much bigger risk than previously imagined. Helmets will never totally prevent concussion, but as helmet materials become more advanced, we may be able to see force dissipation that can clinically, and pathophysiologically, reduce injury. We must keep in mind, however, that it will be virtually impossible to eliminate concussion from sport, because reducing brain–skull impact is difficult.

Research on helmet and other protective equipment, particularly for youth athletes, is desperately needed. Whether the same helmet style can confer similar protection for the adult and child athlete is not known. As the number of children participating in contact sports continues to grow, new models of injury prevention will be needed. Parents of youth athletes are becoming very sensitized to the injury of concussion, and they will often do "whatever it takes" to decrease their child's chance of sustaining a concussion. Because of the potential high financial cost of newer, more technically advanced equipment and training programs, it is imperative that we first obtain data supporting particular prevention methods to make them worthwhile.

Continued research on concussion mechanism in all sports is needed to develop methods that are likely to decrease the injury. Whether introducing helmets to sports not currently using them would be beneficial is yet to be seen and requires research. If helmets decrease concussion risk without changing a sport's culture, we may see some sports (e.g., women's field hockey, women's lacrosse) transition to helmet use in the years to come. However, in some sports, the use of helmets on the playing field would alter the game so severely (e.g., soccer) that their introduction is unlikely.

Strength, Conditioning, and Skill

Appropriate fitness for sport has been shown to prevent musculoskeletal problems such as shoulder instability, muscle strains, low back injuries, and knee pain (Hunt,

2003). There is no such evidence for this prevention effect with concussion, as it has not specifically been studied. Intuitively, one would advise athletes that being "in good shape" and being skilled at their sport and position help with overall injury prevention, and that theory may extend to concussion. Especially with children, the acquisition of sport skills and strength may indeed confer some concussion protection by way of avoiding potentially harmful positions in practice or game situations; this theory needs to be rigorously tested, however, before programs can be designed for injury prevention.

Techniques in sport have been scrutinized for possible ways to reduce concussion risk. Football tackling has been identified as an area that needs to be stressed and changed, as some note that tackling has evolved from traditional techniques involving wrapping an opponent with the arms during the tackle, into "hits" that encourage players to launch themselves at their opponents, primarily leading with their head (Gregory, 2010). Youth football coaches have developed programs that educate young athletes about the risks of improper tackling and teach techniques intended to avoid head injury. Research needs to address the effectiveness of these types of programs to determine if they actually lead to reduced injuries.

CONCLUSION

Although the epidemiology of pediatric mTBI is relatively well understood at this point, few universally effective prevention mechanisms exist. Our understanding of rates and patterns of pediatric mTBI, as well as risk factors for these injuries, should be leveraged to drive development, implementation, and evaluation of targeted, tailored prevention programs. We have finally made great strides in challenging the culture of sport to reject the idea that concussions are just "dings" or "bell ringers"— now we must focus our research efforts on reducing the incidence and severity of these injuries.

REFERENCES

Bakhos, L. L., Lockhart, G. R., Myers, R., & Linakis, J. G. (2010). Emergency department visits for concussion in young child athletes. *Pediatrics*, *126*(3), e550–e556.

Barlow, K. M., Crawford, S., Stevenson, A., Sandhu, S. S., Belanger, F., & Dewey, D. (2010). Epidemiology of postconcussion syndrome in pediatric mild traumatic brain injury. *Pediatrics*, *126*(2), e374–e381.

Bowman, S. M., Bird, T. M., Aitken, M. E., & Tilford, J. M. (2008). Trends in hospitalizations associated with pediatric traumatic brain injuries. *Pediatrics*, *122*(5), 988–993.

Brener, I., Harman, J. S., Kelleher, K. J., & Yeates, K. O. (2004). Medical costs of mild to moderate traumatic brain injury in children. *Journal of Head Trauma Rehabilitation*, *19*(5), 405–412.

Cantu, R. C. (2009). Consensus statement on concussion in sport—the 3rd International Conference on Concussion, Zurich, November 2008. *Neurosurgery*, *64*(5), 786–787.

Carroll, L. J., Cassidy, J. D., Holm, L., Kraus, J., & Coronado, V. G. (2004). Methodological issues and research recommendations for mild traumatic brain injury: The WHO

Collaborating Centre Task Force on Mild Traumatic Brain Injury. *Journal of Rehabilitation Medicine, 43*(Suppl.), 113–125.

Centers for Disease Control and Prevention (CDC), National Center for Injury Prevention and Control. (2003). *Report to Congress on mild traumatic brain injury in the United States: Steps to prevent a serious public health problem.* Atlanta, GA: Author.

Collins, M., Lovell, M. R., Iverson, G. L., Ide, T., & Maroon, J. (2006). Examining concussion rates and return to play in high school football players wearing newer helmet technology: A three-year prospective cohort study. *Neurosurgery, 58*(2), 275–286.

Covassin, T., Swanik, B., & Sachs, M. L. (2003). Sex differences and the incidence of concussions among collegiate athletes. *Journal of Athletic Training, 38*(3), 238–244.

Cross, K. M., & Serenelli, C. (2003). Training and equipment to prevent athletic head and neck injuries. *Clinical Journal of Sports Medicine, 22*(3), 639–667.

Delaney, J. S., Al-Kashmiri, A., Drummond, R., & Correa, J. A. (2008). The effect of protective headgear on head injuries and concussions in adolescent football (soccer) players. *British Journal of Sports Medicine, 42*(2), 110–115.

DeMatteo, C. A., Hanna, S. E., Mahoney, W. J., Hollenberg, R. D., Scott, L. A., Law, M. C., et al. (2010). "My child doesn't have a brain injury, he only has a concussion." *Pediatrics, 125*(2), 327–334.

Dick, R. W. (2009). Is there a gender difference in concussion incidence and outcomes? *British Journal of Sports Medicine, 43*(Suppl. 1), i46–i50.

Faul, M., Xu, L., Wald, M. M., & Coronado, V. G. (2010). *Traumatic brain injury in the United States: Emergency department visits, hospitalizations, and deaths 2002–2006.* Atlanta, GA: Centers for Disease Control and Prevention, National Center for Injury Prevention and Control.

Finkelstein, E., Corso, P., Miller, T., & Associates. (2006). *The incidence and economic burden of injuries in the United States.* New York: Oxford University Press.

Frommer, L. J., Gurka, K. K., Cross, K. M., Ingersoll, C. D., Comstock, R. D., & Saliba, S. A. (2011). Sex differences in concussion symptoms of high school athletes. *Journal of Athletic Training, 46*(1), 76–84.

Ganesalingam, K., Yeates, K. O., Ginn, M. S., Taylor, H. G., Dietrich, A., Nuss, K., et al. (2008). Family burden and parental distress following mild traumatic brain injury in children and its relationship to post-concussive symptoms. *Journal of Pediatric Psychology, 33*(6), 621–629.

Gessel, L. M., Fields, S. K., Collins, C. L., Dick, R. W., & Comstock, R. D. (2007). Concussions among United States high school and collegiate athletes. *Journal of Athletic Training, 42*(4), 495–503.

Gilchrist, J., Thomas, K. E., Wald, M., & Langlois, J. (2007). Nonfatal traumatic brain injuries from sports and recreation activities—United States, 2001–2005. *Morbidity and Mortality Weekly Report, 56*(29), 733–737.

Gordon, K. E., Dooley, J. M., Fitzpatrick, E. A., Wren, P., & Wood, E. P. (2010). Concussion or mild traumatic brain injury: Parents appreciate the nuances of nosology. *Pediatric Neurology, 43*(4), 253–257.

Granito, V. (2002). Psychological response to athletic injury: Sex differences. *Journal of Sports Behavior, 25*, 243–259.

Gregory, S. (2010). The problem with football. *Time, 175*, 36–43.

Guerrero, J. L., Thurman, D. J., & Sniezek, J. E. (2000). Emergency department visits associated with traumatic brain injury: United States, 1995–1996. *Brain Injury, 14*(2), 181–186.

Halstead, M. E. (2010). Contact sports for young athletes: Keys to safety. *Pediatric Annals, 39*(5), 275–278.

Halstead, M. E., Walter, K. D., & Council of Sports Medicine and Fitness. (2010). Sport-related concussion in children and adolescents. *Pediatrics*, 126(3), 597–615.

Hunt, A. (2003). Musculoskeletal fitness: The keystone in overall well-being and injury prevention. *Clinical Orthopaedics and Related Research*, 409, 96–105.

Koh, J. O., Cassidy, J. D., & Watkinson, E. J. (2003). Incidence of concussion in contact sports: A systematic review of the evidence. *Brain Injury*, 17(10), 901–907.

Kutcher, J. S., & Echner, J. T. (2010). At-risk populations in sports-related concussion. *Current Sports Medicine Reports*, 9(1), 16–20.

Lincoln, A. E., Caswell, S. V., Almquist, J. L., Dunn, R. E., Norris, J. B., & Hinton, R. Y. (2011). Trends in concussion incidence in high school sports: A prospective 11-year study. *American Journal of Sports Medicine*, 39, 958–963.

Lincoln, A. E., Hinton, R. Y., Almquist, J. L., Lager, S. L., & Dick, R. W. (2007). Head, face, and eye injuries in scholastic and collegiate lacrosse: A 4-year prospective study. *American Journal of Sports Medicine*, 35(2), 207–215.

Macnab, A. J., Smith, T., Gagnon, F. A., & Macnab, M. (2002). Effect of helmet wear on the incidence of head/face and cervical spine injuries in young skiers and snowboarders. *Injury Prevention*, 8(4), 324–327.

Mansell, J., Tierney, R. T., Sitler, M. R., Swanik, K. A., & Stearne, D. (2005). Resistance training and head–neck segment dynamic stabilization in male and female collegiate soccer players. *Journal of Athletic Training*, 40(4), 310–319.

Marshall, S. W., Loomis, D. P., Waller, A. E., Chalmers, D. J., Bird, Y. N., Quarrie, K. L., et al. (2005). Evaluation of protective equipment for prevention of injuries in rugby union. *International Journal of Epidemiology*, 34(1), 113–118.

McCrory, P., Collie, A., Anderson, V., & Davis, G. (2004). Can we manage sport related concussion in children the same as in adults? *British Journal of Sports Medicine*, 38(5), 516–519.

McIntosh, A. S., McCrory, P., & Finch, C. F. (2004). Performance enhanced headgear: A scientific approach to the development of protective headgear. *British Journal of Sports Medicine*, 38(1), 46–49.

McIntosh, A. S., McCrory, P., Finch, C. F., Best, J. P., Chalmers, D. J., & Wolfe, R. (2009). Does padded headgear prevent head injury in rugby union football? *Medicine and Science in Sports and Exercise*, 41(2), 306–313.

McIntosh, A. S., & McCrory, P. (2001). Effectiveness of headgear in a pilot study of under 15 rugby union football. *British Journal of Sports Medicine*, 35(3), 167–169.

Meehan, W. P., & Mannix, R. (2010). Pediatric concussions in United States emergency departments in the years 2002 to 2006. *Journal of Pediatrics*, 157(6), 889–893.

Ommaya, A. K., Goldsmith, W., & Thibault, L. (2002). Biomechanics and neuropathology of adult and paediatric head injury. *British Journal of Neurosurgery*, 16(3), 220–242.

Pettersen, J. A. (2002). Does rugby headgear prevent concussion?: Attitudes of Canadian players and coaches. *British Journal of Sports Medicine*, 36(1), 19–22.

Powell, J. W., & Barber-Foss, K. D. (1999). Traumatic brain injury in high school athletics. *Journal of the American Medical Association*, 282(10), 958–963.

Queen, R. M., Weinhold, P. S., Kirkendall, D. T., & Yu, B. (2003). Theoretical study of the effect of ball properties on impact force in soccer heading. *Medicine and Science in Sports and Exercise*, 35(12), 2069–2076.

Saleh, S. S., Fuortes, L., Vaughn, T., & Bauer, E. (2001). Epidemiology of occupational injuries and illnesses in a university population: A focus on age and gender differences. *American Journal of Industrial Medicine*, 39(6), 581–586.

Sulheim, S., Holme, I., Ekeland, A., & Bahr, R. (2006). Helmet use and risk of head injuries in alpine skier sand snowboarders. *Journal of the American Medical Association*, 295(8), 919–924.

Terrell, R. T., Bostick, R. M., Abramson, R., Xie, D., Barfield, W., Cantu, R., et al. (2008). APOE, APOE promoter, and TAU genotypes and risk for concussion in college athletes. *Clinical Journal of Sports Medicine*, *18*(1), 10–17.

Thompson, D. C., Rivara, F. P., & Thompson, R. (1999). Helmets for preventing head and facial injuries in bicyclists. *Cochrane Database of Systematic Reviews*, Issue 4, Art. No. CD001855.

Tierney, R. T., Higgins, M., Caswell, S. V., Brady, J., McHardy, K., Driban, J. B., et al. (2008). Sex differences in head acceleration during heading while wearing soccer headgear. *Journal of Athletic Training*, *43*(6), 578–584.

Tierney, R. T., Sitler, M. R., Swanik, C. B., Swanik, K. A., Higgins, M., & Torg, J. (2005). Gender differences in head–neck segment dynamic stabilization during head acceleration. *Medicine and Science in Sports and Exercise*, *37*(2), 272–279.

Viano, D. C., Pellman, E. J., Withnall, C., & Shewchenko, N. (2006). Concussion in professional football: Performance of newer helmets in reconstructed game impacts—Part 13. *Neurosurgery*, *59*(3), 591–606.

Yang, J., Peek-Asa, C., Allareddy, V., Phillips, G., Zhang, Y., & Cheng, G. (2007). Patient and hospital characteristics associated with length of stay and hospital charges for pediatric sports-related injury hospitalizations in the United States, 2000–2003. *Pediatrics*, *119*(4), e813–e820.

Yard, E. E., & Comstock, R. D. (2009). Compliance with return to play guidelines following concussion in U.S. high school athletes, 2005–2008. *Brain Injury*, *23*(11), 888–898.

Biomechanics of Sports Concussion

Jason P. Mihalik

Epidemiological data indicate that young children, particularly those younger than 15 years of age, represent the majority of all cases of traumatic brain injury (TBI; Langlois, Rutland-Brown, & Thomas, 2004). For reasons that are more clearly elucidated in later chapters, adolescents are at an increased risk for secondary—and potentially catastrophic—injuries. Unfortunately, adolescents are often not privy to the same level of medical supervision as their adult counterparts and, ultimately, may often be permitted to prematurely return to activity or full sport participation. Investigators in this area are faced with a number of issues as they pertain to understanding head injury impact mechanics. First, current ethics standards have made the use of primate animal models difficult, as basic research in this area has been limited to the rat and small mammals in recent years. Second, the use of postmortem cadavers does not allow researchers the ability to study impact mechanics in the context of dynamic everyday activities, including sports participation and work. The lack of muscle tonus and decreased volume of cerebrospinal fluid make it difficult to replicate *in vivo* collision scenarios using cadaveric specimens. Last, the ethical implications of randomly assigning study participants into a TBI group or a control group for the purpose of prospective TBI biomechanical studies should be clearly evident. Thus, the biomechanics of TBI remain an area elusive to many researchers (e.g., Guskiewicz & Mihalik, 2011). This chapter describes some basic principles of head impact biomechanics and reviews the historical literature in this area. Additionally, a discussion of how the study of head impact biomechanics may facilitate injury prevention among athletes and of contemporary head impact biomechanics research follows.

BASIC BIOMECHANICAL PRINCIPLES OF TBI

The degree of complexity in quantifying the biomechanics of head injury has led some to question whether a comprehensive understanding of the dynamics of head injury will ever be achieved (Guskiewicz & Mihalik, 2011; Shetter & Demakas, 1979). All mechanisms of head and brain injury involve a near-instant transfer of kinetic energy, which requires either an absorption (acceleration) or release (deceleration). Relevant biomechanical terms are defined in Table 3.1. Although force is the product of mass and acceleration ($F = m \times a$), little tradeoff occurs between the two. For example, a high-velocity bullet may penetrate the skull and brain but not cause a concussion because the mass of the bullet is too small to impart the necessary kinetic energy to the head and brain (Gurdjian, Lissner, Webster, Latimer, & Haddad, 1954). Although the overall force is the same in both conditions, if a somewhat larger projectile—but one that is traveling at a lower speed than the bullet—strikes the head, mild TBI (mTBI) may now ensue. The latter would be representative of most in-sport scenarios, whether due to helmet-to-helmet impact, head-to-ground impact, or any other object-to-head or object-to-body contact. Another property of kinetic energy that follows is that if an athlete's head is not mobile or is in contact with a wall or other surface, the kinetic forces imparted on the head and brain will travel through it and be transmitted elsewhere, often leaving brain function intact. The latter property is believed to play a role in body collisions whereby the young athlete anticipates a body collision. Through cervical muscle contraction, it is believed that forces related to the body collision act over a greater effective mass (head, neck, and trunk), and thus resulting head accelerations are lowered.

Regardless of whether the brain undergoes acceleration or deceleration—a sudden "speeding up" or "slowing down" of the head, respectively—the end result is a collision that produces an impact or impulse. In the context of mTBI, the term *impact* typically denotes a blow making direct contact with the head. An *impulse*, on the other hand, refers to a force that sets the head in motion without directly striking it.

TABLE 3.1. Terminology Related to TBI Biomechanics

Force: The effect one body has on another by way of a push or a pull applied to an object. A force is required to change the state of motion of an object such as that causing acceleration. It is equal to the product of mass and acceleration (F = mass $\times$ acceleration).

Impact: A blow making direct contact with the head. Examples of impacts range from helmet-to-helmet collisions, a player's head being hit with a stick, or a player's head being struck by a projectile used in the sport (e.g., soccer ball, hockey puck).

Impulse: A force that sets the head in motion without directly striking it. Impulsive forces are most commonly caused by tackling or body checking, and are the result of abruptly stopping an opponent's body from traveling in the direction in which it was moving.

Linear (translational) acceleration: The rate of change of linear velocity per unit of time. It is the straight-line acceleration of the head's center of gravity following an impact or impulse. Linear acceleration is traditionally measured in terms of g, gravitational acceleration.

Rotational (angular) acceleration: The rate of change of angular velocity per unit of time. It is the acceleration of the head as it rotates about a set of axes running through the head center of gravity. Rotational acceleration is traditionally measured in radians per second squared (rad/s^2).

g force: Unit of measurement for linear acceleration, expressed relative to gravitational acceleration ($1 g = 9.81$ m/s^2).

rad/s^2: Unit of measurement for rotational acceleration (radians per second squared).

Examples of impacts range from helmet-to-helmet collisions, a player's head being hit with a stick, or a player's head being struck by a projectile used in the sport (e.g., soccer ball, hockey puck). Impulsive forces are most commonly caused by tackling or body checking, and are the result of abruptly stopping an opponent's body from traveling in the direction in which it was moving. An example of an impulsive force in a nonsport setting is the effect experienced by passengers when a car quickly accelerates or decelerates. Impacts and impulses are traditionally linear (translational) or rotational (angular) in nature. In real-world activities, some combination of both linear and angular accelerations is usually associated with impacts and impulses. Ommaya and Gennarelli (1974) argued that impulse injuries are best suited to biomechanical reconstructions of acceleration or deceleration TBI since there is no contamination by impact mechanics. Many factors are thought to play a role in the body's ability to dissipate head impact forces, including individual differences in cerebrospinal fluid level and function, vulnerability to brain tissue injury, relative musculoskeletal strengths and weaknesses, and the anticipation of an oncoming impact or impulse.

The severity of TBI has traditionally been related to the acceleration exerted on the brain in both impact and impulsive mechanisms. Acceleration is typically described in one of two ways: linear or rotational. Linear acceleration of the brain may be defined as movement in a straight line through the brain's center of mass (Shaw, 2002) and is typically represented in the literature as a g force, expressed relative to gravitational acceleration. For example, standing on the earth at sea level imposes 1 g acceleration on a person. The g forces experienced by those on rollercoasters can range from 3.5 to 6.3 g. These g forces are considerably lower than those related to the TBI biomechanics presented later in this chapter. However, the seemingly high g forces related to head impact biomechanics are sustained over very short time durations (e.g., 8–12 ms), and are not sustained over longer periods of time (i.e., seconds) experienced during rollercoasters or aerobatic flying. Rotational acceleration of the brain occurs when the head accelerates on an arc about its center of gravity. The contribution of linear and rotational acceleration to TBI remains a topic of controversy. Initial studies with primates indicated that rotational acceleration forces were most likely responsible for producing a loss of consciousness (Ommaya & Gennarelli, 1974). Forces causing high linear accelerations were more likely to result in brain contusions or hemorrhage. Although true in earlier works surrounding TBI biomechanics, data from more recent sport-related research suggest that a combination of linear and rotational acceleration plays a role in the concussive injury (Guskiewicz et al., 2007; Mihalik, Bell, Marshall, & Guskiewicz, 2007a; Ommaya & Gennarelli, 1974; Shetter & Demakas, 1979).

HISTORICAL TBI BIOMECHANICS RESEARCH

A number of landmark studies has furthered our understanding of head impact biomechanics. These studies were initiated in the 1940s by Denny-Brown and his colleagues (e.g., Denny-Brown & Russell, 1941). Their study sample consisted primarily of cats, although monkeys and dogs were also used. The innovative advance in their line of research was twofold: They used a pendulum hammer to impart head impacts, and they suspended their subjects such that the head was free to move following an experimental impact. Until that time, impacts had been imparted on animals whose heads were fixed, disregarding entirely the actual dynamics of impact situations, such as those occurring in motor vehicle accidents or head impacts sustained on the playing field. Complementing this original work and eliminating the need for the animal model, physical models of the human skull and brain were then constructed (Holbourn, 1943, 1945). In these models the skull was made of wax and the brain within it was composed of a gelatinous structure. This work initially led Holbourn to suggest that rotational motion was likely needed to produce cortical lesions and concussion.

One of the considerable advances in the study of TBI biomechanics occurred when Pudenz and Shelden (1946) removed the top half of monkey skulls and replaced them with transparent plastic domes. Using high-speed cinephotography, the researchers were able to capture the movement of the brain following a head impact. Supporting Holbourn's basic tenet, Pudenz and Shelden documented that the brain noticeably lags behind the skull upon rotational head movement due to inertia. Almost 30 years later, Ommaya and Gennarelli used animal models and confirmed Holbourn's basic theory (Ommaya & Gennarelli, 1974). In their study, they imparted several rotational impacts to squirrel monkeys; the monkeys suffered a concussion as a result. The researchers observed that a direct impact to the head was not a necessary requirement to produce head trauma. This finding eventually led to the realization that inertial nonimpact loading resulting from an impulsive force can provide sufficient force to induce a mTBI following a tackle or with more common whiplash mechanisms associated with motor vehicle accidents (Letcher, Corrao, & Ommaya, 1973; Ommaya, Corrao, & Letcher, 1973; Ommaya & Gennarelli, 1974; Ommaya, Hirsch, Flamm, & Mahone, 1966; Ommaya, Rockoff, & Baldwin, 1964).

Difficulties with these historical works preclude a direct application of their findings to modern-day youth. The most obvious is that earlier definitions of concussion did not formally exist until the Congress of Neurological Surgeons published their definition (Committee on Head Injury Nomenclature of the Congress of Neurological Surgeons, 1966). As a result, Denny-Brown and Russell struggled to clearly delineate the criteria they used to identify concussion. A strength of their work, however, was that they emphasized the importance of head movements in the context of mTBI and, more importantly, how these head movements may or may not elicit concussion. Holbourn (1945) used these findings to justify his theory that angular acceleration of the head propagated movements of the brain within the skull, generating shear strains most prominent at the surface of the brain. These strains usually result in the transient deficits clinicians observe following mTBI, as opposed to the deeper brainstem lesions that result in more severe forms of TBI.

Unfortunately, it is often difficult to assess subtle postimpact cognitive awareness when using animals. Although loss of consciousness and death are obvious markers of TBI in animal subjects, objectively measuring mental status in animals following a given head impact is challenging. Further compounding this issue, most animal studies employed light anesthesia in their animals using substances such as pentobarbital. Pentobarbital is approved for human use to treat seizures and as a preoperative sedative. It functions by depressing the central nervous system (CNS) at all levels, including the sensory cortex, motor activity, and altered cerebellar function (Deglin & Vallerand, 2009). Pentobarbital has also been used to reduce intracranial pressure and lower cerebral oxygen demands in patients with TBI (San Diego Reference

Library, 2008) and is the primary ingredient in both veterinary and human euthanasia compounds. Knowing these uses, it is easy to understand how the presence of pentobarbital and other anesthetics may mask any cognitive declines that could be observed in the animal model.

The information provided to this point has highlighted the historical work in the area of TBI biomechanics. As is evident from this body of work, the majority—if not all—of TBI biomechanics research was performed on animal models. An extensive review of the contemporary animal model research is provided in the next chapter. Although these animal studies have provided excellent insights into modeling TBI biomechanics, questions remain with regard to how these findings relate to the human model.

HUMAN TBI RESEARCH: ARE CHILDREN THE SAME AS "LITTLE ADULTS"?

Although there are some mechanisms of injury common to both pediatric and adult populations (e.g., motor vehicle accidents, athletic participation), other mechanisms occur more frequently in younger populations. For example, the majority of severe TBI among infants less than 1 year of age is the result of abuse (McClelland, Rekate, Kaufman, & Persse, 1980). Further, McClelland et al. (1980) reported that 10% of all TBI among children younger than 5 years of age results from nonaccidental causes. TBI remains the leading cause of death among young children.

Head injury biomechanics also differ between pediatric and adult patients. Several factors contribute to these differences, including, but not limited to, differences in brain hydration status, cerebral vasculature, anthropometrics of the skull and brain, degree of neurostructural development, and the relative size of the head compared to the rest of the body (Bauer & Fritz, 2004; Goldsmith & Plunkett, 2004; Kirkwood et al., 2008). Intuitively, the relative frailty of children seems like it should mean that they are more susceptible to brain injury, with injuries occurring with lower levels of energy. Counter to this hypothesis, biomechanists have demonstrated that lesser forces are required to cause similar TBI in larger brains than in smaller brains with lesser mass (Goldsmith & Plunkett, 2004; Ommaya, Goldsmith, & Thibault, 2002). All postinjury symptoms constant, this phenomenon has caused some to speculate that a greater force is required for the pediatric patient to sustain TBI compared to his or her adult counterpart (McCrory, Collie, Anderson, & Davis, 2004). Even within the pediatric realm, these findings are not consistent, suggesting that the brain and its protective structures vary in their responses across the developmental lifespan. A higher number of early seizures, skull fractures, subdural hematoma, and low-energy-mechanism head injuries—but fewer cases of loss of consciousness—were observed in infants and children younger than 3 years of age, compared to older children (Berney, Froidevaux, & Favier, 1994). Clearly, research data to illustrate the true pediatric TBI biomechanical picture are still lacking. What we do know to date is that children behave very differently from adults. Providing an additional level of complexity to the pediatric TBI problem, early research suggests that tolerances and responses to TBI-causing forces differ across the pediatric spectrum. Studying pediatric TBI biomechanics is quite difficult.

STUDYING ATHLETIC TBI BIOMECHANICS: TOOLS IN THE RESEARCHER'S TOOLBOX

A number of techniques have been employed to study the biomechanics of athletic TBI, such as animal studies and computational modeling. In the area of forensics, it is not uncommon to use specialized equipment (i.e., crash test dummies and other human skull/brain surrogates) to reconstruct injurious events. Although these techniques hold merit in their own right, it has often been difficult to generalize the findings from these studies to *in vivo* human athletic participation. In the past 7 years, technological advancements have permitted the use of telemetrically instrumented helmets capable of measuring characteristics of head impacts sustained by athletes participating in American football and ice hockey.

In earlier work by the National Football League, laboratory reconstruction of concussive injuries captured on video was performed (Pellman, Viano, Tucker, Casson, & Waeckerle, 2003). The investigators reviewed television camera footage of known concussive collisions. They used on-field landmarks such as yard line indicators to determine the moving velocities of the striking player and the player struck. They also identified the location on the head where the impact was delivered or sustained by the players, the angle of impact, and other factors that would be required to reconstruct the collisions. They then reconstructed the collisions using instrumented surrogates in a laboratory setting. The studies were not without scientific limitations. Television cameras operate at much lower frequencies (e.g., 60 Hz or 60 frames per second) compared to other biomechanical motion analysis systems. Thus, the extrapolative errors of player velocities and the ability to accurately identify impact location may be high. The research team only analyzed 31 out of 182 cases, with no clear description as to why the remaining 151 cases were excluded. Thus, conclusions were made based on this very small and selective sample of cases.

Another novel technique that has been employed with the goal of studying TBI biomechanics in the athletic arena is that of real-time accelerometer data collection. Preliminary data that captured techniques for this purpose were limited in design. Naunheim, Standeven, Richter, and Lewis (2000) studied the linear accelerations sustained by four high school athletes: an ice hockey defenseman, a football offensive lineman, a football defensive lineman, and a soccer player. A triaxial accelerometer was inserted within a football and ice hockey helmet, and linear acceleration values were recorded during actual play. The mean linear acceleration measured in the football and ice hockey players was 29.2 g and 35.0 g, respectively. The data obtained from the soccer player lack external validity for two main reasons. First, since there was no method of affixing the accelerometer to the player's head, the soccer player wore an instrumented football helmet. Second, game data were not captured; instead, the soccer player was asked to head 23 balls kicked at a standardized velocity, an acceptable methodological compromise, given participation while wearing a football helmet would not be permitted. This study was the first of its kind to attempt the real-time *in vivo* study of head impacts during athletic participation in young athletes, and to report objective measures to this end.

Our research team at the University of North Carolina at Chapel Hill, along with other research groups (at Virginia Polytechnic Institute and State University, Dartmouth College, and Oklahoma University, among others), has employed the use of more advanced real-time data collection systems capable of monitoring head impacts sustained by our athletes participating in American football and ice hockey. The system is aptly named the Head Impact Telemetry (HIT) System. A major component of the HIT System is the installation of six single-axis accelerometers that are positioned within the open spaces between the helmet padding (see Figure 3.1). The HIT System is capable of measuring the magnitude and direction of the head's—not helmet's—center of gravity acceleration from the accelerometers. Linear acceleration is measured and reported in g, expressed relative to gravitational acceleration, and rotational acceleration is measured in rad/s². For any threshold impact, information from all six accelerometers is collected at 1 kHz for a period of 40 ms; 8 ms are recorded prior to the data collection trigger, and 32 ms of data are collected following the threshold trigger. These data are streamed in real time to a sideline controller. The data are time-stamped on the accelerometer player unit, encoded, and transmitted to a sideline controller via a radio frequency telemetry link. Additional measures, including the Head Impact Technology severity profile (HITsp; Greenwald, Gwin, Chu, & Crisco, 2008) and traditional measures of head impact biomechanics such as the Gadd Severity Index and Head Injury Criterion, are also analyzed and stored at this time. The user interfaces with the Sideline Response System via the HIT Impact Analyzer software on the laptop. The telemetry system is capable of transmitting accelerometer data from as many as 100 players over a distance well in excess of the length of a football field.

Duma and his colleagues (2005) at Virginia Polytechnic Institute and State University were the first to employ acceleration-measuring technology in helmets for large numbers of athletes during normal practice and game situations. Duma et al. reported the magnitude of head impacts to be $32 \pm 25\ g$. This range contrasts with the range of 20–23 g we would later record and report of a similar sample of Division I collegiate football players (Mihalik, Bell, Marshall, & Guskiewicz, 2007b). Does this discrepancy in range of force suggest that college players at one institution sustain head impacts that are considerably different from those at a like institution? Although possible, the explanation for these differences likely rests with how these data were analyzed. Typically, biomechanical measures of head impacts are very positively skewed, with the majority of all head impacts yielding low linear acceleration

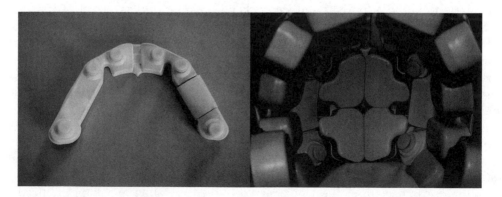

FIGURE 3.1. A major component of the HIT System is the installation of six single-axis accelerometers that are positioned within the open spaces between the helmet padding within Riddell football helmets.

outcomes that do not represent a normal distribution. Our analyses accounted for the skewed data, and we were able to perform statistical transformations that permitted us to present a more conservative point estimate in our sample. Our study also measured all head impacts sustained by each player in every practice and game throughout the season.

How can this same technology be implemented in youth athletics? Insofar as athletes are wearing properly fitting Riddell helmets, the HIT System can be implemented at all levels of football participation. That said, at the time this chapter was written, a PubMed search for *head impacts high school football* yielded only three citations (Broglio et al., 2009, 2010; Schnebel, Gwin, Anderson, & Gatlin, 2007). A summary of linear acceleration values reported in the literature that covers college and high school football, as well as youth ice hockey, is provided in Table 3.2.

Our own work at UNC–Chapel Hill has extended to youth athletics, with a particular emphasis on youth ice hockey. The required modifications to the existing HIT System are unique in this sport in that the protective lining of the helmet must be customized to accept the HIT System instrumentation (see Figure 3.2). Our preliminary data in youth ice hockey players suggest that mean linear accelerations typically do not exceed 19 *g* (Mihalik, Guskiewicz, Jeffries, Greenwald, & Marshall, 2008), a number comparable to that observed in our sample of collegiate football players. Acknowledging that these impacts are subconcussive and may occur with less frequency than for football players, it is still potentially alarming that young 13- and 14-year-old ice hockey players are repetitively sustaining head impacts commensurate with much older, taller, and heavier collegiate football players. While research continues in this area, it is important for researchers to use this novel instrumentation to not only better appreciate the nature of head impacts sustained by athletes, but to understand how players can better protect themselves and their opponents from sustaining high-magnitude impacts, hopefully resulting in lower incidences of mTBI in amateur, collegiate, and professional sports, alike.

TABLE 3.2. Summary of Findings Related to Head Impact Biomechanics Research

Researchers	Population	Frequency	Overall mean linear acceleration	Seasons studied
Broglio et al. (2010)	78 high school football players	54,247	25.1 *g*	4
Schnebel et al. (2007)	40 college football players	54,154 (college)	Not reported	1
	16 high school football players	8,526 (high school)		
Mihalik et al. (2007)	72 college football players	57,024	22.25 *g*	2
Duma et al. (2005)	38 college football players	3,312	32 *g*	1
Brolinson et al. (2006)	52 college football players	11,604	20.9 *g*	2
Mihalik et al. (2008)	14 youth ice hockey players (13 years old)	4,543	18.98 *g*	1
Mihalik et al. (2010)	16 youth ice hockey players (14 years of age)	666	21.5 *g*	1

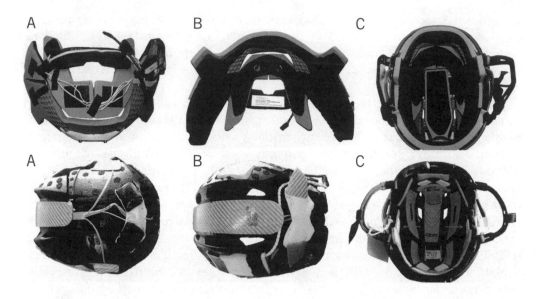

FIGURE 3.2. The protective foam of the ice hockey helmets were removed from the helmet shell (Easton Stealth S9 model depicted on top; RBK 6K/8K model depicted on bottom). Following this, six single-axis accelerometers were fitted into custom holes cut into the foam.

THRESHOLDS TO ATHLETIC TBI

Research on mTBI has provided clinicians with useful information as it pertains to individual pieces of the proverbial concussion puzzle, including, but not limited to, symptomatology, postural stability, and cognitive function. Although these studies have provided us with important information and have changed the way many medical professionals manage injuries, they do very little to help us understand what causes a concussion and how we might best be able to minimize the risk of injury entirely. Numerous studies have investigated impact biomechanics to shed light on proposed injury thresholds for mTBI. Earlier primate work to this end identified very high linear and rotational accelerations needed to result in injury (Hodgson, Thomas, & Khalil, 1983; Ommaya & Gennarelli, 1974). These animal models are unlikely to be representative of threshold values associated with human TBI, however. Discrepancies between the thresholds found in animals and humans are likely due to the fact that monkey skulls and musculoskeletal anthropometrics (e.g., bone density, skull thickness, and musculoskeletal strength) are significantly superior to that of humans. Moreover, the ability of the researchers to accurately measure linear and rotational accelerations more than 25 years ago was quite limited compared to today's standards. Last, operational definitions of concussion employed for research purposes prior to 1997 (American Academy of Neurology, 1997) almost all included some level of loss of consciousness, suggesting that researchers were imparting more serious and severe impacts to the monkey subjects in order to render them *concussed*.

Hugenholtz and Richard (1982) were among the first in the literature to propose an mTBI threshold in humans in terms of linear acceleration *g* forces. In their report, they proposed that an mTBI would likely result from a blow to the head that exceeded 80–90 g and was sustained for greater than 4 milliseconds. In the study conducted by the National Football League described earlier, it was suggested that mTBI in helmeted impacts are likely to occur between 70 and 75 g. Zhang et al. also proposed injury threshold values employing the use of the Wayne State University Brain Injury Model (Zhang, Yang, & King, 2004). They report that the resultant linear accelerations of the head center of gravity exceeding 82 g were associated with a 50% probability of suffering an mTBI event. These values are similar to those proposed by Ono et al., who suggested that impacts of 90 g, sustained for 9 milliseconds or longer, would result in mTBI (Ono, Kikuchi, Nakamura, Kobayashi, & Nakamura, 1980). Although subtle differences exist between these theoretical thresholds for TBI, they are based on adult models. Pediatric TBI thresholds in relation to athletic TBI are virtually nonexistent. Would it matter if pediatric-specific data to this effect existed? Based on our ongoing data, we have not identified any validity to the current theoretical thresholds even with adults. The notion that a "threshold" exists and that one could identify an injury on the basis of some impact measure is elusive to researchers (Guskiewicz & Mihalik, 2011). Our own data indicated that only 7 of 1,858 (less than 0.38%) head impacts exceeding 80 g resulted in a diagnosed case of mTBI (Mihalik et al., 2007b). Using these thresholds in the context of real-time monitoring of athletes, while extremely sensitive, lacks the specificity to make these tools clinically meaningful for this purpose at this time.

INJURY BIOMECHANICS: TRANSLATING CLINICAL RESEARCH TO INJURY PREVENTION

The underlying issue in the management of pediatric TBI remains: How does our understanding of head impact biomechanics translate to the on-field management of our young athletes? The answer, unfortunately, is not yet complete as research in this field is still in its infancy. However, we certainly know more today than we did 20 years ago, or even 5 years ago. The findings of our studies and those conducted by others have provided key evidence supporting the need to change the way our sports are played, with the end goal of protecting our athletes. That said, the implications of foundational biomechanical studies to understanding the detection, prevention, and treatment of mTBI are worthy of discussion. The basic tenet of the injury threshold principle is that there is an increased likelihood an athlete has a TBI if he or she sustains an impact exceeding some threshold. If these thresholds hold true, then head impact monitoring devices should—in theory—be able to detect players who sustain severe head impacts and alert the sideline medical staff, coach, or parent to this injurious event and withhold the athlete from ongoing participation. We sought to study this phenomenon in our sample of collegiate football players. The players completed a full postinjury clinical testing battery within 16–24 hours following the end of the given session in which they sustained an impact greater than 90 g (McCaffrey, Mihalik, Crowell, Shields, & Guskiewicz, 2007). In the absence of a concussion diagnosis at the time of impact, and recruiting participants solely on the basis of head impacts sustained during the practice or competition session, sustaining an impact in excess of 90 g did not result in a clinically observable case of mTBI.

The study of TBI biomechanics in youth ice hockey players has provided some insights into how these findings may translate to *injury prevention* initiatives in youth sports. Playing within the confines of the sport's rules has been identified as a method of reducing injuries through a number of epidemiological studies. Our work with youth ice hockey players was the first to provide objective evidence supporting these findings. We found that more than 17.3% of body collisions (more than one out of every six) incurred some level of infraction, the majority of which were not enforced by officials during competition. These "illegal" body collisions, particularly those involving direct head contact, elbowing to the head, or high sticking to the head, resulted in higher measures of head impact severity than legal collisions (Mihalik et al., 2010b). The obvious take-home message from this study is that athletes and coaches should conform to playing rules. As hockey officials share a responsibility in maintaining a safe playing environment for the players, we would recommend that officials should more stringently enforce existing rules and assess more severe penalties to participants who purposefully attempt to foul an opponent at the youth ice hockey level.

We acknowledge that a young athlete often has no control over what an opponent does during competition. As a result, we recognize the need to identify injury prevention strategies that young athletes can practice to protect themselves from injury. In a follow-up study, we identified an intuitive, but key, finding: Collision anticipation may play a role in minimizing head impact severity (Mihalik et al., 2010a). We found that unanticipated collisions—body collisions the athlete did not see coming and thus was ill prepared for—resulted in higher impact forces than those impacts for which an athlete was prepared to deliver or receive. Further, we found that impacts on the open ice resulted in slightly higher impact forces than impacts along the playing boards. Does this mean that we eliminate all open ice collisions in youth ice hockey? Others have made the argument. We would recommend a more middle-of-the-road approach: Teach our young athletes to recognize areas of the ice that are high risk for severe impacts, and educate them on ways to better anticipate collisions so that they can better dissipate the associated forces and thereby prevent injury. How can this be accomplished? Practically speaking, coaches and athletes should incorporate body-checking exercises in practices, and coaches should spend time educating young athletes on proper checking techniques in order to minimize the risk of injury and increase the safety of ice hockey.

Another proposed avenue for injury prevention has considered the role cervical musculature may play in minimizing head impact severity. The basic underlying principle is as follows: if athletes anticipate oncoming collisions, they will be better able to control head movements by contracting (i.e., tensing) their cervical musculature. Using a Newtonian approach, acceleration is the result of force divided by mass. When the cervical musculature is contracted, it is thought to significantly increase the effective mass of the head–neck–trunk segment, resulting in a lower acceleration of the head. When an impact is unanticipated, and the cervical musculature is not tensed and prepared for a collision, the effective mass is reduced to that of the head. Given an equal force from a body collision, the head would experience a substantially greater acceleration and therefore would more likely sustain an injury. In theory, this point seems rather intuitive; however, there has been a general lack of research in this area. Existing studies have focused primarily on a soccer-heading task, and the findings of these studies are limited and conflicting with respect to head impact biomechanics. Our work with youth ice hockey players does not support absolute cervical muscle strength as a factor in explaining differences in head impact biomechanics (Mihalik et al., 2011). Does this mean that there is no value in strengthening the cervical musculature? This area of research is still in its infancy, and we caution against any firm conclusions being drawn at this time for two reasons. First, the static clinical measures of strength we recorded do not factor in the anticipation level of the athlete during collisions, nor do they factor in the isokinetic properties of muscle tissues undergoing such loads. Second, research has supported the value of strengthening the cervical muscles as part of a general whole-body conditioning program in the context of preventing musculoskeletal and orthopedic injuries. There is still strong support for the role neck musculature may play in reducing the risk of mTBI that is worthy of investigation in a young, at-risk sample. The youth ice hockey study findings reported earlier suggest that studying TBI biomechanics may be useful in influencing rule changes for improving safety in youth sports. We imagine that such changes would prevent collisions in which players may be ill prepared and vulnerable to sustain high-level impacts to the head. Due to limited work in this area, future biomechanical studies in youth sports are needed to better interpret these findings.

THE NEXT FRONTIERS

In reviewing the literature, it is clear that very little is known about the types of forces that cause pediatric mTBI and, perhaps alarmingly, very few suggested methods to reduce head impact forces. Cantu (1996) suggested five methods that can result in a reduction of mTBI: changes in rules (1) and coaching technique (2), improvements in conditioning (3) and equipment (4), and increasing medical supervision (5). These target areas were, in hindsight, very prescient. At the time this chapter was written, USA Hockey was considering a rule change that would increase the age at which youth hockey players could begin body checking from Peewee (11- and 12-year-olds) to Bantam (13- and 14-year-olds). What effect would delaying body checking have on young hockey players? That is, would injury risk decrease since they were hitting at an older age? Or would injury risk increase because the fundamental skills of body checking were no longer taught to young skaters (i.e., skills required to handle the puck while delivering and receiving body checks), thereby predisposing athletes to be less able to protect themselves on the ice? Given the strong influence coaches have on young athletes, the successes of ongoing injury prevention work will likely rest with the quality of coaching athletes receive. Enhancing anticipation drills during practices and reinforcing proper body checking or tackling techniques are realistic aspects of youth sports that our data suggest may lead to marked decreases in the number of injuries young athletes sustain. Aspects of conditioning are worthy of further study, particularly as they relate to dynamic muscle activation during competition. Improvements in player equipment will be important in our ongoing quest to prevent injuries. That said, one acknowledgment that will be repeated throughout this text is that children are not simply "little adults." The equipment standards in place for preventing adult TBI likely should not be extrapolated to youth. Studies to this end should continue to ensure that protective equipment meets the fundamental and unique characteristics of youth athletes. For example, the National Operating Committee on Standards for Athletic Equipment (NOCSAE) is currently studying a new helmet-testing standard that would represent the safety of the young football player.

CONCLUSIONS

In summary, our understanding of the mechanisms of injury is still quite limited in the field of TBI. Why does one 85 *g* head impact result in concussion, whereas another 85 *g* head impact result in no clinically reported or observable signs of concussion? More interestingly, how can a 60 *g* impact cause a concussion when a 160 *g* impact does not? These questions are not rhetorical. Rather, they are the premise for why researchers are seeking to further understand the phenomena of TBI biomechanics. Each aspect of the continuum of care for pediatric TBI can be related back to the ongoing research questions:

> What kind of impact caused this injury?
> What is unique about *that* impact that causes a young patient to clinically present in this way?
> What could a young patient have done differently during participation that would have lessened the severity of the concussion or prevented it entirely?

The answers will not be simple to uncover, but the field of TBI biomechanics will continue to address these and other important research questions in the future.

REFERENCES

American Academy of Neurology. (1997). Practice parameter: The management of concussion in sports (summary statement). Report of the Quality Standards Subcommittee. *Neurology, 48*(3), 581–585.

Bauer, R., & Fritz, H. (2004). Pathophysiology of traumatic injury in the developing brain: An introduction and short update. *Experimental and Toxicologic Pathology, 56*(1–2), 65–73.

Berney, J., Froidevaux, A. C., & Favier, J. (1994). Paediatric head trauma: Influence of age and sex. II. Biomechanical and anatomo-clinical correlations. *Child's Nervous System, 10*(8), 517–523.

Broglio, S. P., Schnebel, B., Sosnoff, J. J., Shin, S., Feng, X., He, X., et al. (2010). Biomechanical properties of concussions in high school football. *Medicine and Science in Sports and Exercise, 42*(11), 2064–2071.

Broglio, S. P., Sosnoff, J. J., Shin, S., He, X., Alcaraz, C., & Zimmerman, J. (2009). Head impacts during high school football: A biomechanical assessment. *Journal of Athletic Training, 44*(4), 342–349.

Cantu, R. C. (1996). Head injuries in sport. *British Journal of Sports Medicine, 30*(4), 289–296.

Committee on Head Injury Nomenclature of the Congress of Neurological Surgeons. (1966). Glossary of head injury, including some definitions of injury to the cervical spine. *Clinical Neurosurgery, 12*, 386–394.

Deglin, J. H., & Vallerand, A. H. (2009). *Davis's drug guide for nurses* (11th ed.). Philadelphia: F. A. Davis.

Denny-Brown, D., & Russell, W. R. (1941). Experimental cerebral concussion. *Brain, 64*(2–3), 93–164.

Duma, S. M., Manoogian, S. J., Bussone, W. R., Brolinson, P. G., Goforth, M. W., Donnenwerth, J. J., et al. (2005). Analysis of real-time head accelerations in collegiate football players. *Clinical Journal of Sport Medicine, 15*(1), 3–8.

Goldsmith, W., & Plunkett, J. (2004). A biomechanical analysis of the causes of traumatic brain injury in infants and children. *American Journal of Forensic Medicine and Pathology, 25*(2), 89–100.

Greenwald, R. M., Gwin, J. T., Chu, J. J., & Crisco, J. J. (2008). Head impact severity measures for evaluating mild traumatic brain injury risk exposure. *Neurosurgery, 62*(4), 789–798.

Gurdjian, E. S., Lissner, H. R., Webster, J. E., Latimer, F. R., & Haddad, B. F. (1954). Studies on experimental concussion: Relation of physiologic effect to time duration of intracranial pressure increase at impact. *Neurology, 4*, 674–681.

Guskiewicz, K. M., & Mihalik, J. P. (2011). Biomechanics of sport concussion: Quest for the elusive injury threshold. *Exercise and Sport Sciences Reviews, 39*(1), 4–11.

Guskiewicz, K. M., Mihalik, J. P., Shankar, V., Marshall, S. W., Crowell, D. H., Oliaro, S. M., et al. (2007). Measurement of head impacts in collegiate football players: Relationship between head impact biomechanics and acute clinical outcome after concussion. *Neurosurgery, 61*(6), 1244–1252.

Hodgson, V. R., Thomas, L. M., & Khalil, T. B. (1983). The role of impact location in reversible cerebral concussion. In *Proceedings of the 27th Stapp Car Crash Conference* (pp. 225–240). Warrendale, PA: Society of Automotive Engineers.

Holbourn, A. H. S. (1943). Mechanics of head injuries. *Lancet, 242*(6267), 438–441.

Holbourn, A. H. S. (1945). The mechanics of brain injuries. *British Medical Bulletin, 3*(6), 147–149.

Hugenholtz, H., & Richard, M. T. (1982). Return to athletic competition following concussion. *Canadian Medical Association Journal, 127*(9), 827–829.

Kirkwood, M. W., Yeates, K. O., Taylor, H. G., Randolph, C., McCrea, M., & Anderson, V. A. (2008). Management of pediatric mild traumatic brain injury: A neuropsychological review from injury through recovery. *Clinical Neuropsychologist, 22*(5), 769–800.

Langlois, J. A., Rutland-Brown, W., & Thomas, K. E. (2004). *Traumatic brain injury in the United States: Emergency department visits, hospitalizations, and deaths.* Atlanta, GA: Centers for Disease Control and Prevention, National Center for Injury Prevention and Control.

Letcher, F. S., Corrao, P. G., & Ommaya, A. K. (1973). Head injury in the chimpanzee: 2. Spontaneous and evoked epidural potentials as indices of injury severity. *Journal of Neurosurgery, 39*(2), 167–177.

McCaffrey, M. A., Mihalik, J. P., Crowell, D. H., Shields, E. W., & Guskiewicz, K. M. (2007). Measurement of head impacts in Division I football players: Clinical measures of concussion following high and low impact magnitudes. *Neurosurgery, 61*(6), 1236–1243.

McClelland, C. Q., Rekate, H., Kaufman, B., & Persse, L. (1980). Cerebral injury in child abuse: A changing profile. *Child's Brain, 7*(5), 225–235.

McCrory, P., Collie, A., Anderson, V., & Davis, G. (2004). Can we manage sport related concussion in children the same as in adults? *British Journal of Sports Medicine, 38*(5), 516–519.

Mihalik, J. P., Bell, D. R., Marshall, S. W., & Guskiewicz, K. M. (2007). Measurement of head impacts in collegiate football players: An investigation of positional and event-type differences. *Neurosurgery, 61*(6), 1229–1235.

Mihalik, J. P., Blackburn, J. T., Greenwald, R. M., Cantu, R. C., Marshall, S. W., & Guskie-wicz, K. M. (2010a). Collision type and player anticipation affect head impact severity among youth ice hockey players. *Pediatrics, 125*(6), e1394–e1401.

Mihalik, J. P., Greenwald, R. M., Blackburn, J. T., Cantu, R. C., Marshall, S. W., & Guskie-wicz, K. M. (2010b). The effect of infraction type on head impact severity in youth ice hockey. *Medicine and Science in Sports and Exercise, 42*(8), 1431–1438.

Mihalik, J. P., Guskiewicz, K. M., Jeffries, J. A., Greenwald, R. M., & Marshall, S. W. (2008). Characteristics of head impacts sustained by youth ice hockey players. *Proceedings of the Institution of Mechanical Engineers, Part P: Journal of Sports Engineering and Technology, 222*(1), 45–52.

Mihalik, J. P., Guskiewicz, K. M., Marshall, S. W., Greenwald, R. M., Blackburn, J. T., & Cantu, R. C. (2010). Does cervical muscle strength in youth ice hockey players affect head impact biomechanics? *Clinical Journal of Sports Medicine, 21*(5), 416–421.

Naunheim, R. S., Standeven, J., Richter, C., & Lewis, L. M. (2000). Comparison of impact data in hockey, football, and soccer. *Journal of Trauma, 48*(5), 938–941.

Ommaya, A. K., Corrao, P., & Letcher, F. S. (1973). Head injury in the chimpanzee: 1. Biody-namics of traumatic unconsciousness. *Journal of Neurosurgery, 39*(2), 152–166.

Ommaya, A. K., & Gennarelli, T. A. (1974). Cerebral concussion and traumatic unconscious-ness: Correlation of experimental and clinical observations of blunt head injuries. *Brain, 97*(4), 633–654.

Ommaya, A. K., Goldsmith, W., & Thibault, L. (2002). Biomechanics and neuropathology of adult and paediatric head injury. *British Journal of Neurosurgery, 16*(3), 220–242.

Ommaya, A. K., Hirsch, A. E., Flamm, E. S., & Mahone, R. H. (1966). Cerebral concussion in the monkey: An experimental model. *Science, 153*(732), 211–212.

Ommaya, A. K., Rockoff, S. D., & Baldwin, M. (1964). Experimental concussion: A first report. *Journal of Neurosurgery, 21*(4), 249–265.

Ono, K., Kikuchi, A., Nakamura, M., Kobayashi, H., & Nakamura, N. (1980). Human head tolerance to sagittal impact: Reliable estimation deduced from experimental head injury using subhuman primates and human cadaver skulls. In *Proceedings of the 24th Stapp Car Crash Conference* (pp. 101–160). Warrendale, PA: Society for Automotive Engineers.

Pellman, E. J., Viano, D. C., Tucker, A. M., Casson, I. R., & Waeckerle, J. F. (2003). Concus-sion in professional football: Reconstruction of game impacts and injuries. *Neurosur-gery, 53*(4), 799–812.

Pudenz, R. H., & Shelden, C. H. (1946). The lucite calvarium: A method for direct observa-tion of the brain. *Journal of Neurosurgery, 3*, 487–505.

San Diego Reference Library. (2008). *Pentobarbital*. Retrieved September 16, 2008, from *www.sdrl.com/druglist/pentobarbital.html*.

Schnebel, B., Gwin, J. T., Anderson, S., & Gatlin, R. (2007). In vivo study of head impacts in football: A comparison of National Collegiate Athletic Association Division I versus high school impacts. *Neurosurgery, 60*(3), 490–495.

Shaw, N. A. (2002). The neurophysiology of concussion. *Progress in Neurobiology, 67*(4), 281–344.

Shetter, A. G., & Demakas, J. J. (1979). The pathophysiology of concussion: A review. *Advances in Neurology, 22*, 5–14.

Zhang, L., Yang, K. H., & King, A. I. (2004). A proposed injury threshold for mild traumatic brain injury. *Journal of Biomechanical Engineering, 126*(2), 226–236.

CHAPTER 4

Animal Models

Andre Obenaus, Lei Huang, Jacqueline S. Coats, Richard Hartman, Jerome Badaut, and Stephen Ashwal

The complex nature of the cause and evolution of traumatic brain injury (TBI) and the wide variety of lesions that occur have made it difficult to develop animal models that accurately reflect the clinical picture. This is particularly true when comparing children to adults. Over the past two decades various experimental approaches have been pursued to develop satisfactory models, initially in larger species, but now more commonly in rodents.

Relevant animal models of TBI must mimic both the injury induction and the short- and long-term neurological deficits seen in human patients. Although no single animal model has all of the desired characteristics, a range of models has been developed that is associated with unique neurological impairments and provides insights into particular injury cascades (see Figure 4.1). As noted by Cernak (2005), experimental models should include the following: (1) the mechanical force used to induce injury must be controlled, reproducible, and quantifiable; (2) the inflicted injury is reproducible, quantifiable, and mimics components of the human condition; (3) the injury outcome, measured by morphological, physiological, biochemical, or behavioral parameters, is related to the mechanical force causing the injury; and (4) the intensity of the mechanical force used to inflict injury should predict outcome severity.

A significant issue of models and their modes of inducing injury is the definition of the degree of injury severity; however, given the numerous experimental models and their differences (Figure 4.1), it is quickly apparent that classification into mild, moderate, or severe TBI is difficult. The clinical criteria for mild TBI (mTBI) have been defined by many clinical specialties and organizations (see Wilde et al., Chapter 1, this volume). What is readily apparent from such criteria is that mTBI is very difficult to model experimentally, in part because of our inability to detect "transient

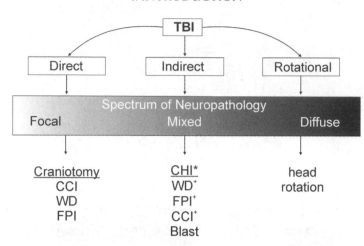

FIGURE 4.1. TBI model schematic. This simplified schema outlines the primary types of injury (direct, indirect, and rotational) and the predominant type of neuropathology that often results. Direct TBI can also be classified as penetrating injuries, whereas indirect TBI can relate to nonpenetrating injuries. The types of models that can induce these injuries are detailed below each type of injury. For more detailed schema, see Cernak (2005) and O'Connor et al. (2011). CCI, cortical contusion injury; WD, weight drop; FPI, fluid percussion injury; CHI, closed head injury. *typically injuries are delivered to the midline; +may include a rotational component.

amnesia" or changes in "consciousness" in animals. This is further exacerbated by mTBI criteria that require the virtual absence of any overt abnormalities on neuroimaging (computed tomography [CT]; magnetic resonance imaging [MRI]). The inability to incorporate lack of consciousness has plagued virtually every animal model, except the fluid percussion injury (FPI) model (Cernak, 2005; Marklund & Hillered, 2011). Additionally, development of animal models that mimic mTBI based on currently used clinical criteria are necessary but problematic, as there often are no overt changes in the animal's physiological function.

We briefly review the major adult and juvenile rodent experimental models of focal and diffuse TBI with a range of injury severities to not only provide the reader with an overview, but also to underscore the virtual dearth of research in pediatric TBI, especially, mTBI. We specifically highlight the ability of MRI to assess injury severity and the temporospatial evolution, the role of different MRI modalities, the effects of single versus repetitive mTBI insults, and finally the behavioral changes seen after pediatric mTBI in rodent and piglet models. We discuss several recent excellent reviews that provide in-depth descriptions and analyses of the different TBI models; their biological rationale, advantages, and limitations; and scientific findings related to the primary and secondary mechanisms of injury (Albert-Weissenberger & Sirén, 2010; Cernak, 2005; Marklund & Hillered, 2011; Morales et al., 2005; Morganti-Kossmann, Yan, & Bye, 2010; O'Connor, Smyth, & Gilchrist, 2011; Ucar, Tanriover, Gurer, Onal, & Kazan, 2006). In addition, an excellent recently published review on the use of MRI in rodent models of brain disorders is included (Denic et al., 2011).

RODENT ADULT TBI MODELS

The biomechanical forces associated with TBI inflict either dynamic or static injury, depending on the amplitude, duration, velocity, and acceleration of the injury (Figure 4.1; Cernak, 2005). Static models are used to focus on morphological and functional processes involved in injury. Dynamic brain trauma includes direct injury whereby trauma is directly imposed on the brain (e.g., nonaccidental trauma, contact sports, falls, etc., where the head is accelerated) and indirect injury whereby the trauma is imposed on the whole body and imparts its effects indirectly on the brain (e.g., motor vehicle accidents where the body is rapidly accelerated/decelerated but the head does not directly strike an object, as in whiplash).

TBI for modeling purposes can be broken into three distinct types of brain injury: direct, indirect, and rotational injuries. "Blast" injuries are not included in this chapter because there is likely little if any relevance to pediatric mTBI. Direct brain injuries can be classified as imparting a more focal injury, whereas at the opposite end of the spectrum, rotational types of TBI result in more diffuse injury (Figure 4.1). Indirect models of TBI can span this continuum, resulting in a more "mixed" type of injury. These head injury models can be further dichotomized depending on whether the head motion is constrained to a single plane or unconstrained and allowed to move freely (Cernak, 2005).

Other investigators have developed alternative classification schemes for experimental TBI. For example, Marklund and Hillered (2011) stratified animal models into five subgroups (focal, mixed, diffuse, complex, and other; see Table 4.1). This organizational schema attempts to reflect clinical measures and brain injuries that occur in humans. It also offers a more practical approach for researchers to determine the most suitable model that fits the research questions being explored. Relevant points emphasized in this review include these considerations: (1) no single animal model can adequately mimic all aspects of human TBI, owing to the heterogeneity of the clinical picture; (2) testing in several TBI models and at different injury severities is crucial to successfully develop therapeutic compounds for clinical TBI; and (3) further refinement of animal models and development of functional outcome measures are important.

TABLE 4.1. Experimental TBI Model Classification Scheme

Focal	Diffuse
Controlled cortical impact (CCI)	Impact/acceleration ("Marmarou") model
Weight-drop injury	Midline (central) fluid percussion injury (CFPI)
Bifrontal contusion	Diffuse TBI models—"CCI-based" models
Acute subdural hematoma	
Epidural hematoma	Complex
	CCI and impact/acceleration models with hypoxia and/or hypotension
Mixed	LFPI model with hypoxia and/or hypotension
Lateral fluid percussion injury (LFPI)	
	Other
	Repetitive models
	Blast injury models
	Penetrating injury models

Note. Based on Markland and Hillered (2011).

With regard to experimental features of TBI models, a number of additional criteria need emphasis, including (1) the importance of being able to precisely grade the severity of injury and that the response must be quantifiable and reproducible between different investigators and laboratories; (2) the model must be able to replicate the type(s) of severity and pathology observed in humans; and (3) the damage produced should represent a component of an injury continuum, increasing in severity as the mechanical forces applied are increased (Morales et al., 2005).

The three most commonly used models of TBI include the weight drop (WD), FPI, and controlled cortical impact (CCI) models and have been extensively reviewed in numerous publications (Albert-Weissenberger & Sirén, 2010; Morales et al., 2005; Ucar et al., 2006; Morganti-Kossmann et al., 2010; O'Connor et al., 2011). Table 4.2 highlights the most important features of these rodent TBI models and their advantages and disadvantages (Albert-Weissenberger & Sirén, 2010). The three primary models are briefly summarized below.

TABLE 4.2. Adult Rodent Models of Head Injury

Model	Species	Injury	Strengths	Weaknesses
Weight-drop (WD)				
Feeney's WD	Rat	Predominantly focal	Injury mechanism and inflicted injury are close to human TBI	High mortality rate due to apnea and skull fractures
Shohami's WD	Rat, mouse	Predominantly focal	Injury severity can be adjusted	Not highly reproducible
Marmarou's WD	Rat, mouse	Predominantly diffuse	Well-characterized neuroscores immediately after injury allow randomization	Reproducibility
Fluid percussion injury (FPI)				
Medial FPI	Rat	Mixed	Injury severity can be adjusted	Requires craniotomy that may compensate for intracranial pressure increases
Lateral FPI	Rat, mouse	Mixed	Inflicted injury is highly reproducible within the same laboratory but variable across laboratories	No immediate postinjury neuroscoring used and injury is variable between laboratories; also a relatively high mortality rate due to apnea
Controlled cortical impact (CCI)				
CCI	Rat, mouse	Predominantly focal	Severity of injury can be adjusted and is highly reproducible	Requires craniotomy; no immediate postinjury neuroscoring usually used

Note. Adapted from Albert-Weissenberger and Sirén (2010).

Weight-Drop Models

The WD impact model produces a number of characteristics consistent with closed-head injury in humans (Albert-Weissenberger & Sirén, 2010; Cernak, 2005; Marklund & Hillered, 2011; Morales et al., 2005; Morganti-Kossmann et al., 2010; O'Connor et al., 2011; Ucar et al., 2006). The advantages of this model include focal and diffuse brain injury, its relative ease in surgically preparing the animals, and the absence of postinjury complicating factors such as infection (Table 4.2; Figure 4.1), but a disadvantage is the variability in the degree of injury severity.

WD models use the gravitational forces of a free-falling weight to produce a focal or diffuse (when closed-head) injury to the brain (Albert-Weissenberger & Sirén, 2010). For focal brain injury, animals are placed on nonflexible platforms to minimize the dissipation of energy, whereas for the creation of a more diffuse brain injury, flexible platforms (i.e., foam) allow the head to accelerate. Severity can be graded by using different weights and/or heights.

This model is easy to reproduce, but some variability exists due to (1) loss of velocity of the weight sliding along a guide tube, and (2) the possibility of a "second hit" induced by the weight rebounding from the skull of the animal resting on the flexible sponge. These shortcomings can be minimized using either an air- or an electromagnetic-driven impact device to mechanically deform the skull (Table 4.2; Cernak, 2005).

Feeney, Boyeson, Linn, Murray, and Dail (1981) used a WD model to impact an intact dura that resulted in a cortical contusion. The pathology included hemorrhage and damage of the blood–brain barrier, subsequent inflammation with microglial and astrocytic activation, neutrophilic and macrophage infiltration, delayed microcirculatory dysfunction, and cortical spreading depression. Despite the focal nature of the injury, widespread axonal injury has been observed. In the Shohami WD model, the skull is impacted laterally, and severity is controlled by weight and height variables (Flierl et al., 2009; Shapira et al., 1988). This model induces an ipsilateral cortical contusion with blood–brain barrier disruption, edema formation, activation of the complement system, progressive cell death, and a postinjury inflammatory response.

A third commonly used WD model is the "impact acceleration" model developed by Marmarou and colleagues (Foda & Marmarou, 1994; Marmarou et al., 1994). The head is placed on a foam bed that allows freedom of movement and acceleration and produces diffuse injury, including hemorrhage, neuronal cell death, astrogliosis, diffuse axonal injury, and cytotoxic brain edema. Others have extensively modified this model by attaching a stainless steel disc to the surface of the skull to allow a more diffuse injury and to prevent potential skull fractures, particularly in mice. In adult rats, a mild diffuse brain injury without local lesion or contusion results in no mortality or skull fractures; stable hemodynamic activity; a brief (5- to 10-second) apneic period; and mild microscopic neuronal, axonal, astrocytic, and small-vessel changes (Foda & Marmarou, 1994; Marmarou et al., 1994).

Tang and colleagues (Tang, Noda, Hasegawa, & Nabeshima, 1997a, 1997b) used acrylic weights combined with a silicon rubber platform to create a mild injury in mice. The device generated concussive-like brain injury without skull fractures eliciting transient behavioral and long-lasting learning and memory impairments in the absence of motor deficits, similar to the reversible loss of consciousness and persistent cognitive deficits observed in human mTBI. A similar approach in adult rats to model cerebral concussion injury also exhibited (1) loss of muscle tone, righting, and corneal reflexes, and whisker responses, that recovered in < 10 minutes; (2) global hemodynamic depression with a short transient decrease of arterial O_2 partial pressure (pO_2), an increase in mean arterial blood pressure, and a reduced heart rate; (3) no visible abnormalities, similar to what has been reported in human mTBI; (4) subtle structural and functional alterations via quantitative MRI analysis despite normal conventional MRI; (5) learning and memory deficits on Morris water maze tests; and (6) cellular neuropathology with cortical and hippocampal neuronal loss (Henninger et al., 2005, 2007).

Fluid Percussion Injury Models

FPI models produce a brain injury by applying a rapid pressure pulse directly onto the dural surface through a craniotomy, either centrally/medially (CFPI/MFPI) over the sagittal suture midway between bregma and lambda, or laterally (LFPI) over the parietal cortex. Graded injury severity can be achieved to produce focal (usually with LFPI) or diffuse (usually with CFPI) injury (Tables 4.2 and Figure 4.1). FPI can result in cortical contusion, hemorrhage, and cytotoxic or vasogenic edema formation in moderate and severe injuries, but little has been reported on mild FPI injures. Immediate physiological responses include changes in blood pressure (transient hypertension), brief respiratory arrest, elevated intracranial pressure, reduced cerebral blood flow, decreased cerebral perfusion pressure, and increased cerebral vascular resistance (Cernak, 2005). FPI models result in cellular alterations in ion homeostasis (e.g., increased intracellular calcium and sodium, decreased intracellular magnesium, reduced potassium homeostasis), reduced cerebral metabolic activity, and depression of EEG activity. A delayed progression of brain damage seen with FPI is accompanied by astrogliosis, diffuse axonal injury, inflammation, cortical spreading depression, and neurodegeneration (Albert-Weissenberger & Sirén, 2010). Moderate LFPI is associated with observable and quantifiable MRI changes that are in stark contrast to those seen in CCI models (Obenaus et al., 2007).

FPI results in testable behavioral abnormalities in rodents that have been used as a model of posttraumatic epilepsy. An important caveat is that even a small shift in the craniotomy site is often associated with marked differences in neurological outcomes and lesion size, indicating that the FPI model requires extensive methodological modification to obtain standardized outcome measures (Albert-Weissenberger & Sirén, 2010). Although FPI still remains one of the most commonly used TBI models, one of its primary limitations is related to increased brainstem injury, which often results in apnea and increased morbidity as well as the development of neurogenic pulmonary edema.

Controlled Cortical Impact Models

CCI models utilize a pneumatic or an electromagnetic piston to deform an exposed dura and the underlying cortex, providing a precise and controlled impact (Albert-Weissenberger & Sirén, 2010; Cernak, 2005; Marklund & Hillered, 2011; Morales et al., 2005). Animals are placed in a stereotactic device allowing accurate cortical deformation; the craniotomy site is often varied laterally and in the rostral caudal direction, allowing injury to the frontal cortex or at sites adjacent to the hippocampus. Dependent on the severity of injury, CCI results in an ipsilateral injury with cortical contusion, hemorrhage, and blood–brain barrier disruption. Extensive cortical tissue loss and hippocampal and thalamic damage can occur (Marklund & Hillered, 2011), particularly in severe CCI (Mac Donald et al., 2007). Typical neuropathological features include neuronal degeneration, astrogliosis, microglial activation, inflammation, and axonal injury. Cytotoxic and vasogenic edema formation are commonly seen after CCI (Obenaus et al., 2007), which makes this an excellent model to study the edema formation and resolution that are well known to occur clinically. Seizures also occur frequently after severe CCI, so it has also been used as a model of posttraumatic epilepsy. We have recently developed a single and repeated mTBI model using an electromagnetic impactor that results in transient observable changes on neuroimaging, with histological and behavioral changes (Huang et al., 2011). Closed-head models can use a similar impactor to induce CHI injury without craniotomy, particularly in mice (Dikranian et al., 2008; Obenaus & Donovan, 2011).

Advantages of the CCI model include its ease of use, reproducibility, and the ability to adjust the degree of injury severity. Drawbacks include the possibility of extensive injury, destruction of large cortical regions, and lack of valid comparisons with the extent of brain injury observed in survivors of human TBI. A large craniectomy is often performed, and if the bone flap is not replaced after injury, the effects of secondary brain swelling may be attenuated, thus mimicking a decompressive craniotomy used in alleviating raised intracranial pressure (ICP) in humans.

PEDIATRIC TBI MODELS

The pediatric brain is not simply a "smaller" adult brain, but rather represents a complex process of development and maturation. The physiological consequences of pediatric TBI are therefore expected to be equally complex and dependent upon the time and location of injury. Identifying the appropriate age in the rodent (i.e., newborn vs. juvenile vs. adolescent) is particularly important in modeling TBI in children. Watson, Desesso, Hurtt, and Cappon (2006) summarized many of the postnatal characteristics that are critical when comparing rodent to human development. For example, in the human brain, aerobic metabolism is mature by 1 year of age, whereas in the rat the same level of maturity is reached by postnatal day 21 (PND21). Similarly, onset of myelination in the rat starts at PND14–17 and within 2–3 months in the human and is complete by PND90 and 20–30 years of age in the rodent and human, respectively (Clancy, Finlay, Darlington, & Anand, 2007; Danzer, 2008; Watson et al., 2006). Although considerable debate continues, some consensus exists that in the rat PND10 is equivalent to the time of birth in humans, whereas others have utilized PND7 (Ikonomidou & Turski, 1996); both PND7 and 10 are combined in our review. The PND35 in the rat is considered equivalent to puberty in the human (Watson et al., 2006). A developmental model in the rat by Prins, Lee, Cheng, Becker, and Hovda (1996) demonstrated significant differences in the evolution of TBI in PND17 and 28, compared to adults (Prins et al., 1996). Thus, many researchers use a broad range of ages to model pediatric TBI; we review these studies based on age and the type of TBI model.

CCI in Rodent Models

PND7–10

Accidental brain injury is the predominant cause of TBI in the human infant, and neonatal mTBI models have been established in the PND7 rat or mouse using closed-head CCI (see above for detailed model description) (Bittigau et al., 1999; Ikonomidou, Qin, Labruyere, Kirby, & Olney, 1996). In these CCI models of mTBI, little evidence of cavitation, distortion, or hemorrhage to the cortical mantle at the impact site or in the contralateral hemisphere was found. mTBI in infant mice resulted in very early and rapidly progressing axonal degeneration in white matter structures, including the cingulum and external capsule. At later time points, substantial apoptotic cell death was observed in the injured cortex and in functionally and anatomically connected neuronal populations between the injury site and the thalamus (Dikranian et al., 2008). Similar injury patterns have been reported in mTBI in the developing rat brain (Bayly et al., 2006).

Although substantial damage to the hippocampal region in these models is not evident, the extrahippocampal circuitry ipsilateral to the injury is selectively and irreversibly damaged, particularly when the injury is delivered to the skull overlying the parietal cortex. Importantly, orientation and spatial learning functions rely on an intact hippocampal circuit relaying information between the hippocampus, the retrosplenial cortex, the subicular complex, the anterior thalamic nuclei, and the mammillary nuclei; thus, damage to these connections results in behavioral and neurological deficits (Aggleton & Brown, 1999; Aggleton, Hunt, Nagle, & Neave, 1996; Aggleton, Neave, Nagle, & Sahgal, 1995; Mitchell, Dalrymple-Alford, & Christie, 2002). These closed-head CCI models of mTBI are useful for studying the long-term consequences of TBI in the developing brain, but additional studies are needed to elucidate the underlying mechanisms.

PND35

Although the incidence of TBI varies with age, particularly in sports-related injury, children 5–14 years of age can account for up to 40% of all brain injuries (Kraus, Rock, & Hemyari, 1990). Using the PND35 rat as a model of the preadolescent human, Prins and colleagues have developed a closed-head injury model of mTBI where the head is placed obliquely in a molded wooden block and the skull is impacted using an electronically controlled pneumatic piston that allows the head to move freely in the direction of the injury (Prins, Hales, Reger, Giza, & Hovda, 2010). Histological assessment showed no axonal death in either the cortex or the hippocampus. However, subtle axonal damage, using β-amyloid precursor protein immunohistochemistry, was observed 24 hours after a single impact with no change in the open-field behavioral tests. When mTBI animals were challenged at 24 hours postinjury by inclusion of a novel object, both the single (and repeated) animals exhibited a significant decrease in the percent of time spent with the novel object relative to sham animals. These results demonstrate that in the PND35 rodent, measurable cognitive deficits can be observed early after mTBI, and in the absence of gross pathology.

PND21 and PND35

More recently we completed a series of preliminary studies evaluating the effects of a single or repetitive mTBI in PND21 and 35 rodents using a model of closed-head CCI (Obenaus & Donovan, 2011). In both groups, neuroimaging for edema (T2 weighed images; T2WI), alterations in water mobility (diffusion weighted imaging; DWI), and determination of the presence of extravascular blood (susceptibility-weighted imaging; SWI) did not demonstrate any overt changes within the parenchyma 1 day post injury (Figure 4.2). Consistent with previous reports and clinical criteria, our mTBI model of closed head injury did not reveal any changes on structural MRI. Even a repetitive injury to the contralateral hemisphere, 2–4 days after the initial mTBI, did not cause observable changes on neuroimaging. These findings suggest that this model, at least from an imaging point of view, does not result in a direct injury to the

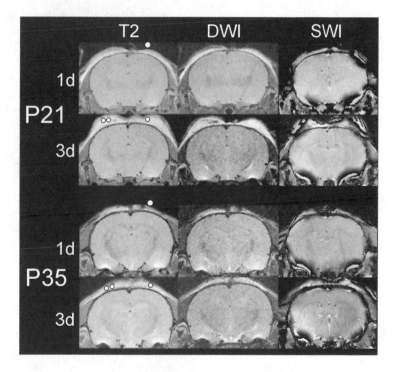

FIGURE 4.2. Neuroimaging of mild juvenile closed-head injury (CHI) at two developmentally sensitive ages. The initial mild CHI (•) was performed in rat pups at PND21 and PND35 followed by the second contralateral mild injury (• •) 2 days after the initial CHI. Multimodal MR imaging was acquired at 24 hours after each impact. In both age groups there were no overt signal intensity changes on any imaging modality (T2, DWI, or SWI). Thus, in a mild CHI conventional MR imaging may not reveal tissue level changes. (PND21 CHI: tip diameter = 4 mm, displacement = 1.5 mm, location = 2 mm lateral, 3 mm posterior from bregma. PND35 CHI: tip diameter = 4 mm, displacement = 3 mm, location = 3 mm lateral, 3 mm posterior from bregma.) • indicates site of impact.

underlying cortical or subcortical tissues. This is in contrast to the kind of injury seen in CCI models wherein brain tissues are directly impacted.

Although structural imaging appeared to be negative in our model, functional imaging, specifically perfusion-weighted imaging (PWI), demonstrated decreased cerebral blood flow and volume (Figure 4.3). When the contralateral cortex was impacted 3 days later, we observed further reductions in cerebral blood flow and volume at the site of the second impact. Notably, since structural imaging is often negative in mTBI, emerging imaging modalities may provide more sensitive indicators of subtle brain injury.

Previous work by Holshouser and colleagues has demonstrated the utility of magnetic resonance spectroscopy (MRS) to evaluate pediatric patients with varying degrees of injury (Ashwal, Holshouser, & Tong, 2006; Ashwal, Wycliffe, & Holshouser, 2010). MRS is technically difficult to do in small animal models, but as shown by Signoretti and colleagues, MRS has the potential to provide significant additional information about an injury that may not be apparent on structural MRI (Belli et al., 2006; Signoretti et al., 2001; Vagnozzi et al., 2005, 2007).

In a PND21 rat model of closed-head injury, using MRS to identify metabolite changes 1 day after the first injury, we found no changes in key brain metabolites, including N-acetylaspartate (NAA, a neuronal marker), choline (Cho, a marker of cell membrane integrity), and creatine (Cre, a marker for cell energy utilization; see Figure 4.4). However, after a second contralateral impact (4 days after the initial

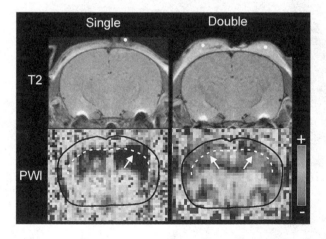

FIGURE 4.3. Perfusion weighted imaging (PWI) after closed-head injury in a PND21 juvenile rat. PWI was performed using an injection of a contrast agent (gadolinium, Gd) to assess perfusion deficits. A reduction (left panel, arrow) in cerebral blood flow (CBF) was observed 24 hours post single mild CHI (tip diameter = 4 mm, displacement = 1.5 mm, location = 2 mm lateral, 3 mm posterior from bregma). At this time point there was a modest decrement in CBF seen on the contralateral side of the brain, consistent with diffuse bilateral changes. A second CHI was induced on the contralateral side 3 days after the first impact. At 14 days after the first single impact (right panel), these initial deficits in perfusion were still observed at the site of single injury (arrow on the right hemisphere). PWI also revealed reduced CBF in the contralateral cortex where the double impact occurred (arrow on the left hemisphere). Additional regions of reduced CBF appeared in subcortical areas. These results suggest that there are long-term deficits in CBF (possibly reflecting metabolic changes) after a mild CHI. • site of impact.

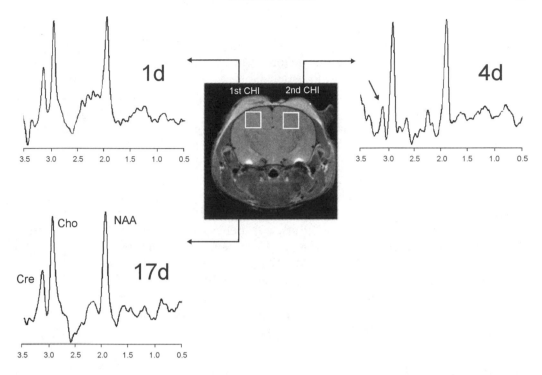

FIGURE 4.4. Magnetic resonance spectroscopy (MRS) after closed head injury (CHI) in a PND21 juvenile rat. MRS was acquired at the site of the first CHI and second CHI (a 3.5 (3.5 cm² voxel), respectively, at variable time points using a PRESS sequence on a 4.7T Bruker MRI. CHI at 24 hours after a single injury (1 day) revealed no overt changes in brain tissue spectral metabolite peaks on the side of the first CHI. The second contralateral CHI (second CHI) was induced 3 days after the first CHI. MRS was performed 1 day later (4 days). At 4 days (arrow) after the first CHI (but 1 day after the second CHI) there was a decrease in the tissue creatine (Cre) peak on the side of second CHI. The reduction in Cre is consistent with the decrements in CBF in our PWI studies (see Figure 4.3). By 17 days after the initial injury there were no observable metabolite changes within brain tissues at the initial injured site.

mTBI), we observed a decreased Cre peak (Figure 4.4). This finding is consistent with reduced energy metabolism/utilization associated with neuronal injury, resulting in an uncoupling between cerebral perfusion and metabolism (Figure 4.3). This cause–effect relation may increase edema or result in other cerebrovascular alterations that reduce cerebral blood flow and results in the spectroscopic changes that we observed. In moderate TBI, clinical studies have shown that patients with the appearance of a lactate peak have worse clinical outcomes (Babikian et al., 2006; Holshouser, Tong, & Ashwal, 2005; Tong et al., 2004). Overall, these preliminary findings suggest that methods such as PWI and MRS may be more sensitive in detecting brain injury after mTBI than conventional (structural) imaging techniques.

Piglet Model of Nonimpact Closed-Head Injury

A critical link for successful translational research is the development of large-animal models of brain injury that provide a platform to correlate meaningful functional outcome measures with well-characterized histological and molecular substrates. Piglets have been used to model acute asphyxial damage to the developing brain resulting from circulatory arrest (Brambrink, Ichord, Martin, Koehler, & Traystman, 1999), cardiopulmonary bypass (Kurth, Priestley, Golden, McCann, & Raghupathi, 1999; Schultz et al., 2004), and TBI (Armstead, 2002; Raghupathi & Margulies, 2002; Raghupathi, Mehr, Helfaer, & Margulies, 2004). Moreover, the histopathology and acute cerebral physiological responses seen in piglets in these injury paradigms more closely resemble those seen in human infants (Hagberg, Peebles, & Mallard, 2002). The piglet brain also more closely resembles human cortical gyral and white matter distribution than the pachygyric rodent brain.

mTBI in piglets is induced by rapid axial head rotations using a pneumatic actuator (Raghupathi & Margulies, 2002; Raghupathi et al., 2004), similar to that described for adult pigs (Smith et al., 2000). Behavioral testing in the piglets with mTBI found a delayed return of the pinch reflex by ~2.4 minutes (Raghupathi & Margulies, 2002; Raghupathi et al., 2004), but serial behavioral testing up to 11 days postinjury, using an open-field paradigm, found no differences between the mTBI and sham groups. Macroscopic and microscopic histological brain examination found no evidence of subarachnoid hemorrhage or ischemia (Friess et al., 2007). These studies have now been extended to repeated TBI (see below).

Weight-Drop Model

Although the weight-drop model has been used in adult models of TBI, it has not yet been reported in pediatric models. Such a model clearly has the potential to be useful, even if comparisons will need to be made to the more commonly used pediatric CCI model.

Repeated Mild-Injury Models

At the present time, only three published reports exist of repeated experimental pediatric mTBI (Friess et al., 2007; Huh, Widing, & Raghupathi, 2007; Prins et al., 2010), each employing different species. Margulies and colleagues, using rotational injury in neonatal piglets (PND3–5), evaluated the effects of two rotational injuries given in quick succession (15 minutes apart). No differences were apparent in cellular density (axonal) measures of diffuse axonal injury (DAI) on histopathology between single or double rotational injuries, but the double rotational injury group showed a wider distribution of axonal swelling (Raghupathi et al., 2004). No measureable neurobehavioral changes were found (Friess et al., 2007).

A follow-up study investigated repeated rotational injuries, either 1 day or 1 week apart (Friess et al., 2009). The 1-day-apart rotational group experienced significantly higher mortality, raising the question of whether this model was a mild injury. Visual-based problem solving was impaired in the 1-day compared to the 1-week-apart group and shams. Also, white matter injury was significantly increased in the 1-week-apart group compared to other groups and correlated with the degree of injury severity.

The effects of recurrent TBI in young rats (PND11) with one, two, and three successive impacts (5 minutes apart) have been reported (Huh et al., 2007). Although the authors did not specify injury severity, based on their previous studies (Huh, Widing, & Raghupathi, 2008, 2011b), we surmise that injury induction in this study was mild due to the lack of skull fractures. Seven days after mTBI, demonstrated graded tissue injuries were found where the two-repeated mTBI resulted in enlarged ventricles and white matter atrophy. The three-repeat mTBI animals exhibited the same neuropathology, but it was visible earlier (i.e., 3 days postinjury). In addition, the three-repeat mTBI group showed evidence of distant injury, within the thalamus. The glial response to repeated mTBI was also increased in a graded fashion. Despite these neuropathological changes, all three groups performed similarly on behavioral testing.

In a closed-head injury model the effects of single and double mTBIs 1 day apart in young rats (PND35; Prins et al., 2010) included a 10% mortality rate, which was lower than that described in the rotational piglet studies (Friess et al., 2009). Behavioral measures from the novel object recognition task revealed increased memory impairment in the repeated mTBI group. Acute axonal injury in the posterior portion of the brain was significantly higher in the repeated mTBI group compared to single mTBI animals, along with a consistent bilateral increase in astrocytic reactivity compared to the single mTBI group (Prins et al., 2010).

Taken together, these studies suggest that repeated mTBIs result in an increase in axonal injury and in proliferation of glial responses (Friess et al., 2009; Huh et al., 2007; Prins et al., 2010; Raghupathi et al., 2004). Although comparison of these findings across species and models is difficult, few differences in behavioral outcomes were found between sham, single, and repeated mTBI groups. Long-term studies during the chronic phase of mTBI have not yet been reported, but likely would provide meaningful and hopefully clinically relevant data.

Direct CCI

Currently no published studies have focused on direct mild mechanical CCI in pediatric-age animals. One potential reason for this lacuna is the difficulty in obtaining reproducible injuries in the pediatric rodent, particularly for mTBI. A large number of tests (see below), from imaging to behavioral indices, are required to reveal the existence of mild deficits. In unpublished experiments, we modeled a single mild CCI to the right frontal cortex (see Figure 4.5) in PND17 rats with a 0.5 millimeter (mm) cortical deformation without rupture of the underlying dura. Assessments 7 days later revealed a small cortical deformation with loss of tissue parenchyma that was very mild, compared to a moderate (i.e., 1.5 mm depth), injury (Ajao et al., 2012).

Neuroimaging of this model revealed early edema formation at 1 day postinjury. Similarly, DWI showed reduced water mobility at the impact site, consistent with swelling of the cortical tissue in the vicinity of the impact (see Figure 4.6). At 3 days postinjury, T2 imaging normalized, but increased water mobility was seen on DWI at the impact site, suggesting mild cell death. The injury at 7 days appeared to have some degree of tissue herniation with a secondary edema phase that was visualized on neuroimaging and is consistent with the onset of delayed vasogenic edema formation.

We also evaluated the potential for extravascular blood deposition in this model, using SWI, which is sensitive to the detection of blood products after TBI (Ashwal

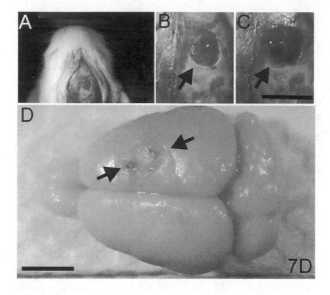

FIGURE 4.5. Induction of juvenile mTBI using the CCI model. The CCI model requires a craniotomy to directly impact the cortex for mTBI induction. (A) Craniotomy site in a juvenile rat pup (PND17) immobilized in a stereotactic device following a right frontal 2.7-mm craniotomy procedure. Care was taken not disrupt the underlying dura. (B) Higher magnification of the craniotomy site prior to CCI induction, illustrating that no injury to the dura occurred. (C) The same craniotomy site immediately after impact with a 2-mm stainless steel tip at a depth of 0.5 mm (duration: 250 ms, speed: 6 m/s) demonstrating a localized contusion site. (D) At 7 days following mild CCI, the injury site is barely visible after perfusion fixation. A small amount of blood is still present within the impact site (arrows), but only minor disruptions are seen in the overlying cortex. (Calibration bar = 0.5 cm.)

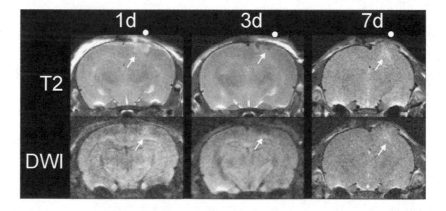

FIGURE 4.6. Temporal neuroimaging of mild juvenile CCI. T2WI and DWI studies in a juvenile rat pup (PND17) after CCI (• indicates injury site) showed the temporal evolution of this mild lesion (arrows). On T2WI, 1 day postinjury, there was development of edema (hyperintensity, arrow) that slowly resolved by 3 days. At 3 days (also on T2WI) extravascular bleeding (hypointensity, arrow) could be observed. By 7 days edema was present again (hyperintensity, arrow) accompanied by tissue deformation within the ipsilateral cortex. DWI, a biomarker for brain water mobility, revealed reduced water mobility (hyperintensity, arrow) corresponding to cytotoxic edema formation and gliosis at 1 and 7 days. Also, at 3 days there was an increase in water mobility (hypointensity, arrow) that could be due to inflammatory processes associated with the extravascular blood that was observed on the T2WI at 3 days postinjury.

et al., 2006). We observed no evidence of hemorrhage early after injury, but we did observe the presence of subtle petechial hemorrhages at 7 days postinjury (see Figure 4.7). Visualization of suspected blood in these tissues, combined with a secondary phase of edema formation, is consistent with neuroinflammation in response to the initial injury. Future studies are required to evaluate these outcomes more rigorously.

These very preliminary studies suggest that cortical deformation using the CCI model of mTBI in pediatric rodents could be useful for studying mechanisms associated with secondary injury in children and that these effects of mTBI can be visualized noninvasively using MRI.

Neurobehavioral Correlates in Pediatric Models

In humans, TBI sustained from birth through adolescence can lead to behavioral deficits (motor, cognitive, affective) that worsen with age and can also result in long-term deficits that are more severe than a similar TBI acquired later in life (Anderson, 2005; Donders & Warschausky, 2007). The behavioral effects of mild or moderate brain injury in animal models are often difficult to detect or interpret, but behavioral observations ultimately offer the most clinically relevant paradigms for testing therapeutic targets. One of the first studies to assess behavioral dysfunction in juvenile rats PND17 used a closed-head weight-drop model (Adelson, Dixon, Robichaud, & Kochanek, 1997; Adelson, Robichaud, Hamilton, & Kochanek, 1996). Testing demonstrated a prolonged recovery time of reflexes as impact severity increased, such that moderately injured rat pups took three times longer than shams to recover, and severely injured pups took five times as long. In more extensive behavioral testing of mild and moderate TBI animals, no changes in grip strength or water maze swim

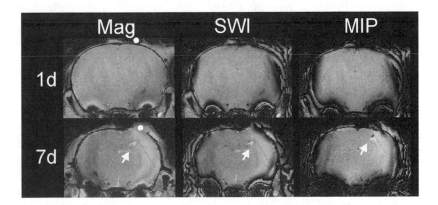

FIGURE 4.7. Susceptibility weighted imaging (SWI) of mild juvenile CCI. SWI in a juvenile rat pup after mild CCI at PND17 revealed no extravascular bleeding within the cortex at 1 day postinjury (• indicates injury site) on either the magnitude image (Mag; raw MRI) or the SWI (phase-corrected) image. The minimum intensity projection (MIP; two slices) images also did not show any extravascular blood at 1 day postinjury. However, at 7 days after mTBI, all three SWI image types (Mag, SWI, MIP) consistently revealed a heterogeneous signal change (hyperintensity and hypointensity, arrows) within the ipsilateral cortical and hippocampal regions, consistent with blood deposition at the injury site.

speed were found, suggesting no differences in motor performance up to 11 days after injury. The severe group showed marked motor deficits 1 day postinjury that persisted for 10 days, as well as water maze performance deficits that lasted for at least 22 days, suggesting possible hippocampal involvement (Adelson et al., 1997). These studies did not have an explicit mTBI group and, if they had had such a group, behavioral deficits would likely have been difficult to ascertain.

Long-term behavioral testing (i.e., 3 months postinjury) was reported in a weight-drop model in PND17 rat pups (Adelson, Dixon, & Kochanek, 2000). The weight used (150 gm) was considered a severe injury in their previous studies (Adelson et al., 1996). Similar to their earlier findings (Adelson et al., 1997), these injured rats exhibited severe motor deficits over the course of the 10 days of testing, although performance improved. Nevertheless, learning deficits were present up to 3 months postinjury. The presence of performance deficits on the cued water maze task (in which the animal can see the escape platform) suggests that the deficits observed in the spatial water maze task (in which the escape platform rests just below the surface of the water) may primarily be due to sensorimotor, rather than spatial, learning deficits.

Behavioral assessment in a weight-drop model with PND7 rat pups evaluated the protective effects of resveratrol, a polyphenolic compound found in grapes and other fruits (Sönmez, Sönmez, Erbil, Tekmen, & Baykara, 2007). Of note, the authors did not state whether this was a mild or moderate injury. TBI rats were hypoactive and performed poorly on the object recognition task, an effect that was reversed by a single injection of resveratrol at 100 mg/kg immediately following the injury. Resveratrol also ameliorated (by ~50%) the detected memory deficits.

In contrast to the findings reported in the weight-drop studies by Adelson et al. (2000), studies by Prins and colleagues using an FPI model in PND17 rats revealed that in moderately injured rat pups no behavioral deficits in Morris water maze learning could be found (Prins & Hovda, 1998). Although the PND17 rat pups did not exhibit behavioral deficits, PND28 injured animals showed transient performance deficits that resolved after the first week of testing, whereas animals injured as adults had subtle performance deficits throughout the 14 days of testing postinjury. These results suggest that a moderate injury produced using the FPI model at PND17 was insufficient to induce long-term learning deficits, but that a brain injury of similar physical magnitude in older juveniles and adult animals did produce deficits.

The effects of an enriched environment (which more closely approximates wild-type living conditions) in juvenile TBI were assessed using behavioral measures in PND19 rat pups (Giza, Griesbach, & Hovda, 2005). A moderate FPI injury to the left parietal cortex did not result in deficits in water maze performance at 30 days postinjury, whereas raising the pups in an enriched environment immediately after injury improved the performance of shams, but not the TBI group. When the enrichment paradigm was delayed until 2 weeks postinjury, spatial learning performance of shams and injured rats improved, but spatial memory, as assessed by the water maze probe trial, only improved for sham rats. These results suggest that moderate TBI in juvenile rats can induce behavioral deficits, but that standard laboratory housing conditions could mask underlying deficits.

The same investigators published an extension of these studies evaluating three different degrees of FPI (2.65, 2.8, and 3.2 atmosphere) in PND19 male rats (Gurkoff,

Giza, & Hovda, 2006). In spite of the lack of neuronal loss in the ipsilateral cortex or CA3 field of the hippocampus, subtle deficits in water maze performance were found 1–10 days later. However, in contrast to the findings of Adelson et al. (1997), no correlation was found between injury severity and the degree of behavioral deficits. In a related study, the effects of using the ketogenic diet (i.e., high-fat, low-protein/carbohydrate) in a closed-head CCI model (PND17, 35, 45, and 60) showed deficits in beam balance testing but only in the PND35 group (Appelberg, Hovda, & Prins, 2009). These beam balance deficits were transient at 3–4 days postinjury and recovered by 5 days postinjury. The behavioral deficits were ameliorated by a ketogenic diet only in younger animals.

What is missing from many of these pediatric TBI studies is the long-term assessment of behavioral outcomes. The longest behavioral assessment in a pediatric study is by Adelson et al. (1997), who measured outcomes at 3 months postinjury. Recently, we examined the emergence of behavioral deficits as early as 30 days that persist until 90 days (Ajao et al., 2012). Perhaps more interesting is that we observed the development of anxiety-like behaviors similar to that reported in humans after TBI (Whelan-Goodinson, Ponsford, Johnston, & Grant, 2009). We are now extending these studies to 6 months postinjury. Given the lack of long-term outcome data, we suggest that other future studies also make a concerted effort to evaluate persistent changes in behavior.

The only nonrodent study to assess behavior in an animal model of juvenile TBI used PND3–5 female piglets (see above; Fricss et al., 2009) subjected to moderate rotational TBI with either a single TBI or double TBI (1 day or 1 week apart). As noted above, piglets subjected to 1-day-apart double TBI had a higher mortality (43%) and more severe visual-based problem-solving deficits compared to piglets with single or 1-week-apart double injury.

In reviewing studies of pediatric mTBI, several limitations are evident, with the most obvious being a dearth of reports using either PND17 or PND35 rodents. In addition, most studies assessed behaviors only acutely or less than 1 month postinjury, with the longest being 3 months. No studies have recorded behavior in older adult animals that were injured as juveniles with the exception of our recent study (Ajao et al., 2012). Also missing from the literature are studies in mice. Although porcine models provide a much more appropriate model of white matter involvement than rodents, transgenic mice can provide valuable tools for therapeutic and mechanistic studies. A broad and comprehensive test battery for behavioral testing in pediatric rodents is also lacking. To more fully characterize the spectrum of behavioral disorders observed in children following TBI, testing of a wide range of behavioral domains, including affective responses, fine and gross motor skills, and learning and memory, by multiple paradigms will likely produce a number of behavioral targets for prognostic and therapeutic studies.

Overall, the above findings demonstrate that rodent closed-head impact models have dominated the field of experimental behavioral testing in pediatric mTBI. Closed-head impact consistently has resulted in acute and relatively long-term (up to 3 months postinjury) behavioral deficits affecting motor and cognitive functions. Open-skull FPI has shown only very subtle, if any, deficits in water maze testing, whereas open-skull CCI has produced clear-cut water maze deficits (Appelberg et al., 2009). Increasing the severity in FPI does not result in increased behavioral deficits

(Gurkoff et al., 2006), but increased severity in closed-head impacts has been associated with worse behavioral deficits (Adelson et al., 1997; Huh, Widing, & Raghupathi, 2011a). In one study of repeated closed-head TBI (PND17), no behavioral differences were observed between animals hit once or twice (Huh et al., 2011a), but in another report (PND35), two hits led to more severe deficits (Prins et al., 2010). The only study of TBI using repeated rotational injury likewise showed that double injury led to more severe deficits than single injury when the second injury was generated within 1 day (Friess et al., 2009). This was the only study to find a relation between neuropathological correlates of injury severity and the degree of behavioral deficits.

Finally, of the studies that assessed TBI at different ages (Appelberg et al., 2009; Huh & Raghupathi, 2007; Prins & Hovda, 1998; Raghupathi & Huh, 2007), only the FPI model induced worse deficits in older (PND35) animals (Prins & Hovda, 1998). The closed-head impact at age of PND11 (Huh & Raghupathi, 2007; Raghupathi & Huh, 2007) and open-skull CCI (Appelberg et al., 2009) models (PND35 and PND75) each corroborated human clinical data suggesting that earlier injury is associated with more severe behavioral outcomes (Anderson, 2005; Donders & Warschausky, 2007). Only the closed-head impact models demonstrated that increasing injury severity produced worse behavioral outcomes (Adelson et al., 1997; Huh et al., 2011a).

SUMMARY

The literature on neonatal, juvenile, and adolescent mTBI animal studies is extremely limited, resulting in very little scientific knowledge about the progression and long-term outcomes of brain injury. Unlike adult models of TBI, virtually no pediatric studies have used neuroimaging as a biomarker to assess disease progression. Behavioral paradigms that reflect functional injury in the adult clearly are not very useful in pediatric models, and more sensitive or perhaps an entirely different battery of neurological and behavioral testing needs to be devised to observe the effects of mTBI. Finally, only a handful of studies has evaluated potential therapeutic compounds in the pediatric population, and additional studies are needed to define the appropriate pediatric mTBI model to test potential therapeutics. Together, significant research needs to be undertaken to fill these knowledge gaps and to ameliorate the clinical consequences of mTBI in human patients.

REFERENCES

Adelson, P. D., Dixon, C. E., & Kochanek, P. M. (2000). Long-term dysfunction following diffuse traumatic brain injury in the immature rat. *Journal of Neurotrauma, 17,* 273–282.

Adelson, P. D., Dixon, C. E., Robichaud, P., & Kochanek, P. M. (1997). Motor and cognitive functional deficits following diffuse traumatic brain injury in the immature rat. *Journal of Neurotrauma, 14,* 99–108.

Adelson, P. D., Robichaud, P., Hamilton, R. L., & Kochanek, P. M. (1996). A model of diffuse traumatic brain injury in the immature rat. *Journal of Neurosurgery, 85,* 877–884.

Aggleton, J. P., & Brown, M. W. (1999). Episodic memory, amnesia, and the hippocampal–anterior thalamic axis. *Behavioral Brain Science*, *22*, 425–444; discussion 444–489.

Aggleton, J. P., Hunt, P. R., Nagle, S., & Neave, N. (1996). The effects of selective lesions within the anterior thalamic nuclei on spatial memory in the rat. *Behavioral Brain Research*, *81*, 189–198.

Aggleton, J. P., Neave, N., Nagle, S., & Sahgal, A. (1995). A comparison of the effects of medial prefrontal, cingulate cortex, and cingulum bundle lesions on tests of spatial memory: Evidence of a double dissociation between frontal and cingulum bundle contributions. *Journal of Neuroscience*, *15*, 7270–7281.

Ajao, D., Pop, V., Kamper, J. E., Adami, A., Rudobeck, E., Huang, L., et al. (2012). *Traumatic brain injury in young rats leads to progressive behavioral deficits coincident with altered myelin in adulthood*. Manuscript submitted for publication.

Albert-Weissenberger, C., & Sirén, A. L. (2010). Experimental traumatic brain injury. *Experimental and Translational Stroke Medicine*, *2*, 16.

Anderson, V. (2005). Functional plasticity or vulnerability after early brain injury? *Pediatrics*, *116*, 1374–1382.

Appelberg, K. S., Hovda, D. A., & Prins, M. (2009). The effects of a ketogenic diet on behavioral outcome after controlled cortical impact injury in the juvenile and adult rat. *Journal of Neurotrauma*, *26*, 497–506.

Armstead, W. M. (2002). Age dependent NMDA contribution to impaired hypotensive cerebral hemodynamics following brain injury. *Brain Research: Developmental Brain Research*, *139*, 19–28.

Ashwal, S., Holshouser, B. A., & Tong, K. A. (2006). Use of advanced neuroimaging techniques in the evaluation of pediatric traumatic brain injury. *Developmental Neuroscience*, *28*, 309–326.

Ashwal, S., Wycliffe, N. D., & Holshouser, B. A. (2010). Advanced neuroimaging in children with nonaccidental trauma. *Developmental Neuroscience*, *32*, 343–360.

Babikian, T., Freier, M. C., Ashwal, S., Riggs, M. L., Burley, T., & Holshouser, B. A. (2006). MR spectroscopy: Predicting long-term neuropsychological outcome following pediatric TBI. *Journal of Magnetic Resonance Imaging*, *24*, 801–811.

Bayly, P. V., Dikranian, K. T., Black, E. E., Young, C., Qin, Y. Q., Labruyere, J., et al. (2006). Spatiotemporal evolution of apoptotic neurodegeneration following traumatic injury to the developing rat brain. *Brain Research*, *1107*, 70–81.

Belli, A., Sen, J., Petzold, A., Russo, S., Kitchen, N., Smith, M., et al. (2006). Extracellular N-acetylaspartate depletion in traumatic brain injury. *Journal of Neurochemistry*, *96*, 861–869.

Bittigau, P., Sifringer, M., Pohl, D., Stadthaus, D., Ishimaru, M., Shimizu, H., et al. (1999). Apoptotic neurodegeneration following trauma is markedly enhanced in the immature brain. *Annals of Neurology*, *45*, 724–735.

Brambrink, A. M., Ichord, R. N., Martin, L. J., Koehler, R. C., & Traystman, R. J. (1999). Poor outcome after hypoxia–ischemia in newborns is associated with physiological abnormalities during early recovery: Possible relevance to secondary brain injury after head trauma in infants. *Experimental and Toxicologic Pathology*, *51*, 151–162.

Cernak, I. (2005). Animal models of head trauma. *NeuroRx*, *2*, 410–422.

Clancy, B., Finlay, B. L., Darlington, R. B., & Anand, K. J. (2007). Extrapolating brain development from experimental species to humans. *Neurotoxicology*, *28*, 931–937.

Danzer, S. C. (2008). Postnatal and adult neurogenesis in the development of human disease. *Neuroscientist*, *14*, 446–458.

Denic, A., Macura, S. I., Mishra, P., Gamez, J. D., Rodriguez, M., & Pirko, I. (2011). MRI in rodent models of brain disorders. *Neurotherapeutics*, *8*, 3–18.

Dikranian, K., Cohen, R., Mac Donald, C., Pan, Y., Brakefield, D., Bayly, P., et al. (2008).

Mild traumatic brain injury to the infant mouse causes robust white matter axonal degeneration which precedes apoptotic death of cortical and thalamic neurons. *Experimental Neurology, 211*, 551–560.

Donders, J., & Warschausky, S. (2007). Neurobehavioral outcomes after early versus late childhood traumatic brain injury. *Journal of Head Trauma Rehabilitation, 22*, 296–302.

Feeney, D. M., Boyeson, M. G., Linn, R. T., Murray, H. M., & Dail, W. G. (1981). Responses to cortical injury: I. Methodology and local effects of contusions in the rat. *Brain Research, 211*(1), 67–77.

Flierl, M. A., Stahel, P. F., Beauchamp, K. M., Morgan, S. J., Smith, W. R., & Shohami, E. (2009). Mouse closed head injury model induced by a weight-drop device. *Nature Protocols, 4*, 1328–1337.

Foda, M. A., & Marmarou, A. (1994). A new model of diffuse brain injury in rats: Part II. Morphological characterization. *Journal of Neurosurgery, 80*, 301–313.

Friess, S. H., Ichord, R. N., Owens, K., Ralston, J., Rizol, R., Overall, K. L., et al. (2007). Neurobehavioral functional deficits following closed head injury in the neonatal pig. *Experimental Neurology, 204*, 234–243.

Friess, S. H., Ichord, R. N., Ralston, J., Ryall, K., Helfaer, M. A., Smith, C., et al. (2009). Repeated traumatic brain injury affects composite cognitive function in piglets. *Journal of Neurotrauma, 26*, 1111–1121.

Giza, C., Griesbach, G. S., & Hovda, D. A. (2005). Experience-dependent behavioral plasticity is disturbed following traumatic injury to the immature brain. *Behavioral Brain Research, 157*, 11–22.

Gurkoff, G. G., Giza, C., & Hovda, D. A. (2006). Lateral fluid percussion injury in the developing rat causes an acute, mild behavioral dysfunction in the absence of significant cell death. *Brain Research, 1077*, 24–36.

Hagberg, H., Peebles, D., & Mallard, C. (2002). Models of white matter injury: Comparison of infectious, hypoxic–ischemic, and excitotoxic insults. *Mental Retardation and Developmental Disabilities Research Reviews, 8*, 30–38.

Henninger, N., Dutzmann, S., Sicard, K. M., Kollmar, R., Bardutzky, J., & Schwab, S. (2005). Impaired spatial learning in a novel rat model of mild cerebral concussion injury. *Experimental Neurology, 195*, 447–457.

Henninger, N., Sicard, K. M., Li, Z., Kulkarni, P., Dutzmann, S., Urbanek, C., et al. (2007). Differential recovery of behavioral status and brain function assessed with functional magnetic resonance imaging after mild traumatic brain injury in the rat. *Critical Care Medicine, 35*, 2607–2614.

Holshouser, B. A., Tong, K. A., & Ashwal, S. (2005). Proton mr spectroscopic imaging depicts diffuse axonal injury in children with traumatic brain injury. *AJNR American Journal of Neuroradiology, 26*, 1276–1285.

Huang, L., Coats, J. S., Mohd-Yusof, A., Neglerio, K., Yin, Y., Assad, S., et al. (2011). *Magnetic resonance imaging assessment of cumulative brain damage in a rat model of repetitive mild traumatic brain injury.* Manuscript submitted for publication.

Huh, J. W., & Raghupathi, R. (2007). Chronic cognitive deficits and long-term histopathological alterations following contusive brain injury in the immature rat. *Journal of Neurotrauma, 24*, 1460–1474.

Huh, J. W., Widing, A. G., & Raghupathi, R. (2007). Basic science: Repetitive mild noncontusive brain trauma in immature rats exacerbates traumatic axonal injury and axonal calpain activation—A preliminary report. *Journal of Neurotrauma, 24*, 15–27.

Huh, J. W., Widing, A. G., & Raghupathi, R. (2008). Midline brain injury in the immature rat induces sustained cognitive deficits, bihemispheric axonal injury and neurodegeneration. *Experimental Neurology, 213*, 84–92.

Huh, J. W., Widing, A. G., & Raghupathi, R. (2011a). Differential effects of injury severity on cognition and cellular pathology after contusive brain trauma in the immature rat. *Journal of Neurotrauma, 28*(2), 245–257.

Huh, J. W., Widing, A. G., & Raghupathi, R. (2011b). Differential effects of injury severity on cognition and cellular pathology after contusive brain trauma in the immature rat. *Journal of Neurotrauma, 28*, 245–257.

Ikonomidou, C., Qin, Y., Labruyere, J., Kirby, C., & Olney, J. W. (1996). Prevention of trauma-induced neurodegeneration in infant rat brain. *Pediatric Research, 39*, 1020–1027.

Ikonomidou, C., & Turski, L. (1996). Prevention of trauma-induced neurodegeneration in infant and adult rat brain: Glutamate antagonists. *Metabolic Brain Disease, 11*, 125–141.

Kurth, C. D., Priestley, M., Golden, J., McCann, J., & Raghupathi, R. (1999). Regional patterns of neuronal death after deep hypothermic circulatory arrest in newborn pigs. *Journal of Thoracic and Cardiovascular Surgery, 118*, 1068–1077.

Mac Donald, C. L., Dikranian, K., Song, S. K., Bayly, P. V., Holtzman, D. M., & Brody, D. L. (2007). Detection of traumatic axonal injury with diffusion tensor imaging in a mouse model of traumatic brain injury. *Experimental Neurology, 205*, 116–131.

Marklund, N., & Hillered, L. (2011). Animal modeling of traumatic brain injury in pre-clinical drug development: Where do we go from here? *British Journal of Pharmacology, 164*(4), 1207–1229.

Marmarou, A., Foda, M. A., van den Brink, W., Campbell, J., Kita, H., & Demetriadou, K. (1994). A new model of diffuse brain injury in rats: Part I. Pathophysiology and biomechanics. *Journal of Neurosurgery, 80*, 291–300.

Mitchell, A. S., Dalrymple-Alford, J. C., & Christie, M. A. (2002). Spatial working memory and the brainstem cholinergic innervation to the anterior thalamus. *Journal of Neuroscience, 22*, 1922–1928.

Morales, D. M., Marklund, N., Lebold, D., Thompson, H. J., Pitkanen, A., Maxwell, W. L., et al. (2005). Experimental models of traumatic brain injury: Do we really need to build a better mousetrap? *Neuroscience, 136*, 971–989.

Morganti-Kossmann, M. C., Yan, E., & Bye, N. (2010). Animal models of traumatic brain injury: Is there an optimal model to reproduce human brain injury in the laboratory? *Injury, 41*(Suppl. 1), S10–S13.

Obenaus, A., & Donovan, V. M. (2011). Closed head injury results in increased ventricular size (unpublished results).

Obenaus, A., Robbins, M., Blanco, G., Galloway, N. R., Snissarenko, E., Gillard, E., et al. (2007). Multi-modal magnetic resonance imaging alterations in two rat models of mild neurotrauma. *Journal of Neurotrauma, 24*, 1147–1160.

O'Connor, W. T., Smyth, A., & Gilchrist, M. D. (2011). Animal models of traumatic brain injury: A critical evaluation. *Pharmacology and Therapeutics, 130*, 106–113.

Prins, M. L., Hales, A., Reger, M., Giza, C. C., & Hovda, D. A. (2010). Repeat traumatic brain injury in the juvenile rat is associated with increased axonal injury and cognitive impairments. *Developmental Neuroscience, 32*, 510–518.

Prins, M. L., & Hovda, D. A. (1998). Traumatic brain injury in the developing rat: Effects of maturation on Morris water maze acquisition. *Journal of Neurotrauma, 15*, 799–811.

Prins, M. L., Lee, S. M., Cheng, C. L., Becker, D. P., & Hovda, D. A. (1996). Fluid percussion brain injury in the developing and adult rat: A comparative study of mortality, morphology, intracranial pressure and mean arterial blood pressure. *Brain Research: Developmental Brain Research, 95*, 272–282.

Raghupathi, R., & Huh, J. (2007). Diffuse brain injury in the immature rat: Evidence for an age-at-injury effect on cognitive function and histopathologic damage. *Journal of Neurotrauma, 24*, 1596–1608.

Raghupathi, R., & Margulies, S. S. (2002). Traumatic axonal injury after closed head injury in the neonatal pig. *Journal of Neurotrauma, 19*, 843–853.

Raghupathi, R., Mehr, M. F., Helfaer, M. A., & Margulies, S. S. (2004). Traumatic axonal injury is exacerbated following repetitive closed head injury in the neonatal pig. *Journal of Neurotrauma, 21*, 307–316.

Shapira, Y., Shohami, E., Sidi, A., Soffer, D., Freeman, S., & Cotev, S. (1988). Experimental closed head injury in rats: Mechanical, pathophysiologic, and neurologic properties. *Critical Care Medicine, 16*, 258–265.

Signoretti, S., Marmarou, A., Tavazzi, B., Lazzarino, G., Beaumont, A., & Vagnozzi, R. (2001). N-acetylaspartate reduction as a measure of injury severity and mitochondrial dysfunction following diffuse traumatic brain injury. *Journal of Neurotrauma, 18*, 977–991.

Smith, D. H., Nonaka, M., Miller, R., Leoni, M., Chen, X. H., Alsop, D., et al. (2000). Immediate coma following inertial brain injury dependent on axonal damage in the brainstem. *Journal of Neurosurgery, 93*, 315–322.

Sönmez, U., Sönmez, A., Erbil, G., Tekmen, I., & Baykara, B. (2007). Neuroprotective effects of resveratrol against traumatic brain injury in immature rats. *Neuroscience Letters, 420*, 133–137.

Tang, Y. P., Noda, Y., Hasegawa, T., & Nabeshima, T. (1997a). A concussive-like brain injury model in mice (I): Impairment in learning and memory. *Journal of Neurotrauma, 14*, 851–862.

Tang, Y. P., Noda, Y., Hasegawa, T., & Nabeshima, T. (1997b). A concussive-like brain injury model in mice (II): Selective neuronal loss in the cortex and hippocampus. *Journal of Neurotrauma, 14*, 863–873.

Tong, K. A., Ashwal, S., Holshouser, B. A., Nickerson, J. P., Wall, C. J., Shutter, L. A., et al. (2004). Diffuse axonal injury in children: Clinical correlation with hemorrhagic lesions. *Annals of Neurology, 56*, 36–50.

Ucar, T., Tanriover, G., Gurer, I., Onal, M. Z., & Kazan, S. (2006). Modified experimental mild traumatic brain injury model. *Journal of Trauma, 60*, 558–565.

Vagnozzi, R., Signoretti, S., Tavazzi, B., Cimatti, M., Amorini, A. M., Donzelli, S., et al. (2005). Hypothesis of the postconcussive vulnerable brain: Experimental evidence of its metabolic occurrence. *Neurosurgery, 57*, 164–171.

Vagnozzi, R., Tavazzi, B., Signoretti, S., Amorini, A. M., Belli, A., Cimatti, M., et al. (2007). Temporal window of metabolic brain vulnerability to concussions: Mitochondrial-related impairment—Part I. *Neurosurgery, 61*, 379–388.

Watson, R. E., Desesso, J. M., Hurtt, M. E., & Cappon, G. D. (2006). Postnatal growth and morphological development of the brain: A species comparison. *Birth Defects Research Part B Developmental and Reproductive Toxicology, 77*, 471–484.

Whelan-Goodinson, R., Ponsford, J., Johnston, L., & Grant, F. (2009). Psychiatric disorders following traumatic brain injury: Their nature and frequency. *Journal of Head Trauma Rehabilitation, 24*, 324–332.

PART II

EVIDENCE-BASED OUTCOMES

CHAPTER 5

Pathophysiological Outcomes

Talin Babikian, John DiFiori, and Christopher C. Giza

Biomechanically, a concussion/mild TBI (mTBI) is defined as a physiological dysfunction of the brain that occurs with or without loss of consciousness that induces a neurometabolic cascade of physiological changes. These changes are presumed to underlie clinical symptoms and potential vulnerability to repeated injuries. In this discussion, the terms *mTBI* and *concussion* are used interchangeably. In general, concussion causes no macroscopic structural damage, computed tomography scans are normal, and in most cases, the acute symptoms resolve within 7–14 days. However, advances in neuroimaging and biomarkers are challenging our current view of concussion by showing evidence of microstructural damage (Mac Donald et al., 2011; Niogi et al., 2008) and by demonstrating functional neural injuries (McAllister et al., 1999; Vagnozzi et al., 2008) that were previously undetected on standard structural neuroimaging. Furthermore, a combination of functional measures and chronic neuropathological evidence has recently raised the concern that an accumulation of small/mild injuries may lead, in select cases, to permanent and significant sequelae such as cognitive and behavioral impairments (De Beaumont et al., 2009; McKee et al., 2009; Talavage et al., in press).

From the perspective of the young brain, understanding the pathophysiology of an injury has particular relevance in several significant ways. These physiological distinctions following pediatric TBI are discussed below and include (1) risk of cell death (particularly via apoptotic mechanisms and after an accumulation of repeated injuries), (2) higher basal levels of metabolism, (3) alterations in neural activation and neural plasticity, (4) vulnerability to axonal injury (since white matter tracts remain incompletely myelinated in some brain regions into early adulthood), and (5) potential effects of genetic susceptibility. Age-dependent differences in these biological mechanisms point out the importance of age-appropriate clinical assessments and longitudinal follow-up, the need for pediatric and younger adolescent clinical data and, quite likely, the requirement for modifications in the management protocols for concussion and recurrent concussion in younger age groups.

BASIC PATHOPHYSIOLOGY

With few exceptions, postconcussive symptoms, including confusion, disorientation, unsteadiness, dizziness, headaches, and visual disturbances, typically resolve fully over time and often do not have identifiable anatomical correlates, suggesting that their pathophysiology is due to a transient disruption in neuronal, axonal, and/or metabolic functioning rather than to cell death (Giza & Hovda, 2001). Although historically the pathophysiology explaining clinical symptomatology following an injury to the brain has been attributed to tearing or shearing of axons, there is convincing evidence in milder injuries that the underlying pathophysiology may be related to neuronal dysfunction, transient in many instances, resulting in a disruptive *process* instead of an *event* (Iverson, Lange, Gaetz, & Zasler, 2007). This disruption can occur at various points in the cycle of normal cellular functions, including ionic fluxes resulting in cellular dysfunction, metabolic abnormalities involving disruption in the use of glucose and mitochondria, alterations in synaptic functions that affect neural activation, and impairments related to axonal connectivity and function.

Following a biomechanical insult to the brain, the rapid and indiscriminate release of excitatory amino acids (EAAs) and extensive efflux of potassium (K^+) trigger a brief period of hyperglycolysis. These events are followed by a period of calcium (Ca^{2+}) influx and mitochondrial dysfunction characterized by diminished oxidative and cerebral glucose metabolism, reduced cerebral blood flow (CBF), as well as axonal injury. Late events in the neurometabolic cascade following a concussive-type brain injury include recovery of glucose metabolism and CBF, delayed cell death, alterations in neurotransmission, and axonal disconnection (Barkhoudarian, Hovda, & Giza, 2011; Giza & Hovda, 2001). The relative time course of these events following experimental concussion is summarized in Figure 5.1 (Giza & Hovda, 2001) and is discussed in greater detail in the sections below.

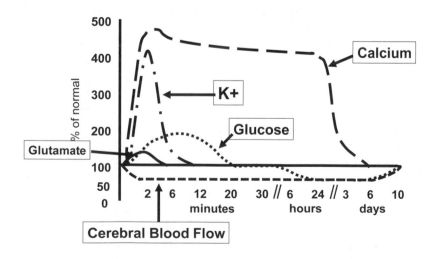

FIGURE 5.1. Neurometabolic cascade following experimental concussion. CBF, cerebral blood flow; CMRgluc, cerebral metabolic rate of glucose; Ca^{2+}, calcium, K^+, potassium.

Further complicating the above cascade of cellular, metabolic, and axonal changes that occur following a concussive brain insult are the ramifications of these disruptions, even if transient, on the developing brain. The young brain is undergoing a series of normal developmental changes in structure and function to support the rapid acquisition of various neurological, cognitive, and behavioral skills that are observed from infancy through adolescence, and beyond. Even if the cascade of neurochemical alterations is transient, these changes, when superimposed upon a period of rapid development, may lead to disruptions in brain plasticity, affecting the ability to acquire developmentally appropriate new skills and connections (Fineman, Giza, Nahed, Lee, & Hovda, 2000; Ip, Giza, Griesbach, & Hovda, 2002). This, in addition to the increasing awareness of the negative effects of repeated concussive injuries, makes it especially important to study the pathophysiology of concussive injuries and their subsequent effects specifically on the developing brain.

CELL DEATH OUTCOMES

Substantial fluctuations in Ca^{2+} in the cellular environment play a critical role in both apoptotic/programmed cell death (Orrenius, Zhivotovsky, & Nicotera, 2003) and necrotic cell death. Although the role of Ca^{2+}-dependent excitotoxicity has long been theoretically implicated in trauma-related cell death, the current understanding is that cell vulnerability due to calcium ionic flux occurs not through a general homeostatic failure in response to excess Ca^{2+}, but rather through its route of entry and its associated molecular infrastructure, such as activation of N-methyl-D-aspartate receptor (NMDAR) associated signaling molecules (Sattler & Tymianski, 2000). Following a sufficiently strong biomechanical force to the head, there is a rapid and relatively indiscriminant release of neurotransmitters and ionic flux. Glutamate, along with other EAAs, binds to NMDA receptors, resulting in an efflux of K^+ and influx of Ca^{2+}. To restore balance, the work of the sodium–potassium pumps is critically important. Postinjury, these pumps need more energy (adenosine triphosphate, or ATP), resulting in a significant increase in energy or glucose metabolism (Giza & Hovda, 2001).

In more severe injuries, trauma to the brain results in apoptotic cell death (Bittigau et al., 1999; Felderhoff-Mueser et al., 2002), with the developing brain having a much lower threshold for this type of pathogenesis (Bittigau et al., 1999). Similarly, in milder injuries, early (first few days) and extensive traumatic axonal injury in subcortical regions have been reported, with reactive astrocytosis noted in the cortex within the second week of injury. This suggests ongoing neuronal and axonal degeneration that correlates with sustained cognitive deficits (Huh, Widing, & Raghupathi, 2008). However, even in milder injuries where gross anatomical pathology is not observed, behavioral deficits can be identified. In a developmental rodent model of "mild" injury (lateral fluid percussion, or LFP), Gurkoff, Giza, and Hovda (2006) showed that following trauma sustained on postnatal day 19 (PND19), no changes were found in the absolute number of neurons 2 weeks postinjury in either the ipsilateral cortex or the CA3 region of the hippocampus. Nonetheless, animals showed acute mild cognitive deficits on the Morris water maze task during the first couple of postinjury training days, but by 10 days postinjury, they were indistinguishable from sham animals with regard to spatial learning (Gurkoff et al., 2006). Similarly, Prins, Hales, Reger, Giza, and Hovda (2010) showed that in an experimental closed-head injury model with juvenile rats (PND35) with an absence of gross pathology, measurable deficits are apparent in working memory as observed by the novel object recognition (NOR) task (Prins et al., 2010).

Repeated Injuries: Animal Data

Experimentally, repeated mild injury that occurs prior to full physiological recovery from an earlier impact can have adverse consequences, sometimes greater than the sum of two independent injuries (for review, see Prins & Giza, in press). Some data suggest that mild axonal injury results in abnormalities in sodium channel functions that exaggerate the pathophysiological response to subsequent injuries (Yuen, Browne, Iwata, & Smith, 2009). Repeated injuries in experimental models, even if mild, are shown to produce anatomical changes, along with behavioral deficits. Huh, Widing, and Raghupathi (2007) subjected 11-day-old rat pups to one, two, or three successive mild impacts. Although skull fractures were not observed, a single impact to the intact skull resulted in petechial hemorrhages in the subcortical white matter, whereas double or triple impacts led to hemorrhagic tissue tears at 1 day postinjury. Two or three consecutive impacts that were minutes apart led to more severe neuropathology at 1 week postinjury; however, neither one nor two impacts resulted in learning deficits on the Morris water maze task (Huh et al., 2007). Prins et al. (2010) observed that the introduction of a second injury 24 hours following the first was associated with an increase in axonal injury, astrocytic reactivity, and memory impairment as measured by the NOR task (Prins et al., 2010). In a larger animal model, Friess et al. (2009) subjected 3- to 5-day-old piglets to single, double (1 day apart), and double (1 week apart) injuries, with more than one injury resulting in poorer neuropathological outcomes (assessed by β-amyloid precursor protein—βAPP staining) and neurobehavioral outcomes. Increased injury severity and mortality were also noted when the two injuries were temporally closer (24 hours vs. 7 days apart) (Friess et al., 2009).

In a model of subthreshold injury in rodents with no apparent damage to brain tissue, repeated daily injuries within the span of a week showed abnormal accumulation of microtubule-associated protein 2 (MAP2) and phosphorylated neurofilament 200 kD (p-NFH) in neuronal perikarya and dendrites ipsilaterally 1 week after the last injury. A month later, these findings were also observed in remote areas, such as the contralateral cortex and the hippocampus. In addition, abnormal accumulation of tau-1 immunoreactivity was observed, with such histological findings being correlated with behavioral deficits characterized by less efficient habituation to a new environment (Kanayama et al., 1996). In another study, repeated injuries resulted in diffuse axonal injury and distant injury bilaterally in the cerebral cortex, subcortical regions, hippocampal CA1, corpus callosum, and striatum. Reactive astrocytosis and edema in the cerebral cortex, brainstem, and cerebellum were reported 10 days following these injuries (Hamberger, Viano, Saljo, & Bolouri, 2009).

Repeated Injuries: Human Studies

Athletes with a history of previous concussions are more likely to have future concussive injuries, with one in 15 players with a concussion incurring additional injuries in the same playing season (Guskiewicz et al., 2003). Furthermore, a history of previous concussions results in slower recovery from symptoms following subsequent injuries (Guskiewicz et al., 2003). There is relatively old literature from boxing showing that repetitive injury can result in progressive neurological deterioration. This was originally termed *dementia pugilistica* but has more recently been referred to as *chronic traumatic encephalopathy* (CTE), which is behaviorally characterized by memory impairments, behavioral/personality changes, parkinsonism, and speech and gait abnormalities (McKee et al., 2009). Neuropathologically, CTE is associated with atrophy of the cerebral hemisphere, medial temporal lobe, thalamus, mammillary bodies, and brainstem. Microscopically, there is also evidence for widespread tau-immunoreactive neurofibrillary tangles, astrocytic tangles, and spindle-shaped and threadlike neuritis. Deposition of β-amyloid is present in fewer than half the cases (McKee et al., 2009).

Recently, postmortem autopsy findings from single cases of National Football League (NFL) players and other professional athletes were used to characterize the presence and extent of microstructural changes to brain tissue subsequent to repeated concussive injuries. Such reports have shown evidence for cerebral tauopathy and CTE, with notable premortem neuropsychiatric impairments, including disinhibited behaviors, mood irregularities extending to major depressive disorder, and suicidality (McKee et al., 2009; Omalu, Bailes, Hammers, & Fitzsimmons, 2010a; Omalu, Hamilton, Kamboh, DeKosky, & Bailes, 2010b).

Increasing concern about the risks associated with sports-related repeated concussive injuries has sparked the attention of both the popular media and the scientific community recently, paving the way to administrative and policy/guideline changes on professional, collegiate, and community youth sports group levels. However, these policy changes are being made with a dearth of age-appropriate clinical data, and a better understanding of the underlying pathophysiology—particularly in the developing brain—may prove invaluable for establishing an evidence-based foundation for the management of pediatric sports concussions.

METABOLIC OUTCOMES

A sharp increase in glucose metabolism follows a head injury, paralleling the higher energy demands needed by the sodium–potassium pumps to restore neurochemical cellular order. This hypermetabolic state is accompanied by a notable decrease in blood flow that puts the brain in an energy crisis, thus potentially making the concussed brain more vulnerable to another insult during this period before the brain has had a chance to recover fully. This phase is followed by a longer period of depressed metabolism. Such dynamic metabolic changes are the hallmark of brain injury across experimental models, and have been observed clinically as well.

In experimental rodent models, fluid percussion (FP) brain injury is characterized by a hyperacute increase, followed by a subacute decrease, in glucose metabolism. After an injury, the rat brain shows an indiscriminate efflux of neurotransmitters and ions (Kawamata, Katayama, Hovda, Yoshino, & Becker, 1992; Osteen, Moore, Prins, & Hovda, 2001) and a transient increase in local metabolic rate of glucose (LCMRglc) in the brain (Sutton, Hovda, Adelson, Benzel, & Becker, 1994; Yoshino, Hovda, Kawamata, Katayama, & Becker, 1991). This increase is due to the increased cellular energy required to restore ionic balance and maintain neuronal membrane potential (Hovda, Villablanca, Chugani, & Phelps, 1996). Following this increase is a longer period of metabolic (glucose) depression that spans between 10 and 14 days postinjury, though the duration of this period varies, to some degree, based on age of the animal, injury severity, and injury type. The specific mechanism for the prolonged decrease in LCMRglc after a brain injury is not well understood, though several suggestions have been made: Ca^{++}-induced mitochondrial disruption (Fineman, Hovda, Smith, Yoshino, & Becker, 1993), ionic flux disruptions (Katayama, Becker, Tamura, & Hovda, 1990), reduced CBF (Cherian, Hlatky, & Robertson, 2004), or lactic acid accumulation (Kawamata et al., 1992).

A similar pattern of glucose metabolic changes is also observed in developing animals following a head injury. Injured preweanling rats (PND17) showed hyperglycolysis immediately after an injury, predominantly in the cortical regions, which primarily subsided within 30 minutes. This initial period of hyperglycolysis was followed by a reduction in metabolism rates within the first 24 hours postinjury, which resolved by day 3. Early resolution of hypoglycolysis in pups is unlike that in adults, where much more prolonged metabolic depression is observed (Thomas, Prins, Samii, & Hovda, 2000). Further, age-related differences in the duration of LCMRglc depression were also observed among PND35 rats after a cortical impact injury. The younger brain shows earlier recovery of glucose metabolic rates than adults (Prins & Hovda, 2009), which suggests age-related differences in metabolic coping strategies or metabolic trafficking.

ALTERNATIVE SUBSTRATES

Cerebral metabolism of any substrate requires both the availability of the substrate and a transport mechanism of the substrate into the brain. The expression of specific transporters of glucose and ketone bodies parallels the developmental switch from a combination of glucose–ketone metabolism in developing (preweanling) rodents to almost exclusive glucose metabolism in the adult brain (Vannucci & Simpson, 2003), with dynamic age-related changes observed after brain injury. Specifically, juvenile rats show changes in the expression of the transporters that are consistent with changes in substrates (Prins & Giza, 2006), whereas no such significant changes are observed in adult rats postinjury (Deng-Bryant, Giza, Hovda, & Prins, 2010). Further, the magnitude of change in transporters early on in the juvenile rat appears to contribute to a greater and more rapid ketone uptake during the critical early changes after a brain injury. This is important after brain injury, including mTBI/concussion, since glucose metabolism may be an inefficient source of energy during this time. Under these conditions, the utilization of alternative substrates, including ketones, has been shown to be neuroprotective. The developmental difference in the brain's ability to shift toward ketone metabolism may ultimately make the juvenile brain the most receptive to alternative substrates as a therapeutic option after a brain injury. Recently, conditions of ketosis (induced by fasting or diet) have been shown to be neuroprotective in both adult and juvenile rats (Appelberg, Hovda, & Prins, 2009; Davis, Pauly, Readnower, Rho, & Sullivan, 2008; Prins, Lee, Fujima, & Hovda, 2004), with administration of ketones revealing age-dependent neuroprotection following an injury (Prins, Fujima,

& Hovda, 2005). PND35 and PND45 rats placed on a ketogenic diet immediately after an injury showed a 58% and 39% decrease, respectively, in cortical contusion volume at 7 days postinjury, with no such beneficial effects observed for injured rats that were younger (PND17) or older (PND75). Administration of ketones has not only preserved cortical histology, but also resulted in decreased motor and cognitive deficits in the juvenile rats (Appelberg et al., 2009). Furthermore, there is emerging but very sparse evidence of other dietary-based supplements that enhance brain function in general, including foods/supplements rich in omega-3 fatty acids (fish, certain nuts), flavonoids (cocoa, green tea, chocolate), vitamins (B, D, and E), and reduction in the intake of saturated fats (animal products) (Gomez-Pinilla, 2008). Dietary supplements have also shown promise as neuroprotective agents in experimental models of TBI (Bailes & Mills, 2010; Mills, Bailes, Sedney, Hutchins, & Sears, 2011).

GLUCOSE METABOLISM IN HUMAN STUDIES

Studies of brain metabolism in children are sparse at best. In studies of human adults, the cerebral metabolic rate of glucose (CMRgluc) was studied using 18F-fluorodeoxyglucose positron emission tomography (FDG-PET) in 42 patients with mild to severe injuries, showing a global reduction in more severe (86%) versus mild/moderate (67%) cases. Further, the extent of reduction was correlated with gross neurological condition in the mildly injured patients ($r = .50$) but not the severely injured patients ($r = -.11$), suggesting a complex and multifactorial etiology for this decrease (Bergsneider et al., 2000). Further investigation of the temporal changes in CMRgluc showed a dynamic profile that was consistent across injury severities (Bergsneider et al., 2001). In moderate to severe injuries, cerebral metabolism of oxygen and arterial lactate levels in the acute phase (first week postinjury) have been reported to be the best predictors of neurological outcome, though the high rate of lactate uptake (regardless of arterial lactate levels) in those with good outcome suggest that lactate may be an alternative fuel in an energy crisis (Glenn et al., 2003).

Following a period of increased glucose metabolism, the injured brain goes through a period of depressed metabolism. Calcium elevations can impair mitochondrial oxidative metabolism, further exacerbating the energy crisis and subsequently leading to cell death. Because free radical production is a normal part of cellular physiology, aerobic organisms have developed various antioxidant defense systems, with the expression of these systems varying by cerebral maturation (Aspberg & Tottmar, 1992; Mavelli, Rigo, Federico, Ciriolo, & Rotilio, 1982). Some studies have indicated that the "underdevelopment" of mitochondrial antioxidant capacity renders the younger brain more susceptible to oxidative challenges (Dreiem, Gertz, & Seegal, 2005). This vulnerability has been experimentally demonstrated after brain injury. Oxidative damage following brain injury in the mature brain (Deng, Thompson, Gao, & Hall, 2007; Hall, Detloff, Johnson, & Kupina, 2004; Singh, Sullivan, Deng, Mbye, & Hall, 2006; Tyurin et al., 2000) has led to many antioxidant treatments that are demonstrated to reduce histopathology (Kawamata et al., 1997; Mori et al., 1998). However, the little evidence for this process in the developing brain has suggested that underdeveloped enzymatic activity (i.e., for that of glutathione peroxidase, or GPx, and superoxide dismutase, or SOD) may be responsible for the higher vulnerability to injury-induced oxidative stress in the immature brain (Fan, Yamauchi, Noble, & Ferriero, 2003).

The early (minutes to hours) effects of a mild closed-head injury on lipid peroxidation and brain energy metabolism were studied using the weight-drop method (450 g from a 1-m height) in the rat. Using high-performance liquid chromatography analysis, measurements of whole-brain malondialdehyde (MDA), ascorbic acid, high-energy phosphates, nicotinic coenzymes, oxypurines, and nucleosides were determined. MDA, an index of lipid peroxidation, which is undetectable in control or sham-operated rats, was observed at 1 minute posttrauma, reaching maximum levels by 2 hours and decreasing slowly thereafter. In contrast, other energy metabolism markers, including ATP, guanosine triphosphate (GTP), and nicotinic coenzyme nicotinamide adenine dinucleotide (NAD) and nicotinamide adenine dinucleotide phosphate (NADP) concentrations, were significantly reduced by 2 hours postinjury, with maximum decreases observed by 2 hours for ATP and GTP and 15 hours for NAD and NADP. These findings suggest that the observed biochemical changes involving lipid peroxidation are directly a result of forces acting on the brain at the time of impact, and may result in the depression of energy metabolism that is caused by peroxidation of the mitochondrial membrane (Vagnozzi et al., 1999). These biochemical modifications have also been shown to be specific to injury severity, with the extent of oxidative stress and alterations in cellular energy metabolism being associated with severity of brain injury (Tavazzi et al., 2005).

In repeat mild injuries in the rat delivered at increasing time intervals (between 1 through 5 days following an initial injury), concentrations of multiple metabolic substrates were measured 48 hours after the last impact. Changes in the metabolic concentrations of these metabolites (including *decreases* in ATP, ATP/ADP, NAA, N-acetylaspartylglutamate, oxidized and reduced NAD, NADP, and acetyl coenzyme A (CoA); and *increases* in NAA acylase expression) were directly associated with the time interval of the repeated impacts, and maximal changes were observed when the two injuries were spaced 3 days apart. The authors concluded that there is a temporal window of brain vulnerability after a mild injury, during which time the presence of a second impact, albeit mild, can have significant effects on mitochondrial-related metabolism. Furthermore, NAA recovery coincided with normalization of all other metabolites (Signoretti, Vagnozzi, Tavazzi, & Lazzarino, 2010; Vagnozzi et al., 2007). NAA is a brain-specific marker (found in 100-fold higher concentrations in the brain vs. other tissue), and is considered both an overall measure of neuronal and axonal health (Ashwal et al., 2000; Hoon & Melhem, 2000) as well as a marker of energy metabolism (Signoretti, et al., 2010). Since NAA is relatively easily measured *in vivo* through MR spectroscopy (MRS), its potential clinical utility in human studies has been raised (Vagnozzi, et al., 2007).

The role of NAA in predicting behavioral outcomes following a head injury in humans, including children, has been recently documented (Ashwal, Holshouser, & Tong, 2006; Babikian et al., 2006). In mild/concussive injuries, MRS for NAA concentrations was examined in 40 athletes (ages 16–35) who had suffered a concussion (Vagnozzi et al., 2010). Compared to healthy controls, the NAA levels in frontal white matter of the athletes showed the largest reductions at day 3 postinjury, with a gradual recovery thereafter, reaching full recovery by day 30. Of note, athletes' self-reported symptoms resolved between 3 and 15 days of injury, although use of a standardized, validated symptom checklist was not reported. A very small sample of this group (n = 3) incurred a second concussive-type injury prior to full normalization. This group showed an identical initial decrease in NAA by day 3, which further decreased by day 15, reaching full recovery by 45 days, and self-report of symptom resolution at 30 days (Vagnozzi et al., 2008). The authors highlighted the potential utility of a relatively safe and easy snapshot presentation of metabolic functioning following a concussive-type brain injury to aid in clinical decision making, including return to play.

SYNAPTIC PLASTICITY AND NEURAL ACTIVATION OUTCOMES

Synaptogenesis is an ongoing developmental process by which activated neural pathways can be strengthened temporarily and even permanently, often in response to experience-dependent neuroplasticity. In the laboratory rat, this process begins preweaning and continues into adolescence (Moss, Meehan, & Salentijn, 1972). In humans, maximum synaptic density and basal cerebral metabolic rates occur in childhood, but cerebral metabolism remains greater than in adults well into the teenage years (Chugani, Phelps, & Mazziotta, 1987). Experience-dependent plasticity is the means by which differences in environment and learning are transformed into long-lasting structural and functional advantages, such as increased numbers of synapses, expanded dendritic arbors (Greenough, Volkmar, & Juraska, 1973; Jacobs, Schall, & Scheibel, 1993), neurogenesis (Kempermann, Kuhn, & Gage, 1997), enhanced learning (Giza, Griesbach, & Hovda, 2005; Tees, Buhrmann, & Hanley, 1990), increased expression of nerve growth factors (Branchi, Francia, & Alleva, 2004), and improved neurotransmission (Irvine, Logan, Eckert, & Abraham, 2006). Laboratory models of experience-dependent plasticity include the enriched environment (EE), where animals reared in special cages with multiple toys and objects and other cage mates show increased cortical thickness, more complex dendritic arbors, and cognitive superiority over rodents reared in standard laboratory conditions (Rosenzweig & Bennett, 1996).

Impaired Plasticity and Neural Activation

Experimental TBI is known to result in abnormal plasticity, including alterations in the regrowth of damaged neural pathways and changes in synaptic structure (Prins, Povlishock, & Phillips, 2003). Furthermore, diffuse concussive experimental TBI (fluid percussion injury) in the immature rat has been shown to alter the responsiveness of the developing brain to rearing in an EE. Specifically, young rats reared in EE immediately following concussive injury do not show overt cortical atrophy or cognitive deficits, but they do show an absence of EE-induced anatomical and cognitive enhancements when tested in adulthood (Fineman et al., 2000; Giza et al., 2005). Some may describe this as if "they went to school but didn't learn properly."

Underlying mechanisms for altered plasticity are complex and likely multifaceted; following experimental TBI, multiple investigators have reported impairments of excitatory neurotransmission through the NMDAR, which may represent a common pathway to this impairment (Biegon et al., 2004; Giza, Maria, & Hovda, 2006;

Kumar, Zou, Yuan, Long, & Yang, 2002; Miller et al., 1990; Osteen, Giza, & Hovda, 2004). Functional impairments of post-TBI neural activation have also been described in animals using electrophysiological (Reeves, Lyeth, & Povlishock, 1995; Sick, Perez-Pinzon, & Feng, 1998; Yaka et al., 2007), metabolic (Ip, Zanier, Moore, Lee, & Hovda, 2003; Passineau et al., 2000), and imaging (Duhaime et al., 2006; Henninger et al., 2007; Santa Maria, Harris, Hovda, & Giza, 2009) modalities.

Functional imaging measures hold particular interest in these experimental models, because they open the potential for translation to human neuroimaging studies. Using evoked somatosensory stimulation in uninjured rats, increases in the blood oxygen-level-dependent (BOLD) signal were significantly attenuated (50%) by administration of an NMDAR antagonist (Gsell et al., 2006). Henninger et al. (2007) showed abnormalities in functional magnetic resonance imaging (fMRI) activation in a rat model that does not result in overt cortical lesions, implying that the injury resulted in functional impairment of neural activity.

In immature animals, loss of BOLD activation was also seen in a piglet model of diffuse TBI; however, this model was associated with significant neuronal damage and so may not reflect solely synaptic dysfunction but perhaps also synaptic/neuronal loss (Duhaime et al., 2006). Of note, using a pharmacological MRI activation paradigm with an NMDAR co-agonist, increased hippocampal cerebral blood volume was seen in young control rats but abolished in the first week after diffuse concussive injury (Santa Maria et al., 2009). This model has not been associated with significant hippocampal cell loss (Gurkoff et al., 2006; Prins, Lee, Cheng, Becker, & Hovda, 1996), and so the absence of drug-induced activation was taken as an indication of synaptic dysfunction.

In humans, substantial evidence exists of altered neural activation patterns after TBI using event-related fMRI. However, in several studies, rather than an overt suppression of activation, a less focused, more dispersed pattern of BOLD activation was seen (Jantzen, Anderson, Steinberg, & Kelso, 2004; McAllister et al., 1999). Interestingly, a drop-off in activation with higher working memory loads has also been found in adults (McAllister et al., 2001). Other investigators report reductions in the level of BOLD activation triggered by neural activity in individuals after mTBI (Chen et al., 2004; Jantzen, 2010). One potential limitation when interpreting post-TBI fMRI studies is the possibility of TBI-induced uncoupling of neural activation from blood flow, which would then result in loss or reduction of BOLD signal even in the presence of intact neural activation. Further investigations using fMRI after mTBI are necessary in several critical areas: (1) combining fMRI with other modalities of neural activation (electrophysiology, magnetic source imaging) to confirm the abnormalities seen using BOLD; (2) better delineating the associations between fMRI BOLD abnormalities and clinically measurable parameters, such as cognitive function and the presence and intensity of symptoms; (3) longitudinal investigations characterizing the recovery time course of normal neural activation and the effects of returning to physical or cognitive activity; (4) fMRI studies of basal cerebral activity (resting state fMRI) after mTBI; (5) using fMRI to determine age-dependent changes in neural activity and recovery from mTBI; and (6) translational functional imaging studies in experimental models, which may allow linkage of altered neural activation directly to underlying neurobiological mechanisms of injury and repair.

Premature Stimulation

One main concern of recovery from concussion/mTBI in young persons is the timing of return to practice/school and return to play. Whereas return to play generally incorporates both the effects of increased neural activity and the potential for reinjury, the return to practice/school may result in increased neural demands without the possibility of direct injury. There are sparse and conflicting clinical data on the effects of postinjury physical and cognitive activation; however, a number of elegant animal studies may shed some light on the underlying pathophysiology.

Physiological activation of the brain may enhance or protect cognitive function, presumably through activation of molecular mechanisms underlying plasticity and neuronal survival (Giza & Prins, 2006; Nithianantharajah & Hannan, 2006). EE rearing (Rosenzweig & Bennett, 1996; Tang, Wang, Feng, Kyin, & Tsien, 2001; Tang & Zou, 2002), nurturing maternal behaviors (Liu, Diorio, Day, Francis, & Meaney, 2000), and voluntary exercise (Griesbach, Hovda, Molteni, Wu, & Gomez-Pinilla, 2004) are some models of physiological activation that have been shown to promote neuroplastic mechanisms and improved cognitive abilities.

After injury, however, premature stimulation may fall upon a neural substrate that is either unresponsive or perhaps even vulnerable to external activation. Thus, the timing of postinjury stimulation may be such that the injured brain is simply unable to activate properly—resulting in slowed reaction time, difficulties in learning, and suboptimal performance. Furthermore, excessive stimulation very early after TBI may even have the potential to exacerbate the underlying neurometabolic energy crisis, acting as a secondary injury to worsen short- or even long-term function.

Unilateral motor cortex lesions in rats result in a contralateral weakness. In studies of forced overuse, lesioned animals had a cast placed upon their good forelimb immediately after the injury, essentially forcing them to use the weakened limb. This type of excessive neural activation in the brain region that was recently injured actually resulted in a larger lesion size and greater functional impairment. Interestingly, though, when the cast was applied in a delayed fashion, 1 week after injury, there was no worsening of the lesion, and functional recovery was improved (Humm, Kozlowski, Bland, James, & Schallert, 1999; Kozlowski, James, & Schallert, 1996). Iverson and colleagues (Chapter 14, this volume) cover in great detail the sports-related relevance of the timing of stimulation in both animal and human models.

CONNECTIVITY/AXONAL FUNCTIONAL OUTCOMES

Diffusion tensor imaging (DTI) is a modification of diffusion-weighted MRI. It measures direction and degree of water diffusion along fibers (as reviewed in Ashwal et al., Chapter 9, this volume), making it a unique tool with which to assess the microstructural changes that occur due to mTBI. Further, because DTI is a quantitative tool, it has the potential to provide a measure of injury severity that can be correlated with clinical assessments of symptom burden and neurocognitive function.

Animal Models

Several studies have used DTI to assess white matter injury from experimentally induced trauma. Mac Donald and colleagues (2007b) obtained baseline (preinjury) DTI in mice, which were then subjected to a CCI injury. DTI was repeated 4–6 hours and 24 hours postinjury, and then compared to the baseline imaging. The DTI findings were also compared to both conventional MRI and direct histological findings of injury as detected with amyloid beta precursor protein (ABPP) and neurofilament immunohistochemistry. In this study, DTI measured axial and radial diffusivity. DTI was also used to report the amount of relative anisotropy (RA), which is a measure of directional asymmetry of diffusion, with higher RA found in anisotropic tissue. This study found that DTI detected histologically proven white matter injury, whereas conventional MRI could not. Further, DTI findings correlated with histological injury. Specifically, RA was found to be decreased near the injury epicenter due to decreased axial diffusivity, and RA was increased (normalized) further from the epicenter, similar to the gradient of injury seen histologically (Mac Donald et al., 2007b).

In a second study of CCI injury in mice, Mac Donald and colleagues (Mac Donald, Dikranian, Bayly, Holtzman, & Brody, 2007a) extended their evaluation to include ultrastructural findings and subacute time points. Specifically, they compared DTI with conventional MRI and histological (ABPP and neurofilament histochemistry) and electron microscopic (EM) findings at 6 hours, 24 hours, 4 days, 1 week, and 4 weeks after trauma. The histological and EM findings demonstrated axonal injury without gliosis in the first 24 hours. At 4 days after injury, gliosis was present along with axonal injury. By the later time points (1 week and 4 weeks), myelin thinning and demyelination were present and gliosis remained, but axonal injury was less than at the earlier time points. DTI was able to detect injury at all time points. Specifically, axial diffusivity (AD) was decreased in the acute phase (first 4 days), then normalized. Conversely, radial diffusivity (RD) was normal in the acute phase, but decreased in the subacute phase. The changes in AD were felt to represent the initial predomination of axonal injury, whereas the later decrease in RD was thought to be due to demyelination, allowing more diffusion to occur perpendicular to the fibers. The RA was diminished at all time points and correctly categorized injured mice from controls at each time point. Further, using mean diffusivity, DTI was able to separate acute from subacute injury. DTI was also correlated with the severity of histological injury, whereas conventional MRI was not.

An important feature of the brain's response to injury is axonal plasticity. Axonal sprouting can occur after injury, and may be part of recovery or could indicate an extension of the original injury (Golarai, Greenwood, Feeney, & Connor, 2001). Kuo et al. (2008) found that DTI was capable of detecting axonal plasticity following induction of status epilepticus in the rat brain *ex vivo*. Recently, Laitinen and colleagues (Laitinen, Sierra, Pitkanen, & Grohn, 2010) evaluated the ability of DTI to identify trauma-induced axonal plasticity in the rat brain using DTI *in vivo* as well as *ex vivo*. In this study, brain injury was produced via status epilepticus that was induced by injection of kainic acid or pilocarpine. DTI was performed no less than 6 months after injury and demonstrated increased fractional anisotropy (FA) that correlated with histological findings of axonal plasticity (mossy fiber sprouting). Thus, DTI appears to be a potential tool for identifying markers of recovery from brain injury.

Another characteristic of the young brain that may affect vulnerability to and recovery from injury is the extent of axon myelination. Reeves and colleagues (Reeves, Phillips, & Povlishock, 2005), using a fluid percussion model of brain injury in rats, assessed injury using compound action potentials (CAP) and ultrastructural analysis. They found that unmyelinated fibers had a greater reduction in CAP than myelinated fibers. Ultrastructural changes were also more extensive in unmyelinated fibers. Moreover, myelinated fibers exhibited a time-dependent recovery in the first week after injury, whereas the unmyelinated fibers did not. Overall, these findings suggest that unmyelinated fibers are more susceptible to brain injury. This vulnerability of unmyelinated fibers to biomechanical injury has direct implications for the developing human brain, where myelination is not complete until well into young adulthood (Giedd et al., 1996; Paus et al., 2001).

Clinical Studies

Studies investigating DTI in individuals with concussion are limited. Most studies of DTI involve adults with non-sports-related injuries. In these studies, DTI findings have consistently demonstrated abnormalities when computed tomography (CT) and conventional MRI have not (Niogi & Mukherjee, 2010). In one of the first clinical studies of DTI, five adults with mTBI had DTI performed within 24 hours after injury. FA was found to be reduced, whereas CT scans and conventional MRI were normal in the respective regions (Arfanakis et al., 2002). Repeat imaging 1 month later showed that DTI findings were improved, though not all regions had normalized (Arfanakis et al., 2002). Importantly, DTI findings in adults may correlate with clinical neurological assessment. Huisman and colleagues studied 20 patients with TBI and found FA to be correlated with the Glasgow Coma Scale (GCS), with lower GCS scores demonstrating a more significant decrease in FA (Huisman et al., 2004).

Bazarian et al. (2007) performed a prospective study of six adult subjects with mTBI (GCS 13–15, brief loss of consciousness or amnesia, normal CT) who underwent DTI and completed a self-reported symptom questionnaire, computerized neurocognitive testing, and quality-of-life measures. The findings were compared to six controls who had suffered a muscular–skeletal injury. During the acute phase, DTI findings correlated with symptom scores and two neurocognitive measures (motor speed and impulse control). The acute phase findings were also correlated with clinical outcome as determined by symptom scores and quality-of-life measures 1 month after injury. In addition, Wilde and colleagues (2008) have reported that increased FA correlated with severity of symptoms in subjects with normal conventional imaging. Importantly, they reported a correlation between increased FA and the Rivermead Post Concussion Symptoms Questionnaire score, a validated clinical marker of concussion symptoms (Wilde et al., 2008).

Niogi and colleagues (2008) evaluated adults with persisting symptoms at least 1 month after mTBI (GCS 13–15, loss of consciousness and amnesia). In a subset of 11 subjects with a normal 3T MRI, reduced FA was found in 10 of the 11. In addition, DTI was significantly correlated with a decline in reaction time. Wozniak et al. (2007) evaluated long-term post-TBI findings in 14 children between 10 and 18 years of age with a history of mild or moderate TBI 6–12 months prior. Each underwent DTI, a neurocognitive battery, and behavioral assessment. The findings were compared to

14 age-matched controls. A decrease in FA was found in the TBI group compared to controls in the inferior frontal, superior frontal, and supracallosal regions. DTI findings were correlated with deficits in executive functioning and motor speed, as well as with behavioral ratings. Two other recent studies of adults with mild to moderate TBI have also linked DTI abnormalities to deficits in executive functioning (Hartikainen et al., 2010; Little et al., 2010).

In a recent prospective study of mTBI, Mayer and colleagues (2010) studied 22 patients with DTI, conventional imaging, and neuropsychological testing, as compared to a control group. In the acute phase, patients with mTBI demonstrated increased FA, despite no apparent differences on traditional imaging or neuropsychological performance between the two groups. In a subset of patients who underwent reimaging 3–5 months later, DTI values were improved, though not completely normalized. Finally, in a recent study of collegiate athletes with symptom duration of a least 1 month following sport-related concussion (no loss of consciousness), DTI found increased mean diffusivity and increased FA (Cubon, Putukian, Boyer, & Dettwiler, 2011).

CONCLUSIONS

mTBI injury results in multiple cerebral physiological changes that are associated with clinical symptoms and outcomes. Better understanding of this pathophysiological cascade of events is critical to more clearly delineate age-related vulnerabilities (or resiliencies), mechanisms that may promote recovery, and the timing of important clinical management decisions regarding these patients. Physiological outcomes described here have been divided into four broad categories: cell death, metabolism, plasticity, and connectivity. Each of these categories is relevant for the injury response of the brain in general; furthermore, the immature brain often has distinctions from the adult brain in these mechanisms. Although overt cell death is not a major part of the concussion response, there is substantial evidence for perturbations of metabolism, neurotransmission, and axonal function, all of which may be exacerbated by repeated injury, particularly when second injuries occur before the brain has had an opportunity to fully recover. Furthermore, the implications of cumulative mild injuries have not been fully elucidated, but are potentially most relevant for children, who may go on to have relatively long exposure to these biomechanical insults.

Advances in noninvasive neuroimaging are affording clinicians a better view of postconcussive pathophysiology, and represent a critical translational bridge that can help connect underlying injury response with clinical sequelae. Although much work remains to be undertaken in children and adolescents, especially those with sport-related concussion, the emerging literature suggests that these new imaging modalities hold promise in assessing the structural/microstructural (MRI/DTI), metabolic (MRS), and functional (fMRI) changes that occur with these injuries. As reviewed in this chapter, these imaging modalities consistently demonstrate a greater sensitivity in identifying structural pathology following mTBI than either CT or conventional MRI, and they correlate with neurobehavioral pathology in the absence of neuroimaging abnormalities on conventional/clinical scans. Thus, these emerging noninvasive imaging technologies may serve as a method that links symptom burden and cognitive deficits to the abnormal cerebral connectivity that occurs with concussion, possibly providing an objective measure to guide management. The growing awareness of developmental differences in concussion biology should certainly be reflected in the clinical approach to these injuries, and may ultimately also result in age-specific management guidelines to protect the young brain.

REFERENCES

Appelberg, K. S., Hovda, D. A., & Prins, M. L. (2009). The effects of a ketogenic diet on behavioral outcome after controlled cortical impact injury in the juvenile and adult rat. *Journal of Neurotrauma*, 26(4), 497–506.

Arfanakis, K., Haughton, V. M., Carew, J. D., Rogers, B. P., Dempsey, R. J., & Meyerand, M. E. (2002). Diffusion tensor MR imaging in diffuse axonal injury. *American Journal of Neuroradiology*, 23(5), 794–802.

Ashwal, S., Holshouser, B. A., Shu, S. K., Simmons, P. L., Perkin, R. M., Tomasi, L. G., et al. (2000). Predictive value of proton magnetic resonance spectroscopy in pediatric closed head injury. *Pediatric Neurology*, 23(2), 114–125.

Ashwal, S., Holshouser, B. A., & Tong, K. A. (2006). Use of advanced neuroimaging techniques in the evaluation of pediatric traumatic brain injury. *Developmental Neuroscience*, 28(4–5), 309–326.

Aspberg, A., & Tottmar, O. (1992). Development of antioxidant enzymes in rat brain and in reaggregation culture of fetal brain cells. *Brain Research: Developmental Brain Research*, 66(1), 55–58.

Babikian, T., Freier, M. C., Ashwal, S., Riggs, M. L., Burley, T., & Holshouser, B. A. (2006). MR spectroscopy: Predicting long-term neuropsychological outcome following pediatric TBI. *Journal of Magnetic Resonance Imaging*, 24(4), 801–811.

Bailes, J. E., & Mills, J. D. (2010). Docosahexaenoic acid reduces traumatic axonal injury in a rodent head injury model. *Journal of Neurotrauma*, 27(9), 1617–1624.

Barkhoudarian, G., Hovda, D. A., & Giza, C. C. (2011). The molecular pathophysiology of concussive brain injury. *Clinics in Sports Medicine*, 30(1), 33–48, vii–viii.

Bazarian, J. J., Zhong, J., Blyth, B., Zhu, T., Kavcic, V., & Peterson, D. (2007). Diffusion tensor imaging detects clinically important axonal damage after mild traumatic brain injury: A pilot study. *Journal of Neurotrauma*, 24(9), 1447–1459.

Bergsneider, M., Hovda, D. A., Lee, S. M., Kelly, D. F., McArthur, D. L., Vespa, P. M., et al. (2000). Dissociation of cerebral glucose metabolism and level of consciousness during the period of metabolic depression following human traumatic brain injury. *Journal of Neurotrauma*, 17(5), 389–401.

Bergsneider, M., Hovda, D. A., McArthur, D. L., Etchepare, M., Huang, S. C., Sehati, N., et al. (2001). Metabolic recovery following human traumatic brain injury based on FDG-PET: Time course and relationship to neurological disability. *Journal of Head Trauma Rehabilitation*, 16(2), 135–148.

Biegon, A., Fry, P. A., Paden, C. M., Alexandrovich, A., Tsenter, J., & Shohami, E. (2004). Dynamic changes in N-methyl-D-aspartate receptors after closed head injury in mice: Implications for treatment of neurological and cognitive deficits. *Proceedings of the National Academy of Sciences of the United States of America*, 101(14), 5117–5122.

Bittigau, P., Sifringer, M., Pohl, D., Stadthaus, D., Ishimaru, M., Shimizu, H., et al. (1999). Apoptotic neurodegeneration following trauma is markedly enhanced in the immature brain. *Annals of Neurology*, 45(6), 724–735.

Branchi, I., Francia, N., & Alleva, E. (2004). Epigenetic control of neurobehavioural plasticity: The role of neurotrophins. *Behavioural Pharmacology*, 15(5–6), 353–362.

Chen, J. K., Johnston, K. M., Frey, S., Petrides, M., Worsley, K., & Ptito, A. (2004). Functional abnormalities in symptomatic concussed athletes: An fMRI study. *NeuroImage*, *22*(1), 68–82.

Cherian, L., Hlatky, R., & Robertson, C. S. (2004). Comparison of tetrahydrobiopterin and L-arginine on cerebral blood flow after controlled cortical impact injury in rats. *Journal of Neurotrauma*, *21*(9), 1196–1203.

Chugani, H. T., Phelps, M. E., & Mazziotta, J. C. (1987). Positron emission tomography study of human brain functional development. *Annals of Neurology*, *22*(4), 487–497.

Cubon, V. A., Putukian, M., Boyer, C., & Dettwiler, A. (2011). A diffusion tensor imaging study on the white matter skeleton in individuals with sports-related concussion. *Journal of Neurotrauma*, *28*(2), 189–201.

Davis, L. M., Pauly, J. R., Readnower, R. D., Rho, J. M., & Sullivan, P. G. (2008). Fasting is neuroprotective following traumatic brain injury. *Journal of Neuroscience Research*, *86*(8), 1812–1822.

De Beaumont, L., Theoret, H., Mongeon, D., Messier, J., Leclerc, S., Tremblay, S., et al. (2009). Brain function decline in healthy retired athletes who sustained their last sports concussion in early adulthood. *Brain*, *132*(Pt. 3), 695–708.

Deng, Y., Thompson, B. M., Gao, X., & Hall, E. D. (2007). Temporal relationship of peroxynitrite-induced oxidative damage, calpain-mediated cytoskeletal degradation and neurodegeneration after traumatic brain injury. *Experimental Neurology*, *205*(1), 154–165.

Deng-Bryant, Y., Giza, C. C., Hovda, D., & Prins, M. L. (2010). *Changes in vascular MCT1 and GLUT1 transporters following traumatic brain injury*. Manuscript submitted for publication.

Dreiem, A., Gertz, C. C., & Seegal, R. F. (2005). The effects of methylmercury on mitochondrial function and reactive oxygen species formation in rat striatal synaptosomes are age-dependent. *Toxicological Sciences*, *87*(1), 156–162.

Duhaime, A. C., Saykin, A. J., McDonald, B. C., Dodge, C. P., Eskey, C. J., Darcey, T. M., et al. (2006). Functional magnetic resonance imaging of the primary somatosensory cortex in piglets. *Journal of Neurosurgery*, *104*(4, Suppl.), 259–264.

Fan, P., Yamauchi, T., Noble, L. J., & Ferriero, D. M. (2003). Age-dependent differences in glutathione peroxidase activity after traumatic brain injury. *Journal of Neurotrauma*, *20*(5), 437–445.

Felderhoff-Mueser, U., Sifringer, M., Pesditschek, S., Kuckuck, H., Moysich, A., Bittigau, P., et al. (2002). Pathways leading to apoptotic neurodegeneration following trauma to the developing rat brain. *Neurobiology of Disease*, *11*(2), 231–245.

Fineman, I., Giza, C. C., Nahed, B. V., Lee, S. M., & Hovda, D. A. (2000). Inhibition of neocortical plasticity during development by a moderate concussive brain injury. *Journal of Neurotrauma*, *17*(9), 739–749.

Fineman, I., Hovda, D. A., Smith, M., Yoshino, A., & Becker, D. P. (1993). Concussive brain injury is associated with a prolonged accumulation of calcium: A 45Ca autoradiographic study. *Brain Research*, *624*(1–2), 94–102.

Friess, S. H., Ichord, R. N., Ralston, J., Ryall, K., Helfaer, M. A., Smith, C., et al. (2009). Repeated traumatic brain injury affects composite cognitive function in piglets. *Journal of Neurotrauma*, *26*(7), 1111–1121.

Giedd, J. N., Rumsey, J. M., Castellanos, F. X., Rajapakse, J. C., Kaysen, D., Vaituzis, A. C., et al. (1996). A quantitative MRI study of the corpus callosum in children and adolescents. *Brain Research: Developmental Brain Research*, *91*(2), 274–280.

Giza, C. C., Griesbach, G. S., & Hovda, D. A. (2005). Experience-dependent behavioral plasticity is disturbed following traumatic injury to the immature brain. *Behavioural Brain Research*, *157*(1), 11–22.

Giza, C. C., & Hovda, D. A. (2001). The neurometabolic cascade of concussion. *Journal of Athletic Training, 36*(3), 228–235.

Giza, C. C., Maria, N. S., & Hovda, D. A. (2006). N-methyl-D-aspartate receptor subunit changes after traumatic injury to the developing brain. *Journal of Neurotrauma, 23*(6), 950–961.

Giza, C. C., & Prins, M. L. (2006). Is being plastic fantastic?: Mechanisms of altered plasticity after developmental traumatic brain injury. *Developmental Neuroscience, 28*(4–5), 364–379.

Glenn, T. C., Kelly, D. F., Boscardin, W. J., McArthur, D. L., Vespa, P., Oertel, M., et al. (2003). Energy dysfunction as a predictor of outcome after moderate or severe head injury: Indices of oxygen, glucose, and lactate metabolism. *Journal of Cerebral Blood Flow and Metabolism, 23*(10), 1239–1250.

Golarai, G., Greenwood, A. C., Feeney, D. M., & Connor, J. A. (2001). Physiological and structural evidence for hippocampal involvement in persistent seizure susceptibility after traumatic brain injury. *Journal of Neuroscience, 21*(21), 8523–8537.

Gomez-Pinilla, F. (2008). Brain foods: The effects of nutrients on brain function. *Nature Reviews Neuroscience, 9*(7), 568–578.

Greenough, W. T., Volkmar, F. R., & Juraska, J. M. (1973). Effects of rearing complexity on dendritic branching in frontolateral and temporal cortex of the rat. *Experimental Neurology, 41*(2), 371–378.

Griesbach, G. S., Hovda, D. A., Molteni, R., Wu, A., & Gomez-Pinilla, F. (2004). Voluntary exercise following traumatic brain injury: Brain-derived neurotrophic factor upregulation and recovery of function. *Neuroscience, 125*(1), 129–139.

Gsell, W., Burke, M., Wiedermann, D., Bonvento, G., Silva, A. C., Dauphin, F., et al. (2006). Differential effects of NMDA and AMPA glutamate receptors on functional magnetic resonance imaging signals and evoked neuronal activity during forepaw stimulation of the rat. *Journal of Neuroscience, 26*(33), 8409–8416.

Gurkoff, G. G., Giza, C. C., & Hovda, D. A. (2006). Lateral fluid percussion injury in the developing rat causes an acute, mild behavioral dysfunction in the absence of significant cell death. *Brain Research, 1077*(1), 24–36.

Guskiewicz, K. M., McCrea, M., Marshall, S. W., Cantu, R. C., Randolph, C., Barr, W., et al. (2003). Cumulative effects associated with recurrent concussion in collegiate football players: The NCAA Concussion Study. *Journal of the American Medical Association, 290*(19), 2549–2555.

Hall, E. D., Detloff, M. R., Johnson, K., & Kupina, N. C. (2004). Peroxynitrite-mediated protein nitration and lipid peroxidation in a mouse model of traumatic brain injury. *Journal of Neurotrauma, 21*(1), 9–20.

Hamberger, A., Viano, D. C., Saljo, A., & Bolouri, H. (2009). Concussion in professional football: Morphology of brain injuries in the NFL concussion model—part 16. *Neurosurgery, 64*(6), 1174–1182; discussion, 1182.

Hartikainen, K. M., Waljas, M., Isoviita, T., Dastidar, P., Liimatainen, S., Solbakk, A. K., et al. (2010). Persistent symptoms in mild to moderate traumatic brain injury associated with executive dysfunction. *Journal of Clinical and Experimental Neuropsychology, 32*(7), 767–774.

Henninger, N., Sicard, K. M., Li, Z., Kulkarni, P., Dutzmann, S., Urbanek, C., et al. (2007). Differential recovery of behavioral status and brain function assessed with functional magnetic resonance imaging after mild traumatic brain injury in the rat. *Critical Care Medicine, 35*(11), 2607–2614.

Hoon, A. H., Jr., & Melhem, E. R. (2000). Neuroimaging: Applications in disorders of early brain development. *Journal of Developmental and Behavioral Pediatrics, 21*(4), 291–302.

Hovda, D. A., Villablanca, J. R., Chugani, H. T., & Phelps, M. E. (1996). Cerebral metabolism following neonatal or adult hemineodecortication in cats: I. Effects on glucose metabolism using [14C]2-deoxy-D-glucose autoradiography. *Journal of Cerebral Blood Flow and Metabolism, 16*(1), 134–146.

Huh, J. W., Widing, A. G., & Raghupathi, R. (2007). Basic science: Repetitive mild noncontusive brain trauma in immature rats exacerbates traumatic axonal injury and axonal calpain activation—a preliminary report. *Journal of Neurotrauma, 24*(1), 15–27.

Huh, J. W., Widing, A. G., & Raghupathi, R. (2008). Midline brain injury in the immature rat induces sustained cognitive deficits, bihemispheric axonal injury, and neurodegeneration. *Experimental Neurology, 213*(1), 84–92.

Huisman, T. A., Schwamm, L. H., Schaefer, P. W., Koroshetz, W. J., Shetty-Alva, N., Ozsunar, Y., et al. (2004). Diffusion tensor imaging as potential biomarker of white matter injury in diffuse axonal injury. *American Journal of Neuroradiology, 25*(3), 370–376.

Humm, J. L., Kozlowski, D. A., Bland, S. T., James, D. C., & Schallert, T. (1999). Use-dependent exaggeration of brain injury: Is glutamate involved? *Experimental Neurology, 157*(2), 349–358.

Ip, E. Y., Giza, C. C., Griesbach, G. S., & Hovda, D. A. (2002). Effects of enriched environment and fluid percussion injury on dendritic arborization within the cerebral cortex of the developing rat. *Journal of Neurotrauma, 19*(5), 573–585.

Ip, E. Y., Zanier, E. R., Moore, A. H., Lee, S. M., & Hovda, D. A. (2003). Metabolic, neurochemical, and histologic responses to vibrissa motor cortex stimulation after traumatic brain injury. *Journal of Cerebral Blood Flow and Metabolism, 23*(8), 900–910.

Irvine, G. I., Logan, B., Eckert, M., & Abraham, W. C. (2006). Enriched environment exposure regulates excitability, synaptic transmission, and LTP in the dentate gyrus of freely moving rats. *Hippocampus, 16*(2), 149–160.

Iverson, G. L., Lange, R. T., Gaetz, M., & Zasler, N. D. (2007). Mild TBI. In N. D. Zasler & D. I. Z. Katz, R. D. (Eds.), *Brain injury medicine: Principles and practice* (pp. 333–371). New York: Demos Medical.

Jacobs, B., Schall, M., & Scheibel, A. B. (1993). A quantitative dendritic analysis of Wernicke's area in humans: II. Gender, hemispheric, and environmental factors. *Journal of Comparative Neurology, 327*(1), 97–111.

Jantzen, K. J. (2010). Functional magnetic resonance imaging of mild traumatic brain injury. *Journal of Head Trauma Rehabilitation, 25*(4), 256–266.

Jantzen, K. J., Anderson, B., Steinberg, F. L., & Kelso, J. A. (2004). A prospective functional MR imaging study of mild traumatic brain injury in college football players. *American Journal of Neuroradiology, 25*(5), 738–745.

Kanayama, G., Takeda, M., Niigawa, H., Ikura, Y., Tamii, H., Taniguchi, N., et al. (1996). The effects of repetitive mild brain injury on cytoskeletal protein and behavior. *Methods and Findings in Experimental Clinical Pharmacology, 18*(2), 105–115.

Katayama, Y., Becker, D. P., Tamura, T., & Hovda, D. A. (1990). Massive increases in extracellular potassium and the indiscriminate release of glutamate following concussive brain injury. *Journal of Neurosurgery, 73*(6), 889–900.

Kawamata, T., Katayama, Y., Hovda, D. A., Yoshino, A., & Becker, D. P. (1992). Administration of excitatory amino acid antagonists via microdialysis attenuates the increase in glucose utilization seen following concussive brain injury. *Journal of Cerebral Blood Flow and Metabolism, 12*(1), 12–24.

Kawamata, T., Katayama, Y., Maeda, T., Mori, T., Aoyama, N., Kikuchi, T., et al. (1997). Antioxidant, OPC-14117, attenuates edema formation and behavioral deficits following cortical contusion in rats. *Acta Neurochirurgica Supplement, 70*, 191–193.

Kempermann, G., Kuhn, H. G., & Gage, F. H. (1997). More hippocampal neurons in adult mice living in an enriched environment. *Nature, 386*(6624), 493–495.

Kozlowski, D. A., James, D. C., & Schallert, T. (1996). Use-dependent exaggeration of neuronal injury after unilateral sensorimotor cortex lesions. *Journal of Neuroscience*, *16*(15), 4776–4786.

Kumar, A., Zou, L., Yuan, X., Long, Y., & Yang, K. (2002). N-methyl-D-aspartate receptors: Transient loss of NR1/NR2A/NR2B subunits after traumatic brain injury in a rodent model. *Journal of Neuroscience Research*, *67*(6), 781–786.

Kuo, L. W., Lee, C. Y., Chen, J. H., Wedeen, V. J., Chen, C. C., Liou, H. H., et al. (2008). Mossy fiber sprouting in pilocarpine-induced status epilepticus rat hippocampus: A correlative study of diffusion spectrum imaging and histology. *NeuroImage*, *41*(3), 789–800.

Laitinen, T., Sierra, A., Pitkanen, A., & Grohn, O. (2010). Diffusion tensor MRI of axonal plasticity in the rat hippocampus. *NeuroImage*, *51*(2), 521–530.

Little, D. M., Kraus, M. F., Joseph, J., Geary, E. K., Susmaras, T., Zhou, X. J., et al. (2010). Thalamic integrity underlies executive dysfunction in traumatic brain injury. *Neurology*, *74*(7), 558–564.

Liu, D., Diorio, J., Day, J. C., Francis, D. D., & Meaney, M. J. (2000). Maternal care, hippocampal synaptogenesis and cognitive development in rats. *Nature Neuroscience*, *3*(8), 799–806.

Mac Donald, C. L., Dikranian, K., Bayly, P., Holtzman, D., & Brody, D. (2007a). Diffusion tensor imaging reliably detects experimental traumatic axonal injury and indicates approximate time of injury. *Journal of Neuroscience*, *27*(44), 11869–11876.

Mac Donald, C. L., Dikranian, K., Song, S. K., Bayly, P. V., Holtzman, D. M., & Brody, D. L. (2007b). Detection of traumatic axonal injury with diffusion tensor imaging in a mouse model of traumatic brain injury. *Experimental Neurology*, *205*(1), 116–131.

Mac Donald, C. L., Johnson, A. M., Cooper, D., Nelson, E. C., Werner, N. J., Shimony, J. S., et al. (2011). Detection of blast-related traumatic brain injury in U.S. military personnel. *New England Journal of Medicine*, *364*(22), 2091–2100.

Mavelli, I., Rigo, A., Federico, R., Ciriolo, M. R., & Rotilio, G. (1982). Superoxide dismutase, glutathione peroxidase and catalase in developing rat brain. *Biochemical Journal*, *204*(2), 535–540.

Mayer, A. R., Ling, J., Mannell, M. V., Gasparovic, C., Phillips, J. P., Doezema, D., et al. (2010). A prospective diffusion tensor imaging study in mild traumatic brain injury. *Neurology*, *74*(8), 643–650.

McAllister, T. W., Saykin, A. J., Flashman, L. A., Sparling, M. B., Johnson, S. C., Guerin, S. J., et al. (1999). Brain activation during working memory 1 month after mild traumatic brain injury: A functional MRI study. *Neurology*, *53*(6), 1300–1308.

McAllister, T. W., Sparling, M. B., Flashman, L. A., Guerin, S. J., Mamourian, A. C., & Saykin, A. J. (2001). Differential working memory load effects after mild traumatic brain injury. *NeuroImage*, *14*(5), 1004–1012.

McKee, A. C., Cantu, R. C., Nowinski, C. J., Hedley-Whyte, E. T., Gavett, B. E., Budson, A. E., et al. (2009). Chronic traumatic encephalopathy in athletes: Progressive tauopathy after repetitive head injury. *Journal of Neuropathology and Experimental Neurology*, *68*(7), 709–735.

Miller, L. P., Lyeth, B. G., Jenkins, L. W., Oleniak, L., Panchision, D., Hamm, R. J., et al. (1990). Excitatory amino acid receptor subtype binding following traumatic brain injury. *Brain Research*, *526*(1), 103–107.

Mills, J. D., Bailes, J. E., Sedney, C. L., Hutchins, H., & Sears, B. (2011). Omega-3 fatty acid supplementation and reduction of traumatic axonal injury in a rodent head injury model. *Journal of Neurosurgery*, *114*(1), 77–84.

Mori, T., Kawamata, T., Katayama, Y., Maeda, T., Aoyama, N., Kikuchi, T., et al. (1998). Antioxidant, OPC-14117, attenuates edema formation, and subsequent tissue damage following cortical contusion in rats. *Acta Neurochirurgica Supplement*, *71*, 120–122.

Moss, M. L., Meehan, M. A., & Salentijn, L. (1972). Transformative and translative growth processes in neurocranial development of the rat. *Acta Anatomica, 81*(2), 161–182.

Niogi, S. N., & Mukherjee, P. (2010). Diffusion tensor imaging of mild traumatic brain injury. *Journal of Head Trauma Rehabilitation, 25*(4), 241–255.

Niogi, S. N., Mukherjee, P., Ghajar, J., Johnson, C., Kolster, R. A., Sarkar, R., et al. (2008). Extent of microstructural white matter injury in postconcussive syndrome correlates with impaired cognitive reaction time: A 3T diffusion tensor imaging study of mild traumatic brain injury. *American Journal of Neuroradiology, 29*(5), 967–973.

Nithianantharajah, J., & Hannan, A. J. (2006). Enriched environments, experience-dependent plasticity and disorders of the nervous system. *Nature Reviews Neuroscience, 7*(9), 697–709.

Omalu, B. I., Bailes, J., Hammers, J. L., & Fitzsimmons, R. P. (2010a). Chronic traumatic encephalopathy, suicides and parasuicides in professional American athletes: The role of the forensic pathologist. *American Journal of Forensic Medicine and Pathology, 31*(2), 130–132.

Omalu, B. I., Hamilton, R. L., Kamboh, M. I., DeKosky, S. T., & Bailes, J. (2010b). Chronic traumatic encephalopathy (CTE) in a National Football League player: Case report and emerging medicolegal practice questions. *Journal of Forensic Nursing, 6*(1), 40–46.

Orrenius, S., Zhivotovsky, B., & Nicotera, P. (2003). Regulation of cell death: The calcium–apoptosis link. *Nature Reviews Molecular Cell Biology, 4*(7), 552–565.

Osteen, C. L., Giza, C. C., & Hovda, D. A. (2004). Injury-induced alterations in N-methyl-D-aspartate receptor subunit composition contribute to prolonged 45calcium accumulation following lateral fluid percussion. *Neuroscience, 128*(2), 305–322.

Osteen, C. L., Moore, A. H., Prins, M. L., & Hovda, D. A. (2001). Age-dependency of 45calcium accumulation following lateral fluid percussion: Acute and delayed patterns. *Journal of Neurotrauma, 18*(2), 141–162.

Passineau, M. J., Zhao, W., Busto, R., Dietrich, W. D., Alonso, O., Loor, J. Y., et al. (2000). Chronic metabolic sequelae of traumatic brain injury: Prolonged suppression of somatosensory activation. *American Journal of Physiology: Heart and Circulatory Physiology, 279*(3), H924–H931.

Paus, T., Collins, D. L., Evans, A. C., Leonard, G., Pike, B., & Zijdenbos, A. (2001). Maturation of white matter in the human brain: A review of magnetic resonance studies. *Brain Research Bulletin, 54*(3), 255–266.

Prins, M. L., Fujima, L. S., & Hovda, D. A. (2005). Age-dependent reduction of cortical contusion volume by ketones after traumatic brain injury. *Journal of Neuroscience Research, 82*(3), 413–420.

Prins, M. L., & Giza, C. C. (2006). Induction of monocarboxylate transporter 2 expression and ketone transport following traumatic brain injury in juvenile and adult rats. *Developmental Neuroscience, 28*(4–5), 447–456.

Prins, M. L., & Giza, C. C. (in press). Repeat traumatic brain injury in the developing brain. *International Journal of Developmental Neuroscience*.

Prins, M. L., Hales, A., Reger, M., Giza, C. C., & Hovda, D. A. (2010). Repeat traumatic brain injury in the juvenile rat is associated with increased axonal injury and cognitive impairments. *Developmental Neuroscience, 32*(5–6), 510–518.

Prins, M. L., & Hovda, D. (2009). The effects of age and ketogenic diet on local cerebral metabolic rates of glucose after controlled cortical impact injury in rats. *Journal of Neurotrauma, 26*(7), 1083–1093.

Prins, M. L., Lee, S. M., Cheng, C. L., Becker, D. P., & Hovda, D. A. (1996). Fluid percussion brain injury in the developing and adult rat: A comparative study of mortality, morphology, intracranial pressure, and mean arterial blood pressure. *Brain Research: Developmental Brain Research, 95*(2), 272–282.

Prins, M. L., Lee, S. M., Fujima, L. S., & Hovda, D. A. (2004). Increased cerebral uptake and oxidation of exogenous betaHB improves ATP following traumatic brain injury in adult rats. *Journal of Neurochemistry, 90*(3), 666–672.

Prins, M. L., Povlishock, J. T., & Phillips, L. L. (2003). The effects of combined fluid percussion traumatic brain injury and unilateral entorhinal deafferentation on the juvenile rat brain. *Brain Research: Developmental Brain Research, 140*(1), 93–104.

Reeves, T. M., Lyeth, B. G., & Povlishock, J. T. (1995). Long-term potentiation deficits and excitability changes following traumatic brain injury. *Experimental Brain Research, 106*(2), 248–256.

Reeves, T. M., Phillips, L. L., & Povlishock, J. T. (2005). Myelinated and unmyelinated axons of the corpus callosum differ in vulnerability and functional recovery following traumatic brain injury. *Experimental Neurology, 196*(1), 126–137.

Rosenzweig, M. R., & Bennett, E. L. (1996). Psychobiology of plasticity: Effects of training and experience on brain and behavior. *Behavioural Brain Research, 78*(1), 57–65.

Santa Maria, N. S., Harris, N. G., Hovda, D. A., & Giza, C. C. (2009). Reduced glutamatergic activation after developmental fluid percussion injury mapped by pharmacological MRI (phMRI). *Journal of Neurotrauma, 36*(8), A44.

Sattler, R., & Tymianski, M. (2000). Molecular mechanisms of calcium-dependent excitotoxicity. *Journal of Molecular Medicine, 78*(1), 3–13.

Sick, T. J., Perez-Pinzon, M. A., & Feng, Z. Z. (1998). Impaired expression of long-term potentiation in hippocampal slices 4 and 48 h following mild fluid-percussion brain injury in vivo. *Brain Research, 785*(2), 287–292.

Signoretti, S., Vagnozzi, R., Tavazzi, B., & Lazzarino, G. (2010). Biochemical and neurochemical sequelae following mild traumatic brain injury: Summary of experimental data and clinical implications. *Neurosurgical Focus, 29*(5), E1.

Singh, I. N., Sullivan, P. G., Deng, Y., Mbye, L. H., & Hall, E. D. (2006). Time course of post-traumatic mitochondrial oxidative damage and dysfunction in a mouse model of focal traumatic brain injury: Implications for neuroprotective therapy. *Journal of Cerebral Blood Flow and Metabolism, 26*(11), 1407–1418.

Sutton, R. L., Hovda, D. A., Adelson, P. D., Benzel, E. C., & Becker, D. P. (1994). Metabolic changes following cortical contusion: Relationships to edema and morphological changes. *Acta Neurochirurgica Supplement (Wien), 60*, 446–448.

Talavage, T. M., Nauman, E., Breedlove, E. L., Yoruk, U., Dye, A. E., Morigaki, K., et al. (in press). Functionally detected cognitive impairment in high school football players without clinically-diagnosed concussion. *Journal of Neurotrauma.*

Tang, A. C., & Zou, B. (2002). Neonatal exposure to novelty enhances long-term potentiation in CA1 of the rat hippocampus. *Hippocampus, 12*(3), 398–404.

Tang, Y. P., Wang, H., Feng, R., Kyin, M., & Tsien, J. Z. (2001). Differential effects of enrichment on learning and memory function in NR2B transgenic mice. *Neuropharmacology, 41*(6), 779–790.

Tavazzi, B., Signoretti, S., Lazzarino, G., Amorini, A. M., Delfini, R., Cimatti, M., et al. (2005). Cerebral oxidative stress and depression of energy metabolism correlate with severity of diffuse brain injury in rats. *Neurosurgery, 56*(3), 582–589.

Tees, R. C., Buhrmann, K., & Hanley, J. (1990). The effect of early experience on water maze spatial learning and memory in rats. *Developmental Psychobiology, 23*(5), 427–439.

Thomas, S., Prins, M. L., Samii, M., & Hovda, D. A. (2000). Cerebral metabolic response to traumatic brain injury sustained early in development: A 2-deoxy-D-glucose autoradiographic study. *Journal of Neurotrauma, 17*(8), 649–665.

Tyurin, V. A., Tyurina, Y. Y., Borisenko, G. G., Sokolova, T. V., Ritov, V. B., Quinn, P. J., et al. (2000). Oxidative stress following traumatic brain injury in rats: Quantitation of biomarkers and detection of free radical intermediates. *Journal of Neurochemistry*, *75*(5), 2178–2189.

Vagnozzi, R., Marmarou, A., Tavazzi, B., Signoretti, S., Di Pierro, D., del Bolgia, F., et al. (1999). Changes of cerebral energy metabolism and lipid peroxidation in rats leading to mitochondrial dysfunction after diffuse brain injury. *Journal of Neurotrauma*, *16*(10), 903–913.

Vagnozzi, R., Signoretti, S., Cristofori, L., Alessandrini, F., Floris, R., Isgro, E., et al. (2010). Assessment of metabolic brain damage and recovery following mild traumatic brain injury: A multicentre, proton magnetic resonance spectroscopic study in concussed patients. *Brain*, *133*(11), 3232–3242.

Vagnozzi, R., Signoretti, S., Tavazzi, B., Floris, R., Ludovici, A., Marziali, S., et al. (2008). Temporal window of metabolic brain vulnerability to concussion: A pilot 1H-magnetic resonance spectroscopic study in concussed athletes—Part III. *Neurosurgery*, *62*(6), 1286–1295.

Vagnozzi, R., Tavazzi, B., Signoretti, S., Amorini, A. M., Belli, A., Cimatti, M., et al. (2007). Temporal window of metabolic brain vulnerability to concussions: Mitochondrial-related impairment—Part I. *Neurosurgery*, *61*(2), 379–388.

Vannucci, S. J., & Simpson, I. A. (2003). Developmental switch in brain nutrient transporter expression in the rat. *American Journal of Physiology: Endocrinology and Metabolism*, *285*(5), E1127–E1134.

Wilde, E. A., McCauley, S. R., Hunter, J. V., Bigler, E. D., Chu, Z., Wang, Z. J., et al. (2008). Diffusion tensor imaging of acute mild traumatic brain injury in adolescents. *Neurology*, *70*(12), 948–955.

Wozniak, J. R., Krach, L., Ward, E., Mueller, B. A., Muetzel, R., Schnoebelen, S., et al. (2007). Neurocognitive and neuroimaging correlates of pediatric traumatic brain injury: A diffusion tensor imaging (DTI) study. *Archives of Clinical Neuropsychology*, *22*(5), 555–568.

Yaka, R., Biegon, A., Grigoriadis, N., Simeonidou, C., Grigoriadis, S., Alexandrovich, A. G., et al. (2007). D-cycloserine improves functional recovery and reinstates long-term potentiation (LTP) in a mouse model of closed head injury. *FASEB Journal*, *21*(9), 2033–2041.

Yoshino, A., Hovda, D. A., Kawamata, T., Katayama, Y., & Becker, D. P. (1991). Dynamic changes in local cerebral glucose utilization following cerebral conclusion in rats: Evidence of a hyper- and subsequent hypometabolic state. *Brain Research*, *561*(1), 106–119.

Yuen, T. J., Browne, K. D., Iwata, A., & Smith, D. H. (2009). Sodium channelopathy induced by mild axonal trauma worsens outcome after a repeat injury. *Journal of Neuroscience Research*, *87*(16), 3620–3625.

CHAPTER 6

Neurological Outcomes

Gavin A. Davis

The neurological outcome following pediatric mild traumatic brain injury (mTBI) is most commonly normal. Put another way, most children with mTBI suffer no neurological deficit. Thus you may ask, why include a chapter on neurological outcomes in a book on mTBI in children? The answer is that some children *do* have neurological consequences following mTBI, and we need to identify these problems, identify children at risk of these adverse outcomes, and determine the clinical implications in these children. Given that most children with mTBI will not suffer from any of the neurological outcomes described in this chapter, the reader should follow this chapter with this caveat in mind. It is also worth noting that the measure of outcome is dependent upon the population studied, the definitions used, the study methodology, and the techniques available. These issues are discussed in detail below, but, given that this chapter assesses evidence-based outcomes, it is important to stress that the evidence is often deficient because of these limitations.

For the purposes of this chapter, pediatric mTBI is defined as children with a Glasgow Coma Scale (GCS) of 13–15 following resuscitation post head injury. The astute reader will also consider the study population. A review of pediatric mTBI in those presenting to a tertiary referral neurosurgical unit will contain a very different patient population from those children presenting to a suburban hospital emergency department or to a general practitioner. Given that many of the study populations are from tertiary referral hospitals, it is apparent that some of the incidence figures presented will apply to the study population and are not necessarily applicable to all children with mTBI. Most children with trivial head injury do not present for medical assessment, and neurological outcomes are assumed to be normal in these children. This chapter therefore focuses primarily on children with mTBI who present for medical attention, about whom we have data available. Some of these children will have sports concussion, and other children will have mTBI from a variety of mechanisms, but all mTBI cases are grouped together for the purposes of this chapter.

CRITICAL REVIEW OF RELEVANT OUTCOME-FOCUSED EMPIRICAL STUDIES IN THE SOMATIC SYMPTOMATOLOGY EXPERIENCED AFTER mTBI

Somatic Symptoms and Postconcussion Syndrome

Following mTBI, it is not uncommon for children to complain of a constellation of symptoms that are often referred to as *postconcussion syndrome* (PCS). An assortment of definitions exists for PCS, including the *International Classification of Diseases*, 10th revision (ICD-10; World Health Organization, 1993) and the *Diagnostic and Statistical Manual of Mental Disorders*—Text Revised (DSM-IV-TR; American Psychiatric Association, 2000). These symptom classifications are described in detail by Wilde et al. (Chapter 1, this volume). PCS symptoms are often divided into three broad groups: somatic, cognitive, and emotional. The somatic group includes headache and dizziness; the cognitive group includes memory and concentration impairments; and the emotional group includes irritability and depression. Is this trichotomous categorization based on clinical utility, prognostic significance, etiological origins, or simplistic convenience? Ayr, Yeates, Taylor, and Browne (2009) address some of these questions in their study, which examined four dimensions of postconcussive symptoms (cognitive, somatic, emotional, and behavioral) and found only two dimensions that demonstrated consistency in child-reported symptoms (cognitive and somatic) and three dimensions that were consistent for parent-reported symptoms (cognitive, somatic, and emotional). Reviewing agreement between child- and parent-reported symptoms, the authors found that the cognitive and somatic dimensions were similar. While providing some evidence for the utility of grouping symptoms, this study did not directly address the issue of mTBI outcomes in children.

Detailed analysis of each symptom can result in confusion. Categorizing dizziness as a somatic complaint implies a somatic cause and consequently suggests pathology within the cerebellum, vestibular apparatus, ocular, or spinal systems. Yet, detailed magnetic resonance imaging (MRI) and neurophysiological assessment of children with mTBI does not usually demonstrate such pathology. Phonophobia, or noise intolerance, although a feature of PCS, is commonly present in a broad range of neurological pathologies, including migraine, subarachnoid hemorrhage, and meningitis. The phonophobia of PCS is obviously a different phenomenon. Is it accurate to describe it as a somatic symptom, or is it an emotional response, or a cognitive response to an altered level of awareness? Although some studies have demonstrated different rates of symptom reports at different times between categories (Taylor et al., 2010), the underlying mechanism of this syndrome is still fiercely debated.

The adult literature is replete with authors discussing the association of PCS and litigation (Hyman, 2001; Landy, 1998)—an association that remains an obstacle to better understanding of this condition. The terms *physiogenic* and *psychogenic* are often used to describe the origins of PCS, with proponents for each cause stating their case. It is apparent that the evidence available is insufficient for us to answer this question, but the truth probably lies in the middle: That is, both physiological and psychological factors may contribute to the etiology of this condition. Anderson, Heitger, and Macleod (2006) describe a combination of hippocampal injury and a secondary maladaptive neuroendocrine stress response reinforcing disability as an etiological concept. The subject of PCS is further complicated by the fact that many PCS symptoms are nonspecific and present in the general pediatric population at any one time. For example, a child presents after mTBI with headache and emotional lability. Is this PCS, or were these symptoms present prior to the injury? Does injury to the brain itself cause these symptoms, or is injury itself, to the brain or any part of the body, associated with the development of such symptoms?

Satz et al. (1999) discuss this issue in detail, expressing their rationale for study methodology; namely, the requirement for not one but *two* control groups in studies of PCS. One control group should consist of children with other injury (i.e., non-brain), and the second control group should consist of children without injury. Thus, comparing the mTBI and other-injury group controls for injury to the brain specifically, and comparison between these two groups and the no-injury group controls for injury per se. It is self-evident, however, that there may be other factors contributing to PCS (e.g., preinjury status, family status, socioeconomic status, school record, psychological and medical history), and these must be controlled for in studies of PCS. Furthermore, two elements of symptom reporting are critical: who and when. *Who* refers to parent, teacher, or child. Child self-report does not always correlate with parent report of symptoms. *When* refers to longitudinal assessment. Symptoms change over time, so assessment at a single point in time may not truly reflect the PCS condition (Yeates et al., 2009). The Yeates study focused on classifying children based on change. However, to characterize the natural history of PCS in children with mTBI compared to children with other injuries, the same group of researchers (Taylor et al., 2010) published further data on the same group of patients. They demonstrated differences between duration of somatic and cognitive symptoms, as well as differences according to child self-reports and the parent report of symptoms. With regard to somatic symptoms in the children with mTBI, they found that parents reported higher initial symptoms compared to parents of children with other injuries, and resolution at 12 months, whereas children with other injuries reported resolution at 3 months. Similar to other studies, they also found that there was a greater tendency to higher levels of PCS with a number of markers of brain insult, including loss of consciousness (LOC), computed tomography (CT), or MRI abnormality, hospitalization, motor vehicle accidents, and injuries to other body regions.

Barlow et al. (2010) compared PCS in a group with mTBI (670 children less than 18 years old, GCS 13–15) with another group with extracranial injuries (197 children) and followed children monthly until symptom resolution. These researchers found that 3 months postinjury, 11% of children with mTBI were symptomatic compared with 0.5% of the extracranial injury group. This percentage was significantly lower than the incidence of symptoms at 1 month (58.5% and 38.5%, respectively). The most common symptoms that had increased following injury, compared to the preinjury level, were fatigue, emotionality, irritability, and headache. The study also demonstrated that the older the child and the more severe the mTBI, the more likely the child was to remain symptomatic over time. Of children with mTBI, 15 children remained symptomatic longer than 12 months, and 9 children reported chronic post-traumatic headaches. However, it should be noted that in assessing preinjury symptoms, 1% of the mTBI group and 3% of the extracranial injuries group reported pre-injury headaches. Therefore, it may be concluded from this study that the incidence of persistent somatic symptoms 12 months after injury is similar to baseline. Obviously there are many confounding variables in such studies, including selection bias (only included children presenting to a tertiary referral hospital), preexisting family dysfunction, recall bias in retrospective preinjury symptom assessment, and the absence of a noninjury control group.

Given that different studies use different patient populations (e.g., hospital inpatients, emergency department presentations, sports clinics), different definitions of mTBI (e.g., GCS, LOC duration, posttraumatic amnesia [PTA]), different methods of assessing symptoms (e.g., parent vs. child report, telephone vs. personal interview, different symptom checklists and scales), it is not surprising that there is a lack of consistency in published incidence, severity, and duration of somatic symptoms in pediatric mTBI. Hooper et al. (2004) examined children with all severities of head injury, and compared 272 children managed in the emergency department (ED) and 409 children admitted to the hospital. Whereas there were more children with severe and moderate head injury in the inpatient group, 98.5% of children in the ED group had a mild head injury. Assessing symptoms following injury in the ED group, the authors demonstrated that headache was the main complaint in 20%, 16.4%, and 6.7% of children with mTBI at 1, 4, and 10 months, respectively. Not surprisingly, the incidence of symptoms was significantly greater in the children with moderate and severe injuries. However, the absence of a control group and no preinjury symptom data significantly limit these results.

It should be apparent to the reader that studies assessing somatic complaints following mTBI have utilized symptom scales—that is, a subjective patient-parent-reported symptom—rather than an objective measure of the somatic pathology. If somatic signs could be measured, then limitations of symptom reporting would be obviated. Of all the somatic symptoms, one has been studied objectively: balance. The interested reader is referred to Grubenhoff and Provance (Chapter 10, this volume) for more details on balance testing.

The persistent grouping of all PCS symptoms under a single umbrella term restricts detailed research into individual somatic symptoms. Although there is ongoing research into cognitive symptoms using a broad range of tools (e.g., computerized neuropsychological tests, functional MRI, and diffusion tensor imaging), the physiological mechanism for true somatic symptoms following mTBI still eludes us. Methods to distinguish true somatic symptoms from cognitive and emotional symptoms are still required.

Intracranial Hemorrhage

One of the complexities involved in reviewing the literature on mTBI is the broad definition of *mild* TBI, which includes everything from the most trivial bump to the head, to concussion, to intracranial hemorrhage. Accepting that GCS 13–15 is the all-inclusive diagnostic criterion for mTBI, the issue arises as to whether there are differences in outcome in the more complex, or complicated, forms of mTBI. As such, mTBI is often divided into uncomplicated and complicated, with the CT imaging of the brain being normal in the former and abnormal in the latter. Clinicians managing children with mTBI in the acute stages direct much of their efforts toward determining which children may have an intracranial hemorrhage, as this may indicate a risk of significant complications.

Intracranial hemorrhage is classified by the anatomical location of the blood: namely, its relationship to the meningeal layers, the brain tissue itself (parenchyma), and the cerebral ventricles. The outermost layer of the meninges is the dura mater; hemorrhage between the dura and the skull is known as an epidural hematoma (EDH). These are commonly, but not always, associated with a skull fracture, and although many EDHs may be subclinical, substantial EDH may result in rapid deterioration in neurological function and subsequent death if not surgically treated urgently (see Figure 6.1). A clinical latent period may occur before deterioration (the "talk and die" scenario); this is the group of children who need to be identified before deterioration. Schutzman, Barnes, Mantello, and Scott (1993) reviewed a series of children with EDH and found that only 40 of 53 children with EDH were diagnosed with EDH within 24 hours of injury, and two infants were asymptomatic at presentation. Thirty-eight percent of children with EDH were alert with normal vital signs and normal neurological examination at presentation, and 40% of children with EDH had an acute neurological deterioration within 24 hours in all but one child.

The next layer of the meninges is the arachnoid mater. Hemorrhage occurring between the dura and the arachnoid is known as *subdural hematoma* (SDH). Although SDH is much more common in children with severe head injury, there is a small subset of children with mTBI who develop SDH, and as with EDH, clinical detection before deterioration is critical in the early management.

The next layer of meninges is the pia mater. Hemorrhage occurring between the arachnoid and the pia is known as *subarachnoid hemorrhage* (SAH). Although traumatic SAH rarely exerts mass effect and compression of vital brain structures, as do SDH and EDH, SAH is usually a marker that the brain has sustained a significant impact force. Occasionally, traumatic SAH may induce cerebral vasospasm, which can result in stroke.

Below the pia mater is the brain itself, or the parenchyma. Bleeding within the parenchyma may be due to small contusions (bruising in the brain secondary to

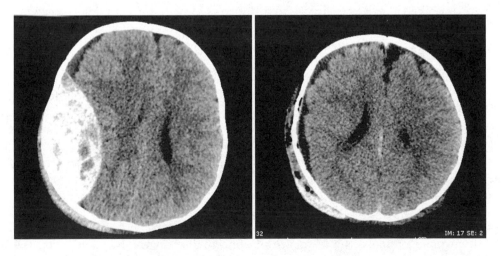

FIGURE 6.1. Left: Large acute epidural hematoma causing significant mass effect on the underlying brain. Right: Following surgical evacuation of the epidural blood clot, the brain has reexpanded with resolution of the mass effect. Image courtesy of Dr. Greg Fitt.

leakage of blood from small blood vessels) or to large hematomas. Contusions are often classified as *coup* or *contrecoup*. Coup contusions occur directly beneath the area of impact, whereas contrecoup contusions are located in areas remote from the site of impact, usually within the frontal or temporal lobes. Small contusions are often asymptomatic, although they can be associated with an increased risk of seizures. Large intracerebral hematomas are rarely associated with mTBI, but when they do develop, they exert mass effect on the brain that may require surgical evacuation.

The deepest layer of the intracranial structures, the ependymal layer, lines the cerebral ventricles. Bleeding into the ventricles (intraventricular hemorrhage, IVH) may cause mass effect, especially by obstruction of the cerebrospinal fluid (CSF) pathways and subsequent hydrocephalus. This condition may occur acutely or develop slowly over time.

This brief overview of intracranial hemorrhage is somewhat simplistic. Although each type of hemorrhage may occur in isolation, it is also common to see multiple types of hemorrhage within the same individual. For example, many children with a cerebral contusion may also have an SAH. Many with an intracerebral hematoma may also have SDH and IVH. The more severe the injury, the more likely that one will identify bleeding within multiple layers. To determine the incidence of each type of hemorrhage within the pediatric mTBI population is difficult because of study methodologies and definitions. Of 695 children admitted with mTBI (GCS 14–15) who underwent CT scan, Stein and Doolin (1995) found contusion in 4%, SAH/IVH in 4%, parenchymal hematoma in 1%, SDH in 4%, and EDH in 2%. In a population-based study of children younger than 15 years transported by emergency medical services (EMS) in Los Angeles County (Wang, Griffith, Sterling, McComb, & Levy, 2000), 209 children out of 8,488 had a GCS of 13 or 14. Of these, there were 157 children for whom complete information was available; 19.1% had intracranial hemorrhage, and 3.2% or five children required surgery for evacuation of intracranial hematoma (SDH in one, EDH in three, and combined SAH/SDH/EDH/contusion in one).

As described above, the clinical importance of identifying a child with an expanding intracranial hemorrhage cannot be overemphasized. Given that CT is the imaging modality of choice in identifying intracranial hemorrhage, the key question that needs to be addressed is, *which children with mTBI require a CT brain?*

In a study of 42,412 children with mTBI (GCS 14–15) presenting to EDs, Kuppermann et al. (2009) obtained CT scans on 14,969 (35.3%) children and found that 376 children had clinically important TBI (e.g., hemorrhage identified on CT). Based on their analysis of the data, they suggested algorithms for CT in children with mTBI. Included in the variables in their algorithm are GCS, mental status, signs of skull base fracture, LOC, vomiting, mechanism of injury, and severe headache. A review of the patient data using their algorithm demonstrated that all neurosurgically treated patients would have been identified with their algorithm. Similarly, Dunning et al. (2006) prospectively studied all children less than 16 years presenting to EDs with head injury. Of 22,772 children enrolled in the study, 97.9% had mTBI (GCS 13–15). Of all enrolled patients, the incidence of abnormality on CT included EDH 0.4%, SDH 0.2%, cerebral contusion 0.4%, and SAH 0.1%, although these figures include children with all categories of head injury severity. The authors used the children's head injury algorithm for the prediction of important clinical events, and found a

98% sensitivity and 87% specificity for the prediction of clinically important head injury, requiring a CT scan rate of 14%.

The National Emergency X-Radiography Utilization Study II (NEXUS II) included 1,666 children. Oman et al. (2006) analyzed the NEXUS II variables and determined that significant intracranial injury was extremely unlikely in children who do not exhibit any of the following: evidence of significant skull fracture, altered level of consciousness, neurological deficit, persistent vomiting, presence of scalp hematoma, abnormal behavior, or coagulopathy. However, using these criteria, the authors note that two injuries would have been missed in the 1,666 children, but none of the missed injuries resulted in delayed clinical deterioration. There is a number of other published guidelines for use of CT in mTBI, but many of these papers excluded children from their study, such as the Canadian CT Head Rule (Stiell et al., 2001).

Posttraumatic Headache and Migraine

Posttraumatic headache (PTH) is one of the most common symptoms following head injury. Headache is also common in the general pediatric population. When a child complains of headache following mTBI, the following questions arise:

- Did the brain injury cause the headache?
- Was the patient symptomatic of headaches prior to the mTBI?
- Is the headache a marker of significant cerebral injury or hemorrhage?
- Is this migraine?
- Did the brain injury cause migraine or expose the migraine in an at-risk individual?
- Is there another cause for the headache, such as cervical spine injury?

The International Headache Society classifies headache after head and neck trauma into subtypes, according to criteria such as acute (< 3 months)/chronic (> 3 months), injury severity (based on GCS and duration of LOC), onset within 7 days of head trauma, and underlying structural abnormality.

In a study of children ages 6 months to 14 years, Casey, Ludwig, and McCormick (1986) identified 340 children with minor head injury (no LOC, GCS 15) and found that 7% of children complained of headache 1 month after injury; however, no control group was used. Control groups are required to ascertain the population incidence of headache over the same period, and the incidence of headache in those with extracranial injuries (demonstrating a response to injury per se, not specific to brain injury). Callaghan and Abu-Arafeh (2001) assessed children presenting to a headache clinic over a 4-year period and identified 21 children with a history of head trauma and 507 children with no history of head trauma. Of the 21 children with PTH, 5 had migraine, 6 had episodic tension headache, 7 had chronic tension headache, and 3 had mixed headaches. They found that none of the children with PTH had a history of headache prior to the injury. As described in the section on PCS, reported PTH incidence varies greatly, depending upon the definitions used, population studied, time at assessment, method of symptom assessment, and age of the children.

Table 6.1 shows a selection of four published studies with headache incidence ranging from 8.4 to 71.6%. It is apparent that the incidence is greatest acutely and

TABLE 6.1. A Selection of Studies Demonstrating the Wide Range of Incidence Figures for Posttraumatic Headache in Children

Reference	Population studied	Headache incidence	Control group incidence	Time after injury of assessment
Rutherford, Merrett, & McDonald (1979)	1-year follow-up of 108 children from earlier study of admitted children	8.4%	—	1 year
Nacajauskaite, Endziniene, Jureniene, & Schrader (2006)	102 (of 301) children admitted with brain concussion	61%	55%	Mean = 27 months All > 1year
Hooper et al. (2004)	272 children presenting to emergency department (98.5% mTBI)	20% 16.4% 6.7%	—	1 month 4 months 10 months
Blinman, Houseknecht, Snyder, Wiebe, & Nance (2009)	116 children admitted with mTBI	71.6% 31.8%	—	During admission 2–3 weeks

diminishes over time. However, control groups are required to compare this rate to the population prevalence of headache. Furthermore, these incidence figures do not provide any information regarding the incidence of preinjury headaches in these children. Only a population-based, longitudinal, prospective study with baseline symptom evaluation will provide accurate information on the incidence and natural history of PTH.

Migraine is a common condition characterized by recurrent unilateral or bilateral throbbing headache that may last for days and is frequently associated with nausea, vomiting, photophobia or phonophobia, and is exacerbated by physical exertion. A number of theories exists as to the cause of migraine, including the vasogenic theory (vascular dysregulation and rebound vasodilatation), the neurogenic theory (neuronal dysfunction causes the vascular changes), and cortical spreading depression (cortical excitatory phase followed by a phase of depressed cortical activity). The clinical features of migraine are due to recurrent activation of the trigeminocervical pain system, but no single mechanism accounts for migraine in all sufferers. A genetic cause for migraine has been identified in some families, and it is most likely that migraine is the manifestation of a diverse, heterogeneous group of abnormalities (Cutrer, 2010).

In the review by Haas and Lourie (1988) it was demonstrated that the clinical symptoms of posttraumatic migraine are identical to classical migraine, except that they follow a head injury. Trauma-triggered migraine usually appears 1–10 minutes following the head trauma, but may not appear for up to 4 hours following injury. The clinical features may include visual disturbance, hemiparesis, seizures, and transient global amnesia. The majority of attacks of posttraumatic migraine resolve within 24 hours, often within a few hours. Haas and Lourie also note that 70% of children with posttraumatic migraine have a first-degree relative with migraine. It was suggested that trauma triggers the clinical presentation of migraine in children who were already predisposed to developing migraine.

Although PTH is common, posttraumatic migraine in children is rarer, but the literature does not provide reliable incidence figures. Children with posttraumatic migraine present to a wide spectrum of clinicians, from general practitioners to pediatric neurologists. Obtaining both the numerator and denominator for incidence figures is fraught with difficulty. However, it is apparent that management of posttraumatic migraine is identical to that of classic nontraumatic migraine.

Posttraumatic Seizures

The association between seizures and severe head injury is well defined (Jennett, 1973). In relation to mTBI, however, there is less clarity because of problems with definitions; the frequency of trivial, underreported injuries; confounding risk factors; and variable times of onset. Definitions of mTBI and posttraumatic seizures (PTSs) vary within the literature. PTSs are broadly classified as early or late. Early PTS occurs within 1 week of brain injury, and late PTS occurs after the first week. Subclassification of early PTS includes terms such as *impact seizures, concussive seizures*, and *immediate seizures*. The use of the term *impact seizure* is useful; it refers to those seizures that occur within 2 seconds of concussion, have a typical brief tonic phase, followed by bilateral myoclonic jerking with asymmetrical posturing, and resolve within 150 seconds. Impact seizures are nonepileptic phenomenon and have a universally good outcome (McCrory, Bladin, & Berkovic, 1997). Different authors define concussive and immediate seizures differently, varying between seconds and 24 hours after impact (see Table 6.2). For the purposes of this chapter, the classification is restricted to the terms *early* and *late seizures*, unless otherwise specified. It must also be noted that there is a difference between the terms *seizure* and *epilepsy*. Epilepsy is defined as two or more unprovoked seizures. Thus, a single, early PTS does not imply that the child has epilepsy.

Annegers and Coan (2000) reviewed the records of the Rochester Epidemiology Project at the Mayo Clinic, including inpatients, outpatients, and ED presentations, between 1935 and 1984 and found 5,984 patients with TBI, ages 0–85 years. They classified mTBI as patients with no fractures and LOC or PTA less than 30 minutes. For those with mTBI, the standardized incidence ratio for early seizures was 3.1 in the first year after injury and 2.1 for the next 4 years. None of the patients with mTBI subsequently developed late seizures. Within the group of children under 5 years of age, the presence of a linear skull fracture was associated with a slightly higher seizure rate (relative risk 1.5). Although this paper did not provide an overall breakdown by age groups, given the fact that the only subgroup analysis reported was for children under 5 years, an assumption could be made that the results for children over 5 years did not differ from the adult group, but there is no other evidence to support this. In an earlier publication by the same group, using the same study population, they report the age breakdown as 0–4 years (542 patients), 5–14 years (1,184 patients), and 15+ years (2,815 patients) (Annegers, Hauser, Coan, & Rocca, 1998). Thus, children comprise approximately one-third of their study population. It is worth noting that whereas the standardized incidence ratio for mTBI and PTS is only 1.5, the increased risk does persist for many years following brain injury.

TABLE 6.2. Differences in Definitions and Populations Studied in Publications Reviewing Seizures in mTBI in Children

Reference	Age group	mTBI definition	Seizure types definition	Population	Number of children	Early PTS	Late PTS	Comments
Annegers & Coan (2000)	Children and adults	No fractures; LOC < 30 minutes; PTA < 30 minutes	Early ≤ 1 week	Rochester Epidemiology Project—inpatients, outpatients, ED visits	mTBI not stated (5,984 TBI in total—all ages)	$n = 36$ SIR = 1.5 1st year = 3.1 Year 1–4 = 2.1 Year 5–9 = 0.9 Year 10+ = 1.1	$n = 0$	In children < 5 years, slight increased risk with linear fracture.
Emmanuelson & Uvebrant (2009)	0–18 years	GCS 13–15	Immediate < 24 hours; early ≤ 1 week	210 with TBI 1987–1991	109 available (28 mTBI)	Not stated	2	
Hahn et al. (1988)	0–16 years	GCS 13–15	Early ≤ 1 week	Admitted 1980–1986	937 total (791 mTBI)	47/791 (5.9%)	—	
Chiaretti et al. (2000)	Mean age 6.68 (± 4.46) years	GCS 13–15	Immediate < 24 hours; early ≤ 1 week	Admitted 1992–1998	125 total (48 mTBI)	1/48	—	
Holmes et al. (2004)	< 18 years	Minor TBI = GCS 15	Immediate = onset before arrival in ED	Presenting to ED 1998–2001	2,043 total (mTBI not stated)	Immediate PTS 63	—	
Dias et al. (1999)	0–18 years	GCS 13–15 at presentation	Immediate < 24 hours	Children with mTBI and PTS presenting to ED 1992–1996	71 children mTBI	Immediate PTS 71	—	mTBI = GCS on presentation 13–15. May have been lower at the scene.
Christensen et al. (2009)	Children and young adults	GCS 14–15 (ACRM definition)	N/S	All children born 1977–2002	1,605,216	—	1,017	Increased risk of epilepsy with age, family history of epilepsy.

Note. ED, Emergency Department; GCS, Glasgow Coma Scale score; LOC, loss of consciousness; PTA, posttraumatic amnesia; PTS, posttraumatic seizure; SIR, standardized incidence ratio.

Emmanuelson and Uvebrant (2009) reviewed survivors from an earlier TBI study with a minimum 10-year follow-up. All patients had been under 18 years at the time of injury. Of the original 210 children, 109 were available for review. Of the 109, 28 had mTBI, and of these, two developed posttraumatic epilepsy, which they defined as at least two unprovoked seizures after the first week following TBI and up to 10 years postinjury. The authors did not state whether or not these children had early PTS before the onset of epilepsy.

Hahn, Fuchs, Flannery, Barthel, and McLone (1988) reviewed 937 children admitted with head injury, of which 791 were classified as mTBI. Forty-seven (5.9%) of the children with mTBI developed early seizures. For children with severe and moderate TBI, the early seizure rates were 35.3% and 26.9%, respectively. Although they reported risk factors for seizures, such as diffuse cerebral edema and acute SDH, data were not presented to differentiate which children with mTBI or more severe TBI had these complicating risk factors. In a small retrospective study of 125 hospitalized children, Chiaretti et al. (2000) identified 1 of 48 children with mTBI who developed an early seizure (compared to 22.7% with severe TBI and 12% with moderate TBI).

In an attempt to identify which children with early PTS require admission to hospital, Holmes, Palchak, Conklin, and Kuppermann (2004) examined 2,043 children with TBI, of which 63 (3.1%) had seizures that they classified as immediate (occurring before presentation to the ED). They did not provide the absolute numbers with mTBI, but did state that the median GCS was 15 (interquartile range 11–15). Those children with PTS and a normal brain CT scan were followed for 1 week, and none had further seizures or neurological decline. Similarly, Dias, Carnevale, and Li (1999) sought to clarify necessity for hospitalization by retrospectively reviewing the records of 71 children with mTBI and immediate PTS (they defined *immediate* as occurring within 24 hours of injury). Nearly 50% of these children had the seizure within 5 minutes of the impact, which suggests that many of these may in fact have been impact seizures. None of the children with PTS suffered any further seizures or other complications during the hospitalization.

In the landmark study on the risk of epilepsy after TBI, Christensen et al. (2009) identified 1,605,216 children born in Denmark between 1977 and 2002. Because inpatient and outpatient treatments in Denmark are recorded on a national register, they reviewed the records of 78,572 people who had had at least one TBI and 17,470 people who developed epilepsy. They identified 1,017 people with epilepsy who had had a preceding brain injury and calculated the relative risk of 2.2 for epilepsy after mTBI. This risk was highest in the first few years after injury, but remained high for more than 10 years postinjury. This risk increased with age and was highest among those older than 15 years at the time of injury. The relative risk (RR) was also increased in those with a family history of epilepsy. Children with no family history of epilepsy but a history of mTBI had an RR of 2.24; a family history of epilepsy and no history of mTBI had an RR of 3.37; and a family history of epilepsy and a history of mTBI had an RR of 5.75.

It is apparent from these studies that the inconsistent definitions make comparison between studies difficult. Many impact seizures may be labeled as early PTS, but as described above, they represent a different entity. The published incidence of early PTS in children with mTBI varies between 2 and 5%, but many variables confound these figures. Most published studies select the cases from hospital data, and as such, do not include the large number of children with mTBI who never present to hospital. Many benign early PTSs may be unwitnessed, and not all episodes witnessed by the lay public are true seizures. The two studies assessing need for hospitalization in children with early PTS (Dias et al., 1999; Holmes et al., 2004) raise the interesting point that most early PTSs do not portend significant risk of late sequelae, but it must be stressed that many of those children had impact seizures, not early PTS. The excellent population-based study from the Danish group demonstrates the increased risk of developing epilepsy over many years following mTBI, and this risk is significantly increased if there is also a family history of epilepsy.

Cerebral Edema and "Talk and Die"

Children with brain injury are at risk of developing cerebral edema. Onset of cerebral edema may be immediate following impact or may be delayed by some hours. There is much debate about the risk factors for developing malignant cerebral edema and whether incomplete recovery from one concussion predisposes the child to cerebral edema following a second concussion; the so-called *second-impact syndrome*. The literature supporting this notion is not conclusive (Cantu, 1998; McCrory, 2001). There is no doubt that some children develop malignant cerebral edema following mTBI. The doubt exists as to whether an earlier concussive injury is a requisite criterion for this condition, or is the second impact, on its own, significant enough to result in cerebral edema?

Bruce et al. (1981) reviewed 214 children ages 6–18 years admitted with head injury who underwent CT brain. Sixty-three of these children demonstrated CT evidence of diffuse cerebral swelling. Their classification system utilized the GCS, but moderate and mild brain injury (GCS > 8) were grouped together in the analysis. However, 23 children (37% of the group) displayed a clear lucid interval following the trauma, in which the children had "a period of talking and complete consciousness for minutes to hours after injury," before subsequent deterioration from cerebral swelling (p. 174). One can infer from this that a significant proportion of these children would have been classified as having mTBI at the scene, prior to the subsequent deterioration. The authors identified that this group of children with a lucid interval all made a good recovery, compared to a significant number of children without a lucid interval who had poor clinical outcomes (death or disability). It remains a point of contention as to the pathophysiology in these children:

> Were the CT findings secondary to vascular engorgement and hyperaemia (increased cerebral blood flow), or was there true cerebral edema (increased cerebral interstitial fluid)?
> Were the children with and without lucid intervals displaying similar or different pathological processes?

The pathophysiology of altered cerebral autoregulation in mTBI has been difficult to investigate because of the invasive nature of definitive tests. Nevertheless, Vavilala et al. (2004) assessed cerebral autoregulation in 36 children with TBI, of which one-third had mTBI. Although some of the measurements performed were indirect measures (e.g., transcranial doppler), they did find that cerebral autoregulation may be impaired following mild, moderate, and severe pediatric TBI; hyperaemia was associated with impaired cerebral autoregulation; and impaired cerebral autoregulation was associated with poor outcome. Similar findings in adults have also been reported (Junger et al., 1997). Metabolic changes reported in children following mTBI include alterations in levels of glucose, potassium, and sodium (Lazar, Erez, Gutermacher, & Katz, 1997).

In cases of purported second-impact syndrome, Cantu proposes loss of autoregulation and vascular engorgement as the underlying pathophysiological mechanism. He reviewed five cases that he suggested illustrate the second-impact syndrome (Cantu, 1998). The five cases all involved boxers, ages 17–24 years. In one case, there was no CT or postmortem performed, so it is uncertain whether death was secondary to intracranial hemorrhage or edema. In two of the cases, the boxers sustained multiple significant blows to the head, resulting in multiple 8 counts, before the onset of cerebral edema and death. It is highly probable that any of the blows that triggered an 8-count interlude was of sufficient force to induce acute malignant cerebral edema, without needing to invoke the concept of second-impact syndrome. Finally, the other two cases both demonstrated brain swelling and subdural hematoma on CT. Although the report suggests that the final impact to the head was "minor," this is highly improbable given that the CT demonstrated traumatic intracranial hemorrhage in addition to the cerebral edema.

Similarly, Cantu and Gean (2010) reviewed the cases of 10 teenagers playing American football (ages 13–19 years) who all developed small SDH and cerebral edema. In nearly every case, a significant impact to the head preceded the injury, and the outcome was universally poor, with five dead and the other five left with severe neurological deficit. Once again, it should be stated that although Cantu and Gean proposed that these cases are examples of second-impact syndrome, it is more likely that the magnitude of force required to produce the SDH was sufficient to induce cerebral edema, independent of any earlier concussive injury. Cantu and Gean's case 6 was described in the court case *Melka v. OAW* (Stevens, 2009), in which the court found that the patient had not actually sustained an initial concussion, and that the injury was due solely to a single, significant force to the head. That is, the court ruled that this case was not one of second-impact syndrome.

Whether one considers cerebral edema in childhood the same as diffuse cerebral swelling, and whether one considers it a primary injury or dependent upon a second impact, it is important to know what the outcome is in children with mTBI, and if this outcome differs from that of adults. Lang, Teasdale, Macpherson, and Lawrence (1994) studied 118 patients with diffuse brain swelling. The study group comprised 59 adults and 59 children ages less than 15 years. The initial GCS scores were not reported, although the authors did report that eight patients did not lose consciousness. Therefore it is not possible to ascertain what proportion of the children had mTBI rather than more severe TBI. Furthermore, some patients had varying degrees of intracranial hemorrhage in addition to diffuse brain swelling, but the overall outcome figures demonstrated that 78% of children made a good or moderate recovery compared with 41% of adults.

Delayed-onset brain swelling is one potential cause of the fatal outcome in the child who is lucid following the brain injury, but subsequently deteriorates and dies— the so-called "talk-and-die" phenomenon. A child presenting for medical attention during the lucid period will frequently have a GCS of 15, and thus presents as an mTBI. But the child's brain may be brewing a sinister pathological process that results in death. This is the complication most feared by all practitioners treating children with mTBI. Although the most common and well-recognized cause of the talk-and-die phenomenon is an expanding intracranial hematoma, there are several other causes, including delayed cerebral edema and seizures.

In the CT era, the classic paper by Snoek, Minderhoud, and Wilmink (1984) reviewed reports of 967 children with head injury and identified 40 children who had no immediate LOC and two children with a very brief LOC (less than 5 minutes), followed by a lucid interval. These 42 children all developed delayed deterioration, and three died. The authors grouped the children into convulsive and nonconvulsive cases, then subclassified the latter group into rapid and slow deterioration. There was one death in the rapid deterioration group, that of an 8-year-old boy who fell from a slowly moving cart, and immediately following the head injury, stood up, walked to his father, and complained of a headache. He soon deteriorated and rapidly died. In the slow deterioration group, there were two deaths. The first was a 13-year-old girl who fell off her bicycle, with no LOC; 3 hours later she was neurologically intact but complained of nausea; she was discharged home but returned several hours later with hemiparesis and drowsiness; CT of her brain demonstrated compression of the ventricles with hemispheric shift, but no hemorrhage identified; the child died the next day. The second case was a 9-year-old boy who fell off a skateboard without LOC, and continued to skateboard before watching TV for several hours and going to bed. The next morning he complained of headache before he acutely deteriorated with loss of consciousness; he underwent bilateral burr holes that demonstrated swollen brain without hematoma; he died 15 hours following admission.

Humphreys, Hendrick, and Hoffman (1990) presented four cases of children who expired via the talk-and-die phenomenon, but three presented with moderate head injury, and only one with mTBI. The latter case was a 14-year-old boy who, while sleepwalking, fell 3 meters, hit his head on the piano, and lost consciousness. At presentation his GCS was 13; brain CT demonstrated a small intracerebral hematoma. He remained stable for 24 hours, then developed apneic episodes requiring intubation and intracranial pressure (ICP) monitoring; he developed malignant elevation of ICP and died 72 hours post admission. Postmortem examination demonstrated extensive intracerebral contusions and cerebral herniation.

In a review of 211 patients who talked before deterioration into coma, Lobato et al. (1991) examined both adults and children. Although the authors did not specifically analyze the childhood population separately, they did note that of the 41 patients without mass lesion on brain CT, "the remaining patients, most of whom were children, showed variable degrees of basal cistern collapse indicative of generalized brain swelling in their admission or follow-up CT," and that these findings support the conclusion "that diffuse brain swelling is the most frequent cause of secondary deterioration in children showing a lucid period after a head injury" (p. 259).

Examining this topic from a different perspective, Graham et al. (1989) reviewed all full necropsies performed between 1968 and 1982 of patients who had been managed by a neurosurgical department. Of the 635 fatal nonmissile head injuries, 87 were children ages 2–15 years, and the causes of death in these children included intracranial hemorrhage and cerebral edema. Fourteen children (16%) had talked after the head injury. Three children who talked after the injury died from "idiopathic brain swelling," and one of the children who "talked and died" was found to have diffuse axonal injury.

The records of children ages 15 years and younger, admitted to hospital with a GCS of 14 or 15, were reviewed by Keskil, Baykaner, Ceviker, and Kaymaz (1995). Of the 257 children admitted with mTBI, 9 died. The most common cause of death was intracranial hematoma, but the authors did describe the case of one child, a 6-year-old boy, who presented with a GCS of 15 and was symptom free, with normal neurological examination and normal skull X-ray. On the second day post mTBI, he suddenly deteriorated and subsequently died. His CT scan demonstrated diffuse cerebral edema.

Of all children with mTBI, malignant cerebral edema affects only a very small proportion of such children but has the most devastating outcomes. The critical questions, are how can we prevent the onset of edema, or can we predict which children are at risk of developing edema and treat them aggressively to reduce the morbidity and mortality? To date, we do not have the answers to these questions. It is likely that a genetic susceptibility to altered cerebral autoregulation is the underlying mechanism in most of these cases. However, the rarity of this condition leads to a significant barrier to effective clinical and genetic research to identify the exact cause. In the interim, it is inherent upon all those involved in the treatment of children following mTBI to be aware of the potential for delayed deterioration, and to have at their disposal the appropriate facilities and personnel to manage this condition in a timely fashion.

Stroke and Dural Sinus Thrombosis

Stroke and dural sinus thrombosis are rare complications of mTBI in children, but appreciation of the clinical condition and outcome is important for all those managing children with mTBI. Posttraumatic stroke may be caused by arterial dissection or by injury to deep, perforating cerebral vessels. Dharker, Mittal, and Bhargava (1993) reported on 23 children, ages 8 months to 6 years, who presented with unilateral weakness following mTBI. Ten children also demonstrated facial weakness, six had aphasia, and three had generalized seizures. CT imaging demonstrated basal ganglia infarction; 22 of 23 children had complete clinical recovery by 4 months. The proposed mechanism of infarction is the acute angle of the perforating branches of the middle cerebral artery in very young children. Similarly, Shaffer, Rich, Pohl, and Ganesan (2003) reported on five children ages 1–6 years with acute hemiparesis following mTBI. On MRI, all had striatocapsular infarction. Three children made complete neurological recovery, and two showed mild or minimal residual neurological signs.

Although Dharker et al. (1993) and Shaffer et al. (2003) demonstrated good clinical outcome in most young children with post mTBI striatocapsular stroke, Kieslich, Fiedler, Heller, Kreuz, and Jacobi (2002) reported on eight children, ages 3–7 years, with symptom onset between 15 minutes and 72 hours post mTBI. All developed hemiparesis secondary to perforating artery infarction. Two children had prothrombotic risk factors. Unlike the other cases, only one child in this report made a com plete recovery; four children had moderate residual disability, and two children had severe disability.

Thus, the clinical presentation of perforating artery stroke following mTBI is restricted to children 7 years and under, with clinical onset between a few minutes and a few days postinjury. Most children present with hemiparesis, but the clinical outcome is highly variable, from complete recovery to severe disability.

Stroke secondary to arterial dissection also occurs after mTBI. In a review of arterial dissection and stroke by Fullerton, Johnston, and Smith (2001), trivial trauma (GCS 15) preceded the arterial dissection in 33% of 118 patients, and the time from trauma to onset of neurological signs ranged from immediate to weeks, with most occurring within 1 week of injury. The most common presentation was hemiparesis, occurring in 97% with anterior circulation dissection, and in 57% with posterior circulation dissection. The mortality rate from arterial dissection was 33% for anterior circulation dissection, and 2% for posterior circulation dissection. Unlike adults with arterial dissection, anterior circulation dissection was more commonly intracranial than extracranial in children.

Unlike arterial injury, venous sinus thrombosis commonly presents with non-specific symptoms such as headache, vomiting, irritability, and impaired balance. These symptoms are common after uncomplicated mTBI, and diagnosis of venous sinus thrombosis requires a high index of suspicion. Five children with posttraumatic sigmoid sinus thrombosis were reported by Taha, Crone, Berger, Becket, and Prenger (1993). The children's age range was 1–7 years, and four of the five had a mild head injury. All the children had delayed onset of neurological symptoms, or a worsening of existing symptoms, 1–4 days following the injury. Diagnosis was made on CT and/ or MRI brain. In the four children with mTBI and sigmoid sinus thrombosis, symptoms improved within 1 week and resolved completely between 2 and 14 weeks following injury. Case reports of right sigmoid sinus thrombosis occurring after mTBI in children ages 4 and 9 years both demonstrated complete neurological recovery (Lakhkar, Singh, & Agrawal, 2010; Yuen, Gan, Seow, & Tan, 2005). Similarly, an 11-year-old boy with protracted vomiting after mTBI was found to have thrombosis of the left transverse and sigmoid sinus, and recovered completely 10 days after the injury (Luerssen, 1991).

Cranial Nerve Injury

The cranial nerves (CN) are peripheral nerves that originate in the brain and brain-stem, rather than in the spinal cord. They are predominantly distributed to the head and neck. In their course from the brain to their extracranial destination, cranial nerves travel a variable distance through the basal cisterns (CSF-filled subarach-noid spaces), and then exit the skull through bony formena. In the context of head injury, the cranial nerves can be damaged within the basal cisterns or within the bony foramena. Mechanisms such as raised ICP and skull base fractures account for many cases of CN injury, but not all. Although CN injury is more common in severe head injury, it is well recognized in mTBI. In adults with mTBI, injuries to all 12 cranial nerves have been described, with CN I (olfactory nerve) and CN VII (facial nerve) being the most commonly injured (Coello, Canals, Gonzalez, & Martin, 2010). Many cases of cranial neuropathy are mild and recover spontaneously, so the true incidence of cranial neuropathy in pediatric mTBI is unknown. Unless the treating doctor specifically looks for symptoms and signs of cranial neuropathy, many will be missed.

Anosmia (the loss of the sense of smell due to injury to CN I) is commonly under-diagnosed in head injury, with many patients unaware of a problem. If not specifically tested for, it will be missed. In a study examining 20 children with mTBI and 20 with severe TBI, Roberts and Simcox (1996) found that 9 (45%) of the children with mTBI demonstrated impaired sense of smell on formal testing, compared with 15 (75%) of the children with severe TBI. Sandford et al. (2006) examined a highly selected cohort of 36 children with varying degrees of head injury, and found that 3 children were hyposmic (failure to correctly identify all odors); however, only one of the 3 children had an mTBI (which the researchers defined as GCS 14–15). Examining 741 children with head injury (mild, moderate, and severe), Jacobi, Ritz, and Emrich (1986) found that 3.2% of children had temporary anosmia, and 1.2% had permanent anosmia. Many studies on olfaction and mTBI suffer from similar methodological problems, such as selection bias, inconsistency in definitions, and mode of olfactory assessment.

Although not a CN injury, internuclear ophthalmoplegia (INO) shares some clinical features with a CN injury to the eye. The nuclei of cranial nerves III, IV, and VI are connected with each other and with the parapontine reticular formation (the lateral gaze center in the pons) via the medial longitudinal fasciculus (MLF). Injury to the MLF causes inability to adduct the ipsilateral eye, and nystagmus with abduction of the contralateral eye, known as INO. Case reports of children with bilateral INO following mTBI have demonstrated an abnormal signal within the pons on MRI and complete remission of symptoms over 2–12 months. (Mueller, Koch, & Toifl, 1993; Muthukumar, Veerarajkumar, & Madeswaran, 2001). These cases highlight the fact that any cerebral structure may sustain injury, even with mTBI, and careful clinical assessment is warranted. Although the true incidence of CN injury in pediatric mTBI is unknown, there is no doubt that it is commonly underreported and worthy of further investigation.

Transient Cortical Blindness

The development of acute blindness following mTBI is extremely distressing to the child and parents. Although very uncommon, transient cortical blindness is well described in children following mTBI, and is usually followed by complete recovery. Cortical blindness is defined as blindness with retention of the pupillary light reflex. Yamamoto and Bart (1988) presented seven cases of children with transient blindness following mTBI. All seven children were between 3 and 6 years of age, and all had mTBI with no LOC. The pupillary response was normal in six children, with one child demonstrating fixed dilated pupils. The duration of blindness lasted between 1 and 6 hours, and all seven children made a complete recovery with normal vision. Similar findings were reported by Snoek et al. (1984): Two children presented with acute blindness within the first hour after injury, and the duration of blindness was less than 1 hour. In their review of the literature up to 1988, Yamamoto and Bart (1988) identified 39 additional cases and suggested that the following factors are associated with a better neurological outcome:

- Pediatric age group
- Mild head trauma
- LOC usually does not occur but is brief if it does
- Mild nausea and vomiting may be present
- Onset of blindness occurs within several hours of head injury
- Optokinetic nystagmus is absent
- Duration of blindness is less than 24 hours
- Agitation and restlessness are common presenting features
- Absence of skull fracture or visible cerebral injury on CT
- Absence of other neurological findings such as seizures, sensory or motor deficits
- EEG initially shows slowing; follow-up EEG is normal
- Fixed and dilated pupils, if present, are transient and not associated with other neurological deficits. This finding should be viewed cautiously by clinicians.

Gleeson and Beattie (1994) presented four cases of children with transient cortical blindness following mTBI, with children ages 1–9 years. Their findings were identical to those described above, with very brief or no LOC, rapid-onset blindness, and complete resolution over a period of some hours. The authors of both series propose that vasospasm may be the underlying mechanism of this condition. Normal brain imaging with CT scan does not provide any assistance in providing an explanation for the etiology of this condition.

Pituitary Dysfunction

The pituitary gland is connected to the hypothalamus by the pituitary stalk, and is responsible for producing many hormones critical to growth and regulation of the human body. The pituitary stalk is frequently injured in severe head injury, but less commonly in cases of mTBI. In cases of pituitary injury, there may be disruption of a single hormone or, occasionally, all pituitary hormones. Hypopituitarism may present with delayed or arrested puberty, secondary amenorrhea, lack of energy, reduced lean body mass, muscle fatigue, decreased exercise capacity, and reduced bone mineral density. If detected early, treatment with hormone replacement provides excellent long-term results. The adult literature has established the prevalence and outcome data for posttraumatic pituitary dysfunction, but the same cannot be said of the pediatric literature (Acerini & Tasker, 2007; Acerini et al., 2006).

Yamanaka et al. (1993) reported the cases of 3- and 11-year-old boys, both of whom struck their head after falling down a few stairs. Neither boy lost consciousness. Several years later, both boys presented for investigation of short stature, and endocrine assessment demonstrated growth hormone deficiency. Both children underwent MRI of the brain, which demonstrated transection of the pituitary stalk. The authors highlighted that reduced growth rate following mTBI in children may be a sign of pituitary injury and should be considered by those managing such injuries. Although pituitary dysfunction following mTBI in children is extremely rare, lack of awareness of this condition may result in an unwanted outcome: Some children will not receive appropriate treatment in a timely fashion.

MAJOR METHODOLOGICAL AND CONCEPTUAL ISSUES RELEVANT TO UNDERSTANDING/CONDUCTING RESEARCH IN THE AREA

This evidence-based review provides a summary of the current published evidence on neurological outcomes in children with mTBI. It is evident that few researchers have specifically studied this topic in totality; rather, most of this information is a by-product of research into other aspects of head injury and some of the individual domains. Given the rarity of significant neurological dysfunction in mTBI, small, single-center studies are often unsuited to perform appropriate research on this subject with the rigorous methodological requirements necessary. Recommendations to address some of these methodological concerns are presented in a review from the WHO task force (Carroll, Cassidy, Holm, Kraus, & Coronado, 2004) and include:

- Appropriate and consistent definitions of mTBI.
- Appropriate study populations and sampling.
- Appreciation and measure of baseline (preinjury) symptoms and signs.
- Appropriate study design, follow-up, analysis strategies, control groups.
- Adequate means to eliminate confounding variables such as recall bias.
- Relevant outcome measures and techniques.

The difficulty with many of the neurological outcomes discussed in this chapter is that there is no objective measure of the outcome or consistency in definitions and diagnosis. For example, headache is a symptom, not a sign. How should one measure headache? How does one assess headache quality and severity? How is a posttraumatic headache different from the common tension headache of childhood? What is the clinical significance of persistent headache? Why do some children develop headache and/or migraine following the same type of injury as those children who do not develop such symptoms?

At the other extreme is a condition such as cerebral edema, where there are objective measures of the condition (e.g., CT scan), but also important doubts about the mechanism of onset, association with previous head injury, and pathophysiological changes. Hyperaemia (increased cerebral blood flow) and true cerebral edema (increased cerebral interstitial fluid) have many similar clinical and radiological features, but significant differences in potential outcome. How can we easily investigate this phenomenon without invasive brain monitoring and/or biopsy?

Neurological, cognitive, and psychological problems are not mutually exclusive. Although there is research evidence supporting the separate grouping of somatic and cognitive symptoms following pediatric mTBI, it has yet to be established whether symptoms labeled somatic are truly somatic in nature. The symptoms allocated as *somatic* on a postconcussive symptom checklist are assumed to be somatic because they correlate with symptoms that occur in many other somatic diseases. But is this assumption valid? Does it affect the neurological outcome or treatment paradigm? If it were demonstrated that many somatic symptoms were, in fact, emotional/psychologically based, would this alter the pharmacotherapy? If symptoms described as emotional were actually somatic, would this have the same impact on treatment strategies? Given the medical and medical–legal protagonists for and against PCS, this issue will likely remain contentious for some time yet.

The child is not merely a small adult, but physiologically, a growing, developing person with a maturing brain. This fact results in significant differences between pediatric and adult mTBI. The baseline, preinjury function of an adult is usually easier to establish than that of the ever-changing, developing child. Alterations in a child's symptoms have to be considered within the spectrum of childhood development, which is quite different from the stable, developed adult. Family dynamics, parental biases, school background, educational difficulties, and congenital problems are some of the many factors that complicate assessment of the individual child and the pediatric population in general. Many, if not most, studies in pediatric head injury are focused on cognitive changes and therefore exclude children with a background of neurological disease, learning disability, or previous neurosurgery. Yet children with these conditions do also suffer head injury. Are we justified in inferring application of results from studies in mTBI to these children who have been excluded from such studies? Are our sample populations truly representative of the general pediatric population that we treat? These questions take on greater significance when considering that most children with mTBI never seek medical attention. The majority of studies published with regard to neurological outcomes derive from populations presenting to hospital EDs, neurosurgical units, or neurology outpatient clinics. How can we generalize these findings to the entire spectrum of pediatric mTBI? Or are we somewhat blasé in grouping all children with GCS 13–15 into the category of mild brain injury? The GCS is a wonderful tool for helping to identify children in need of acute neurosurgical treatment, and for monitoring changes in the conscious state over time; however it has many limitations in the milder end of the spectrum. The child with a head injury and a GCS of 15 who has a small temporal lobe contusion and who develops epilepsy is defined as having an mTBI. A child who has a head injury with 5 seconds LOC with full recovery and no ongoing symptoms or sequelae is also defined as having an mTBI. The child with a GCS of 13 and a small epidural hematoma is also defined as having an mTBI. Is this useful? Why do we group head injuries into categories? Is it to guide triage, treatment, prognosis, research protocols, or hospital funding? As these examples demonstrate, treatment and prognosis are markedly different within the single category of mTBI. Is there a smarter approach that we should be using?

IMPLICATIONS OF THE RESEARCH FINDINGS FOR CLINICAL MANAGEMENT

As stated at the beginning of this chapter, most children with mTBI do not suffer adverse neurological outcomes. Therefore, the key question that many of these studies address is in trying to identify the child at risk of an adverse outcome, in order to guide that child's management appropriately. The question of which child to scan with CT in order to identify or exclude intracranial hemorrhage has been well addressed with a number of large studies, particularly those presented by Dunning et al. (2006) and Kuppermann et al. (2009). The issue of post mTBI headache remains a more difficult issue to address because of the variable background prevalence of headache in the pediatric population, difficulties in measuring the quality and severity of headache, and differentiating the many subtypes of headache and migraine from the many potential causes, including physical (e.g., neck strain) and psychological.

Seizures in mTBI also suffer from the problems with definitions and difficulties with identifying true seizures from the myriad of other phenomena associated with mTBI. However, the Danish population-based study provides excellent data on the relative risk of epilepsy in the pediatric population, indicating an increased risk in those with a history of mTBI, and more so in those with a family history of epilepsy. But this population-based study does not provide the clinician with the answer to the question of whether the child sitting in front of him or her will or won't develop epilepsy following a recent mTBI.

Cerebral edema and the second-impact syndrome remain key questions when it comes to semantics, but there is no doubt that some children will develop sudden, malignant brain swelling after an mTBI. There are no clinical predictors of this condition, but there is no doubt from the literature that symptomatic children must not return to the field following concussion, and all concussed children must be assessed by a medical practitioner. The variable outcome following acute cerebral swelling suggests that the availability of acute resuscitation equipment and trained personnel are critical in managing this potentially lethal condition.

The rare neurological conditions described above, including cranial neuropathy, stroke, and cortical blindness, have variable neurological outcomes, but it is clear from the data that awareness of these conditions, and expedient management, provide the best possible clinical outcomes.

TRENDS AND FUTURE RESEARCH DIRECTIONS

The future looks brighter than the past because this hitherto oft-neglected topic is now receiving significant research attention. The international community has now set some minimum standards for future research (Carroll et al., 2004), and books such as this will help to promote interest and debate within the medical and research communities.

Lack of control groups or inadequate control groups have been a significant limitation in the past. Future research in pediatric mTBI will require a noninjured control group and an other-injuries control group. These added controls will improve our understanding of the mechanism of injury itself causing symptoms, in addition to brain-specific injury. However, the population studied will need to represent the general pediatric population, and not merely those children presenting to tertiary referral hospitals. Baseline, preinjury characteristics of children are also critical in addressing many of these issues, as are appropriate methods of measuring the relevant variables. Objective measures are the ideal goal in neurological outcomes. Subjective interpretation of symptoms and signs has limited much of the research to date. Association with important risk factors, particularly genetic markers, is most likely the way of the future. Brain imaging, including functional imaging, will undoubtedly cast a new light on this topic. However, although functional imaging is an excellent research tool, difficulties with its clinical application in the general community may be a significant limitation (Davis, Iverson, Guskiewicz, Ptito, & Johnston, 2009).

Identification of the child at risk for neurological sequelae following mTBI remains the long-term goal, but to study the risk factors, an understanding of all the neurological sequelae is critical. This chapter provides a unique insight into the extensive range of neurological conditions that have been reported to result from mTBI in children. The true incidence of most of these conditions is unknown because of the numerous limitations outlined earlier. Applying this knowledge to future research protocols will assist in establishing accurate epidemiological data, and subsequently, risk stratification and improved management and/or prevention of these many serious conditions.

REFERENCES

Acerini, C. L., & Tasker, R. C. (2007). Traumatic brain injury induced hypothalamic–pituitary dysfunction: A paediatric perspective. *Pituitary, 10*(4), 373–380.

Acerini, C. L., Tasker, R. C., Bellone, S., Bona, G., Thompson, C. J., & Savage, M. O. (2006). Hypopituitarism in childhood and adolescence following traumatic brain injury: The case for prospective endocrine investigation. *European Journal Endocrinology, 155*(5), 663–669.

American Psychiatric Association. (2000). *Diagnostic and statistical manual of mental disorders* (4th ed., text rev.). Arlington, VA: Author.

Anderson, T., Heitger, M., & Macleod A. D. (2006). Concussion and mild head injury. *Practical Neurology, 6*, 342–357.

Annegers, J. F., & Coan, S. P. (2000). The risks of epilepsy after traumatic brain injury. *Seizure, 9*(7), 453–457.

Annegers, J. F., Hauser, W. A., Coan, S. P., & Rocca, W. A. (1998). A population-based study of seizures after traumatic brain injuries. *New England Journal of Medicine, 338*(1), 20–24.

Ayr, L. K., Yeates, K. O., Taylor, H. G., & Browne, M. (2009). Dimensions of postconcussive symptoms in children with mild traumatic brain injuries. *Journal of the International Neuropsychological Society, 15*(1), 19–30.

Barlow, K. M., Crawford, S., Stevenson, A., Sandhu, S. S., Belanger, F., & Dewey, D. (2010). Epidemiology of postconcussion syndrome in pediatric mild traumatic brain injury. *Pediatrics, 126*(2), e374–e381.

Blinman, T. A., Houseknecht, E., Snyder, C., Wiebe, D. J., & Nance, M. L. (2009). Postconcussive symptoms in hospitalized pediatric patients after mild traumatic brain injury. *Journal Pediatric Surgery, 44*(6), 1223–1228.

Bruce, D. A., Alavi, A., Bilaniuk, L., Dolinskas, C., Obrist, W., & Uzzell, B. (1981). Diffuse cerebral swelling following head injuries in children: The syndrome of "malignant brain edema." *Journal of Neurosurgery, 54*(2), 170–178.

Callaghan, M., & Abu-Arafeh, I. (2001). Chronic posttraumatic headache in children and adolescents. *Developmental Medicine and Child Neurology, 43*(12), 819–822.

Cantu, R. C. (1998). Second-impact syndrome. *Clinical Sports Medicine, 17*(1), 37–44.

Cantu, R. C., & Gean, A. D. (2010). Second-impact syndrome and a small subdural hematoma: An uncommon catastrophic result of repetitive head injury with a characteristic imaging appearance. *Journal of Neurotrauma, 27*(9), 1557–1564.

Carroll, L. J., Cassidy, J. D., Holm, L., Kraus, J., & Coronado, V. G. (2004). Methodological issues and research recommendations for mild traumatic brain injury: The WHO Collaborating Centre Task Force on Mild Traumatic Brain Injury. *Journal of Rehabilitation Medicine, 43*(Suppl.), 113–125.

Casey, R., Ludwig, S., & McCormick, M. C. (1986). Morbidity following minor head trauma in children. *Pediatrics*, *78*(3), 497–502.

Chiaretti, A., De Benedictis, R., Polidori, G., Piastra, M., Iannelli, A., & Di Rocco, C. (2000). Early post-traumatic seizures in children with head injury. *Child's Nervous System*, *16*(12), 862–866.

Christensen, J., Pedersen, M. G., Pedersen, C. B., Sidenius, P., Olsen, J., & Vestergaard, M. (2009). Long-term risk of epilepsy after traumatic brain injury in children and young adults: A population-based cohort study. *Lancet*, *373*(9669), 1105–1110.

Coello, A. F., Canals, A. G., Gonzalez, J. M., & Martin, J. J. (2010). Cranial nerve injury after minor head trauma. *Journal of Neurosurgery*, *113*, 547–555.

Cutrer, F. M. (2010). Pathophysiology of migraine. *Seminars in Neurology*, *30*(2), 120–130.

Davis, G. A., Iverson, G. L., Guskiewicz, K. M., Ptito, A., & Johnston, K. M. (2009). Contributions of neuroimaging, balance testing, electrophysiology and blood markers to the assessment of sport-related concussion. *British Journal of Sports Medicine*, *43*(Suppl. 1), i36–i45.

Dharker, S. R., Mittal, R. S., & Bhargava, N. (1993). Ischemic lesions in basal ganglia in children after minor head injury. *Neurosurgery*, *33*(5), 863–865.

Dias, M. S., Carnevale, F., & Li, V. (1999). Immediate posttraumatic seizures: Is routine hospitalization necessary? *Pediatric Neurosurgery*, *30*(5), 232–238.

Dunning, J., Daly, J. P., Lomas, J. P., Lecky, F., Batchelor, J., & Mackway-Jones, K. (2006). Derivation of the children's head injury algorithm for the prediction of important clinical events: Decision rule for head injury in children. *Archives of Disease in Childhood*, *91*(11), 885–891.

Emmanuelson, I., & Uvebrant, P. (2009). Occurrence of epilepsy during the first 10 years after traumatic brain injury acquired in childhood up to the age of 18 years in the south western Swedish population-based series. *Brain Injury*, *23*(7), 612–616.

Fullerton, H. J., Johnston, S. C., & Smith, W. S. (2001). Arterial dissection and stroke in children. *Neurology*, *57*(7), 1155–1160.

Gleeson, A. P., & Beattie, T. F. (1994). Post-traumatic transient cortical blindness in children: A report of four cases and a review of the literature. *Journal of Accident and Emergency Medicine*, *11*(4), 250–252.

Graham, D. I., Ford, I., Adams, J. H., Doyle, D., Lawrence, A. E., McLellan, D. R., et al. (1989). Fatal head injury in children. *Journal of Clinical Pathology*, *42*(1), 18–22.

Haas, D. C., & Lourie, H. (1988). Trauma-triggered migraine: An explanation for common neurological attacks after mild head injury—review of the literature. *Journal of Neurosurgery*, *68*(2), 181–188.

Hahn, Y. S., Fuchs, S., Flannery, A. M., Barthel, M. J., & McLone, D. G. (1988). Factors influencing posttraumatic seizures in children. *Neurosurgery*, *22*(5), 864–867.

Holmes, J. F., Palchak, M. J., Conklin, M. J., & Kuppermann, N. (2004). Do children require hospitalization after immediate posttraumatic seizures? *Annals of Emergency Medicine*, *43*(6), 706–710.

Hooper, S. R., Alexander, J., Moore, D., Sasser, H. C., Laurent, S., King, J., et al. (2004). Caregiver reports of common symptoms in children following a traumatic brain injury. *NeuroRehabilitation*, *19*(3), 175–189.

Humphreys, R. P., Hendrick, E. B., & Hoffman, H. J. (1990). The head-injured child who "talks and dies": A report of 4 cases. *Child's Nervous System*, *6*(3), 139–142.

Hyman, H. A. (2001). Neurolitigation of the mTBI case without loss of consciousness: Using somatic complaints to make your case. *NeuroRehabilitation*, *16*(2), 103–108.

International Classification of Headache Disorders: 2nd edition. (2004). *Cephalalgia*, *24*(Suppl. 1), 9–160.

Jacobi, G., Ritz, A., & Emrich, R. (1986). Cranial nerve damage after paediatric head trauma: A long-term follow-up study of 741 cases. *Acta Paediatrica Hungarica*, 27(3), 173–187.

Jennett, B. (1973). Epilepsy after non-missile head injuries. *Scottish Medical Journal*, 18(1), 8–13.

Junger, E. C., Newell, D. W., Grant, G. A., Avellino, A. M., Ghatan, S., Douville, C. M., et al. (1997). Cerebral autoregulation following minor head injury. *Journal of Neurosurgery*, 86(3), 425–432.

Keskil, I. S., Baykaner, M. K., Ceviker, N., & Kaymaz, M. (1995). Assessment of mortality associated with mild head injury in the pediatric age group. *Childs Nervous System*, 11(8), 467–473.

Kieslich, M., Fiedler, A., Heller, C., Kreuz, W., & Jacobi, G. (2002). Minor head injury as cause and co-factor in the aetiology of stroke in childhood: A report of eight cases. *Journal of Neurology, Neurosurgery, and Psychiatry*, 73(1), 13–16.

Kuppermann, N., Holmes, J. F., Dayan, P. S., Hoyle, J. D., Jr., Atabaki, S. M., Holubkov, R., et al. (2009). Identification of children at very low risk of clinically-important brain injuries after head trauma: A prospective cohort study. *Lancet*, 374(9696), 1160–1170.

Lakhkar, B., Singh, B. R., & Agrawal, A. (2010). Traumatic dural sinus thrombosis causing persistent headache in a child. *Journal of Emergencies, Trauma and Shock*, 3(1), 73–75.

Landy, P. J. (1998). Neurological sequelae of minor head and neck injuries. *Injury*, 29(3), 199–206.

Lang, D. A., Teasdale, G. M., Macpherson, P., & Lawrence, A. (1994). Diffuse brain swelling after head injury: More often malignant in adults than children? *Journal of Neurosurgery*, 80(4), 675–680.

Lazar, L., Erez, I., Gutermacher, M., & Katz, S. (1997). Brain concussion produces transient hypokalemia in children. *Journal of Pediatric Surgery*, 32(1), 88–90.

Lobato, R. D., Rivas, J. J., Gomez, P. A., Castaneda, M., Canizal, J. M., Sarabia, R., et al. (1991). Head-injured patients who talk and deteriorate into coma: Analysis of 211 cases studied with computerized tomography. *Journal of Neurosurgery*, 75(2), 256–261.

Luerssen, T. G. (1991). Head injuries in children. *Neurosurgery Clinics of North America*, 2(2), 399–410.

McCrory, P. (2001). Does second impact syndrome exist? *Clinical Journal of Sport Medicine*, 11(3), 144–149.

McCrory, P. R., Bladin, P. F., & Berkovic, S. F. (1997). Retrospective study of concussive convulsions in elite Australian rules and rugby league footballers: Phenomenology, aetiology, and outcome. *British Medical Journal*, 314, 171–174.

Mueller, C., Koch, S., & Toifl, K. (1993). Transient bilateral internuclear ophthalmoplegia after minor head-trauma. *Developmental Medicine and Child Neurology*, 35(2), 163–166.

Muthukumar, N., Veerarajkumar, N., & Madeswaran, K. (2001). Bilateral internuclear ophthalmoplegia following mild head injury. *Childs Nervous System*, 17(6), 366–369.

Nacajauskaite, O., Endziniene, M., Jureniene, K., & Schrader, H. (2006). The validity of post-concussion syndrome in children: A controlled historical cohort study. *Brain and Development*, 28(8), 507–514.

Oman, J. A., Cooper, R. J., Holmes, J. F., Viccellio, P., Nyce, A., Ross, S. E., et al. (2006). Performance of a decision rule to predict need for computed tomography among children with blunt head trauma. *Pediatrics*, 117(2), e238–e246.

Roberts, M. A., & Simcox, A. F. (1996). Assessing olfaction following pediatric traumatic brain injury. *Applied Neuropsychology*, 3(2), 86–88.

Rutherford, W. H., Merrett, J. D., & McDonald, J. R. (1979). Symptoms at one year following concussion from minor head injuries. *Injury*, 10(3), 225–230.

Sandford, A. A., Davidson, T. M., Herrera, N., Gilbert, P., Magit, A. E., Haug, K., et al. (2006). Olfactory dysfunction: A sequela of pediatric blunt head trauma. *International Journal of Pediatric Otorhinolaryngology, 70*(6), 1015–1025.

Satz, P. S., Alfano, M. S., Light, R. F., Morgenstern, H. F., Zaucha, K. F., Asarnow, R. F., et al. (1999). Persistent post-concussive syndrome: A proposed methodology and literature review to determine the effects, if any, of mild head and other bodily injury. *Journal of Clinical and Experimental Neuropsychology, 21*(5), 620–628.

Schutzman, S. A., Barnes, P. D., Mantello, M., & Scott, R. M. (1993). Epidural hematomas in children. *Annals of Emergency Medicine, 22*(3), 535–541.

Shaffer, L., Rich, P. M., Pohl, K. R., & Ganesan, V. (2003). Can mild head injury cause ischaemic stroke? *Archives of Disease in Childhood, 88*(3), 267–269.

Snoek, J. W., Minderhoud, J. M., & Wilmink, J. T. (1984). Delayed deterioration following mild head injury in children. *Brain, 107*(Pt. 1), 15–36.

Stein, S. C., & Doolin, E. J. (1995). Management of minor closed head injury in children and adolescents. *Pediatric Surgery International, 10*(7), 465–471.

Stevens, J. (2009). Jury: AHS not negligent in Melka case. Retrieved April 2, 2011, from *www.allbusiness.com/legal/evidence-testimony/13004457-1.html.*

Stiell, I. G., Wells, G. A., Vandemheen, K., Clement, C., Lesiuk, H., Laupacis, A., et al. (2001). The Canadian CT Head Rule for patients with minor head injury. *Lancet, 357*(9266), 1391–1396.

Taha, J. M., Crone, K. R., Berger, T. S., Becket, W. W., & Prenger, E. C. (1993). Sigmoid sinus thrombosis after closed head injury in children. *Neurosurgery, 32*(4), 541–545; discussion, 545–546.

Taylor, H. G., Dietrich, A., Nuss, K., Wright, M., Rusin, J., Bangert, B., et al. (2010). Post-concussive symptoms in children with mild traumatic brain injury. *Neuropsychology, 24*(2), 148–159.

Vavilala, M. S., Lee, L. A., Boddu, K., Visco, E., Newell, D. W., Zimmerman, J. J., et al. (2004). Cerebral autoregulation in pediatric traumatic brain injury. *Pediatric Critical Care Medicine, 5*(3), 257–263.

Wang, M. Y., Griffith, P., Sterling, J., McComb, J. G., & Levy, M. L. (2000). A prospective population-based study of pediatric trauma patients with mild alterations in consciousness (Glasgow Coma Scale score of 13–14). *Neurosurgery, 46*(5), 1093–1099.

World Health Organization. (1993). *The international classification of mental and behavioural disorders diagnostic criteria for research* (10th ed.). Geneva: Author.

Yamamoto, L. G., & Bart, R. D., Jr. (1988). Transient blindness following mild head trauma. Criteria for a benign outcome. *Clinical Pediatrics (Philadelphia), 27*(10), 479–483.

Yamanaka, C., Momoi, T., Fujisawa, I., Kikuchi, K., Kaji, M., Sasaki, H., et al. (1993). Acquired growth hormone deficiency due to pituitary stalk transection after head trauma in childhood. *European Journal of Pediatrics, 152*(2), 99–101.

Yeates, K. O., Taylor, H. G., Rusin, J., Bangert, B., Dietrich, A., Nuss, K., et al. (2009). Longitudinal trajectories of postconcussive symptoms in children with mild traumatic brain injuries and their relationship to acute clinical status. *Pediatrics, 123*(3), 735–743.

Yuen, H. W., Gan, B. K., Seow, W. T., & Tan, H. K. (2005). Dural sinus thrombosis after minor head injury in a child. *Annals of the Academy of Medicine Singapore, 34*(10), 639–641.

CHAPTER 7

Neurobehavioral Outcomes

Keith Owen Yeates and H. Gerry Taylor

Mild traumatic brain injuries (mTBI) are common in children and adolescents. Annually, at least 700,000 youth ages 0–19 sustain TBI that require hospital-based medical care in the United States, and the large majority of these injuries are mild in severity (Bazarian et al., 2005; Faul, Xu, Wald, & Coronado, 2010; see Comstock & Logan, Chapter 2, this volume). Even if only a small proportion of children with mTBI suffer persistent negative outcomes, then mTBI is a serious public health problem.

The outcomes of mTBI in children and adolescents are controversial (McKinlay, 2009; Yeates, 2010). Research on the outcomes of mTBI has been identified as a pressing need in both national and international consensus conferences (Carroll, Cassidy, Holm, Kraus, & Comstock, 2004a; Centers for Disease Control and Prevention, 2003; NIH Consensus Panel on Rehabilitation of Persons with Traumatic Brain Injury, 1999; Seidel et al., 1999). The need for additional research is particularly acute given the decreasing rate of hospitalization for children with mTBI (Bowman, Bird, Aitken, & Tilford, 2008). This trend places a burden on health care providers in emergency medicine and outpatient care settings to make informed decisions regarding the management of mTBI in children and adolescents (Kamerling, Lutz, Posner, & Vanore, 2003).

This chapter summarizes the existing literature regarding the neurobehavioral outcomes of mTBI in children and adolescents, focusing on the ongoing debate regarding postconcussive symptoms. Conceptual and methodological issues that arise in research on the outcomes of mTBI are discussed, and the chapter concludes with suggestions for future research directions.

DEFINITIONAL CONCERNS

Many different terms have been used to refer to mTBI, including *minor closed-head injury* (American Academy of Pediatrics, 1999), *mild traumatic brain injury* (American Congress of Rehabilitation Medicine, 1993), and *concussion* (McCrory et al., 2009). Differences in terminology are a frequent cause of confusion and hamper comparisons of findings across research studies (Bodin, Yeates, & Klamar, 2012; see Wilde et al., Chapter 1, this volume). The World Health Organization (WHO) Collaborating Centre Task Force on Mild Traumatic Brain Injury (Carroll et al., 2004a) offered the following consensus definition of mTBI:

> MTBI is an acute brain injury resulting from mechanical energy to the head from external physical forces. Operational criteria for clinical identification include: (i) 1 or more of the following: confusion or disorientation, loss of consciousness for 30 minutes or less, post-traumatic amnesia for less than 24 hours, and/or other transient neurological abnormalities such as focal signs, seizure, and intracranial lesion not requiring surgery; (ii) Glasgow Coma Scale score of 13–15 after 30 minutes post-injury or later upon presentation for healthcare. (p. 115)

Notably, this definition includes injuries ranging from the mildest of concussions, presenting with brief alterations in mental status, to so-called "complicated" mTBI (i.e., those with trauma-related lesions on neuroimaging, not requiring surgery).

Variability in terminology and associated criteria hampers the accurate identification and diagnosis of children with mTBI (Powell, Ferraro, Dikmen, Temkin, & Bell, 2008). Epidemiological studies of mTBI are also hindered by the use of the *International Classification of Diseases, 10th Revision* (ICD-10; World Health Organization, 1992) diagnostic codes employed in most clinical settings (CDC, National Center for Injury Prevention and Control, 2003). The ICD includes multiple codes that are potentially applicable to mTBI, but they are not limited to injuries that are exclusively mild in severity, and they also encompass external trauma to the head that is not necessarily associated with any alteration in brain function or structure. Obviously, inaccuracies and inconsistencies in diagnostic criteria and classification will impede research on the outcomes of mTBI.

NEUROBEHAVIORAL OUTCOMES OF mTBI

Cognitive Outcomes

Cognitive tests tend to be sensitive to mTBI only acutely, at least when children are studied as a group (Satz, 2001; Satz, Zaucha, McCleary, Light, & Asarnow, 1997). High school athletes with concussions display deficits on cognitive testing immediately postinjury, particularly in processing speed, reaction time, and memory, but the deficits tend to resolve within 1–2 weeks, albeit perhaps more slowly than in college-age athletes (Field, Collins, Lovell, & Maroon, 2003). Little or no evidence is available regarding cognitive outcomes following concussions in younger athletes, and future studies are needed to determine if they display more prolonged cognitive deficits.

In the general population, both epidemiological and clinical studies provide little evidence of persistent cognitive deficits resulting from mTBI, especially in studies that are methodologically rigorous (e.g., Babikian et al., 2011; Babikian & Asarnow, 2009; Bijur & Haslum, 1995; Fay et al., 1993). One caveat to this finding is that previous research has focused largely on school-age children. The cognitive outcomes of mTBI in infants, toddlers, and other preschool children have not been studied to the same extent, although some studies suggest the possibility of more extended deficits, at least in children whose injuries fall on the more severe end of the spectrum of mTBI (Gronwall, Wrightson, & McGinn, 1997; McKinlay, Dalrymple-Alford, Horwood, & Fergusson, 2002; McKinley et al., 2010a).

Postconcussive Symptoms

Research using broad-based measures of adjustment has generally not found significant differences between children with mTBI and those with injuries not involving the head (Light et al., 1998). However, broad-based measures focus predominantly on emotional and behavioral problems and hence tend not to be sensitive to medical disorders such as mTBI (Drotar, Stein, & Perrin, 1995).

Relatively few studies of mTBI in children have focused specifically on what are commonly referred to as "postconcussive symptoms," and which include a range of somatic (e.g., headache, fatigue), cognitive (e.g., inattention, forgetfulness, slowed processing), and affective (e.g., irritability, disinhibition) complaints (Yeates et al., 1999, 2001). Although not specific to mTBI, postconcussive symptoms are more common and severe in children with mTBI than in children with injuries not involving the head or in healthy children matched for demographics (Barlow et al., 2010; Hawley, 2003; Mittenberg, Wittner, & Miller, 1997; Ponsford et al., 1999; Taylor et al., 2010; Yeates et al., 1999, 2009).

Postconcussive symptoms tend to be most pronounced shortly after injury and to resolve over time (Barlow et al., 2010; Nacajauskaite, Endziniene, Jureniene, & Schrader, 2006; Ponsford et al., 1999; Taylor et al., 2010), but some children with mTBI experience persistent symptoms, with potentially negative consequences for long-term psychosocial functioning and quality of life (McKinlay et al., 2002; Moran et al., in press; Overweg-Plandsoen et al., 1999; Yeates et al., 2009). We recently examined reliable change in postconcussive symptoms in children with mTBI, as compared to those with orthopedic injuries (Yeates et al., in press-a). Analyses of reliable change permit a determination of whether an individual displays a statistically reliable change in scores across two occasions. Reliable increases in somatic symptoms occurred in 44% of children with complicated mTBI shortly after injury and in 20% at 3 months postinjury, as compared to 7% at both times among children with orthopedic injuries. Similarly, reliable increases in cognitive symptoms occurred in 20% of children with mTBI who displayed a loss of consciousness shortly after injury, in 15% at 3 months postinjury, and in 17% at 12 months postinjury, as compared to 4–6% among children with orthopedic injuries. Among children with mTBI, reliable increases in postconcussive symptoms at 3 months postinjury were associated with significant declines in physical and psychosocial quality of life, as well as with an increased likelihood of educational intervention for children who were not receiving such intervention at the time of their injuries.

The persistent postconcussive symptoms that sometimes occur following mTBI may constitute a coherent syndrome or disorder (Brown, Fann, & Grant, 1994). The diagnosis of post-concussion syndrome is included in the ICD-10 (World Health Organization, 1992), and research criteria for postconcussional disorder are contained in the fourth edition of the *Diagnostic and Statistical Manual of Mental Disorders* (DSM-IV; American Psychiatric Association, 1994). However, the ICD-10 and DSM-IV have different diagnostic criteria, which differ in their apparent assumptions about the etiology of post-concussion syndrome, result in different incidence estimates, yield limited diagnostic agreement, and may not be specific to TBI (Boake et al., 2004, 2005; Yeates & Taylor, 2005). Recent research has shown that postconcussive symptoms form reliable and stable dimensions in children with mTBI (Ayr, Yeates, Taylor, & Browne, 2009), suggesting a potential basis for refining the symptom criteria for post-concussion syndrome in both the ICD-10 and DSM-IV.

Postconcussive symptoms often occur in the absence of objective evidence of brain injury. This absence has engendered disputes in the adult literature about whether the etiology of post-concessive symptoms reflects "psychogenesis" or "physiogenesis" (Alexander, 1997; Bigler, 2008; Lishman, 1988). Proponents of psychogenesis argue that postconcussive symptoms reflect premorbid differences, postinjury psychological factors, or outright malingering, rather than any alteration in brain function (Binder, 1986). In contrast, proponents of physiogenesis point to experimental studies of nonhuman animals and clinical research with humans suggesting that mTBI can result in acute neuropathology and other abnormalities in brain function (Giza & Hovda, 2001). They also cite studies showing that postconcussive symptoms can be associated with deficits on standardized cognitive testing and abnormalities on neuroimaging (Levin et al., 2008; Wilde et al., 2008). Of course, these explanations are not mutually exclusive. Indeed, research with adults shows that both injury characteristics and non-injury-related variables help account for the outcomes of mTBI (Kashluba, Paniak, & Casey, 2008; Luis, Vanderploeg, & Curtiss, 2003; Ponsford et al., 2000).

This debate can be readily extended to pediatric populations. Research is needed to identify both injury and non-injury-related factors that predict persistent postconcussive symptoms in children and adolescents (Satz, 2001; Yeates & Taylor, 2005). Our studies of mTBI clearly indicate that both types of factors are operative. For instance, we have found that postconcussive symptoms are more persistent and severe when mTBI is associated with abnormalities on neuroimaging, loss of consciousness, and other indicators of severity (Taylor et al., 2010; Yeates et al., 2009, in press-a). However, we have also found that children are at greater risk for postconcussive symptoms following mTBI, relative to orthopedic injury (OI), if they have lower overall cognitive ability or rely on avoidance or wishful thinking to cope with their injuries (Fay et al., 2009; Woodrome et al., 2011).

More recently, we found that children from families that were higher functioning and had more environmental resources were more likely to demonstrate somatic symptoms following mTBI than those from poorer functioning homes with fewer resources (Yeates et al., in press-b). This finding runs counter to previous research among children with severe TBI, showing that the effects of TBI are exacerbated in the context of poorer premorbid child and family functioning (Yeates et al., 1997). We offered several potential explanations for the findings: Family adversity may obscure the effects of mTBI for parents, making them less likely to perceive changes in postconcussive symptoms; parents of children from higher-functioning families with more resources may be more attentive to changes in their children's health, making them more likely to perceive increased symptoms following mTBI; children from higher-functioning families with more resources may be more sensitive to the effects of mTBI, perhaps because they face higher demands or expectations in their daily environment or are more closely monitored; or the effects of mTBI may be masked by other, more powerful causes of cognitive and somatic symptoms among children from lower-functioning families or those with lower resources.

Psychiatric Outcomes

A limited amount of research has focused specifically on psychiatric disorders following mTBI in children. The rate of psychiatric disorders in children with mTBI varies widely, ranging from 10 to upward of 100% across studies (e.g., Bloom et al., 2001; Brown, Chadwick, Shaffer, Rutter, & Traub, 1981; Massagli et al., 2004). Two large prospective studies of mTBI are especially noteworthy: The first involved a birth cohort (McKinlay et al., 2002), and the second involved a review of computerized medical data pertaining to children consecutively treated for mTBI (Massagli et al., 2004). Both studies showed that children with mTBI had significantly more new-onset behavioral symptoms than controls. However, the outcome measures in these studies were not generated from standardized psychiatric interviews, and the studies lacked control groups of children with injuries not involving the head.

The range of psychiatric disorder reported in studies of consecutively treated children with mTBI using standardized assessments is narrower than that in the overall literature (i.e., 10–40%). In such studies, children with mTBI have shown increased rates of new-onset psychiatric disorders relative to both injured controls and to uninjured controls, although the differences have not always been statistically significant (Brown et al., 1981; Luis & Mittenberg, 2002; Max et al., 1998). Among the more common disorders that are identified in such studies are attention-deficit/hyperactivity disorder, oppositional defiant disorder/conduct disorder, personality change due to TBI, depressive disorder, and anxiety disorder. However, no specific disorder has a particularly high incidence when considered in isolation.

Long-Term Adult Outcomes

Research on the long-term adult outcomes of mTBI occurring during childhood is extremely limited. One early study reported on very-long-term consequences 23 years after mainly mTBI in children (Klonoff, Clark, & Klonoff, 1993). Severity of injury was determined by unconsciousness, neurological status, skull fracture, electroencephalography (EEG), posttraumatic seizures, and a composite measure that combined those factors. Outcomes included physical, cognitive, and emotional symptoms. Severity of TBI, as determined by the composite measure of neurological variables, was the best predictor of long-term sequelae. Measures of IQ obtained during the postacute phase were also found to predict long-term outcome. The occurrence of subjective symptom complaints was associated with a heightened incidence of grade failure/retention, unemployment, and strained relationships with family members.

Two more recent papers have focused on very-long-term neuropsychological and psychosocial outcomes after mTBI in children (Hessen, Anderson, & Nestvold, 2008; Hessen, Nestvold, & Sundet, 2006). Both papers were based on a prospective study conducted in Norway (Nestvold, Lundar, Blikra, & Lønnum, 1988) beginning in 1974. All patients referred to a teaching hospital because of injuries to the head, face, and neck over a 12-month period were invited to participate. Because the study took place before the introduction of the Glasgow Coma Scale (Teasdale & Jennett, 1974), severity of injury was primarily classified according to duration of posttraumatic amnesia (PTA). Additionally, within the first 24 hours of admission, all the patients underwent a neurological examination and a standard EEG. Most of the patients in the original sample were considered to have suffered an mTBI, consistent with epidemiological studies. The diagnostic criteria for mTBI encompassed a spectrum of severity, ranging from uncomplicated injuries with no signs of neurological insult to more complicated injuries with PTA, loss of consciousness, EEG abnormalities, focal neurological signs, and fractures.

Approximately 23 years after their initial participation, all patients still living near the site of the original study were invited to take part in a follow-up, and 70% agreed. In one paper (Hessen et al., 2006), follow-up data were reported for 45 out of the 62 participants who were 15 years old or less at the time of their injuries. They completed an extensive neuropsychological test battery. On the basis of normative data, their performance on all neuropsychological tests was in the normal range. However, neuropsychological deficits were apparent in the subgroup of patients who had displayed a combination of PTA greater than 30 minutes and an abnormal EEG within the first 24 hours postinjury. The results suggest that complicated mTBI in children and adolescents may be associated with persistent, if mild, neuropsychological dysfunction.

In another paper (Hessen et al., 2008), the Minnesota Multiphasic Personality Inventory–2 (MMPI-2) profiles of patients 15 years or less at the time of their injury were examined. Overall, participants had scores on the MMPI-2 very close to normative means. However, complicated mTBI, defined as the presence of a skull fracture and both PTA greater than 30 minutes and abnormal EEG within 24 hours of injury, was associated with significant elevations on subscales reflecting somatic complaints, fatigue, worry about health problems, and negative expectations about the ability to work. The findings indicate that children and adolescents with complicated mTBI may be at risk for chronic postconcussive symptoms, and again suggest a potentially differential impact of uncomplicated versus complicated mTBI.

RESEARCH ISSUES

Definition of mTBI

Previous research on mTBI suffers from a variety of methodological shortcomings (Dikmen & Levin, 1993). One major limitation involves the definition of mTBI, which has varied substantially across studies, along with associated inclusion/exclusion criteria (Williams, Levin, & Eisenberg, 1990). Most studies have defined mTBI based on Glasgow Coma Scale (Teasdale & Jennett, 1974) scores ranging from 13 to 15, but they have been inconsistent in applying other criteria, such as presence or duration of unconsciousness or PTA. Studies can often be criticized for not defining both the lower and upper limits of severity of mTBI, which can range from brief alterations in mental status without loss of consciousness to more severe signs and symptoms, including loss of consciousness, PTA, transient neurological abnormalities, and positive neuroimaging findings. Some studies have defined mTBI based on the persistence of postconcussive symptoms, but this requirement confounds the injury itself with its outcomes. Issues of definition and classification are especially problematic in studies of infants and younger children, for whom traditional measures of injury severity, such as the Glasgow Coma Scale, may not be valid (Durham et al., 2000).

Some previous studies have included children who sustained a head trauma without any acute signs or symptoms of concussion, and excluded children with more severe injuries. These practices have engendered potentially erroneous conclusions about the outcomes of mTBI. The WHO Collaborating Centre Task Force on Mild Traumatic Brain Injury reviewed the prognosis of mTBI (Carroll et al., 2004b) and cited two studies to justify their conclusion that postconcussive symptoms in children "are usually transient in nature" (p. 88) and "appear to be largely resolved within 2–3 months of the injury" (p. 85). However, both of the cited studies excluded children with neuroimaging abnormalities, despite the inclusion of such abnormalities in the Task Force's operational definition of mTBI. Studies including children with more severe injuries have found more pronounced and persistent postconcussive symptoms, as compared to children with orthopedic injuries or healthy children (Fay et al., 2009; Mittenberg et al., 1997; Taylor et al., 2010; Yeates et al., 2009, in press-a).

Comparison Groups

Previous studies can be criticized for the absence of appropriate comparison groups (Dikmen & Levin, 1993). Many early studies did not include comparison groups, relying on normative data to determine the effects of mTBI. Noninjured children matched on demographic variables also have been used as a comparison group (e.g., Fay et al., 1993). However, noninjured children are not equated to children with mTBI in terms of the experience of a traumatic injury or ensuing medical treatment. Research also suggests that children who sustain traumatic injuries are more likely to display premorbid behavioral disorders and differ in other ways from noninjured children (Gerring et al., 1998; McKinlay et al., 2010b).

In one of the larger studies of mTBI (Asarnow et al., 1995; Babikian et al., 2011; Light et al., 1998), the cognitive test performance of children with mTBI was worse than that of children who were matched demographically but not injured. In contrast, the cognitive and behavioral functioning of children with mTBI did not differ from that of children with injuries not involving the head. Comparison groups comprising children who have sustained mild injuries not involving the head and who have undergone acute medical treatment are desirable in research on mTBI.

Outcome Measurement

The measurement of postconcussive symptoms has typically been limited to questionnaires and rating scales, usually completed only by parents. Parent–child agreement regarding postconcussive symptoms is significant but modest (Gioia, Schneider,

Vaugh, & Isquith, 2008; Hajek et al., 2011), suggesting that both child and parent reports should be explored in studies of mTBI. Of course, in infants and younger children, only parent ratings may be available, but the validity of ratings in that age range warrants further investigation. The reporting of postconcussive symptoms may also depend on the format for symptom reporting. For example, in adults, rating scales elicit reports of more symptoms than do open-ended structured interviews (Iverson, Brooks, Ashton, & Lange, 2010; Nolin, Villemure, & Heroux, 2006).

Previous research has also treated postconcussive symptoms as if they occur along a single dimension. However, our research indicates that postconcussive symptoms are multidimensional, with a clear distinction being drawn between somatic and cognitive symptoms (Ayr et al., 2009). The dimensions not only can be distinguished psychometrically, but also follow distinct trajectories post mTBI (Taylor et al., 2010). They also appear to be distinct from other kinds of symptoms, such as those associated with posttraumatic stress disorder (Bryant & Harvey, 1999; Hajek et al., 2010).

Assessment of Risk Factors

The assessment of risk factors that predict outcomes following mTBI has been problematic. Most studies have not adequately characterized the severity of children's injuries. Children with mTBI are often treated as a homogeneous group, without regard to whether factors such as loss of consciousness or abnormalities on neuroimaging increase the risk of negative outcomes. Few studies have explored existing schemes for grading mTBI, such as those set forth by the American Academy of Neurology (1997), or used neuroimaging to distinguish between complicated and uncomplicated mTBI. Advanced neuroimaging techniques, such as susceptibility-weighted and diffusion tensor imaging, may also provide a more sensitive assessment of injury severity in mTBI (Ashwal, Tong, Obenaus, & Holshouser, 2010; Beauchamp et al., 2011). For instance, diffusion tensor imaging may provide continuous, quantitative measures of white matter integrity that can detect abnormality even in brain tissue that appears healthy to visual inspection (Chu et al., 2010).

Research also needs to incorporate measures of non-injury-related risk factors as possible predictors. In many cases, children with premorbid learning or behavior problems are omitted from studies, although they may be at particular risk for persistent postconcussive symptoms. As noted earlier, we have shown that children's premorbid cognitive ability moderates the outcomes of mTBI (Fay et al., 2009). Parent and family functioning also can be affected by mTBI (Ganesalingam et al., 2008) and moderates outcomes, as it does in children with more severe TBI (Yeates et al., in press-a). In the long run, models are needed that capture the interplay of injury-related and non-injury-related child and family factors in predicting postconcussive symptoms (see Figure 7.1).

Alternative Explanations

Previous research has not yet conclusively ruled out a variety of potential alternative explanations for the deleterious effects purportedly associated with mTBI. These would include children's effort or motivation, pain, and symptom exaggeration.

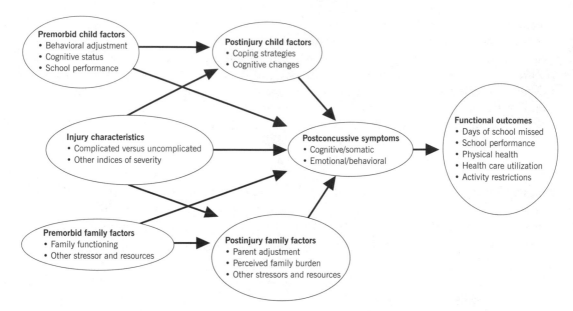

FIGURE 7.1. Model for the study of postconcussive symptoms in children with mild traumatic brain injury. From Yeates and Taylor (2005). Copyright 2005 by Informa Medical and Pharmaceutical Science Journals. Reprinted by permission.

Future research should incorporate tests of effort, such as the Medical Symptom Validity Test (Green, 2004), which has been shown to account for substantial variance in cognitive test performance among children with mTBI (Kirkwood, Yeates, Randolph, & Kirk, 2012). Pain should also be examined more closely, because it is a very common consequence of TBI and may contribute to poor cognitive test performance and also exacerbate related symptom complaints (Nampiaparampil, 2008). Finally, some children or parents may be prone to symptom exaggeration, perhaps because of the lay expectations associated with mTBI (Mittenberg et al., 1992). Research that incorporates indices such as the F Index from the Behavior Assessment System for Children—Second Edition (BASC-2; Reynolds & Kamphaus, 2004) may help to determine whether reports of postconcussive symptoms after mTBI are influenced by such expectations. For instance, a recent study (described in Kirkwood, 2012) found that a small percentage (2.5%) of children with mTBI exceeded cutoffs on the BASC F Index, based on self-reports.

Timing of Assessment

Research on mTBI has often been cross-sectional and focused on relatively short-term outcomes. This problem is compounded in some studies by retrospective recruitment of participants from among clinical referrals, creating a significant ascertainment bias. Prospective and longitudinal studies of unselected samples are needed to examine the sequelae of mTBI over time, as well as how the relationship of risk factors to postconcussive symptoms varies postinjury (Ponsford et al., 1999).

In longitudinal studies, decisions regarding the timing of assessments are critical (Taylor & Alden, 1997). Acute postinjury assessments are often desirable, not only to document the immediate effects of mTBI, but also to obtain retrospective measures of children's premorbid functioning as soon after the injury as possible, and thereby increase the validity of parent recall. The timing of subsequent assessments will be based in part on the expected course of outcomes following mTBI. The DSM-IV criteria for postconcussive syndrome, for instance, require that symptoms persist for at least 3 months, so an assessment at that time is often desirable (American Psychiatric Association, 1994). However, even longer-term assessments may be needed to determine whether mTBI results in significant impairment in children's social or academic functioning.

Prediction of Individual Outcomes

Studies of mTBI have focused on group outcomes, in part because most common statistical techniques yield results that are based on group data. Thus, most analyses are variable-centered and inform us only of group trends. In clinical practice, however, we want to know whether the occurrence of mTBI accounts for postconcussive symptoms in a particular patient, because we recognize that the importance of risk factors is likely to vary across individuals. One way to focus more on individual outcomes is to divide groups into subgroups based on certain characteristics and then determine if outcomes are different for persons in different subgroups. Parsing a sample of children with mTBI into those with versus without loss of consciousness exemplifies this approach (Taylor et al., 2010). A second approach is to identify individuals with a given outcome, such as persistent postconcussive symptoms, and then determine the combinations of risk factors linked to this outcome. An advantage of the latter, person-centered method is that it permits the researcher to identify combinations of risk factors associated with the outcome (Laursen & Hoff, 2006).

In studies of longitudinal change, growth curve modeling permits the investigation of change at an individual level in relation to multiple risk factors (Francis et al., 1991; Taylor et al., 2010). Mixture modeling, in contrast, is used to empirically identify latent classes of individuals based on different developmental trajectories (Nagin, 2005). Figure 7.2 provides an example of this approach; it shows developmental trajectories of postconcussive symptoms in children with mTBI and in those with orthopedic injuries (Yeates et al., 2009). In this study, children with mTBI were more likely than those with orthopedic injuries to demonstrate trajectories involving high acute levels of symptoms. Moreover, children with mTBI whose acute clinical presentation reflected more severe injury were especially likely to demonstrate such trajectories, in contrast to those with mTBI with less severe acute presentations. Finally, analyses of reliable change also can be used to identify individual children who display unusually large increases in postconcussive symptoms and to study the risk factors associated with such increases (McCrea et al., 2005; Yeates et al., in press-a).

FUTURE DIRECTIONS

No comprehensive theories are available at this time to guide research on the outcomes of mTBI. However, future research on mTBI in children should reflect advances in our understanding of biological, behavioral and psychological, and social factors that are likely to affect outcomes. At the biological level, genetic factors may help explain

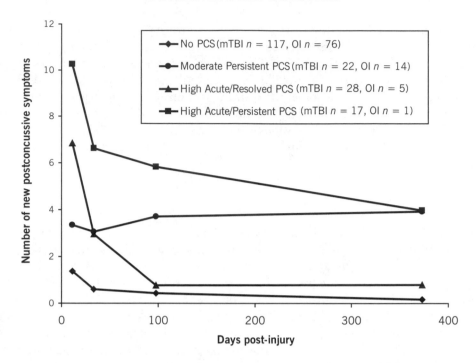

FIGURE 7.2. Illustration of developmental trajectory analysis of postconcussive symptoms (PCS) in children with mTBI or orthopedic injuries (OI). Four latent groups were identified on the basis of the number of new postconcussive symptoms reported at four occasions postinjury, irrespective of whether participants were in the mTBI or OI group. Adapted from Yeates et al. (2009). Copyright 2009 by the American Academy of Pediatrics. Adapted by permission.

variability in outcomes. The apolipoprotein E gene has not been found to predict outcomes of mTBI in children (Moran et al., 2009), but many other candidate genes should be examined (Jordan, 2007). Research at a biological level also is likely to yield more sensitive measures of brain injury. For instance, various biomarkers are under study as possible indicators of underlying brain injury in mTBI (Berger, Hayes, Wang, & Kochanek, 2010).

At the behavioral and psychological levels, future research may offer more refined and sensitive outcome measures. Computerized testing has the advantage of being able to assess reaction time, which has been shown to be sensitive to concussion soon after injury (Iverson, Brooks, Collins, & Lovell, 2006). Existing measures of postconcussive symptoms are also in need of additional refinement, so that they accurately reflect underlying dimensions of symptom type (Ayr et al., 2009). Ideally, screening instruments could be developed that physicians in emergency department and outpatient settings would use to assess children with mTBI to determine whether to refer for more extensive neuropsychological evaluation (Gioia et al., 2008).

Investigators should also consider broadening assessments to include domains other than cognitive functioning and postconcussive symptoms. For instance, research in sports concussion has identified simple measures of balance and postural stability that differentiate concussed athletes from those without concussion, but such measures have not been incorporated in broader studies of mTBI in children (Ellemberg, Henry, Macciocchi, Guskiewicz, & Broglio, 2009; Guskiewicz, 2001).

Outcome research should also incorporate measures of constructs such as quality of life and psychiatric disorder. In choosing outcome measures, investigators might consider efforts to establish common data elements in studies of TBI outcomes across a range of severity (McCauley et al., 2012).

Finally, at a social level, research is needed to clarify which aspects of the family and broader social environment influence outcomes and to delineate the mechanisms by which they do so. Recent studies have shown that the family and social environment are related to children's functioning following mTBI (Yeates et al., in press-b). Future research will benefit from the consideration of more sophisticated models of the relationship between contextual factors and developmental outcomes (Steinberg & Avenevoli, 2000).

A key long-term goal for research on the outcomes of mTBI should be to develop a biopsychosocial model that incorporates developmental considerations and allows for individual variability in the importance of different risk factors. A comprehensive, integrated model should provide a clearer picture of risk and resiliency in children with mTBI, and thereby foster more effective clinical management (Kirkwood et al., 2008). For instance, the provision of anticipatory guidance can prevent the onset of postconcussive symptoms (Ponsford et al., 2001), and active rehabilitation can ameliorate symptoms when they do occur (Gagnon, Galli, Friedman, Grilli, & Iverson, 2009). Future research will enable health care providers to offer parents and children evidence-based information regarding the effects of mTBI and to identify those children who are most at risk for demonstrating negative outcomes. Health care providers can then target at-risk children and their families for appropriate management.

ACKNOWLEDGMENTS

The preparation of this chapter was supported by Grant Nos. HD44099 and HD39834 from the National Institutes of Health to Keith Owen Yeates.

REFERENCES

Alexander, M. P. (1997). Minor traumatic brain injury: A review of physiogenesis and psychogenesis. *Seminars in Clinical Neuropsychiatry, 2,* 177–187.

American Academy of Neurology. (1997). Practice parameter: The management of concussion in sports (summary statement). Report of the Quality Standards Subcommittee. *Neurology, 48,* 581–585.

American Academy of Pediatrics. (1999). The management of minor closed head injury in children. *Pediatrics, 104,* 1407–1415.

American Congress of Rehabilitation Medicine. (1993). Definition of mild traumatic brain injury. *Journal of Head Trauma Rehabilitation, 8,* 86–87.

American Psychiatric Association. (1994). *Diagnostic and statistical manual of mental disorders* (4th ed.). Washington, DC: Author.

Asarnow, R. F., Satz, P., Light, R., Zaucha, K., Lewis, R., & McCleary, C. (1995). The UCLA study of mild head injury in children and adolescents. In M. E. Michel & S. Broman (Eds.), *Traumatic head injury in children* (pp. 117–146). New York: Oxford University Press.

Ashwal, S., Tong, K. A., Obenaus, A., & Holshouser, B. A. (2010). Advanced neuroimaging techniques in children with traumatic brain injury. In V. A. Anderson & K. O. Yeates

(Eds.), *New directions in pediatric traumatic brain injury: Multidisciplinary and translational perspectives* (pp. 68–93). New York: Oxford University Press.

Ayr, L. K., Yeates, K. O., Taylor, H. G., & Browne, M. (2009). Dimensions of post-concussive symptoms in children with mild traumatic brain injuries. *Journal of the International Neuropsychological Society, 15*, 19–30.

Babikian, T., & Asarnow, R. (2009). Neurocognitive outcomes and recovery after pediatric TBI: Meta-analytic review of the literature. *Neuropsychology, 23*, 283–296.

Babikian, T., Satz, P., Zaucha, K., Light, R., Lewis, R. S., & Asarnow, R. F. (2011). The UCLA longitudinal study of neurocognitive outcomes following mild pediatric traumatic brain injury. *Journal of the International Neuropsychological Society, 17*, 1–10.

Barlow, K. M., Crawford, S., Stevenson, A., Sandhu, S. S., Belanger, F., & Dewey, D. (2010). A prospective epidemiological study of post-concussion syndrome in pediatric mild traumatic brain injury. *Pediatrics, 126*, e374–e381.

Bazarian, J. J., McClung, J., Shah, M. N., Cheng, Y. T., Flesher, W., & Kraus, J. (2005). Mild traumatic brain injury in the United States, 1998–2000. *Brain Injury, 19*, 85–91.

Beauchamp, M. H., Ditchfield, M., Babl, F. E., Kean, M., Catroppa, C., Yeates, K. O., et al. (2011). Detecting traumatic brain lesions in children: CT vs. MRI vs. susceptibility weighted imaging (SWI). *Journal of Neurotrauma, 28*, 915–927.

Berger, R. P., Hayes, R. L., Wang, K. K. W., & Kochanek, P. (2010). Using serum biomarkers to diagnose, assess, treat and predict outcome after pediatric TBI. In V. A. Anderson & K. O. Yeates (Eds.), *New directions in pediatric traumatic brain injury: Multidisciplinary and translational perspectives* (pp. 36–53). New York: Oxford University Press.

Bigler, E. D. (2008). Neuropsychology and clinical neuroscience of persistent post-concussive syndrome. *Journal of the International Neuropsychological Society, 14*, 1–22.

Bijur, P. E., & Haslum, M. (1995). Cognitive, behavioral, and motoric sequelae of mild head injury in a national birth cohort. In S. Broman & M. E. Michel (Eds.), *Traumatic head injury in children* (pp. 147–164). New York: Oxford University Press.

Binder, L. M. (1986). Persisting symptoms after mild head injury: A review of the postconcussive syndrome. *Journal of Clinical and Experimental Neuropsychology, 8*, 323–346.

Bloom, D. R., Levin, H. S., Ewing-Cobbs, L., Saunders, A. E, Song, J., & Kowatch, R. A. (2001). Lifetime and novel psychiatric disorders after pediatric traumatic brain injury. *Journal of the American Academy of Child and Adolescent Psychiatry, 40*, 572–579.

Boake, C., McCauley, S. R., Levin, H. S., Contant, C. F., Song, J. X., Brown, S. A., et al. (2004). Limited agreement between criteria-based diagnoses of postconcussional syndrome. *Journal of Neuropsychiatry and Clinical Neurosciences, 16*, 493–499.

Boake, C., McCauley, S. R., Levin, H. S., Pedroza, C., Contant, C. F., Song, J. X., et al. (2005). Diagnostic criteria for postconcussional syndrome after mild to moderate traumatic brain injury. *Journal of Neuropsychiatry and Clinical Neurosciences, 17*, 350–356.

Bodin, D., Yeates, K. O., & Klamar, K. (2012). Definition and classification of concussion. In J. N. Apps & K. D. Walter (Eds.), *Pediatric and adolescent concussion: Diagnosis, management, and outcome* (pp. 9–20). New York: Springer.

Bowman, S. M., Bird, T. M., Aitken, M. E., & Tilford, J. M. (2008). Trends in hospitalizations associated with pediatric traumatic brain injuries. *Pediatrics, 122*, 988–993.

Brown, G., Chadwick, O., Shaffer, D., Rutter, M., & Traub, M. (1981). A prospective study of children with head injuries: III. Psychiatric sequelae. *Psychological Medicine, 11*, 63–78.

Brown, S. J., Fann, J. R., & Grant, I. (1994). Postconcussional disorder: Time to acknowledge a common source of neurobehavioral morbidity. *Journal of Neuropsychiatry and Clinical Neurosciences, 6*, 15–22.

Bryant, R. A., & Harvey, A. G. (1999). Postconcussive symptoms and posttraumatic stress disorder after mild traumatic brain injury. *Journal of Nervous and Mental Disease, 187*, 302–305.

Carroll, L. J., Cassidy, J. D., Holm, L., Kraus, J., & Coronado, V. G. (2004a). Methodological issues and research recommendations for mild traumatic brain injury: The WHO Collaborating Centre Task Force on Mild Traumatic Brain Injury. *Journal of Rehabilitation Medicine* (Suppl. 43), 113–125.

Carroll, L. J., Cassidy, J. D., Peloso, P. M., Borg, J., von Holst, H., Holm, L., et al. (2004b). Prognosis for mild traumatic brain injury: Results of the WHO Collaborating Centre Task Force on Mild Traumatic Brain Injury. *Journal of Rehabilitation Medicine* (Suppl. 43), 84–105.

Centers for Disease Control and Prevention (CDC), National Center for Injury Prevention and Control. (2003). *Report to Congress on mild traumatic brain injury in the United States: Steps to prevent a serious public health problem.* Atlanta, GA: Author.

Chu, Z., Wilde, E. A., Hunter, J. V., McCauley, S. R., Bigler, E. D., Troyanskaya, M., et al. (2010). Voxel-based analysis of diffusion tensor imaging in mild traumatic brain injury in adolescents. *American Journal of Neuroradiology, 31,* 340–346.

Dikmen, S. S., & Levin, H. S. (1993). Methodological issues in the study of mild head injury. *Journal of Head Trauma Rehabilitation, 8,* 30–37.

Drotar, D., Stein, R. E. K., & Perrin, E. C. (1995). Methodological issues in using the Child Behavior Checklist and its related instruments in clinical child psychology research. *Journal of Clinical Child Psychology, 24,* 184–192.

Durham, S. R., Clancy, R. R., Leuthardt, E., Sun, P., Kamerling, S., Dominquez, T., et al. (2000). CHOP Infant Coma Scale ("Infant Face Scale"): A novel coma scale for children less than 2 years of age. *Journal of Neurotrauma, 17,* 729–737.

Ellemberg, D., Henry, L. C., Macciocchi, S. N., Guskiewicz, K. M., & Broglio, S. P. (2009). Advances in sports concussion assessment: From behavioral to brain imaging measures. *Journal of Neurotrauma, 26,* 2365–2382.

Faul, M., Xu, L., Wald, M. M., & Coronado, V. G. (2010). *Traumatic brain injury in the United States: Emergency department visits, hospitalizations, and deaths 2002–2006.* Atlanta, GA: Centers for Disease Control and Prevention, National Center for Injury Prevention and Control.

Fay, G. C., Jaffe, K. M., Polissar, N. L., Liao, S., Martin K. M., Shurtleff, H. A., et al. (1993). Mild pediatric traumatic brain injury: A cohort study. *Archives of Physical Medicine and Rehabilitation, 74,* 895–901.

Fay, T. B., Yeates, K. O., Taylor, H. G., Bangert, B., Dietrich, A., Nuss, K. E., et al. (2009). Cognitive reserve as a moderator of postconcussive symptoms in children with complicated and uncomplicated mild traumatic brain injury. *Journal of the International Neuropsychological Society, 16,* 94–105.

Field, M., Collins, M. W., Lovell, M. R., & Maroon, J. (2003). Does age play a role in recovery from sports-related concussion?: A comparison of high school and collegiate athletes. *Journal of Pediatrics, 142,* 546–553.

Francis, D. J., Fletcher, J. M., Stuebing, K. K., Davidson, K. C., & Thompson, N. M. (1991). Analysis of change: Modeling individual growth. *Journal of Consulting and Clinical Psychology, 59,* 27–37.

Gagnon, I., Galli, C., Friedman, D., Grilli, L., & Iverson, G. L. (2009). Active rehabilitation for children who are slow to recover following sport-related concussion. *Brain Injury, 23,* 956–964.

Ganesalingam, K., Yeates, K. O., Ginn, M. S., Taylor, H. G., Dietrich, A., Nuss, K., et al. (2008). Family burden and parental distress following mild traumatic brain injury in children and its relationship to post-concussive symptoms. *Journal of Pediatric Psychology, 33,* 621–629.

Gerring, J. P., Brady, K. D., Chen, A., Vasa, R., Grados, M., Bandeen-Roche, K. J., et al. (1998). Premorbid prevalence of ADHD and development of secondary ADHD after closed head injury. *Journal of the American Academy of Child and Adolescent Psychiatry, 37,* 647–654.

Gioia, G. A., Collins, M., & Isquith, P. K. (2008). Improving identification and diagnosis of mild traumatic brain injury with evidence: Psychometric support for the Acute Concussion Evaluation. *Journal of Head Trauma Rehabilitation, 23,* 230–242.

Gioia, G. A., Schneider, J. C., Vaughan, C. G., & Isquith, P. K. (2009). Which symptom assessments and approaches are uniquely appropriate for paediatric concussion? *British Journal of Sports Medicine, 43*(Suppl. I), i13–i22.

Giza, C. C., & Hovda, D. A. (2001). The neurometabolic cascade of concussion. *Journal of Athletic Training, 36,* 228–235.

Green, P. (2004). *Manual for Green's Medical Symptom Validity Test (MSVT).* Edmonton Alberta, Canada: Green's Publishing.

Gronwall, D., Wrightson, P., & McGinn, V. (1997). Effect of mild head injury during the preschool years. *Journal of the International Neuropsychological Society, 3,* 592–597.

Guskiewicz, K. M. (2001). Postural stability assessment following concussion: One piece of the puzzle. *Clinical Journal of Sports Medicine, 11,* 182–189.

Hajek, C. A., Yeates, K. O., Taylor, H. G., Bangert, B., Dietrich, A., Nuss, K., et al. (2010). Relationships among postconcussive symptoms and symptoms of PTSD in children following mild traumatic brain injury. *Brain Injury, 24,* 100–109.

Hajek, C. A., Yeates, K. O., Taylor, H. G., Bangert, B., Dietrich, A., Nuss, K. E., et al. (2011). Agreement between parents and children on ratings of postconcussive symptoms following mild traumatic brain injury. *Child Neuropsychology, 17,* 17–33

Hawley, C. A. (2003). Reported problems and their resolution following mild, moderate, and severe traumatic brain injury amongst children and adolescents in the UK. *Brain Injury, 17,* 105–129.

Hessen, E., Anderson, V., & Nestvold, K. (2008). MMPI-2 profiles 23 years after pediatric mild traumatic brain injury. *Brain Injury, 22,* 39–50.

Hessen, E., Nestvold, K., & Sundet, K. (2006). Neuropsychological function in a group of patients 25 years after sustaining minor head injuries as children and adolescents. *Scandinavian Journal of Psychology, 47,* 245–251.

Iverson, G. L., Brooks, B. L., Ashton, V. L., & Lange, R. T. (2010). Interview versus questionnaire symptom reporting in people with the postconcussion syndrome. *Journal of Head Trauma Rehabilitation, 25,* 23–30.

Iverson, G. L., Brooks, B. L., Collins, M. W., & Lovell, M. R. (2006). Tracking neuropsychological recovery following concussion in sport. *Brain Injury, 20,* 245–252.

Jordan, B. D. (2007). Genetic influences on outcome following traumatic brain injury. *Neurochemical Research, 32,* 905–915.

Kamerling, S. N., Lutz, N., Posner, J. C., & Vanore, M. (2003). Mild traumatic brain injury in children: Practice guidelines for emergency department and hospitalized patients. *Pediatric Emergency Care, 19,* 431–440.

Kashluba, S., Paniak, C., & Casey, J. E. (2008). Persistent symptoms associated with factors identified by the WHO Task Force on Mild Traumatic Brain Injury. *The Clinical Neuropsychologist, 22,* 195–208.

Kirkwood, M. W. (2012). Overview of tests and techniques to detect negative response bias in children. In E. M. S. Sherman & B. L. Brooks (Eds.), *Pediatric forensic neuropsychology* (pp. 136–161). New York: Oxford University Press.

Kirkwood, M. W. Yeates, K. O., Randolph, C., & Kirk, J. (2012). The implications of symptom validity test failure for ability-based test performance in a pediatric sample. *Psychological Assessment, 24,* 36–45.

Kirkwood, M. W., Yeates, K. O., Taylor, H. G., Randolph, C., McCrea, M., & Anderson, V. A. (2008). Management of pediatric mild traumatic brain injury: A neuropsychological review from injury through recovery. *The Clinical Neuropsychologist, 22,* 769–800.

Klonoff, H., Clark, C., & Klonoff, P. S. (1993). Long-term outcome of head injuries: A 23-year follow-up study of children with head injuries. *Journal of Neurology, Neurosurgery, and Psychiatry, 56*, 410–415.

Laursen, B., & Hoff, E. (2006). Person-centered and variable-centered approaches to longitudinal data. *Merrill–Palmer Quarterly, 52*, 377–389.

Levin, H. S., Hanten, G., Roberson, G., Li, X., Ewing-Cobbs, L., Dennis, M., et al. (2008). Prediction of cognitive sequelae based on abnormal computed tomography findings in children following mild traumatic brain injury. *Journal of Neurosurgery: Pediatrics, 1*, 461–470.

Light, R., Asarnow, R., Satz, P., Zucha, K., McCleary, C., & Lewis, R. (1998). Mild closed-head injury in children and adolescents: Behavior problems and academic outcomes. *Journal of Consulting and Clinical Psychology, 66*, 1023–1029.

Lishman, W. A. (1988). Physiogenesis and psychogenesis in the post-concussion syndrome. *British Journal of Psychiatry, 153*, 460–469.

Luis, C. A., & Mittenberg, W. (2002). Mood and anxiety disorders following pediatric traumatic brain injury: A prospective study. *Journal of Clinical and Experimental Neuropsychology, 24*, 270–279.

Luis, C. A., Vanderploeg, R. D., & Curtiss, G. (2003). Predictors of postconcussion symptom complex in community dwelling male veterans. *Journal of the International Neuropsychological Society, 9*, 1001–1015.

Massagli, T. L., Fann, J. R., Burington, B. E., Jaffe, K. M., Katon, W. J., & Thompson, R. S. (2004). Psychiatric illness after mild traumatic brain injury in children. *Archives of Physical Medicine and Rehabilitation, 85*, 1428–1434.

Max, J. E., Koele, S. L., Smith, W. L., Jr., Sato, Y., Lindgren, S. D., Robin, D. A., et al. (1998). Psychiatric disorders in children and adolescents after severe traumatic brain injury: A controlled study. *Journal of the American Academy of Child and Adolescent Psychiatry, 37*, 832–840.

McCauley, S. R., Wilde, E. A., Anderson, V. A., Bedell, G., Beers, S. R., Campbell, T. F., et al. (2012). Recommendations for the use of common outcome measures in pediatric traumatic brain injury research. *Journal of Neurotrauma, 29*, 678–705.

McCrea, M., Barr, W. B., Guskiewicz, K., Randolph, C., Marshall, S. W., Cantu, R., et al. (2005). Standard regression-based methods for measuring recovery after sport-related concussion. *Journal of the International Neuropsychological Society, 11*, 58–69.

McCrory, P., Meeuwisse, W., Johnston, K., Dvorak, J., Aubry, M., Molloy, M., et al. (2009). Consensus statement on concussion in sport 3rd international conference on concussion in sport held in Zurich, November 2008. *Clinical Journal of Sports Medicine, 19*, 185–195.

McKinlay, A. (2009). Controversies and outcomes associated with mild traumatic brain injury in childhood and adolescence. *Child: Care, Health, and Development, 36*, 3–21.

McKinlay, A., Dalrymple-Alford, J. C., Horwood, L. J., & Fergusson, D. M. (2002). Long-term psychosocial outcomes after mild head injury in early childhood. *Journal of Neurology, Neurosurgery, and Psychiatry, 73*, 281–288.

McKinlay, A., Grace, R. C., Horwood, L. J., Fergusson, D. M., & MacFarlane, M. R. (2010a). Long-term behavioural outcomes of pre-school mild traumatic brain injury. *Child: Care, Health, and Development, 36*, 22–30.

McKinlay, A., Kyonka, E. G. E., Grace, R. C., Horwood, L. J., Fergusson, D. M., & MacFarlane, M. R. (2010b). An investigation of the pre-injury risk factors associated with children who experience traumatic brain injury. *Injury Prevention, 16*, 31–35.

Mild Traumatic Brain Injury Committee of the Head Injury Interdisciplinary Special Interest Group of the American Congress of Rehabilitation Medicine. (1993). Definition of mild traumatic brain injury. *Journal of Head Trauma Rehabilitation, 8*, 86–87.

Mittenberg, W., DiGiulio, D. V., Perrin, S., & Bass, A. E. (1992). Symptoms following mild head injury: Expectation as aetiology. *Journal of Neurology, Neurosurgery, and Psychiatry, 55,* 200–204.

Mittenberg, W., Wittner M. S., & Miller, L. J. (1997). Postconcussion syndrome occurs in children. *Neuropsychology, 11,* 447–452.

Moran, L. M., Taylor, H. G., Ganesalingam, K., Gastier-Foster, J. M., Frick, J., Bangert, B., et al. (2009). Apolipoprotein E4 as a predictor of outcomes in pediatric mild traumatic brain injury. *Journal of Neurotrauma, 26,* 1489–1495.

Moran, L. M., Taylor, H. G., Rusin, J., Bangert, B., Dietrich, A., Nuss, K. E., et al. (in press). Quality of life in pediatric mild traumatic brain injury and its relationship to post-concussive symptoms. *Journal of Pediatric Psychology.*

Nacajauskaite, O., Endziniene, M., Jureniene, K., & Schrader, H. (2006). The validity of post-concussion syndrome in children: A controlled historical cohort study. *Brain and Development, 28,* 507–514.

Nagin, D. S. (2005). *Group-based modeling of development.* Cambridge, MA: Harvard University Press.

Nampiaparampil, D. E. (2008). Prevalence of chronic pain after traumatic brain injury: A systematic review. *Journal of the American Medical Association, 300,* 711–719.

Nestvold, K., Lundar, T., Blikra, G., & Lønnum, A. (1988). Head injuries during one year in a Central Hospital in Norway: A prospective study. *Neuroepidemiology, 7,* 134–144.

NIH Consensus Panel on Rehabilitation of Persons with Traumatic Brain Injury. (1999). Rehabilitation of persons with traumatic brain injury. *Journal of the American Medical Association, 282,* 974–983.

Nolin, P., Villemure, R., & Heroux, L. (2006). Determining long-term symptoms following mild traumatic brain injury: Method of interview affects self-report. *Brain Injury, 20,* 1147–1154.

Overweg-Plandsoen, W. C. G., Kodde, A., van Straaten, M., van der Linden, E. A. M., Neyens, L. G. J., Aldenkamp, A. P., et al. (1999). Mild closed head injury in children compared to traumatic fractured bone: Neurobehavioural sequelae in daily life 2 years after the accident. *European Journal of Pediatrics, 158,* 249–252.

Ponsford, J., Willmott, C., Rothwell, A., Cameron, P., Ayton, G., Nelms, R., et al. (1999). Cognitive and behavioral outcomes following mild traumatic head injury in children. *Journal of Head Trauma Rehabilitation, 14,* 360–372.

Ponsford, J., Willmott, C., Rothwell, A., Cameron, P., Ayton, G., Nelms, R., et al. (2001). Impact of early intervention on outcome after mild traumatic brain injury in children. *Pediatrics, 108,* 1297–1303.

Ponsford, J., Willmott, C., Rothwell, A., Cameron, P., Kelly, A.-M., Nelms, R., et al. (2000). Factors influencing outcome following mild traumatic brain injury in adults. *Journal of the International Neuropsychological Society, 6,* 568–579.

Powell, J. M., Ferraro, J. V., Dikmen, S. S., Temkin, N. R., & Bell, K. R. (2008). Accuracy of mild traumatic brain injury diagnosis. *Archives of Physical Medicine and Rehabilitation, 89,* 1550–1555.

Reynolds, C. R., & Kamphaus, R. W. (2004). *Behavior Assessment System for Children—Second Edition manual.* Circle Pines, MN: AGS Publishing.

Satz, P. (2001). Mild head injury in children and adolescents. *Current Directions in Psychological Science, 10,* 106–109.

Satz, P., Zaucha, K., McCleary, C., Light, R., & Asarnow, R. (1997). Mild head injury in children and adolescents: A review of studies (1970–1995). *Psychological Bulletin, 122,* 107–131.

Seidel, J. S., Henderson, D., Tittle, S., Jaffe, D. M., Spalte, D., Dean, J. M., et al. (1999). Priorities for research in emergency medical services for children: Results of a consensus conference. *Annals of Emergency Medicine, 33,* 206–210.

Steinberg, L., & Avenevoli, S. (2000). The role of context in the development of psychopathology: A conceptual framework and some speculative propositions. *Child Development*, *71*, 66–74.

Taylor, H. G., & Alden, J. (1997). Age-related differences in outcome following childhood brain injury: An introduction and overview. *Journal of the International Neuropsychological Society*, *3*, 555–567.

Taylor, H. G., Dietrich, A., Nuss, K., Wright, M., Rusin, J., Bangert, B., et al. (2010). Postconcussive symptoms in children with mild traumatic brain injury. *Neuropsychology*, *24*, 148–159.

Teasdale, G., & Jennett, B. (1974). Assessment of coma and impaired consciousness: A practical scale. *Lancet*, *2*, 81–84.

Wilde, E. A., McCauley, S. R., Hunger, J. V., Bigler, E. D., Chu, Z., Wang, Z. J., et al. (2008). Diffusion tensor imaging of acute mild traumatic brain injury in adolescents. *Neurology*, *70*, 948–955.

Williams, D. H., Levin, H. S., & Eisenberg, H. M. (1990). Mild head injury classification. *Neurosurgery*, *27*, 422–428.

Woodrome, S. E., Yeates, K. O., Taylor, H. G., Rusin, J., Bangert, B., Dietrich, A., et al. (2011). Coping strategies as a predictor of post-concussive symptoms in children with mild traumatic brain injury versus mild orthopedic injury. *Journal of the International Neuropsychological Society*, *17*, 317–326.

World Health Organization. (1992). *The ICD-10 classification of mental and behavioural disorders: Clinical descriptions and diagnostic guidelines*. Geneva: Author.

Yeates, K. O. (2010). Mild traumatic brain injury and postconcussive symptoms in children and adolescents. *Journal of the International Neuropsychological Society*, *16*, 953–960.

Yeates, K. O., Kaizar, E., Rusin, J., Bangert, B., Dietrich, A., Nuss, K., et al. (in press-a). Reliable change in post-concussive symptoms and its functional consequences among children with mild traumatic brain injury. *Archives of Pediatrics and Adolescent Medicine*.

Yeates, K. O., Luria, J., Bartkowski, H., Rusin, J., Martin, L., & Bigler, E. D. (1999). Postconcussive symptoms in children with mild closed-head injuries. *Journal of Head Trauma Rehabilitation*, *14*, 337–350.

Yeates, K. O., & Taylor, H. G. (2005). Neurobehavioural outcomes of mild head injury in children and adolescents. *Pediatric Rehabilitation*, *8*, 5–16.

Yeates, K. O., Taylor, H. G., Barry, C. T., Drotar, D., Wade, S. L., & Stancin, T. (2001). Neurobehavioral symptoms in childhood closed-head injuries: Changes in prevalence and correlates during the first year post injury. *Journal of Pediatric Psychology*, *26*, 79–91.

Yeates, K. O., Taylor, H. G., Drotar, D., Wade, S. L., Klein, S., Stancin, T., et al. (1997). Pre-injury family environment as a determinant of recovery from traumatic brain injuries in school-age children. *Journal of the International Neuropsychological Society*, *3*, 617–630.

Yeates, K. O., Taylor, H. G., Rusin, J., Bangert, B., Dietrich, A., Nuss, K., et al. (in press-b). Premorbid child and family functioning as predictors of post-concussive symptoms in children with mild traumatic brain injuries. *International Journal of Developmental Neuroscience*.

Yeates, K. O., Taylor, H. G., Rusin, J., Bangert, B., Dietrich, A., Nuss, K., et al. (2009). Longitudinal trajectories of post-concussive symptoms in children with mild traumatic brain injuries and their relationship to acute clinical status. *Pediatrics*, *123*, 735–743.

PART III

CLINICAL EVALUATION

CHAPTER 8

Biochemical Markers

Rachel P. Berger and Noel Zuckerbraun

A *biomarker* is an objectively measured and evaluated characteristic that is an indicator of normal biological processes, pathogenic processes, or pharmacological responses to a therapeutic intervention (Biomarkers Definitions Working Group, 2001). Physicians routinely use biomarkers in clinical practice to diagnose disease, assess disease severity, assist in disease prognosis, and evaluate treatment efficacy. Many types of biomarkers are used and depend on the organ being evaluated. For children with traumatic brain injury (TBI), for example, there are electrophysiological biomarkers (e.g., the absence of evoked potentials as a predictor of poor outcome after cardiac arrest; Fisher, Peterson, & Hicks, 1992), radiological biomarkers (e.g., *N*-acetylaspartate as an indicator of neuronal death; Giroud et al., 1996), and physiologic biomarkers (e.g., the Pediatric Risk of Mortality Score [PRISM] as predictor of mortality; Pollack, Ruttimann, & Getson, 1988). Although these biomarkers can be highly sensitive and specific, their measurement can be expensive, time-consuming, and invasive. In contrast, serum biomarkers offer the possibility of obtaining data through noninvasive and inexpensive means. Generally, injury and/or cell death results in increased concentrations of a given serum biomarker, either due to the release of that biomarker from the injured cell (e.g., creatine phosphokinase [CPK] in patients with myocardial infarction) or due to the lack of excretion of a normally excreted chemical that results in its accumulation (e.g., blood urea nitrogen in renal failure). In some cases, a decrease rather than an increase in a biomarker concentration indicates pathology (e.g., albumin in patients with liver failure).

For over 30 years, researchers have sought to develop serum brain biomarkers that could be used in the same way that serum markers of cardiac, liver, or renal injury are used. Development of a clinically acceptable brain biomarker, however, has proven much more difficult than the development of biomarkers for other organs. The difficulty is likely multifaceted and includes anatomical and physiological barriers as well as regulatory and legal barriers. The complexity of the brain and the concomitant complexity of its response to injury, for example, have been a formidable barrier to development of an accurate biomarker. The presence of the blood–brain barrier, which limits the amount and size of biomarkers that can cross into the serum, has also been a challenge. The current regulatory environment and the related process of obtaining Food and Drug Administration (FDA) approval for clinical use of novel biomarkers have also slowed the progression of potentially scientifically acceptable markers from the bench to the bedside (Oli et al., 2007; Rifai, Gillette, & Carr, 2006).

Initial studies related to serum biomarkers of brain injury were published in the late 1970s and described increases in two biomarkers: myelin-basic protein (MBP) and the brain-specific fraction of CPK, CPK-BB, in adults with severe TBI (Harwood, Catrou, & Cole, 1978; Karpman, Weinstein, Finley, & Karst-Sabin, 1981; Thomas, Palfreyman, & Ratcliffe, 1978). In the 1980s and even 1990s, adults with severe TBI remained the population of interest, although the biomarkers being studied changed. MBP and CPK-BB virtually disappeared from the literature and neuron-specific enolase (NSE) and S100B became the biomarkers of interest (Raabe et al., 1998; Raabe, Grolms, & Seifert, 1999; Woertgen, Rothoerl, Holzschuh, Metz, & Brawanski, 1997). With increasing awareness of the potential short- and long-term effects of mild TBI (mTBI) on adults, as well as the limitations of the Glasgow Coma Scale (GCS) and head computed tomography (CT) in the areas of diagnosis and assessment of injury severity and outcome prediction in mTBI, researchers began to shift their focus to adults with milder TBI. Interestingly, despite the change in the patient population from patients with severe TBI to those with mTBI, the biomarkers being studied remained the same (de Boussard et al., 2005; Ingebrigtsen et al., 2000; Mussack et al., 2000; Stalnacke, Tegner, & Sojka, 2003).

As with many aspects of medicine, interest in and investigation of serum biomarkers of brain injury in the pediatric population lagged significantly behind that in adults, and the earliest studies of serum brain biomarkers in children with TBI of any severity were not published until the early 2000s (Berger, Pierce, Wisniewski, Adelson, & Kochanek, 2002; Spinella et al., 2003). The literature related specifically to serum biomarkers in pediatric mTBI is limited and can be discussed almost in its entirety in this chapter. The goals of the current chapter are, therefore, to (1) discuss the potential clinical uses of serum biomarkers in children with mTBI, (2) review the existing pediatric literature as well as selected adult studies related to these clinical uses, and (3) propose future research questions and directions in this field.

It is helpful to divide the potential clinical uses of serum biomarkers in pediatric mTBI into categories that parallel the way in which the relevant clinical questions arise during the care of a child with possible mTBI. The clinical uses discussed below are areas in which some clinical research has been done; it is easy to foresee additional clinical scenarios in which biomarkers might be of use. The four clinical scenarios in which biomarkers may be helpful are (1) determining when an infant or young child with soft neurological signs (e.g., vomiting) but without a history of trauma needs to be evaluated for TBI (e.g., the biomarker as a "point-to-the-brain" test); (2) discriminating patients with a head injury (i.e., general trauma to the head without injury to the brain necessarily) from those with mTBI; (3) identifying children with mTBI who have a skull fracture and/or intracranial injury; and (4) predicting which children with mTBI are at greatest risk of developing long-term sequelae/ postconcussion syndrome.

Given the limited number of serum biomarkers that have been evaluated, a brief review of these biomarkers would be instructive prior to discussing the current literature (see Table 8.1). As mentioned above, the earliest serum biomarkers evaluated were MBP and CPK-BB. These markers were soon displaced by NSE and S100B. NSE is a glycolytic enzyme localized primarily to neuronal cytoplasm that is released when neurons are irreversibly injured or die. NSE is also present in small quantities in platelets and red blood cells. As a result, hemolysis of blood samples—a common occurrence in pediatrics—can result in false positive NSE concentrations. This remains an important limitation of this biomarker, although a recently published study reported on a methodology for adjusting NSE concentrations to account for the degree of hemolysis (Berger & Richichi, 2009).

The most well-studied biomarker in adults and children with TBI of all severities is S100B, the major low-affinity calcium-binding protein in astrocytes. It is released when astrocytes are irreversibly injured or die. The half-life of serum S100B is less than 100 minutes, and as a result, increases in serum S100B after mTBI are transient. Perhaps the most important limitation of S100B is its high normative concentrations in young children, particularly those less than 2 years of age (Berger et al., 2005, 2006; Portela et al., 2002). Because many healthy young children have S100B concentrations that, in adults, would be considered pathological, interpreting a single S100B concentration measured in a young child is difficult.

The only other brain-specific protein that has been measured in adults with mTBI is cleaved tau protein (c-tau; Bazarian, 2004; Begaz, Kyriacou, Segal, & Bazarian, 2006). Tau is a protein found in the axons of healthy neurons that binds to microtubules. TBI results in proteolysis of tau to c-tau. To date, no studies related to c-tau in children with mTBI have been published.

While the biomarkers discussed above are the only ones that have been studied in children, interest has recently focused on structural markers of axonal injury after mTBI, specifically, α-II spectrin and its degradation products, spectrin breakdown

TABLE 8.1. Characteristics of the Most Commonly Studied Biomarkers

Biochemical marker	Abbreviation	Location
Myelin-basic protein	MBP	Myelin
Creatine phosphokinase–brain-specific isoform	CPK-BB	Brain, lungs
Neuron-specific enolase	NSE	Neurons, platelets, red blood cells, neuroendocrine cells
S100β	NA	Astrocytes, chondrocytes, adipocytes
Cleaved tau	c-tau	Axons of central nervous system neurons, proteolytically cleaved after release to form c-tau
αII spectrin/spectrin breakdown degradation products 120, 145, and 150	SBDP 120, 145, and 150	Cortical membrane cytoskeletal protein breakdown products generated by calpain or caspase

products (SBDP) 120, 145, and 150. Although serum data for these markers are limited to several abstracts (Oli et al., 2007; Robicsek et al., 2007), the markers may hold potential for use in mTBI because impaired axonal function as well as ultrastructural axonal shearing changes are likely to be important in the pathophysiology of mTBI (Bazarian, Blyth, & Cimpello, 2006; Maxwell, Povlishock, & Graham, 1997).

USE OF SERUM BIOMARKERS AS A "POINT-TO-THE-BRAIN" TEST

In children who are old enough to communicate, in those whose head injury (HI) is witnessed and proximal to the time of the medical evaluation, and in cases in which there is obvious injury to the head/face, the diagnosis of HI can be made without difficulty. When there have been no witnesses to the HI and there are no obvious injuries to the head or face, however, occult HI must be considered in the differential diagnosis. In these situations, serum biomarkers would serve as a "point-to-the-brain" test, much the same way that liver function tests can direct the treating physician to the liver as a possible source of the patient's symptoms. For example, in cases of abusive head trauma (e.g., shaken baby syndrome), the caretaker may bring a child to medical attention for signs of HI such as vomiting or irritability, but without a history of trauma. The caretaker may not provide a history of trauma either because he or she is being deliberately evasive or because he or she is unaware that trauma has occurred. Without a history of trauma or external evidence of trauma, a physician is unlikely to even consider HI in the differential diagnosis of a vomiting or fussy infant. Yet if the diagnosis of abusive head trauma is missed and an infant is inadvertently returned to a violent environment, he or she may be reinjured or even killed (Jenny, Hymel, Ritzen, Reinert, & Hay, 1999). Alternatively, in cases in which a known HI occurred days or even weeks prior to presentation, it is often unclear whether the symptoms may be related to the HI or due to a separate and unrelated viral syndrome, which can also present with the same nonspecific symptoms.

Several studies have demonstrated that even well-appearing children with abusive head trauma have increases in serum biomarker concentrations. Berger et al. (2006) measured serum concentrations of NSE, S100B, and MBP in children < 1 year of age who presented to an emergency department (ED) for evaluation of a symptom that would be considered a soft neurological sign. These symptoms included vomiting without diarrhea, an apparent life-threatening event, irritability/fussiness, lethargy, or seizure-like activity. Head CT was performed at the discretion of the treating physician. All subjects were tracked until 1 year of age to evaluate for subsequent evidence of possible child abuse. Of the 98 subjects enrolled, 76% were not diagnosed with abusive head trauma at enrollment or during the follow-up period, 14% were diagnosed with abusive head trauma at the time of enrollment in the study, and 5% were diagnosed with nontraumatic brain injuries (e.g., hydrocephalus) at the time of enrollment. The remaining 5% of subjects were not diagnosed with abusive head trauma at the time of enrollment, but re-presented during the tracking period for possible child abuse. Overall, 11 of the 14 (79%) subjects with recognized abusive head trauma had an increase in either serum NSE or MBP, even though all these children were well appearing (GCS 15) and had no history of trauma. Interestingly, 80% (4/5) of the subjects who re-presented with possible abuse during the follow-up period had an increased serum NSE concentration at enrollment, suggesting that these may have been missed cases of HI. Using previously derived cutoffs for abnormal biomarker concentrations (Berger et al., 2005), NSE was 76% sensitive and 66% specific, and MBP was 36% sensitive and 100% specific for abusive head trauma. S100B was neither sensitive nor specific for abusive head trauma in this population.

In a more recent study that explored the possibility of using a panel of biomarkers to "point to the brain" (Berger, Ta'asan, Rand, Lokshin, & Kochanek, 2009), multiplex bead technology was used to evaluate the concentrations of 44 different serum biomarkers in children diagnosed with abusive head trauma who had a GCS score of 15 at presentation (cases) and in children of the same age who presented with the same symptoms but had a normal head CT (controls). There were significant group differences in the concentrations of 9 of the 44 markers screened: vascular cellular adhesion molecule, interleukin-12, matrix metallopeptidase-9, intracellular adhesion molecule, eotaxin, hepatocyte growth factor, tumor necrosis factor receptor 2, interleukin-6 and fibrinogen. A combination of interleukin-6, and vascular cellular adhesion molecule—the two markers with the most significant group differences—discriminated children with brain injury from those without brain injury with a sensitivity of 87% and a specificity of 90%. Unlike previous studies that focused exclusively on brain-specific markers of injury, this study explored non-brain-specific markers. The results suggest that differences exist in the biochemical profile between children in whom HI is the etiology of their symptoms and children with the same symptoms but with a noncranial etiology.

DISCRIMINATING HI FROM mTBI

An HI is defined very generally as trauma to the head. It includes injuries caused by falls from beds, falls down steps, and collisions between children. An HI may or may not result in any signs of impact, such as bruising or swelling to the scalp or face, or any symptoms. In the majority of cases, it does not even prompt medical attention. Only a fraction of children who have HI sustain mTBI. The ability to identify the small number of children with HI who have mTBI has important implications for sports and school and for risk of postconcussive symptoms/syndrome. Although identifying mTBI when it occurs is important, it is also important that every HI is not labeled as mTBI. In cases in which mTBI is a possibility, acute injury characteristics (if witnessed) and patient-reported symptoms are an integral part of the decision-making process. Neurocognitive testing can improve the diagnostic yield, but is often impractical in the acute clinical setting. Perhaps most importantly, all of these indicators are difficult to assess in young children because they cannot describe amnesia, nausea, or even headache. In these cases, an objective marker of mTBI would be helpful to clinicians evaluating children.

In the sole study that has specifically evaluated the ability of biomarkers to distinguish HI from mTBI, Geyer, Ulrich, Grafe, Stach, and Till (2009) measured serum S100B and NSE concentrations in 148 children, ages 6 months to 15 years, who were clinically diagnosed as having HI ($n = 53$) or mTBI ($n = 95$). Children were diagnosed with mTBI if they had an HI that was accompanied by symptoms such as loss of consciousness, amnesia, nausea, vomiting, somnolence, or dizziness. The authors found no significant difference in either NSE or S100B concentrations between the children with HI compared with mTBI. The authors concluded that NSE and S100B have "low sensitivity for detecting mTBI in children." This conclusion, however, may not be entirely accurate; the study did not have a control group (e.g., age-matched children without a history of any HI), and the NSE concentrations in both study groups were markedly higher than the reported normal values in adults and children.

IDENTIFICATION OF INTRACRANIAL INJURY IN CHILDREN WITH mTBI

Using biomarkers to identify intracranial injury after mTBI has been an area of active research for almost a decade (Biberthaler et al., 2001, 2006; Muller et al., 2007; Mussack et al., 2002; Romner, Ingebrigtsen, Kongstad, & Borgesen, 2000; Savola et al., 2004). In the largest multicenter study to date, 1,309 adults with mTBI—defined as a history of TBI, a GCS score of 13–15, and one or more clinical risk factors such as vomiting or severe headache—underwent head CT and measurement of serum S100B. S100B identified the subset with intracranial injury with 99% sensitivity and 30% specificity using a previously derived cutoff for S100B (Biberthaler et al., 2006). The authors concluded that the negative predictive value of an undetectable S100B serum level was 99% (i.e., there was a 99% probability that a patient with a normal S100B did not have intracranial injury). The authors also concluded that use of S100B in this context could result in a 30% decrease in the use of head CT without missing any cases of intracranial injury. As a result of this study and several others with similar findings, S100B is currently used in clinical practice in Europe in adults with mTBI (Unden & Romner, 2010).

The use of serum biomarkers in this clinical context is perhaps even more important in children than adults because of concerns about radiation risk from head CT in children (Brenner, Elliston, Hall, & Berdon, 2001; Brody, Frush, Huda, & Brent, 2007; Kirpalani & Nahmias, 2008). In the largest and most well-designed study to date, Castellani et al. (2009) measured serum S100B concentrations in 109 children with mTBI who underwent head CT as part of their clinical evaluation. An abnormal S100B concentration was set a priori. Thirty-six patients had either an intracranial injury or a skull fracture on head CT. The negative predictive value of a normal S100B was 100%, meaning that all children with an abnormal head CT had an abnormal S100B concentration. There were also 42 children with a normal head CT who had an abnormal S100B concentration. Therefore, use of S100B as a screening tool in this group of 109 children could have reduced the number of head CTs by 28%; of the 109 subjects enrolled, 31 (28%) had a negative S100B concentration and would not have needed to undergo head CT if S100B was used as a screening tool. This number is remarkably similar to the adult data described above, in which use of S100B would have reduced head CT use by 30%. The inclusion of skull fracture in the definition of an abnormal head CT and in the calculation of the sensitivity and negative predictive value of S100B in the study by Castellani and colleagues should be recognized.

In a study by Bechtel, Frasure, Marshall, Dziura, and Simpson (2009), serum S100B concentrations were measured in 152 children. Most of these children had mTBI, although some had more severe TBI. Twenty-four of these children had intracranial injury. Mean S100B concentrations were higher in children with intracranial injury compared to those without intracranial injury. They determined that at a concentration of 50 ng/L, there was a sensitivity of 75%, specificity of 56%, positive predictive value of 20%, and negative predictive value of 90% for detection of intracranial injury. Although these data suggest a possible use of S100B to identify intracranial injury in children with TBI, the way in which the data were presented does not allow for analysis of the subgroup of children with mTBI. Since almost all children with a GCS score < 15 would undergo head CT because of the known increased risk of intracranial injury in this population, S100B would not be needed to determine which children needed to undergo head CT. Another significant limitation of this study was the decision to maximize accuracy, rather than focusing on maximizing sensitivity. When used in this context, the negative predictive value of S100B would need to be at least 99% to be clinically acceptable. Therefore, the 90% negative predictive value reported in the study would not be acceptable in the clinical scenario in which a biomarker would determine which patients do *not* need to undergo head CT.

In the only pediatric study to date evaluating the use of NSE to predict intracranial injury, Fridriksson, Kini, Walsh-Kelly, and Hennes (2000) measured NSE concentration in 50 children ages 0–18 years with TBI. Not all of these children had mTBI; however, 45% of the subjects had intracranial injury. In this population, an increased serum NSE concentration was 77% sensitive and 52% specific for intracranial injury. Unfortunately, the authors did not report on the specificity of NSE at a sensitivity of 100% or provide the negative predictive value of a normal NSE. In addition, as mentioned above, not all subjects had mTBI. Table 8.2 summarizes the research in this area.

When reviewing studies related to the ability of biomarkers to identify intracranial injury, two important issues need to be considered: first, the way in which intracranial injury is defined; and second, what type of intracranial injury is important to identify. The majority of studies has defined intracranial injury by head CT, since this is the current gold standard for evaluation of intracranial injury. However, serum brain biomarkers are likely to be more sensitive than head CT for identification of subtle intracranial injury. The high sensitivity of serum markers would not be unique to brain injury; serum biomarkers are currently the reference standard for diagnosis of cardiac injury, for example (Lewandrowski, Chen, & Januzzi, 2002). As with heart or liver, the threshold for cellular brain injury is likely well below the threshold of imaging. In one of the earliest studies of biomarkers in adults with mTBI, Ingebrigtsen and colleagues measured serum S100B concentrations in 50 adults with mTBI and normal CT scans. In this study, 14 subjects (28%) had abnormal concentrations of serum S100B. Of these 14 patients, 4 had brain contusions visualized on MRI, leading the investigators to question whether S100B may be more sensitive than head CT (Ingebrigtsen, Waterloo, Jacobsen, Langbakk, & Romner, 1999). In the only pediatric study to address this issue, Akhtar Spear, Senac, Peterson, and Diaz (2003) measured serum S100B concentrations in 15 children with mTBI. All had a normal head CT. S100B concentrations were increased in 13 of the 15 children. Brain MRI was abnormal in 7 patients. The authors did not find a difference in the mean S100B concentration among subjects with an abnormal versus normal MRI. The authors concluded that S100B did not appear to be helpful in identifying those

TABLE 8.2. Identification of Children with Intracranial Injury after mTBI

Author (year)	Biomarker evaluated	Conclusions	Significant strengths	Significant weaknesses
Castellani et al. (2009)	S100B	NPV of a normal S100B was 100%—no children with skull fracture or ICI would have been missed.	Overall sample size large ($n = 109$) with 36 outcome events (abnormal head CT); all subjects underwent head CT; cutoff for abnormal S100B set a priori	None
Bechtel, Frasure, Marshall, Dziura, & Simpson (2009)	S100B	Mean S100B concentration higher in children with ICI vs. those without; at S100B concentration of 50 ng/L, there was a sensitivity of 75%, specificity of 56%, PPV of 20%, and NPV of 90% for identification of ICI.	Larger study ($n = 152$)	Not all subjects had mTBI; only 24 outcome events (ICI); statistical calculations maximized accuracy rather than the more clinically relevant NPV.
Fridriksson, Kini, Walsh-Kelly, & Hennes (2000)	NSE	An increased serum NSE concentration was 77% sensitive and 52% specific for ICI.	Sample size ($n = 50$); 45% with outcome of interest (ICI)	Not all subjects had mTBI; no calculation of specificity of NSE at a sensitivity of 100% or NPV of a normal NSE.

Note. ICI, intracranial injury; NPV, negative predictive value; NSE, neuron-specific enolase; PPV, positive predictive value.

patients with an abnormal brain MRI, although an accompanying editorial raised the issue of whether more sensitive imaging, such as diffusion tensor imaging, might better reflect the increases in serum S100B concentrations (Berger, 2003).

The second important issue is what type of intracranial injury is necessary to identify. In the study by Castellani and colleagues (2009) described above, isolated skull fractures were grouped with intracranial injury and considered abnormal for the purposes of identifying which children should undergo head CT. This methodology is in contrast to adult studies, which have not considered skull fracture to be an abnormality that needs to be identified. There are developmental reasons why identification of a skull fracture might be important in young children. Leptomeningeal cysts, for example, are a rare but well-recognized and potentially life-threatening complication of a skull fracture that are unique to young children (Scarfo, Mariottini, Tomaccini, & Palma, 1989). Identification of skull fracture is also important in the context of abusive head trauma. The type and/or location of skull fracture may be the only clue to the physician that the history of injury provided by the caretaker is not consistent with the injuries identified and that the child needs additional evaluation for possible child abuse. In the case of children with sports injuries, the presence of a skull fracture may alter return-to-play recommendations; return to play after a skull fracture routinely occurs 6 weeks after injury and is not dependent on mTBI symptoms. As a result, the recognition of skull fractures is crucial, so that return-to-play guidelines can be implemented appropriately to minimize the possibility of future injury.

OUTCOME PREDICTION AFTER mTBI

Although most children with mTBI recover with simple cognitive rest and a regulated return to sports, some children still have persistent or even worsening symptoms 1 year after injury and are at high risk for postconcussion syndrome. The ability to predict which children are at highest risk of having long-term sequelae would allow for initial selection of children for whom early rehabilitation would be most helpful. As a result, the potential use of biomarkers to predict complications and, specifically, postconcussion syndrome has been an active area of research. A recent review article identified 11 adult studies in which the ability of biomarkers to predict postconcussive symptoms was assessed (Begaz et al., 2006). The authors of the review article concluded that "no biomarker has consistently demonstrated the ability to predict post-concussive symptoms after mTBI" (p. 1201).

The pediatric literature specifically evaluating the ability of biomarkers to predict outcome after mTBI is limited. Berger, Beers, Richichi, Wiesman, and Adelson (2007) measured serial NSE, S100B, and MBP concentrations in children with TBI of all severities and assessed their ability to predict outcome as assessed by the Glasgow Outcome Scale (GOS). The results suggest that higher peak NSE, S100B, and MBP concentrations are associated with worse outcome. However, subjects with mTBI comprised only a subset of the study populations and were not analyzed independently of subjects with more severe injury. Importantly, all subjects in the study had intracranial injury. A study by Beers, Berger, and Adelson (2007) evaluated the ability of NSE, S100B, and MBP to predict neurocognitive outcome in children < 3 years of age with TBI. As with the previously discussed studies, children with mTBI made up only a subset of the subjects of the study. The results of the Beers study, however, are consistent with the study by Berger and colleagues and demonstrate that higher biomarker concentrations are associated with poorer neurocognitive outcome. In the only other pediatric study that included children with mTBI, Bandyopadhyay, Hennes, Gorelick, Wells, and Walsh-Kelly (2005) evaluated the ability of NSE to predict poor outcome (defined by GOS) after TBI. Of 86 children enrolled, 7 had poor outcome. An increased serum NSE concentration predicted poor outcome with 86% sensitivity and 74% specificity. There are no studies, to our knowledge, that have specifically investigated the ability of serum biomarkers to predict postconcussion symptoms after mTBI.

It is instructive to consider the way in which serum biomarkers would be used to predict outcome compared to the way in which they would be used in the context of predicting intracranial injury. In the context of predicting intracranial injury, the negative predictive value (i.e., the ability of a normal biomarker concentration to *exclude* intracranial injury) is the most relevant statistic. In the case of outcome prediction after mTBI, one might expect that the positive predictive value (i.e., the ability of an abnormal biomarker to *predict* postconcussive symptoms) would be a more relevant statistic since current standard of care is that patients receive additional rehabilitation only if they exhibit postconcussive symptoms. When comparing studies that address the same clinical scenario, it is important to recognize which statistic is being presented and which is most relevant in that specific situation.

There may also be biomarkers that confer a genetic predisposition to poor outcome after mTBI. Apolipoprotein E (ApoE) is produced by glial cells, including astrocytes, which are contained in the blood–brain barrier. Several adult studies have suggested that the ApoE ε4 allele is associated with poor prognosis and unfavorable outcome after TBI of all severities (Alexander et al., 2007; Chiang, Chang, & Hu, 2003; Sundstrom et al., 2004).

Two pediatric studies have investigated whether there may be a similar relationship between ApoE and outcome in children. A study by Brichtova and Kozak (2008) included 70 children with TBI of differing severities, including 15 children with mTBI. Outcome was assessed by the GOS score 1 year after injury. The authors concluded that children with the ApoE ε4 genotype were more likely to have unfavorable outcome. The authors did not specifically discuss the differences in outcome between the children with mTBI without the ε4 allele ($n = 10$) and those with the allele ($n = 5$), although in their discussion they did state that "in less severe head injuries, the ApoE ε4 genotype can indicate possible neuropsychological deficit and thus allow for establishment of early neuropsychological care" (p. 355).

A study by Moran and colleagues (2009) evaluated the relationship between ApoE ε4 and outcome at 2 weeks, 3 months, and 12 months after mTBI. Ninety-nine children between the ages of 8 and 15 years with mTBI were enrolled; 28 children had the ε4 allele. The authors found that children with the ε4 allele exhibited better performance on a test of constructional skill, but did not differ on any other neuropsychological tests or on measurements of postconcussive symptoms. Based on the data from these two studies, it is unclear whether ApoE genotyping may be helpful in identifying the subset of children with mTBI who are most likely to have long-term sequelae. Additional research is clearly needed. Table 8.3 summarizes this body of research.

One of the significant limitations in evaluating the ability of biomarkers to predict outcome after mTBI is the difficulty assessing outcome, particularly in preverbal children. If outcome cannot be accurately assessed, any correlation between biomarker concentrations and outcome will be difficult to interpret. For this reason, studies requiring assessment of outcome have focused on children 8 years of age and older, in whom postconcussive symptoms can be assessed using validated measures (Yeates et al., 1999, 2009).

OTHER ISSUES RELATED TO BIOMARKERS IN PEDIATRIC mTBI

Challenges for Future Research

Given the prevalence and morbidity of pediatric mTBI, the number of clinical studies related to biomarkers is surprisingly limited. The reasons for this are likely multifaceted, ranging from issues relevant to pediatric research in general to those related to research in the field of pediatric TBI overall. These issues include the relatively small

TABLE 8.3. Use of Biomarkers to Predict Outcome after mTBI

Author (year)	Biomarker(s) studied	Conclusions	Significant strengths	Significant weaknesses
Beers, Berger, & Adelson (2007)	NSE, S100B, MBP	Peak NSE and MBP concentration and time to peak NSE inversely correlated with GOS, VABS, and IQ 6 months after injury; time to peak S100B inversely correlated with IQ and VABS at 6 months.	More refined outcome criteria; multiple markers measured at > 1 time point	Not all subjects had mTBI; all children < 3 years of age; small sample size (*n* = 30)
Berger, Beers, Richichi, Wiesman, & Adelson (2007)	NSE, S100B, MBP	Higher peak NSE, S100B, and MBP concentrations are associated with worse outcome.	Large sample size (*n* = 152), multiple biomarkers measured at > 1 time point	Not all subjects had mTBI; gross outcome measure (GOS)
Bandyopadhyay, Hennes, Gorelick, Wells, & Walsh-Kelly (2005)	NSE	Significant difference in NSE between good and poor outcome groups.	Larger study (*n* = 86)	Single marker; gross outcome measure (GOS)
Brichtova & Kozak (2008)	ApoE	Children with ApoE ε4 genotype more likely to have unfavorable outcome.	First pediatric study, outcome assessed 1 year after injury	Sample size (*n* = 15 with mTBI within a larger population); outcome measure was gross (GOS score)
Moran et al. (2009)	ApoE	Better performance on test of constructional skill in children with ε4 allele; no other differences on neuropsychological tests or measures of postconcussive symptoms.	Large sample size (*n* = 99, 28 with ε4 allele), outcome assessed at 3 time points	Limited to ages 8–15 years

Note. GOS, Glasgow Outcome Scale; MBP, myelin-basic protein; NSE, neuron-specific enolase; VABS, Vineland Adaptive Behavior Scale score.

number of researchers and mentors in pediatric clinical research, the lack of a pediatric research infrastructure in many hospitals, ongoing issues related to the lack of funding for pediatric research, and Institutional Review Board concerns related to head CT and brain MRI that are often part of TBI-related research. The interested reader is referred to the pediatric section of a recent NIH Roundtable publication entitled, "Opportunities to Advance Research on Neurologic and Psychiatric Emergencies," which discusses these issues in more detail (D'Onofrio et al., 2010).

Some barriers are specific to pediatric biomarker research. Perhaps the most important one is the need to collect an adequate volume of serum to measure serum biomarkers. While collection of 5–10 mL of blood in adults is not difficult, this volume is unattainable in children, except perhaps in older teenagers. There are strict rules based on both subject weight and hemoglobin that dictate the amount of blood that can be collected. For example, in a 4-kg child, the total allowable blood volume in a single blood draw for research and clinical care is 8 mL; the total allowable blood volume is 16 mL in a 30-day period, for a combination of research and clinical care.

Obtaining parental and/or subject permission to collect blood can also be difficult. Since blood is not routinely collected as part of clinical care in children with mTBI, for example, it is necessary to obtain both consent and assent (when the child is old enough to participate in the consenting process) for blood to be drawn to measure biomarkers as part of a research study. Not surprisingly, the consent rate for blood collection for research is, anecdotally, low; parents of infants and young children are very hesitant to allow their child to undergo phlebotomy as part of a research study, and older children often do not assent.

There are also scientific issues related to biomarker research in children. Because children's brains are actively developing, biomarkers that are useful in infants may be different from those in school-age children or teenagers, and normative values may vary significantly by age. S100B is the most sensitive serum biomarker in adults. The inability to use it in young children because of high normative values, is just one example of the differences between children and adults (Berger et al., 2006). Furthermore, the types of injuries sustained by infants, toddlers, school-age children, and teenagers vary widely in their pathophysiology. As a result, the biomarkers that are useful in detecting abusive head trauma in infants are unlikely to be the same as the biomarkers that predict outcome after sports-related concussion in teenagers. For these reasons, clinical studies should be designed to include children of all ages and to age-match cases and controls.

Direction of Future Research

Future research in pediatric brain biomarkers is likely to focus on two primary areas: introduction of novel biomarkers and development of biomarker panels. Although the studies described in the current review article were performed over more than a decade, the number of different biomarkers that were evaluated is remarkably small. The biomarkers discussed above were initially pursued as possible markers of mTBI because their concentrations were increased after severe TBI and could be easily measured using an enzyme-linked immunoassay. The biochemical mechanisms that produced the biomarker changes were not, and in some cases are still not, well understood. Novel proteomic techniques, though technically difficult and markedly expensive, have greatly improved the ability to directly identify novel serum biomarkers of brain injury. Though significantly more research is needed, these new techniques have the potential to revolutionize the field of biomarker discovery. Details about the techniques used in neuroproteomics are beyond the scope of this chapter, but the interested reader is referred to two excellent review articles on the topic (Ottens et al., 2007; Wang et al., 2005). Over the next 10 years, growth in the field of neuroproteomics will likely result in a marked increase in the number of brain biomarkers that can be evaluated in both adults and children with mTBI.

As is clear from the current literature review, almost every study of biomarkers after pediatric and adult mTBI has focused on a single biomarker, most commonly S100B. Given the heterogeneity and complexity of mTBI, the different clinical scenarios in which biomarkers may be useful, and all the developmental issues discussed above, a single biomarker is unlikely to fulfill all of the clinical needs for children of all ages with mTBI. It is much more likely that several different types of biomarkers with varying kinetics and specificities for different parts of the brain will be needed. The strategy of using a panel of markers is being employed in adults to identify stroke (Lynch et al., 2004; Reynolds et al., 2003; Sotgiu et al., 2006) and cardiac disease (McCann et al., 2009). The only pediatric biomarker study of children with mTBI that evaluated combinations of biomarkers is the study by Berger et al. (2009).

In conclusion, the field of biomarkers in pediatric mTBI is in its infancy. The number of studies, the number of subjects, and the number of biomarkers that have been evaluated are all very limited. Although advances in the field of biomarkers in adult mTBI can help to advance the field considerably, more pediatric-specific studies are badly needed. Issues related to developmental changes in the pediatric brain, differences in outcome assessment in children versus adults, and differences in etiology of injuries between adults and children all need to be addressed in pediatric studies. Finally, the relatively new field of neuroproteomics has the potential to bring novel pediatric-specific biomarkers to the research arena and, eventually, to children as part of clinical care.

ACKNOWLEDGMENT

We would like to thank Haley Stutz for her assistance in formatting and revising the chapter.

REFERENCES

Akhtar, J. I., Spear, R. M., Senac, M. O., Peterson, B. M., & Diaz, S. M. (2003). Detection of traumatic brain injury with magnetic resonance imaging and S-100B protein in children, despite normal computed tomography of the brain. *Pediatric Critical Care Medicine*, 4(3), 322–326.

Alexander, S., Kerr, M. E., Kim, Y., Kamboh, M. I., Beers, S. R., & Conley, Y. P. (2007). Apolipoprotein E4 allele presence and functional outcome after severe traumatic brain injury. *Journal of Neurotrauma*, 24(5), 790–797.

Bandyopadhyay, S., Hennes, H., Gorelick, M. H., Wells, R. G., & Walsh-Kelly, C. M. (2005). Serum neuron-specific enolase as a predictor of short-term outcome in children with closed traumatic brain injury. *Academic Emergency Medicine*, 12(8), 732–738.

Bazarian, J. (2004). The accuracy of mild traumatic brain injury surveillance using retrospective case ascertainment by ICD-9 codes. *Academic Emergency Medicine*, 11(5), 568.

Bazarian, J. J., Blyth, B., & Cimpello, L. (2006). Bench to bedside: Evidence for brain injury after concussion—looking beyond the computed tomography scan. *Academic Emergency Medicine*, 13(2), 199–214.

Bechtel, K., Frasure, S., Marshall, C., Dziura, J., & Simpson, C. (2009). Relationship of serum S100B levels and intracranial injury in children with closed head trauma. *Pediatrics*, 124(4), e697–e704.

Beers, S. R., Berger, R. P., & Adelson, P. D. (2007). Neurocognitive outcome and serum biomarkers in inflicted versus non-inflicted traumatic brain injury in young children. *Journal of Neurotrauma*, 24(1), 97–105.

Begaz, T., Kyriacou, D. N., Segal, J., & Bazarian, J. J. (2006). Serum biochemical markers for post-concussion syndrome in patients with mild traumatic brain injury. *Journal of Neurotrauma, 23*(8), 1201–1210.

Berger, R. P. (2003). Biomarkers or neuroimaging in central nervous system injury: Will the real "gold standard" please stand up? *Pediatric Critical Care Medicine, 4*(3), 391–392.

Berger, R. P., Adelson, P. D., Pierce, M. C., Dulani, T., Cassidy, L. D., & Kochanek, P. M. (2005). Serum neuron-specific enolase, S100B, and myelin basic protein concentrations after inflicted and noninflicted traumatic brain injury in children. *Journal of Neurosurgery, 103*(1, Suppl.), 61–68.

Berger, R. P., Beers, S. R., Richichi, R., Wiesman, D., & Adelson, P. D. (2007). Serum biomarker concentrations and outcome after pediatric traumatic brain injury. *Journal of Neurotrauma, 24*(12), 1793–1801.

Berger, R. P., Dulani, T., Adelson, P. D., Leventhal, J. M., Richichi, R., & Kochanek, P. M. (2006). Identification of inflicted traumatic brain injury in well-appearing infants using serum and cerebrospinal markers: A possible screening tool. *Pediatrics, 117*(2), 325–332.

Berger, R. P., Pierce, M. C., Wisniewski, S. R., Adelson, P. D., & Kochanek, P. M. (2002). Serum S100B concentrations are increased after closed head injury in children: A preliminary study. *Journal Neurotrauma, 19*(11), 1405–1409.

Berger, R. P., & Richichi, R. (2009). Derivation and validation of an equation for adjustment of neuron-specific enolase concentrations in hemolyzed serum. *Pediatric Critical Care Medicine, 10*(2), 260–263.

Berger, R. P., Ta'asan, S., Rand, A., Lokshin, A., & Kochanek, P. (2009). Multiplex assessment of serum biomarker concentrations in well-appearing children with inflicted traumatic brain injury. *Pediatric Research, 65*(1), 97–102.

Biberthaler, P., Linsenmeier, U., Pfeifer, K. J., Kroetz, M., Mussack, T., Kanz, K. G., et al. (2006). Serum S-100B concentration provides additional information for the indication of computed tomography in patients after minor head injury: A prospective multicenter study. *Shock, 25*(5), 446–453.

Biberthaler, P., Mussack, T., Wiedemann, E., Gilg, T., Soyka, M., Koller, G., et al. (2001). Elevated serum levels of S-100B reflect the extent of brain injury in alcohol intoxicated patients after mild head trauma. *Shock, 16*(2), 97–101.

Biomarkers Definitions Working Group. (2001). Biomarkers and surrogate endpoints: Preferred definitions and conceptual framework. *Clinical Pharmacology and Therapeutics, 69*, 89–95.

Brenner, D., Elliston, C., Hall, E., & Berdon, W. (2001). Estimated risks of radiation-induced fatal cancer from pediatric CT. *American Journal of Roentgenology, 176*(2), 289–296.

Brichtova, E., & Kozak, L. (2008). Apolipoprotein E genotype and traumatic brain injury in children: Association with neurological outcome. *Child's Nervous System, 24*(3), 349–356.

Brody, A. S., Frush, D. P., Huda, W., & Brent, R. L. (2007). Radiation risk to children from computed tomography. *Pediatrics, 120*(3), 677–682.

Castellani, C., Bimbashi, P., Ruttenstock, E., Sacherer, P., Stojakovic, T., & Weinberg, A. M. (2009). Neuroprotein S-100B: A useful parameter in paediatric patients with mild traumatic brain injury? *Acta Paediatrica, 98*(10), 1607–1612.

Chiang, M. F., Chang, J. G., & Hu, C. J. (2003). Association between apolipoprotein E genotype and outcome of traumatic brain injury. *Acta Neurochirurgica, 145*(8), 649–653; discussion, 653–654.

de Boussard, C. N., Lundin, A., Karlstedt, D., Edman, G., Bartfai, A., & Borg, J. (2005). S100 and cognitive impairment after mild traumatic brain injury. *Journal of Rehabilitation Medicine, 37*(1), 53–57.

D'Onofrio, G., Jauch, E., Jagoda, A., Allen, M. H., Anglin, D., Barsan, W. G., et al. (2010).

NIH roundtable on opportunities to advance research on neurologic and psychiatric emergencies. *Annals of Emergency Medicine, 56*(5), 551–564.

Fisher, B., Peterson, B., & Hicks, G. (1992). Use of brainstem auditory-evoked response testing to assess neurologic outcome following near drowning in children. *Critical Care Medicine, 20*(5), 578–585.

Fridriksson, T., Kini, N., Walsh-Kelly, C., & Hennes, H. (2000). Serum neuron-specific enolase as a predictor of intracranial lesions in children with head trauma: A pilot study. *Academic Emergency Medicine, 7*(7), 816–820.

Geyer, C., Ulrich, A., Grafe, G., Stach, B., & Till, H. (2009). Diagnostic value of S100B and neuron-specific enolase in mild pediatric traumatic brain injury. *Journal of Neurosurgery–Pediatrics, 4*(4), 339–344.

Giroud, M., Walker, P., Bernard, D., Lemesle, M., Martin, D., Baudouin, N., et al. (1996). Reduced brain N-acetyl-aspartate in frontal lobes suggests neuronal loss in patients with amyotrophic lateral sclerosis. *Neurological Research, 18*(3), 241–243.

Harwood, S. J., Catrou, P. G., & Cole, G. W. (1978). Creatine phosphokinase isoenzyme fractions in the serum of a patient struck by lightning. *Archives of Internal Medicine, 138*(4), 645–646.

Ingebrigtsen, T., Romner, B., Marup-Jensen, S., Dons, M., Lundqvist, C., Bellner, J., et al. (2000). The clinical value of serum S-100 protein measurements in minor head injury: A Scandinavian multicentre study. *Brain Injury, 14*(12), 1047–1055.

Ingebrigtsen, T., Waterloo, K., Jacobsen, E. A., Langbakk, B., & Romner, B. (1999). Traumatic brain damage in minor head injury: Relation of serum S-100 protein measurements to magnetic resonance imaging and neurobehavioral outcome. *Neurosurgery, 45*(3), 468–475; discussion, 475–476.

Jenny, C., Hymel, K. P., Ritzen, A., Reinert, S. E., & Hay, T. C. (1999). Analysis of missed cases of abusive head trauma. *Journal of the American Medical Association, 281*(7), 621–626.

Karpman, R. R., Weinstein, P. R., Finley, P. R., & Karst-Sabin, B. (1981). Serum CPK isoenzyme BB as an indicator of brain tissue damage following head injury. *Journal of Trauma, 21*(2), 148–151.

Kirpalani, H., & Nahmias, C. (2008). Radiation risk to children from computed tomography. *Pediatrics, 121*(2), 449–450.

Lewandrowski, K., Chen, A., & Januzzi, J. (2002). Cardiac markers for myocardial infarction: A brief review. *American Journal of Clinical Pathology, 118*(Suppl.), S93–S99.

Lynch, J. R., Blessing, R., White, W. D., Grocott, H. P., Newman, M. F., & Laskowitz, D. T. (2004). Novel diagnostic test for acute stroke. *Stroke, 35*(1), 57–63.

Maxwell, W. L., Povlishock, J. T., & Graham, D. L. (1997). A mechanistic analysis of nondisruptive axonal injury: A review. *Journal of Neurotrauma, 14*(7), 419–440.

McCann, C. J., Glover, B. M., Menown, I. B., Moore, M. J., McEneny, J., Owens, C. G., et al. (2009). Prognostic value of a multimarker approach for patients presenting to hospital with acute chest pain. *The American Journal of Cardiology, 103*(1), 22–28.

Moran, L. M., Taylor, H. G., Ganesaligam, K., Gastier-Foster, J. M., Frick, J., Bangert, B., et al. (2009). Apolipoprotein E4 as a predictor of outcomes in pediatric mild traumatic brain injury. *Journal of Neurotrauma, 26*(9), 1489–1495.

Muller, K., Townend, W., Biasca, N., Unden, J., Waterloo, K., Romner, B., et al. (2007). S100B serum level predicts computed tomography findings after minor head injury. *Journal of Trauma, 62*(6), 1452–1456.

Mussack, T., Biberthaler, P., Wiedemann, E., Kanz, K. G., Englert, A., Gippner-Steppert, C., et al. (2000). S-100b as a screening marker of the severity of minor head trauma (MHT)—a pilot study. *Acta Neurochirurgica Supplementum, 76*, 393–396.

Mussack, T., Biberthaler, P., Kanz, K. G., Heckl, U., Gruber, R., Linsenmaier, U., et al. (2002). Immediate S-100B and neuron-specific enolase plasma measurements for rapid evaluation of primary brain damage in alcohol-intoxicated, minor head-injured patients. *Shock, 18*(5), 395–400.

Oli, M., Akinyi, L., Mo, J., Scharf, D., Robicsek, S., Gabrielli, A., et al. (2007). *Development and validation of novel brain biomarker assays.* St. Pete Beach, FL: Advanced Technology for Combat Casualty Care (ATACCC).

Ottens, A. K., Kobeissy, F. H., Fuller, B. F., Liu, M. C., Oli, M. W., Hayes, R. L., et al. (2007). Novel neuroproteomic approaches to studying traumatic brain injury. *Progress in Brain Research, 161,* 401–418.

Pollack, M. M., Ruttimann, U. E., & Getson, P. R. (1988). Pediatric risk of mortality (PRISM) score. *Critical Care Medicine, 16*(11), 1110–1116.

Portela, L. V., Tort, A. B., Schaf, D. V., Ribeiro, L., Nora, D. B., Walz, R., et al. (2002). The serum S100B concentration is age dependent. *Clinical Chemistry, 48*(6, Pt. 1), 950–952.

Raabe, A., Grolms, C., Keller, M., Dohnert, J., Sorge, O., & Seifert, V. (1998). Correlation of computed tomography findings and serum brain damage markers following severe head injury. *Acta Neurochirurgica, 140*(8), 787–791; discussion, 791–792.

Raabe, A., Grolms, C., & Seifert, V. (1999). Serum markers of brain damage and outcome prediction in patients after severe head injury. *British Journal of Neurosurgery, 13*(1), 56–59.

Reynolds, M. A., Kirchick, H. J., Dahlen, J. R., Anderberg, J. M., McPherson, P. H., Nakamura, K. K., et al. (2003). Early biomarkers of stroke. *Clinical Chemistry, 49*(10), 1733–1739.

Rifai, N., Gillette, M. A., & Carr, S. A. (2006). Protein biomarker discovery and validation: The long and uncertain path to clinical utility. *Nature Biotechnology, 24*(8), 971–983.

Robicsek, S., Gabrielli, A., Layon, A., Wishin, J., Akinyi, L., Mo, J., et al. (2007). BANDITS: A novel clinical platform to validate the utility of potential brain injury biomarkers: Case study #1. *25th National Neurotrauma Symposium, 18.*

Romner, B., Ingebrigtsen, T., Kongstad, P., & Borgesen, S. E. (2000). Traumatic brain damage: Serum S-100 protein measurements related to neuroradiological findings. *Journal of Neurotrauma, 17*(8), 641–647.

Savola, O., Pyhtinen, J., Leino, T. K., Siitonen, S., Niemela, O., & Hillbom, M. (2004). Effects of head and extracranial injuries on serum protein S100B levels in trauma patients. *Journal of Trauma, 56*(6), 1229–1234.

Scarfo, G. B., Mariottini, A., Tomaccini, D., & Palma, L. (1989). Growing skull fractures: Progressive evolution of brain damage and effectiveness of surgical treatment. *Child's Nervous System, 5*(3), 163–167.

Sotgiu, S., Zanda, B., Marchetti, B., Fois, M. L., Arru, G., Pes, G. M., et al. (2006). Inflammatory biomarkers in blood of patients with acute brain ischemia. *European Journal of Neurology, 13*(5), 505–513.

Spinella, P. C., Dominguez, T., Drott, H. R., Huh, J., McCormick, L., Rajendra, A., et al. (2003). S-100beta protein-serum levels in healthy children and its association with outcome in pediatric traumatic brain injury. *Critical Care Medicine, 31*(3), 939–945.

Stalnacke, B. M., Tegner, Y., & Sojka, P. (2003). Playing ice hockey and basketball increases serum levels of S-100B in elite players: A pilot study. *Clinical Journal of Sport Medicine, 13*(5), 292–302.

Sundstrom, A., Marklund, P., Nilsson, L. G., Cruts, M., Adolfsson, R., Van Broeckhoven, C., et al. (2004). APOE influences on neuropsychological function after mild head injury: Within-person comparisons. *Neurology, 62*(11), 1963–1966.

Thomas, D. G., Palfreyman, J. W., & Ratcliffe, J. G. (1978). Serum-myelin-basic-protein assay in diagnosis and prognosis of patients with head injury. *Lancet, 1*(8056), 113–115.

Unden, J., & Romner, B. (2010). Can low serum levels of S100B predict normal CT findings after minor head injury in adults?: An evidence-based review and meta-analysis. *Journal of Head Trauma Rehabilitation, 25*(4), 228–240.

Wang, K. K., Ottens, A. K., Liu, M. C., Lewis, S. B., Meegan, C., Oli, M. W., et al. (2005). Proteomic identification of biomarkers of traumatic brain injury. *Expert Review of Proteomics, 2*(4), 603–614.

Woertgen, C., Rothoerl, R. D., Holzschuh, M., Metz, C., & Brawanski, A. (1997). Comparison of serial S-100 and NSE serum measurements after severe head injury. *Acta Neurochirurgica, 139*(12), 1161–1164; discussion, 1165.

Yeates, K. O., Taylor, H. G., Rusin, J., Bangert, B., Dietrich, A., Nuss, K., et al. (2009). Longitudinal trajectories of postconcussive symptoms in children with mild traumatic brain injuries and their relationship to acute clinical status. *Pediatrics, 123*(3), 735–743.

Yeates, K. O., Luria, J., Bartkowski, H., Rusin, J., Martin, L., & Bigler, E. D. (1999). Postconcussive symptoms in children with mild closed head injuries. *Journal of Head Trauma Rehabilitation, 14*(4), 337–350.

CHAPTER 9

Neuroimaging

Stephen Ashwal, Karen A. Tong, Brenda Bartnik-Olson, and Barbara A. Holshouser

The role of neuroimaging in the evaluation of children with mild traumatic brain injury (mTBI) has evolved over the past decade as computed tomography (CT) and magnetic resonance imaging (MRI) are increasingly utilized. CT was initially used to determine whether a child had an intracranial injury (ICI) that required neurosurgical management. Subsequently, CT helped determine whether a child could safely be discharged from the emergency department or required hospitalization for continued observation as well as to assess a risk of long-term deficits. This application of CT technology led to an increasing number of scans, questions about their cost-effectiveness, and development of decision rules (i.e., tools designed to help clinicians make bedside diagnostic and therapeutic decisions) to increase the diagnostic yield for ICI, although no consensus has been reached as to which set(s) of rules is optimal. In this chapter, we review recent data regarding the yield of CT, particularly related to clinical decision rules for ordering a scan. We also review the limited data regarding the use of MRI in cases of pediatric mTBI, in particular, advanced imaging sequences such as diffusion weighted imaging (DWI), diffusion tensor imaging (DTI), MR spectroscopy, and susceptibility weighted imaging (SWI). We conclude the chapter with a discussion of the roles of CT and MRI in helping to define subcategories of mTBI within the context of a proposed imaging algorithm.

COMPUTED TOMOGRAPHY

Although the role of CT is well established for children who have moderate to severe TBI (Ashwal, Holshouser, & Tong, 2006; Klig & Kaplan, 2010; Kuppermann, 2008), its application for infants and children with mTBI continues to be explored. At issue is the possibility that children presenting to the emergency department may appear normal or have relatively minor neurological or neuropsychological complaints and limited, if any, neurological findings on examination. Yet a small but definite percentage of these children (4–7%) will have imaging abnormalities that, on occasion, prompt neurosurgical management (0.5%) or hospitalization, or are associated with some degree of long-term neuropsychological or neurological impairment (Haydel, 2005; Osmond et al., 2010). For all pediatric patients, CT has been recommended for children with Glasgow Coma Scale (GCS) scores reflecting moderate or severe injury (i.e., GCS < 13), but to date, no agreement has been reached as to which children with mTBI (GCS 13–15) require CT scanning.

Decision Rule Algorithms for Children with mTBI

Although some studies have suggested that clinical findings may identify children at low risk for ICI as detected by CT, other investigators have suggested that specific clinical findings may be insufficient for this purpose and that CT may be underutilized (Palchak et al., 2003). However, there has been increasing concern about the use of CT scans because of long-term risks of malignancy associated with radiation exposure from CT (Klig & Kaplan, 2010). Studies have estimated that the lifetime risk of mortality from leukemia or solid organ malignancy from a single pediatric head CT ranges from approximately 1:2,000 for infants to 1:5,000 for older children (Brenner, 2002). In addition, there are frequently forgotten potential life-threatening risks in the transportation and sedation of children for procedures. Costs generated from increased staff time for observation and monitoring of sedated children cannot be disregarded as well. Additional concerns have been raised that some of the decision rules have been applied to very young (preverbal) children under age 2 years, but rely on variables (e.g., eliciting a history of amnesia, headache, or loss of consciousness) which may not be applicable in this age group (Beaudin, Saint-Vil, Ouimet, Mercier, & Crevier, 2007).

Several studies have investigated the use of decision rules for children with "all," "moderate/severe," or "mild" TBI, and these data have been reviewed by Maguire and colleagues (Maguire, Boutis, Uleryk, Laupacis, & Parkin, 2009). As they highlight, rules derived from children who have a range of injury severity have limited utility, because in the setting of major head trauma, pediatric emergency physicians are likely to order CT scanning regardless of the recommendations of a clinical prediction rule, and thus decision rules are potentially more useful for children with mTBI. However, recent studies from the Pediatric Emergency Care Applied Research Network (PECARN) clearly showed that decision rules can be highly accurate and valuable for children with all degrees of injury severity (Jones, Patrick, & Hickner, 2010; Kuppermann et al., 2009). This study, for children under 2 years of age, demonstrated a 100% negative predictive value and 100% sensitivity for a clinically important TBI; and for children older than age 2 years, the negative predictive value was 99.95%, with a sensitivity of 96.8%.

At least five studies (presented in Table 9.1) contain data applying different sets of decision rules to children with mTBI (Atabaki et al., 2008; Dunning et al., 2006; Haydel, 2005; Haydel & Shembekar, 2003; Osmond et al., 2010; Palchak et al., 2003). Overall, use of these screening algorithms had a positive diagnostic yield between 4.1

TABLE 9.1. Studies That Developed Performance Rules in Children with mTBI

Author (year)	Study design	Study definition of mTBI	Definition of intracranial injury	Rule elements[a]	% children with ICI on CT scan when CT done	% ICI correctly predicted by rule
Haydel and Shembekar (2003)	Prospective (N = 175). Study dates: not given but duration of 30 months. Level I trauma center. Mean age = 12.8 years.	Blunt head trauma with loss of consciousness and a GCS 15.	Any acute traumatic intracranial lesion, including subdural, epidural, or parenchymal hematoma; subarachnoid hemorrhage; cerebral contusion; or depressed skull fractures.	• Headache • Vomiting • Drug or alcohol intoxication • Short-term memory deficits • Posttraumatic seizure • Physical evidence of trauma above the clavicles	8%	100%
Palchak et al. (2003)	Prospective (N = 1,098). Study dates: 7/98–9/01. Peds ED from a Level I trauma center. Mean age = 8.3 years.	History of nontrivial blunt head trauma, with history or physical examination findings consistent with head trauma and GCS 14–15.	ICI defined by the presence of intracranial hemorrhage, hematoma, or cerebral edema.	• Abnormal mental status • Clinical signs of skull fracture • Scalp hematoma in children ages ≤ 2 years • A history of vomiting	7.7%	94.9%
Dunning et al. (2006)	Prospective (N = 22,298) with GCS scores in the 13–15 range. Study dates: 2/00–8/02. 10 hospitals in the northwest of	mTBI included any child with a history or signs of head injury with GCS 13–15.	Any new, acute, traumatic intracranial pathology as reported by the consultant radiologist, including intracranial hematomas of any size, cerebral	*History* Witnessed loss of consciousness of > 5 minutes' duration. History of amnesia (either anterograde or retrograde) of > 5 minutes' duration. Abnormal drowsiness (defined as drowsiness in excess of that expected by the	5.44%	97.6%

164

(cont.)

England. Mean age = 5.7 years. Study not limited to mTBI but to all patients. Used CHALICE rule.

contusion, diffuse cerebral edema, and depressed skull fractures.

examining doctor). ≥ 3 vomits after head injury (a vomit is defined as a single, discrete episode of vomiting). Suspicion of nonaccidental injury (NAI, defined as any suspicion of NAI by the examining doctor). Seizure after head injury in a patient who has no history of epilepsy.

Examination

GCS < 14, or if < 1 year old GCS < 15. Suspicion of penetrating or depressed skull injury or tense fontanel. Signs of a basal skull fracture (defined as evidence of blood or cerebrospinal fluid from ear or nose, panda eyes, Battle's sign, hemotympanum, facial crepitus, or serious facial injury). Positive focal neurology (defined as any focal neurology, including motor, sensory, coordination, or reflex abnormality). Presence of bruise, swelling, or laceration > 5 cm if < 1 year old.

Mechanism

High-speed road traffic accident as pedestrian, cyclist or occupant (defined as accident with speed > 40 miles/hour). Fall of > 3 meters in height. High-speed injury from a projectile or an object.

TABLE 9.1. (cont.)

Author (year)	Study design	Study definition of mTBI	Definition of intracranial injury	Rule elements[a]	% children with ICI on CT scan when CT done	% ICI correctly predicted by rule
Atabaki et al. (2008)	Prospective (N = 1,000). Study dates: 3/97–3/00. Four Level I Peds trauma centers. Mean age = 8.9 years.	GCS 13–15	Presence of subdural, epidural, subarachnoid, intraparenchymal, and intraventricular hemorrhages, as well as contusions and cerebral edema.	• Dizziness • Skull defect • Sensory deficit • Mental status change • Bicycle-related injury • Age younger than 2 years • GCS < 15 • Evidence of a basilar skull fracture	6.5%	95.4%
Osmond et al. (2010)	Prospective (N = 3,866) patients. Mean age = 9.2 years. Study dates: 7/01–11/05. 10 Canadian Peds teaching institutions. Used CATCH rule.	History of (1) blunt head trauma resulting in witnessed loss of consciousness, definite amnesia, witnessed disorientation, persistent vomiting (two or more distinct episodes of vomiting 15 minutes apart) or persistent irritability in ED (for children under 2 years of age); (2) initial GCS ED score of at least 13; (3) injury within the past 24 hours.	ICI defined as any acute CT finding attributable to acute injury, including closed depressed skull fracture (i.e., depressed past the inner table) and pneumocephalus, but excluding nondepressed skull fractures and basilar skull fractures	*High risk* (need for neurologic intervention) • GCS < 15 at 2 hours after injury • Suspected open or depressed skull fracture • History of worsening headache • Irritability on examination *Medium risk* (brain injury on CT scan) • Any sign of basal skull fracture (e.g., hemotympanum, "raccoon" eyes, otorrhea or rhinorrhea of the cerebrospinal fluid, Battle's sign) • Large, boggy hematoma of the scalp • Dangerous mechanism of injury (e.g., motor vehicle crash, fall from elevation ≥ 3 feet [≥ 91 cm] or five stairs, fall from bicycle with no helmet)	4.1%	98.1%

Note. Data based on Maguire, Boutis, Uleryk, Laupacis, and Parkin (2009). Peds, pediatric; ED, emergency department; GCS, Glasgow Coma Scale; ICI, intracranial injury.
[a] A CT scan is required if any of the criteria are present. If none are present, the patient is at low risk of intracranial pathology.

and 8.0%, with sensitivities ranging between 94.9 and 100%. These studies demonstrate that different rules are helpful in detecting children with mTBI who have ICI. In the study of Atabaki and colleagues, sensory deficit, GCS less than 15, palpable skull defect, mental status change, age younger than 2 years, and signs of basilar skull fracture were associated with higher risk for ICI than other signs or symptoms of concern such as loss of consciousness (LOC), amnesia, headache, or vomiting (Atabaki et al., 2008). Likewise, in the study by Dunning and colleagues (2006) there was a strong association between the presence of skull fracture and increased ICI. The study by Palchak and colleagues (2003) also showed that the presence of skull fracture was a high risk factor but further demonstrated that abnormal mental status or the occurrence of vomiting was important. Haydel and Shembekar reported similar criteria but also noted that the presence of posttraumatic seizures, drug or alcohol intoxication, deficits in short-term memory, or physical evidence of trauma above the clavicles increased the risk of ICI (Haydel, 2005; Haydel & Shembekar, 2003). Other studies that were not prospective and that did not develop decision rules did not find a reliable association between LOC and ICI, although scalp lacerations and neurological deficits were significant risk factors (Davis, Hughes, Gubler, Waller, & Rivara, 1995; Falimirski, Gonzalez, Rodriguez, & Wilberger, 2003). Several studies also have suggested that children younger than age 2 years are at increased risk for ICI, with as many as 48% of injuries being occult or asymptomatic (Atabaki et al., 2008; Greenes & Schutzman, 2001).

Value of a Negative CT Scan in Children with mTBI

Multiple studies have shown that in children with mTBI who have a normal clinical examination, the presence of a normal CT scan suggests that it is safe to discharge them from the ED and that they are at very low risk for delayed ICI or neurological sequelae (Schutzman & Greenes, 2001; Thiessen & Woolridge, 2006). Likewise, in a related group of studies of children with mTBI who had a skull fracture but no ICI, none showed delayed clinical worsening (Greenes & Schutzman, 1997, 1999; Schutzman et al., 2001; Shane & Fuchs, 1997). One of the obvious advantages of being able to discharge children with mTBI is that it is more cost-effective than hospital observation for several days (Davis et al., 1995).

CT Abnormalities Reported in mTBI

Table 9.2 summarizes data on the specific CT imaging abnormalities reported in previous studies of children with mTBI in which greater than 100 cases were studied. The definition of mTBI varied, with some using a GCS-based algorithm whereas other studies used a set of clinical criteria either with/without LOC. In contrast to the CT yield based on decision rules (Part A of Table 9.2), a separate group of retrospective studies (Part B) reported on the number of children with mTBI who had an ICI and the types of lesions observed. In this group, the percentage of patients with ICI ranged from 7.6 to 14% and averaged 9.8%. For both groups combined, 44% had contusions, 37.5% had epidural hematomas, 27% had subdural hematomas, 17.7% had subarachnoid hemorrhage, 1.7% had parenchymal hematomas, 24.0% had cerebral edema, and 17.9% had "other" types of abnormalities, including pneuomocephalus,

TABLE 9.2. Types of CT-Determined Intracranial Injury Reported in Children with Mild Head Injury (GCS ≥ 13)

Author (year)	N	No. (%) patients with ICI in whom a CT was done	Types of ICI with no. of patients having that type of ICI[a]						
			SDH	SAH	EDH	Parenchymal hematoma	Contusion	Cerebral edema	Misc.[c]
A. Diagnostic yield of ICI in studies in which CT was done based on a decision rule with number of specific ICI observed									
Haydel & Shembekar (2003)	175	13[b] (7.4)	3	2	2	0	7	0	1
Palchak et al. (2003)	1,098	98 (7.7)	31	24	16	0	50	17	0
Dunning et al. (2006)	22,759	281 (5.4)	54	28	91	0	83	58	0
Atabaki et al. (2008)	1,000	65 (6.5)	26	15	0	0	18	2	8
Osmond et al. (2010)	3866	159 (4.1)	32	19	55	10	41	6	48
B. Diagnostic yield of ICI in studies in which CT done in all patients with mTBI									
Simon et al. (2001)	429	62 (14)	12	19	14	0	22	0	0
Boran et al. (2006)	421	32 (7.6)	5	0	11	0	16	0	5
Melo et al. (2008)[d]	1,888	174 (9.2)	NA	NA	37	0	28	62	47
Mean percentage of different types of ICI in children with mTBI who had CT done			27.0	17.7	37.5	1.7%	44.0	24.0	17.9

Note. SDH, subdural hematoma; SAH, subarachnoid hemorrhage; EDH, epidural hematoma; Misc., miscellaneous causes; NA, not available or data listed under "others" category.
[a]In some studies, patients had more than one type of lesion.
[b]Fourteen patients reported, but only 13 had ICI. Remaining patient just had a skull fracture.
[c]"Others" category contained findings such as pneuomocephalus, extraaxial hematoma (undifferentiated), cerebellar hematoma, mass effect, skull fractures.
[d]In this study, of the 205 patients listed as having an abnormal CT scan, findings included 118 with a simple linear skull fracture and 36 with a depressed skull fracture. The total number of patients listed with ICI was 174.

extra-axial hematoma (undifferentiated), cerebellar hematoma, mass effect, or skull fractures. One interesting point about CT scan interpretation is that scans evaluated by ED physicians as showing no intracranial injury may underestimate radiological findings (Davis et al., 1995).

Although we now have improved algorithms to detect ICI, several critical questions remain unanswered (Atabaki et al., 2008):

- What is the significance of positive CT findings in patients who do not require neurosurgical intervention?
- Is the detection of a clinically insignificant intracranial hemorrhage or contusion worth the risks of irradiation and sedation?
- How useful are negative CT findings in symptomatic children?

CT Abnormalities in Children with mTBI and the Need for Neurosurgical Intervention

The need for neurosurgical intervention in children with mTBI is extremely rare. Less than 0.5% of patients require surgery for lesions found on CT scan (Osmond et al., 2010). This need for surgical intervention is typically associated with clinical deterioration. In some patients, a second CT scan is done to see if the findings on the initial scan have progressed (see section below). On rare occasions, children with mTBI who are discharged from the ED or hospital develop slowly progressive symptoms that require reevaluation, rescanning, and hospital admission for surgical treatment, typically an epidural or subdural hematoma (Connors, Ruddy, McCall, & Garcia, 2001; Davis et al., 1995). In one pediatric mTBI study, the incidence of neurosurgical intervention was quite high, and differences were noted between the GCS group of 13–14 (6.7%) compared to the GCS 15 group (2.3%) (Melo et al., 2008).

Indications for Repeating a CT in Children with mTBI

Although three recent studies have examined the need for repeating a CT scan in children with TBI (Durham, Liu, & Selden, 2006; Schnellinger, Reid, & Louie, 2010), only one has data on children with mTBI (Hollingworth et al., 2007). In this study 20% (50 of 257) of children with mTBI had worsening CT findings, and three patients (1%) required subsequent neurosurgical intervention (Hollingworth et al., 2007). This was in contrast to children with moderate and severe head injuries, in whom 43% had worsening of CT findings and 6% required surgery. In most surgical patients, repeat CT was preceded by rapid decline in neurological status or elevated intracranial pressure. They also found that stratification based on four factors (initial head injury severity, any intraparenchymal finding on initial CT, normal findings on initial CT, or coagulopathy) identified 89% of patients with worsening ICI on the repeat CT and 100% of the surgical patients. In some cases, repeat scanning with MRI may be more useful than CT. Figure 9.1 shows an example of a small extra-axial hemorrhage that was initially misinterpreted as a subdural hemorrhage. A follow-up MRI showed expansion of blood and clarification of the hemorrhage as epidural in location.

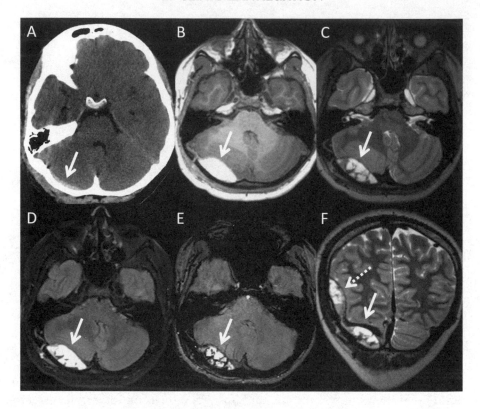

FIGURE 9.1. Images from a 13-year-old boy who fell from a horse, had brief loss of consciousness, one episode of emesis, and amnesia for the event. In the ED, he was alert, oriented, and had no neurological deficits. Initial CT (A) showed small crescentic extra-axial hemorrhages along the posterior right cerebellum (solid arrow) and right occipital lobe (not shown) that were interpreted as subdural bleeds. He was discharged home 2 days after admission, but had a follow-up MRI (B–E) 9 days after injury, which showed enlargement of the posterior fossa hemorrhage (solid arrow), now with a lentiform shape. On T1 images (B), the bright signal was indicative of subacute blood. The T2 (C), FLAIR (D), and SWI (E) images show T2 hyperintense signal with internal septation, particularly on the latter sequences. Coronal T2 images (F) revealed a communication between the infratentorial hemorrhage and the supratentorial hemorrhage (dashed arrows), consistent with a single epidural hematoma that was likely due to injury of the transverse sinus. However, he remained asymptomatic and had a normal clinical examination. CT, computed tomography; ED, emergency department; FLAIR, fluid-attenuated inversion recovery; SWI, susceptibility-weighted imaging.

MAGNETIC RESONANCE IMAGING

Reports in the literature with respect to the use of MRI in the mTBI population are limited, despite the increased sensitivity of this technique, compared to CT, to identify ICI. MRI in the pediatric and adolescent TBI population has focused on the moderate–severely injured, or more recently in patients with mTBI who suffer from "postconcussion syndrome" or persistent cognitive, emotional, or behavioral deficits.

Conventional MRI

MRI is able to detect lesions that are not visible on CT, and as such, has the potential to improve diagnosis of mild TBI. Conventional MRI, including T1-weighted (T1WI), T2-weighted (T2WI), and T2 FLAIR (fluid-attenuated inversion recovery) sequences, as well as T2* (gradient echo) and diffusion-weighted imaging (DWI), are used in routine clinical practice for patients with TBI. Compared with CT, these techniques often provide additional information, including evidence of subtle hemorrhage and extra-axial collections as well as demonstration of early ischemia. In addition, with the increasing recognition of radiation risks from CT, MRI may be more prudent to use than CT in the evaluation of such patients.

Prasad and colleagues prospectively studied 60 children less than 6 years of age with inflicted or noninflicted TBI, using acute CT and conventional MRI (Prasad, Ewing-Cobbs, Swank, & Kramer, 2002). Hierarchical multiple regression analyses indicated that the number of lesions on CT or MRI, as well as clinical variables (e.g., GCS, duration of coma), were predictive of outcomes (modified Glasgow Outcome Scale [GOS]) up to 1 year. In a recent study of 40 children with TBI, our group was also able to show that MRI (specifically T2WI, FLAIR, and susceptibility-weighted imaging [SWI]) provided more precise lesion detection and prediction of 6- to 12-month outcomes than CT (Sigmund et al., 2007). T2WI is a standard technique that is generally able to detect a wide range of parenchymal lesions, including edema, infarction, and moderate to large hemorrhages. FLAIR is a more specialized technique that suppresses the T2 signal of cerebrospinal fluid (CSF) and is usually more sensitive in detecting parenchymal lesions near the cortex or ventricles. SWI is a highly specialized gradient echo sequence that is very sensitive in detecting small hemorrhagic lesions often associated with diffuse axonal injury (DAI; Tong et al., 2008). Whether intraparenchymal edema and hemorrhage differ in their prediction of adverse outcome is uncertain. In our study, T2WI, FLAIR, and SWI showed significant differences in lesion volumes between normal and poor, as well as mild and poor outcome groups, whereas CT showed no significant differences in lesion volume between any groups. Our findings suggest that T2WI, FLAIR, and SWI MRI sequences provide a more accurate assessment of injury severity and detection of outcome-influencing lesions than CT in children with TBI. However, CT currently remains an essential part of the acute TBI workup to assess the need for neurosurgical intervention.

Susceptibility-Weighted Imaging

Of the various MRI techniques, SWI has the greatest potential to identify hemorrhagic lesion location and lesion burden. SWI is a high spatial resolution 3D gradient echo MRI technique with unique phase-subtraction postprocessing that is sensitive to magnetic susceptibility differences between tissues and substances, and accentuates the paramagnetic properties of blood products. It is very sensitive for detection of intravascular venous deoxygenated blood as well as extravascular blood products (Haacke, Xu, Cheng, & Reichenbach, 2004; Sehgal et al., 2005). SWI has been used at our institution since 2001, and in a recent review we described its role in providing additional imaging information in neonates, infants, and children with a wide variety of neurological conditions, including TBI (Tong et al., 2008).

SWI has been shown to be much more sensitive in detecting hemorrhagic DAI lesions after TBI in children compared to a conventional gradient echo (GRE) sequence. In an early study, we examined seven children with TBI (5 ± 3 days after injury) and demonstrated that the number of hemorrhagic DAI lesions seen on SWI was 6 times greater than on conventional GRE imaging, and that the volume of hemorrhage was approximately twofold greater (Tong et al., 2003). SWI can visualize smaller and more numerous hemorrhages than conventional MRI, and by inference, much more than that seen with CT (see Figures 9.2 and 9.3).

In an expanded SWI study, we examined 40 children and adolescents with mild to severe TBI and DAI, on average 1 week after injury (Tong et al., 2004). The number and volume of hemorrhagic lesions were compared to long-term neurological outcome assessed using the Pediatric Cerebral Performance Category Scale (PCPCS) score, which is modified from the Glasgow Outcome Scale (GOS) score and quantifies the overall functional neurological morbidity and cognitive impairment of infants and children. We found that children with lower GCS scores (≤ 8, $n = 30$) or prolonged

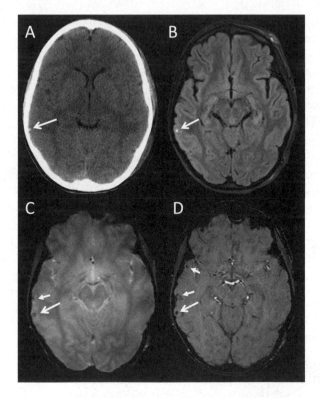

FIGURE 9.2. Selected slices from CT (A), MRI FLAIR (B), MRI standard GRE (C), and SWI (D) demonstrate a small hemorrhagic contusion in the right temporal lobe cortex (long arrow) in a 9-year-old boy who fell off his ATV, briefly lost consciousness, and was subsequently normal. Standard GRE and SWI are more sensitive for hemorrhagic lesions and show additional lesions (short arrows), but SWI can detect even more abnormalities than standard GRE sequences. CT, computed tomography; FLAIR, fluid-attenuated inversion recovery; GRE, gradient echo; MRI, magnetic resonance imaging; SWI, susceptibility-weighted imaging.

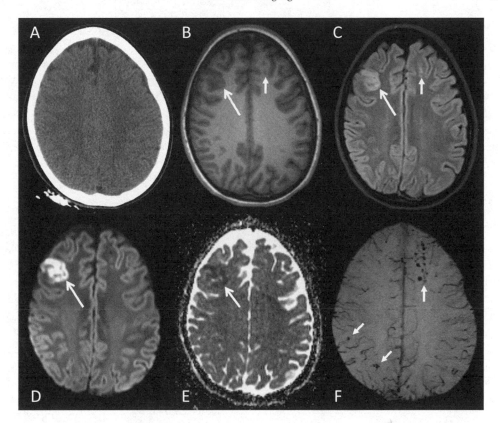

FIGURE 9.3. Images from a 13-year-old girl who was involved in a motor vehicle accident with transient loss of consciousness, was awake and responsive in the ED, and had a normal neurological examination. Her initial CT (A) was normal, but on MRI FLAIR (C), a hyperintense contusion (large arrow) was visible in the right frontal cortex, which was also bright on diffusion images (D) and dark on corresponding ADC (E) images. The SWI (F) images showed numerous small hypointense hemorrhagic shearing injuries (small arrows) in the gray–white matter junctions of the left frontal lobe and right parietal lobe. Note that the left frontal shearing injuries (small arrow) are faintly hyperintense on FLAIR and faintly hypointense on T1 images (B). The right frontal contusion is not well seen on T1 images. ADC, apparent diffusion coefficient; CT, computed tomography; ED, emergency department; FLAIR, fluid-attenuated inversion recovery; MRI, magnetic resonance imaging; SWI, susceptibility-weighted imaging.

coma (> 4 days, n = 20) had a significantly greater average number and volume of hemorrhagic lesions. Also, children with normal outcomes or mild neurological disability at 6–12 months after injury had significantly fewer number and volume of hemorrhagic DAI lesions than those who were moderately or severely disabled or in a vegetative state. We also determined that there were regional differences in DAI injury. Over 90% of patients had lesions in the parietal–temporal–occipital gray matter, parietal–temporal–occipital white matter, and frontal white matter. Four regions were less commonly affected (i.e., < 65% of patients): thalamus, brainstem, cerebellum, and basal ganglia. Of the 40 patients, 12 (30%) had lesions in all nine of the brain regions examined, of which 42% had poor outcomes. In contrast, there were 14 patients who had lesions in six or fewer regions, and all had good outcomes at

6–12 months. Only patients with involvement of seven or more regions had poor outcomes.

In a subgroup of these patients, Babikian and colleagues (2005) performed neuropsychological testing of 18 children and adolescents, 1–4 years after injury and compared results to initial SWI findings. Negative correlations between lesion number/volume and neuropsychological functioning were shown. Because SWI is more sensitive in detecting hemorrhagic DAI, more precise data can be obtained to objectively assess the severity of acute injury, which may provide more accurate long-term neurological and neuropsychological prognostic information.

Diffusion Weighted Imaging

DWI is a highly specialized MRI sequence that can detect the diffusion of water, specifically the protons bound to water in various tissues and fluids (Huisman, 2003). Diffusion represents the random thermal movement of molecules (i.e., Brownian motion). Image contrast on DWI is related to differences in the diffusion rate of water molecules rather than to changes in total tissue water. DWI can differentiate between lesions with decreased or increased diffusion compared to normal brain tissue. Restricted diffusion is believed to reflect cytotoxic edema in contrast to increased diffusion that typically occurs with vasogenic edema (Schaefer, Huisman, Sorensen, Gonzalez, & Schwamm, 2004). DWI has proven to be sensitive in the early detection of acute cerebral ischemia and seems promising in the evaluation of TBI, potentially revealing pathology when conventional MRI is normal (Huisman, 2003; Schaefer et al., 2004).

DWI can be used to show shearing injuries not visible on T2WI or FLAIR but is less sensitive than T2* imaging in detecting hemorrhagic lesions. The potential usefulness of DWI was analyzed in a study of adults with TBI by Hergan and colleagues (Hergan, Oser, & Langle Jun, 2002). DWI was obtained in 98 adults with TBI and DAI, and lesions were classified into three categories depending on their DWI signal and apparent diffusion coefficient (ADC) characteristics. *Type 1* lesions were DWI hypointense and ADC hyperintense, most likely representing lesions with vasogenic edema. *Type 2* lesions were DWI hyperintense and ADC hypointense, likely reflecting cytotoxic edema. *Type 3* lesions were central hemorrhagic lesions surrounded by an area of increased diffusion. In addition, lesions were classified according to their size and extent into three groups: *group A*, focal injury; *group B*, regional/confluent injury; and *group C*, extensive/diffuse injury. In another study, these investigators studied 25 adult patients with TBI and DAI, and found that the ADC values of DWI hyperintense lesions were reduced in 64% of lesions, were elevated in 24%, and were similar to the ADCs of normal brain tissue in 12% (Huisman, Sorensen, Hergan, Gonzalez, & Schaefer, 2003).

These investigators have also reported that DWI identifies the largest number of overall lesions, as well as the largest volume of trauma-related signal abnormalities in DAI, when compared with conventional MRI sequences that include T2-weighted fast-spin-echo, FLAIR, and T2*-weighted GRE sequences (although this was prior to the introduction of SWI) (Huisman et al., 2003). They have shown that the total volume of DWI signal abnormalities encountered in DAI correlates better than other imaging variables with the acute GCS score and the subacute Rankin scale score in adults with TBI (Schaefer et al., 2004).

Although less is known about DWI in pediatric TBI, recent studies have suggested that DWI may be a sensitive indicator of TBI, particularly in the setting of nonaccidental trauma (Ashwal, Wycliffe, & Holshouser, 2010). In one study, 89% of 18 children with presumed nonaccidental trauma showed abnormalities on DWI and ADC maps, and in 81% of the positive cases, DWI revealed more extensive injury than conventional MRI or showed injuries when MRI appeared normal (Biousse et al., 2002; Suh, Davis, Hopkins, Fajman, & Mapstone, 2001). Several studies have also suggested that hypoxia and ischemia are common mechanisms of intraparenchymal injury in children with nonaccidental trauma, possibly due to reactive vasospasm adjacent to hemorrhagic lesions, strangulation, cervicomedullary injuries, or apnea (Ashwal et al., 2010). All of these mechanisms, alone or in combination, could likely cause cerebral ischemic injury that would be manifest by changes in DWI.

Other case reports also have demonstrated DWI changes in white matter after nonaccidental trauma, suggesting that DWI is more sensitive than conventional MRI and more likely to detect lesions earlier in the evolution of injury (Chan, Chu, Wong, & Yeung, 2003; Parizel et al., 2003). These reports also described large areas of dramatic diffusion restriction, which support the belief that ischemia is a major component of brain injury in nonaccidental trauma, probably more so than DAI.

In a recent study, we evaluated the role of DWI and ADC for outcome prediction after pediatric TBI ($n = 37$ TBI, $n = 10$ control subjects) (Galloway, Tong, Ashwal, Oyoyo, & Obenaus, 2008). Fifteen regions of interest (ROIs) were manually drawn on ADC maps that were grouped for analysis into peripheral gray matter, peripheral white matter, deep gray and white matter, and posterior fossa. All ROIs excluded areas that appeared abnormal on T2-weighted images. Acute injury severity was measured using the GCS, and 6- to 12-month outcomes were assessed using the PCPCS. Patients were categorized into five groups: (1) controls; (2) all patients with TBI; (3) patients with mild/moderate TBI and good outcomes; (4) patients with severe TBI and good outcomes; and (5) patients with severe TBI and poor outcomes. ADC values in the peripheral white matter were significantly reduced in children with severe TBI and poor outcomes (72.8 ± 14.4 (10^{-3} mm^2/s) compared to those with severe TBI and good outcomes ($82.5 + 3.8$ (10^{-3} mm^2/s; $p < .05$). We also found that the average total brain ADC value alone had the greatest ability to predict outcome and could correctly predict outcome in 84% of cases. This study demonstrated that assessment of DWI and ADC values in pediatric TBI was useful in evaluating injury, particularly in brain regions that appear normal on conventional imaging. DWI may be useful in evaluating children with mTBI, although no published reports have yet examined this possibility.

Diffusion Tensor Imaging

DTI of brain white matter reflects the integrity of myelinated fibers and cell membranes in white matter tracts and relies on the fact that water diffusion is highly anisotropic in these regions. Diffusion is considered isotropic when motion is equal and unconstrained in all directions. In contrast, the structure and organization of myelin sheaths in the white matter tracts cause a greater restriction of water mobility perpendicular, rather than parallel, to the fiber tracts and is termed *anisotropic diffusion* (Klingberg, Vaidya, Gabrieli, Moseley, & Hedehus, 1999).

A common way to summarize diffusion tensor measurements is to calculate diffusivity and anisotropy. Mean diffusivity (MD) is derived by dividing the trace, or sum, of the three eigenvalues of the diffusion tensor by 3. Anisotropy is represented by fractional anisotropy (FA) and relative anisotropy (RA). FA is a measure of the portion of the diffusion tensor due to anisotropy, where a value of 0 represents completely isotropic (free) diffusion and a value of 1 represents anisotropic diffusion that is restricted to one direction (Le Bihan et al., 2001; Niogi & Mukherjee, 2010). Typically, FA maps are color-coded depending on the tracts' fiber direction (red for left–right, blue for superior–inferior, and green for anterior–posterior), which is indicated by the tensor's main eigenvector (Plate 9.1). The RA is derived from a ratio between the anisotropic and isotropic portions of the diffusion tensor.

DTI and TBI

As a consequence of TBI, shear strain deformation results in axonal injury scattered throughout the white matter, notably the subcortical white matter, corpus callosum, and upper brainstem. Histological studies have shown that axonal injury is believed to begin as a focal neurofilament misalignment, which can appear as early as 6 hours after injury (Povlishock & Christman, 1995). A second phase of DAI includes impaired axoplasmic transport, local accumulation of organelles, and local swelling and expansion of the axonal cylinder. Over time, lobulation of regions of axonal swelling occur and are followed by a disconnection of the axon.

Many of the early DTI studies in the mTBI population have focused on characterizing changes in diffusivity and anisotropy in the context of the structural changes in injured axons. In the adult population, DTI studies have shown increased mean diffusivity and reduced FA in various white matter regions, including the corpus callosum, internal and external capsule, at both subacute (1–30 days) and chronic time points (> 30 days postinjury) (Arfanakis et al., 2002). The authors proposed that these changes were due to the misalignment of the axonal membrane, causing diffusion restriction parallel to the axon with increased diffusion in directions perpendicular to the axon. It was further hypothesized that a subsequent impaired axoplasmic transport, local accumulation of organelles, and local swelling and expansion of the axonal cylinder would cause further diffusion restriction parallel to the main axis of the fibers and decrease FA (Arfanakis et al., 2002). In contrast, a later study of adult subjects with mTBI, imaged within the first 72 hours after injury, showed a significantly lower trace value and increase in FA values in a composite region made up of the anterior and posterior internal capsule, anterior and posterior corpus callosum, and external capsule (Bazarian et al., 2007). The authors suggested that these very early findings were the result of increased axonal permeability and the net movement of water from the extracellular space into the axon, thereby reducing the interstitial space between axons and increasing directionality. Overall these early studies suggest that there is likely a time course for changes in anisotropy and diffusivity, where the acute and early subacute phases are characterized by increases in FA and

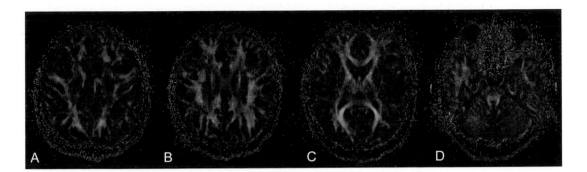

PLATE 9.1. Color-coded fractional anisotropy (FA) maps from a 30-direction diffusion tensor imaging (DTI) study acquired in a healthy 17-year-old male at 3.0 Tesla (TR/TE = 5700/101 msec; b = 0 and 1,000 sec/mm^2; number of averages = 2; slice thickness = 3 mm) through the level (approximate) of the centrum semiovale (A), body of the corpus callosum (B), internal capsule (C), and cerebral peduncles (D). FA maps are color-coded depending on the fiber tract orientation: green for anterior–posterior, blue for superior–inferior, and red for left–right.

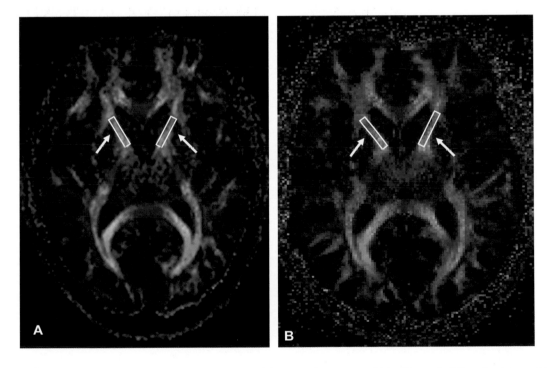

PLATE 9.2. Representative fractional anisotropy (FA) maps of a 15-year-old healthy male (A) and subject with mTBI (B) acquired using a 12-direction DTI sequence (TR/TE = 5600/98 msec; b = 0 and 1,000 sec/mm^2; number of averages = 3; slice thickness = 3 mm). In a cohort of 10 subjects with mTBI, quantitative analysis using regions of interest (arrows) showed increased FA in the anterior internal capsules, compared to a group of 8 age-matched control subjects (mTBI FA = 0.74 vs. 15-year-old healthy male FA = 0.67; p = 0.01).

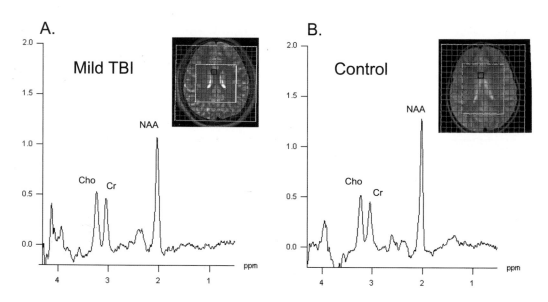

PLATE 9.3. (A) A 3D-MRSI acquisition (PRESS; TR/TE = 1700/144 msec; 3T) shows reduced NAA but normal levels of Cr and Cho in the normal-appearing genu from a symptomatic (persistent headaches) 13-year-old female with mTBI taken 213 days after injury compared to (B) a normal age-matched control subject. Cho, choline; Cr, creatine; NAA, *N*-acetylaspartate.

decreased diffusivity associated with free water dispersion, whereas a decrease in FA and increase in diffusivity reflect degenerative changes more common in long-term or chronic periods postinjury (Levin et al., 2008b).

In the pediatric population, Wilde and colleagues first demonstrated that the anterior commissure, like the corpus callosum, was vulnerable to white matter degenerative changes after TBI (Wilde, Bigler, et al., 2006). A companion study in 16 children demonstrated that higher FA values in the corpus callosum correlated with increased cognitive processing speed, faster interference resolution on an inhibition task, and better functional outcome, as measured by the GOS score (Wilde et al., 2006b), suggesting that changes in white matter microstructural integrity measured by DTI can account for variations in cognitive performance and predict outcome. In a study including six pediatric patients with mTBI, decreased cortical white matter FA correlated with changes in processing speed, working memory, executive function, and behavioral dysregulation at 6–12 months postinjury, indicating that DTI measures are also sensitive to long-term changes in white matter and cognitive function following mild injury (Wozniak et al., 2007). In a later study of 10 adolescents with acute mTBI (GCS score of 15; negative CT; 1–6 days postinjury), 8 of 10 subjects had increased FA values and decreased ADC and RD in the corpus callosum, which correlated with more intense postconcussion symptoms and emotional distress (Wilde et al., 2008). The increase in FA was thought to be the result of axonal swelling, which restricts overall diffusion by restricting the interstitial space surrounding axons. Moreover, decreases in ADC likely reflect trauma-induced cytotoxic edema and inflammation (see DWI section above), whereas decreased radial diffusivity (RD) reflects myelin damage. Interestingly, 2 of the 10 subjects with the longest interval between injury and imaging (4 and 6 days) had decreased FA and increased diffusivity (Wilde et al., 2008). In a small cohort of adolescent mTBI subjects studied at our institution (age range 8–16 years; 1–6 months postinjury), an increase in FA was measured in the anterior limb of the internal capsule, compared to age-matched controls (Plate 9.2). Like the adult population with mTBI, these studies suggest that changes in anisotropy and diffusivity in the pediatric population with mTBI follow a time course.

More recent studies have continued to focus on the relation between DTI metrics and neurocognitive status. In a study of 10 adolescent subjects with mTBI and 10 demographically matched controls, voxel-based statistical analysis showed a significant decrease in ADC and RD in five white matter regions that correlated with increases on the Rivermead Post Concussion Symptoms Questionnaire (RPCSQ) scale, which includes indices of cognitive, emotional, and somatic systems (Chu et al., 2010). In a study evaluating the relation between memory function and DTI changes in the cingulum bundles following acute mTBI, a bilateral decrease in ADC and increase in FA were detected (Wu et al., 2010). In the mTBI group, the increase in FA in the left cingulum bundle correlated with findings on a 30-minute delayed recall test, suggesting that injury to the cingulum bundles contributes to neurocognitive problems following mTBI.

Although only a few DTI studies have been conducted in the pediatric population with mTBI, findings to date implicate subclinical axonal injury that is not readily detected by routine CT or imaging studies as a contributing factor in persistent neurocognitive deficits.

MAGNETIC RESONANCE SPECTROSCOPY

Magnetic resonance spectroscopy (MRS) is a noninvasive neuroimaging tool that allows *in vivo* analysis of neurochemicals and their metabolites in humans. MRI uses the strong signals from proton nuclei of water and their spatial location to reconstruct anatomical images. In contrast, 1H-MRS focuses on protons located on neurochemicals present in much lower concentrations than water within tissues. The low signal-to-noise ratio necessitates the use of water suppression techniques and lower spatial resolution necessary in order to measure them. 1H-MRS is the most widely used application of *in vivo* MRS in humans and will be exclusively discussed in this review, but other atoms that can be used include 31P, 13C, 14N, 19F, and 23Na.

Several key brain metabolites are measured with 1H-MRS using both short (i.e., TE = 20–40 ms) and long (i.e., TE = 135–270 ms) echo delay time MRS techniques. Each metabolite resonates at a particular frequency dependent on the structure of the molecule and the strength of interaction between the nucleus and the electronic cloud within the particular molecule. The size of the change in frequency is known as the chemical shift (measured in parts per million [ppm]). After Fourier analysis, the plot of signal amplitude versus frequency in ppm is known as the MR spectrum. N-acetylaspartate (NAA; 2.01 ppm), an amino acid synthesized in mitochondria, is a neuronal and axonal marker that decreases with neuronal loss or dysfunction (Moffett, Ross, Arun, Madhavarao, & Namboodiri, 2007). In white matter, the NAA peak includes a greater contribution from N-acetylaspartylglutamate (NAAG) than in gray matter. Total creatine (Cr; 3.0 ppm), comprised of creatine and phosphocreatine, is a marker for intact brain energy metabolism. Total choline (Cho; 3.02 ppm), primarily consisting of phosphoryl and glycerophosphoryl choline, is a marker for membrane synthesis or repair, inflammation, or demyelination (Bluml, 1999). Lactate (Lac; 1.33 ppm) accumulates as a result of anaerobic glycolysis and in the setting of TBI may be a response to release of glutamate (Alessandri et al., 2000). Short echo time acquisitions allow for measurement of additional metabolites with short T2 relaxation times that cannot be detected using long echo time acquisitions because their signals decay too rapidly. Specifically, glutamate and immediately formed glutamine comprise two groups of multiple overlapping resonances (β,γ-Glx; 2.07–2.5 ppm and α-Glx; 3.6–3.8 ppm) and are excitatory amino acid neurotransmitters released to the extracellular space after brain injury that play a major role in neuronal death (Bullock et al., 1998). Myoinositol (Ins; 3.56 ppm), an organic osmolyte located in astrocytes, increases as a result of glial proliferation (Garnett et al., 2000). Lipids and macromolecules (LipMM) produce broad peaks at 0.9 ppm and 1.3 ppm (often overlapping with lactate) and may increase as a result of severe brain injury due to a breakdown of cell membrane and release of fatty acids (Panigrahy, Nelson, & Bluml, 2010).

MRS in the Evaluation of Pediatric TBI

Neuroimaging methods capable of identifying brain abnormalities after mTBI are critical for accurate diagnosis and to identify patients at risk for long-term effects. Understanding the underlying pathophysiology that occurs in the brain after mTBI is also critical to the development of effective treatments. MRS holds great promise for mTBI research because it provides a sensitive, noninvasive assessment of neurochemical alterations after brain injury and has shown metabolic abnormalities in regions of the brain that appear normal on conventional MRI sequences (Garnett et al., 2000; Holshouser, Tong, & Ashwal, 2005). Reports using 1H-MRS in adults and children have predominantly studied moderate to severe TBI and have found similar key neurometabolic alterations after injury. Typically, NAA is reduced as a result of neuronal loss or dysfunction and Cho is elevated due to shearing of myelin and cellular membranes (DAI) and/or repair. Cr is assumed to be fairly constant; however, recent studies have shown that Cr levels are altered in various disease states (Hattingen et al., 2008; Inglese et al., 2003), including after mTBI (Gasparovic et al., 2009).

As discussed below, many studies using 1H-MRS have shown potential for providing early prognostic information regarding clinical outcome in pediatric patients with accidental and nonaccidental head injury. These studies, although performed in a "mixed" population of TBI patients, including patients with a wide age and injury severity range, showed that MRS is sensitive to metabolite changes after TBI.

One of our first studies of pediatric brain injury recognized that patient data had to be compared to age-matched control values for proper interpretation (see Figure 9.4) (Holshouser et al., 1997). The study reported that elevated lactate and decreased NAA ratios in occipital gray matter predicted poor long-term (6–12 months) outcome, as determined by the PCPCS score in all age groups. This study showed that MRS was very useful for studying different etiologies of pediatric brain injury in all age groups and led to other studies that concentrated only on TBI.

A later study from our group in infants and children (GCS 3–15; 1.5T) with TBI found significantly lower NAA/Cr or NAA/Cho and higher Cho/Cr in patients with poor outcome (Ashwal et al., 2000). Lactate was present in 91% of infants and 80% of children with poor outcomes, and along with NAA ratios, was useful for predicting long-term outcome. The correlation between lactate and outcome was strongest in infants with nonaccidental trauma or child abuse, rather than accidental trauma, as confirmed in later studies (Aaen et al., 2010; Makoroff, Cecil, Care, & Ball, 2005), and may likely be due to multiple factors (e.g., age, secondary insult, delayed medical treatment). This study also demonstrated that spectra from brain areas that did not appear visibly injured showed altered metabolite ratios, suggesting widespread metabolite changes that correlated with injury severity and long-term outcome. In addition, NAA ratios in a subset of these patients were strongly associated with long-term (1–3 years) neuropsychological outcomes (Babikian et al., 2006; Brenner, Freier, Holshouser, Burley, & Ashwal, 2003). A comparison study showed that long echo time acquisitions were slightly better at detecting and quantifying lactate without the interference of short T2 relaxation time metabolites such as lipids (Holshouser, Ashwal, Shu, & Hinshaw, 2000). A longitudinal study evaluating neurometabolite changes using quantitative single voxel spectroscopy (SVS) (TE = 144 ms; 3T) during the late phase (1–3 years) of mostly young pediatric patients with mild TBI (ages 3–6 years) found that NAA levels in the left frontal white matter and NAA, Cr, and Cho levels in the medial frontal gray matter were strongly and positively correlated with the GCS score at the time of injury, and correlated somewhat with certain neuropsychological, academic, and social measures (Walz, Cecil, Wade, & Michaud, 2008). These findings were compared to other studies that found long-term decreases in NAA and Cho after more severe injury (Parry et al., 2004), attributed to neuronal

Occipital Gray Matter

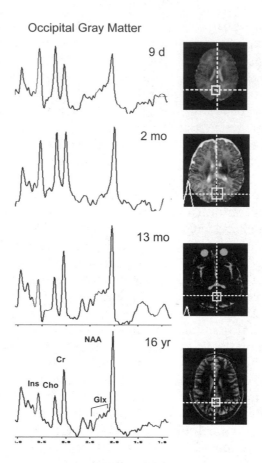

FIGURE 9.4. Normal age-related changes in single voxel MRS spectra (STEAM; TR/TE = 3000/20 ms; 1.5T) from mid-occipital gray matter show lower levels of NAA and creatine (Cr), and higher levels of choline (Cho) and myoinositol (Ins) in a term neonate compared to older children. As the brain develops, NAA and Cr increase and Cho and Ins decrease rapidly through the first year of life, leveling off to adolescent levels by 18–24 months of age. MRS, magnetic resonance spectroscopy; NAA, *N*-acetylaspartate.

loss/dysfunction and atrophy. Both studies suggested that quantitative MRS is needed to monitor and report metabolite concentrations rather than ratios.

Changes in excitatory neurotransmitters such as glutamate and glutamine (Glx) and Ins have been studied after pediatric TBI with quantitative SVS (Ashwal et al., 2004a, 2004b). Ins from occipital gray matter was 22% higher in children with TBI compared to controls and 35% higher in patients with poor outcomes in a study of 38 children. Increased Ins in patients with TBI and poor long-term neurological outcome was postulated to be due to astrogliosis or to a disturbance in osmotic function. Glx from occipital gray matter was significantly increased in children with TBI compared to controls, but did not correlate with injury severity or outcome. This finding was attributed by the authors to the delay from the time of injury to imaging in patients with severe TBI as compared to those with mild–moderate TBI, for the former often needed to be medically stabilized for transport to the scanner.

According to the literature, Glx levels most likely peak early after injury and fall rapidly (Schumann, Stiller, Thomas, Brinker, & Samii, 2000); therefore, the fact that Glx was elevated longer in severely injured patients makes Glx measurements potentially useful for evaluating injury severity and studying the pathophysiology of injury. Improved spectral resolution and quantitation of the Glx peaks at higher clinical field strengths of 3.0 Tesla could prove useful, particularly for studying changes in mTBI.

Multivoxel magnetic resonance spectroscopic imaging (MRSI), which allows simultaneous evaluation of multiple brain regions, has also been used to study TBI in children. In one study, 2D-MRSI (PRESS, TE = 60 ms; 1.5T) in normal-appearing brains of school-age children studied up to 3 years after TBI (mild–severe) showed that NAA was lower in patients with TBI than in control subjects and had the strongest correlations with cognitive (intellectual and arithmetic) measures (Hunter et al., 2005). Another study used 2D-MRSI in children (ages 2–18 years) to measure metabolite ratios from visibly injured (lesions seen on SWI) versus normal-appearing brains (no abnormalities on SWI or MRI) within 2 weeks of injury (Holshouser et al., 2005). Proton MRSI (PRESS, TE = 144 ms; 1.5T) in 40 pediatric patients with TBI (GCS 3–15) was acquired in a transverse plane through the level of the corpus callosum. T2-weighted, FLAIR, and SWI were used to identify voxels as normal-appearing or with nonhemorrhagic or hemorrhagic injury. A significant decrease in NAA/Cr and increase in Cho/Cr (evidence of DAI) were observed in normal-appearing and visibly injured (hemorrhagic) brains compared to controls. NAA/Cr was decreased more in normal-appearing brains for patients with poor outcome compared to patients with good outcomes or controls. Reduction of NAA in visibly injured brain is most likely caused by the primary impact, whereas reduction of NAA in normal-appearing brain may reflect DAI and Wallerian degeneration (Garnett et al., 2000) and captures the diffuse nature of TBI. A plot of the percentage of voxels from normal-appearing brain in which NAA/Cr ratios were at least two standard deviations of normal for age in

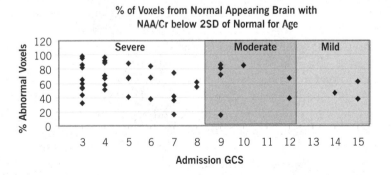

FIGURE 9.5. A plot of the percentage of voxels from normal-appearing brain (voxels with no hemorrhage or contusion on MRI) in which the NAA/Cr ratios are decreased below two standard deviations (SD) of normal for age, grouped by admission Glasgow Coma Scale score (GCS) shows that pediatric patients categorized in the mild injury range (GCS = 13–15) also have decreased NAA/Cr ratios in up to 60% of voxels sampled, although overall still less than the severely injured. Spectra were acquired with MRSI (PRESS; TR/TE = 3000/144 ms); 1.5T) in a 10-mm thick slab through the level of the corpus callosum. Cr, creatine; MRI, magnetic resonance imaging; NAA, N-acetylaspartate.

each patient is shown in Figure 9.5, grouped by admission GCS. Approximately 50% of voxels from normal-appearing brain taken at the level of the corpus callosum in children who were categorized as mildly injured, had decreased NAA/Cr ratios early after injury. This percentage was higher than many children who had more severe injuries and suggests that NAA may be a marker of patients with mTBI who are at risk for cognitive or neurological deficits. Neuropsychological follow-up (1–3 years) showed that the pooled NAA/Cr and NAA/Cr decrease in the corpus callosum had the strongest correlations with intellectual and memory deficits (Babikian et al., 2006). This finding is in agreement with another study reporting that a majority of patients with mild to severe brain injury showed diminished NAA/Cr levels in the splenium compared with normal control volunteers (Cecil et al., 1998). A more recent longitudinal study of 36 children (6–18 years old, GCS = 3–15) used MRSI (PRESS, TE = 62 ms; 1.5T) and found that NAA/Cr was reduced and Cho/Cr increased in TBI patients as compared to controls (Yeo et al., 2006). The researchers also found that overall performance, as well as language and visual–motor skills, were positively correlated with NAA/Cr and negatively correlated with Cho/Cr. These studies demonstrate that proton MRSI is extremely sensitive for detecting metabolic injury in brain that appears normal on neuroimaging and helps explain why global neuropsychological deficits are often seen in patients with normal imaging findings.

Although no studies have been published that deal exclusively with the pediatric mTBI population, several studies have used MRS in adults with mTBI (GCS = 13–15) or in a mixed population of adolescents and young adults who experienced sports-related concussions. Some of these studies suggest that NAA change is a discriminating factor in mTBI and may be a suitable biochemical marker for monitoring the cerebral metabolic status of the brain following injury (Cohen et al., 2007; Henry, Tremblay, Boulanger, Ellemberg, & Lassonde, 2010; Vagnozzi et al., 2008). One study evaluated nonlocalized whole-brain NAA (WBNAA) in mildly injured adult patients and found significant WBNAA deficits (12%) relative to controls that were not associated with focal injuries, suggesting that mTBI produced diffuse neuronal injury (Cohen et al., 2007). Other studies concentrated on concussed athletes. One particular study at 3T evaluated the time course of metabolite recovery (Vagnozzi et al., 2008). The main finding showed an initial decrease in NAA (18.5%) in the frontal lobes that recovered by 3% at 15 days and returned to normal, relative to controls, within 30 days after injury, although the athletes declared full resolution of symptoms at 3 days. If a second injury occurred before 15 days (three subjects), the NAA/Cr ratio took longer to normalize (45 days), and symptoms did not resolve until 30 days postinjury. The authors suggested that NAA measurements may be a valid tool for determining when athletes should return to play after concussion.

A second study of concussed male collegiate athletes was conducted using quantitative SVS (PRESS, TE = 20 ms; 3T) in multiple regions within 7 days of injury in order to evaluate changes in Ins and Glu as well as NAA (Henry et al., 2010). The researchers found a combination of decreased NAA and Glu in primary motor (M1) cortex. Another study found alterations in intracortical inhibition in concussed athletes (De Beaumont, Lassonde, Leclerc, & Theoret, 2007). Both studies together suggest that the motor system may be particularly vulnerable to the effects of sports-inflicted concussions.

Other studies in adults with mTBI from a variety of causes reported significant regional and global metabolite changes, including decreased NAA as well as increased Cho, using whole-brain echo planar MRSI (TE = 70 ms; 1.5T) in the sub-acute period; however, results did not correlate with 6-month outcomes (Govindaraju et al., 2004). One study aimed to quantitatively measure brain neurotransmitters, glutamate and glutamine (as Glx), in adult patients with mTBI within 19 days of injury with 2D-MRSI (PRESS, TE = 40 ms; 3T) (Gasparovic et al., 2009). These researchers found lower levels of gray matter Glx and higher levels of white matter Cr in subjects with mTBI, relative to controls, suggesting tissue-specific metabolite responses to mTBI. An additional study from the same investigators utilizing a larger sample of patients confirmed these results and also acquired longitudinal data with neuropsychological assessments (Yeo et al., 2006). The researchers found that metabolite changes normalized over a 3- to 5-month interval following injury. They also found no significant correlations with traditional measures of attention, memory, processing speed, etc., and they suggested that these measures may have less than optimal sensitivity to mTBI. This is an important finding also reported in previous studies, suggesting that other cognitive or behavioral tests may be more useful for evaluating patients with mTBI. In some of our own work with pediatric patients who have mild injury (GCS 15), we have seen metabolite changes months after injury, particularly in the corpus callosum and frontal white matter, when compared to age-matched normal subjects. Plate 9.3 is an example of reduced NAA but normal levels of Cr and Cho in the normal-appearing genu from a symptomatic (headaches) patient with mTBI studied 213 days after injury.

Absence of structural injury after mTBI is common, yet recent literature, as reviewed in previous sections of this chapter and other sections of this book, support observations that mild brain injury may have considerable detrimental effects. As discussed above, MRS is potentially very useful for detecting injury in a brain that appears normal on CT and MRI. Studies directed exclusively at the pediatric population with mTBI, however, are needed to determine if MRS can be used as a routine clinical tool to determine injury and monitor recovery.

THE ROLE OF CT AND MRI
IN THE EVALUATION OF CHILDREN WITH mTBI

Numerous clinical definitions of mTBI have been proposed and are discussed elsewhere in this book. Irrespective of clinical criteria, a proportion of symptomatic as well as asymptomatic children with mTBI have ICI. One recent study in children (ages 5–15 years) with mTBI compared serial neuropsychological outcomes in 32 children with abnormal initial CT scans (24 hours postinjury) to 48 children with mTBI whose CT scans were normal (Levin et al., 2008a). Children with ICI had significantly worse episodic memory, slower cognitive processing, diminished recovery in managing cognitive interference, and poorer performance in calculating and reading than patients in the mTBI group without ICI. Because such studies show that a significant proportion of children with mTBI and ICI (regardless of whether they are initially clinically symptomatic) have long-term sequelae, CT and MRI may play an important role in categorizing children with mTBI into subgroups.

Figure 9.6 presents an algorithm for the proposed use of CT and MRI in the evaluation of children with mTBI. This algorithm was developed by us and is not evidence-based but derived from our experience and opinion. It is a starting point

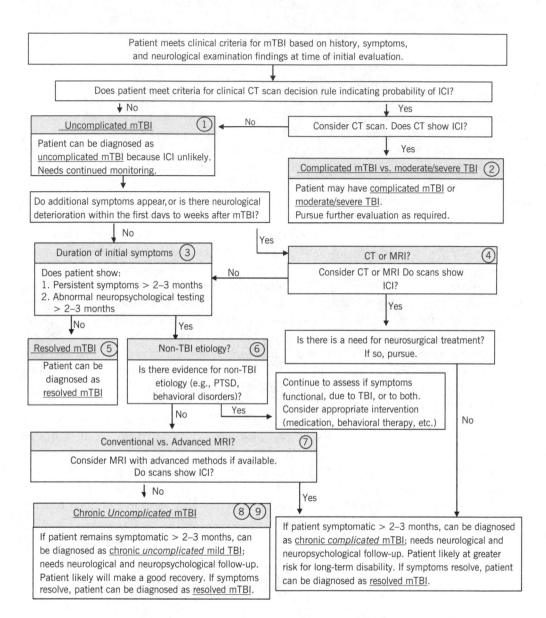

FIGURE 9.6. Algorithm for the proposed use of neuroimaging in children with mild TBI. This algorithm was prepared by us, based on our experience and is not evidence-based. There are 9 points along the pathway that raise questions about terminology, if and when imaging should be done, and what kind of imaging might be most appropriate. These issues are further discussed in the text. In this pathway, the diagnosis of mTBI is presumably established by the clinician using a set of diagnostic criteria. A decision rule can then be used to determine if a CT scan should/should not be obtained. If the decision rule is negative, the child can be diagnosed as having uncomplicated mTBI, as the probability of having an ICI is very low. If the rule is positive, then a CT scan should be obtained, and if there is no ICI, the child can be diagnosed as having uncomplicated mTBI; but if it shows ICI, the child can be considered to have complicated mTBI or moderate/severe TBI. Both groups will require careful follow-up. In the uncomplicated mTBI group (i.e., those without ICI), serial observation will determine if symptoms resolve or whether new symptoms develop subacutely that might be an indication for MRI. In other children, symptoms may not completely resolve after 2–3 months or there may be abnormalities on neuropsychological testing. Evaluation for behavioral disorders should also be considered. MRI could be performed in these children, and advanced MRI methods, if available, may be advantageous, as they are more sensitive in detecting injury. If no imaging abnormalities are detected, the diagnosis of chronic uncomplicated mTBI can be made; but if imaging abnormalities are present, the diagnosis of chronic complicated mTBI can be made. CT, computed tomography; ICI, intracranial injury; MRI, magnetic resonance imaging.

for an approach to evaluating children with mTBI. We have identified nine areas of uncertainty and controversy that require further research.

1. Uncomplicated versus Complicated mTBI

Decision rules used acutely after mTBI can predict which children with mTBI are at low risk for ICI. It may be reasonable to provisionally diagnose these low-risk children, when first seen, as having *uncomplicated mTBI* on a clinical basis without the "gold standard" of having a negative CT scan. Alternatively, the majority of initially asymptomatic children with mTBI children who have not been scanned but who have ICI will likely develop symptoms within the first week postinjury. Development of symptoms would prompt the ordering of a CT scan that presumably would show ICI, requiring a change in diagnosis to *complicated mTBI*. In the original publication that brought attention to this issue, complicated mTBI was limited to three types of injury (i.e., depressed skull fractures, intracerebral contusions/hematomas, and epidural/subdural hematomas) (Williams, Levin, & Eisenberg, 1990). As noted in Table 9.3, no imaging criteria currently exist for what constitutes complicated mTBI. Most studies do not state the imaging criteria used to diagnose complicated mTBI, and studies that list criteria do not state the actual imaging abnormalities present in the study patients. These lesions are all impact related and would be present at the time of injury, or, in the case of subdural/epidural hematomas, within several days to 1 week after injury. Thus, children with uncomplicated mTBI who remain asymptomatic for longer than 1 week are unlikely to develop new intracranial lesions. Diagnosing these children as having uncomplicated mTBI would seem appropriate and consistent as long as they are monitored and, although at risk, they are less likely than the group with complicated mTBI to have long-term sequelae.

2. Complicated mTBI versus Moderate–Severe TBI

At least two distinct interpretations of the significance of ICI in individuals with mTBI have been suggested in relation to whether they have complicated mTBI or moderate–severe TBI (Malec et al., 2007; Williams et al., 1990). This controversy developed because of the limitations of the GCS score in assessing severity and the unresolved question of the clinical significance of ICI in terms of acute management and long-term prognosis. The approach taken by those favoring use of the term *complicated mTBI* required a GCS score of 13–15 with ICI as defined above (i.e., depressed skull fractures, intracerebral contusions/hematomas, or epidural/subdural hematomas) (Williams et al., 1990). In contrast, Malec and colleagues proposed the Mayo Clinic classification system for TBI severity (Malec et al., 2007). Specifically, they proposed that if a patient with TBI met any one of five criteria, he or she could be classified as moderate–severe TBI. The fifth criteria is relevant to the issue of imaging mTBI, as they recommended that if a patient has one of eight CT criteria, he or she should be diagnosed as moderate–severe TBI. They also proposed that if the criteria do not apply, then the patient could be considered as *mild (probable) TBI*.

In the original study on complicated mTBI versus moderate TBI by Williams and colleagues (215 subjects ages 16–50), the distinction between the three types of ICI that they observed in the patients with mTBI had relevance to their outcomes. The

TABLE 9.3. Case Definitions of Complicated mTBI

Author (year)	Case definition of complicated mTBI
CT studies	
Williams et al. (1990)	GCS of 13–15 and depressed skull fractures, intracerebral contusions/hematomas, or epidural/subdural hematomas. This was original study defining complicated TBI
Borgaro, Prigatano, Kwasnica, & Rexer (2003)	Complicated mTBI defined as the presence of a space-occupying lesion. No imaging data given.
Iverson (2006)	Day-of-injury CT that was considered abnormal but no definition of what "abnormal" meant nor data on CT scan findings.
Kennedy et al. (2006)	No definition given but referred to paper by Williams et al. (1990) and stated "positive neuroimaging findings." Reported cortical contusions in 74%, as well as extra-axial fluid collections (60%), subarachnoid hemorrhages (49%), punctate/petechial hemorrhages (23%), intraventricular hemorrhages (14%), and noncortical contusions (12%).
Levin et al. (2008a)	Complicated mTBI included patients with parenchymal contusion, intracerebral or extra-axial hemorrhage, brain swelling, shearing injury, or a depressed or basilar skull fracture and were compared to an mTBI group defined as patients whose CT findings were normal or limited to a linear skull fracture. Children with complicated mTBI had significantly poorer episodic memory, slower cognitive processing, diminished recovery in managing cognitive interference, and poorer performance in calculating and reading than those with uncomplicated mTBI.
Kashluba, Hanks, Casey, & Millis (2008)	GCS score of 13–15 and an intracranial brain lesion documented by CT. No imaging data included.
Hessen & Nestvold (2009)	Presence of posttraumatic amnesia > 30 minutes and EEG pathology within 24 hours after TBI. Imaging criteria not included in definition.
Lange, Iverson, & Franzen (2009)	No stated definition of complicated mTBI but referred to paper by Williams et al. (1990). No data on imaging findings.
Fay et al. (2010)	Trauma-related intracranial abnormalities on MRI. No imaging data given.
MRI studies	
Hofman et al. (2000)	No definition given but found that 12/21 patients with mTBI (GCS of 14–15, loss of consciousness for less than 20 minutes, and posttraumatic amnesia for less than 6 hours) had MRI abnormalities. No a priori definition of what an MRI lesion was, nor quantification of the types and number of MRI lesions. Found no difference in neurocognitive performance between patients with normal and abnormal MRI findings.
Hughes et al. (2004)	MRI abnormalities classified as definitely traumatic if hemorrhage or local mass effect. Nonspecific areas of T2 signal change (deep white matter hyperintensities) were identified and patients put in two groups (> or < 5 lesions). There was weak correlation between MRI and neuropsychological tests for attention in the acute period and no significant correlation with a questionnaire for postconcussion symptoms or return to work status.

Note. GCS, Glasgow Coma Scale; CT, computed tomography; EEG; electroencephalography; MRI, magnetic resonance imaging.

patients with depressed skull fractures and no other lesions had similar neuropsychological outcomes as the patients with uncomplicated mTBI, whereas patients with intracerebral contusions/hematomas or subdural/epidural hematomas had outcomes more similar to the moderate TBI group. Such studies need to be replicated in children, as it may be possible to use more specific clinical and CT criteria to better delineate what should be considered a complicated mTBI versus a moderate–severe TBI.

3. Symptom Duration

There remains limited knowledge and ongoing controversy regarding the natural history of mTBI in children. The knowledge acquired depends on whether one is relying on patient/caregiver data, the results of standardized neuropsychological test batteries, or the clinical neurological examination. In order to decide whether to obtain a CT or MRI study, better information is needed as to when a child with mTBI returns to baseline. In addition, better assessments are needed regarding the added diagnostic and prognostic value of imaging in a child with mTBI who has persistent symptoms. In the algorithm (Figure 9.6), we selected 2–3 months as the time point after which one should consider imaging. This time frame was based on a 2004 report from the World Health Organization Collaborating Centre Task Force on Mild Traumatic Brain Injury (Carroll et al., 2004) that analyzed data from 28 longitudinal, 1 cross-sectional, and 1 case series studies of children with mTBI. From this analysis, two phase-II cohort studies indicated that postconcussion symptoms are largely resolved within 2–3 months (Farmer, Singer, Mellits, Hall, & Charney, 1987; Ponsford et al., 1999).

4. CT or MRI for Imaging Evaluation of Subacute Symptoms?

For the acute evaluation of a child with TBI, CT is the preferred modality to detect ICI that may require neurosurgical intervention or hospitalization, whereas MRI (e.g., T2WI, FLAIR, and SWI) provides a better assessment of injury severity and detection of outcome-influencing lesions (Sigmund et al., 2007). Depending on the severity, nature, and timing of new symptoms, or if previous symptoms worsen after injury, a decision will need to be made whether imaging should be performed, and if so, what kind. If there are clinical concerns for increasing mass effect, increased intracranial pressure, or need for possible neurosurgical intervention, a CT scan is appropriate. Because of the greater awareness of the potential long-term risks of CT radiation injury and the recognition that MRI provides greater anatomical and functional imaging information, preference is increasing for MRI rather than CT when children with TBI develop new symptoms or if previous symptoms worsen. These same guidelines likely apply to children with mTBI, but requires further investigation. Another issue that requires further study relates to the optimum timing of MRI. Early MRI may detect abnormalities (e.g., using DWI or MRS) that are not found if performed several weeks or months later.

5. Resolved mTBI

Symptoms in most children with mTBI resolve within days to weeks, particularly if sports-related, with recovery of neuropsychological function to baseline within 2–3 months. The term *resolved mTBI* could be used to describe these patients. Application of this term will depend on the nature of the original symptoms and how they are followed. Additional studies are needed to correlate initial CT findings with resolution of mTBI symptoms.

6. Non-TBI Etiology in a Child with mTBI and Chronic Symptoms

As with many acute neurological disorders (e.g., stroke), it may be difficult to differentiate chronic symptoms due to brain injury versus a post TBI psychological reactive disorder (e.g., posttraumatic stress disorder, anxiety, depression, hyperactivity). This difficulty is particularly likely in children and adolescents, especially when the injury is mild. A decision must be made as to which should be performed first: imaging or psychological testing. An electroencephalogram may be helpful. Demonstration of significant cerebral dysfunction (e.g., generalized or focal slowing, suppression or epileptiform discharges) may suggest underlying structural nervous system injury that is causing chronic symptoms rather than a functional disorder. Even when imaging detects an abnormality, it remains uncertain whether this is triggering symptoms. Establishing a psychological or psychiatric diagnosis and treatment plan may be beneficial. Without additional investigation of these issues, we cannot state a preference for imaging or behavioral evaluation as the initial diagnostic approach.

7. Conventional versus Advanced MRI?

CT may be helpful in the acute stage after mTBI in children who meet decision rules that place them at greater risk for ICI. MRI may be more helpful for children with subacute symptoms. Children with chronic symptoms (of greater than 2–3 months' duration) may have (1) persistent unchanged symptoms, (2) some improvement but no return to baseline, or (3) abnormal neuropsychological testing. Conventional MRI or advanced MRI techniques can detect brain injury when CT, and even when some MRI techniques, are normal (see Figure 9.3). This has been well demonstrated in children with accidental as well as nonaccidental trauma (Ashwal et al., 2006, 2010). As more MRI studies are published of children with mTBI, sufficient data may show that MRI findings are more likely to be associated with long-term neuropsychological, behavioral, or neurological disability. Additional studies are needed to assess the prognostic potential of MRI for identifying risk for long-term neurobehavioral disorders. Further research in the pediatric mTBI population is needed as to whether conventional MRI methods (e.g., T2WI, FLAIR) are sufficiently sensitive to detect subtle injury or whether newer imaging methods (e.g., MRSI, DTI) would have greater diagnostic and prognostic yield.

8. Chronic Uncomplicated versus Chronic Complicated mTBI

In children with chronic symptoms, further diagnostic refinement may be possible using MRI. The presence of conditions such as DAI, subtle contusions, volumetric loss, or functional changes (e.g., associated with reduced fractional anisotropy) all suggest nervous system injury. In some individuals, the initial CT scan may have been normal but the MRI shows subtle ICI. Just as the terms *complicated* and *uncomplicated* have been suggested for categorizing patients with acute mTBI based on CT results, we suggest that the same approach could be considered for children with chronic mTBI symptoms. For example, those with MRI abnormalities, detected with conventional or advanced methods, could be diagnosed as having *chronic complicated mTBI*, and presumably this group would be at greater risk for long-term cognitive impairments. Those children with normal MRI could be diagnosed with *chronic uncomplicated mTBI* and presumably would be at lower risk. Both groups would need neurological and neuropsychological follow-up. However, two studies in adult patients with mTBI who did have MRI abnormalities failed to find significant long-term cognitive impairments, so clearly further studies of this issue in children are required (Hofman, Nelemans, Kemerink, & Wilmink, 2000; Hughes et al., 2004).

9. Chronic mTBI: Delayed Evaluation

Although the proposed algorithm begins at the time of injury, another group of children to be considered are those with mTBI who are not formally evaluated immediately after injury, but are seen for an initial neurological, neuropsychological, or psychiatric evaluation weeks or months after injury due to persistent or worsening postconcussive symptoms. The status of these children can be ascertained retrospectively if information obtained in the acute period is available (e.g., acute medical evaluation and CT or MRI reports). Depending on the individual's symptoms, findings on neurological examination, or the results of neuropsychological testing, brain dysfunction may be suspected. Neuroimaging should be considered for these individuals. However, the decision to obtain neuroimaging is confounded by the fact that many of these children may also have some reactive behavioral disorders, making it difficult to separate structural from functional components. As in subacute imaging, MRI is likely more useful than CT in the delayed evaluation of chronic mTBI, particularly using advanced imaging methods such as MRS and DTI. Further research in this group of children with mTBI is required to determine if imaging is helpful to diagnose underlying post mTBI impairments and whether this might have late therapeutic or prognostic implications.

REFERENCES

Aaen, G. S., Holshouser, B. A., Sheridan, C., Colbert, C., McKenney, M., Kido, D., et al. (2010). Magnetic resonance spectroscopy predicts outcomes for children with nonaccidental trauma. *Pediatrics*, *125*(2), 295–303.

Alessandri, B., al-Samsam, R., Corwin, F., Fatouros, P., Young, H. F., & Bullock, R. M. (2000). Acute and late changes in N-acetyl-aspartate following diffuse axonal injury in rats: An MRI spectroscopy and microdialysis study. *Neurology Research*, *22*(7), 705–712.

Arfanakis, K., Haughton, V. M., Carew, J. D., Rogers, B. P., Dempsey, R. J., & Meyerand, M. E. (2002). Diffusion tensor MR imaging in diffuse axonal injury. *American Journal of Neuroradiology*, *23*(5), 794–802.

Ashwal, S., Holshouser, B. A., Shu, S. K., Simmons, P. L., Perkin, R. M., Tomasi, L. G., et al. (2000). Predictive value of proton magnetic resonance spectroscopy in pediatric closed head injury. *Pediatric Neurology*, *23*(2), 114–125.

Ashwal, S., Holshouser, B. A., & Tong, K. A. (2006). Use of advanced neuroimaging techniques in the evaluation of pediatric traumatic brain injury. *Developmental Neuroscience, 28*(4–5), 309–326.

Ashwal, S., Holshouser, B. A., Tong, K. A., Serna, T., Osterdock, R., Gross, M., et al. (2004a). Proton MR spectroscopy detected glutamate/glutamine is increased in children with traumatic brain injury. *Journal of Neurotrauma, 21*(11), 1539–1552.

Ashwal, S., Holshouser, B. A., Tong, K. A, Serna, T., Osterdock, R., Gross, M., et al. (2004b). Proton spectroscopy detected myoinositol in children with traumatic brain injury. *Pediatric Research, 56*(4), 630–638.

Ashwal, S., Wycliffe, N. D., & Holshouser, B. A. (2010). Advanced neuroimaging in children with nonaccidental trauma. *Developmental Neuroscience, 32*(5–6), 343–360.

Atabaki, S. M., Stiell, I. G., Bazarian, J. J., Sadow, K. E., Vu, T. T., Camarca, M. A., et al. (2008). A clinical decision rule for cranial computed tomography in minor pediatric head trauma. *Archives of Pediatric and Adolescent Medicine, 162*(5), 439–445.

Babikian, T., Freier, M. C., Ashwal, S., Riggs, M. L., Burley, T., & Holshouser, B. A. (2006). MR spectroscopy: Predicting long-term neuropsychological outcome following pediatric TBI. *Journal of Magnetic Resonance Imaging, 24*(4), 801–811.

Babikian, T., Freier, M. C., Tong, K. A., Nickerson, J. P., Wall, C. J., Holshouser, B. A., et al. (2005). Susceptibility weighted imaging: Neuropsychologic outcome and pediatric head injury. *Pediatric Neurology, 33*(3), 184–194.

Bazarian, J. J., Zhong, J., Blyth, B., Zhu, T., Kavcic, V., & Peterson, D. (2007). Diffusion tensor imaging detects clinically important axonal damage after mild traumatic brain injury: A pilot study. *Journal of Neurotrauma, 24*(9), 1447–1459.

Beaudin, M., Saint-Vil, D., Ouimet, A., Mercier, C., & Crevier, L. (2007). Clinical algorithm and resource use in the management of children with minor head trauma. *Journal of Pediatric Surgery, 42*(5), 849–852.

Biousse, V., Suh, D. Y., Newman, N. J., Davis, P. C., Mapstone, T., & Lambert, S. R. (2002). Diffusion-weighted magnetic resonance imaging in shaken baby syndrome. *American Journal of Ophthalmology, 133*(2), 249–255.

Bluml, S. (1999). In vivo quantitation of cerebral metabolite concentrations using natural abundance 13C MRS at 1.5 T. *Journal of Magnetic Resonance, 136*(2), 219–225.

Boran, B. O., Boran, P., Barut, N., Akgun, C., Celikoglu, E., & Bozbuga, M. (2006). Evaluation of mild head injury in a pediatric population. *Pediatric Neurosurgery, 42*(4), 203–207.

Borgaro, S. R., Prigatano, G. P., Kwasnica, C., & Rexer, J. L. (2003). Cognitive and affective sequelae in complicated and uncomplicated mild traumatic brain injury. *Brain Injury, 17*(3), 189–198.

Brenner, D. J. (2002). Estimating cancer risks from pediatric CT: Going from the qualitative to the quantitative. *Pediatric Radiology, 32*(4), 228–223; discussion, 228–233.

Brenner, T., Freier, M. C., Holshouser, B. A., Burley, T., & Ashwal, S. (2003). Predicting neuropsychologic outcome after traumatic brain injury in children. *Pediatric Neurology, 28*(2), 104–114.

Bullock, R., Zauner, A., Woodward, J. J., Myseros, J., Choi, S. C., Ward, J. D., et al. (1998). Factors affecting excitatory amino acid release following severe human head injury. *Journal Neurosurgery, 89*(4), 507–518.

Carroll, L. J., Cassidy, J. D., Peloso, P. M., Borg, J., von Holst, H., Holm, L., et al. (2004). Prognosis for mild traumatic brain injury: Results of the WHO Collaborating Centre Task Force on Mild Traumatic Brain Injury. *Journal of Rehabilitation Medicine, 43* (Suppl.), 84–105.

Cecil, K. M., Hills, E. C., Sandel, M. E., Smith, D. H., McIntosh, T. K., Mannon, L. J., et al. (1998). Proton magnetic resonance spectroscopy for detection of axonal injury in the splenium of the corpus callosum of brain-injured patients. *Journal of Neurosurgery*, *88*(5), 795–801.

Chan, Y. L., Chu, W. C., Wong, G. W., & Yeung, D. K. (2003). Diffusion-weighted MRI in shaken baby syndrome. *Pediatric Radiology*, *33*(8), 574–577.

Chu, Z., Wilde, E. A., Hunter, J. V., McCauley, S. R., Bigler, E. D., Troyanskaya, M., et al. (2010). Voxel-based analysis of diffusion tensor imaging in mild traumatic brain injury in adolescents. *American Journal of Neuroradiology*, *31*(2), 340–346.

Cohen, B. A., Inglese, M., Rusinek, H., Babb, J. S., Grossman, R. I., & Gonen, O. (2007). Proton MR spectroscopy and MRI-volumetry in mild traumatic brain injury. *American Journal of Neuroradiology*, *28*(5), 907–913.

Connors, J. M., Ruddy, R. M., McCall, J., & Garcia, V. F. (2001). Delayed diagnosis in pediatric blunt trauma. *Pediatric Emergency Care*, *17*(1), 1–4.

Davis, R. L., Hughes, M., Gubler, K. D., Waller, P. L., & Rivara, F. P. (1995). The use of cranial CT scans in the triage of pediatric patients with mild head injury. *Pediatrics*, *95*(3), 345–349.

De Beaumont, L., Lassonde, M., Leclerc, S., & Theoret, H. (2007). Long-term and cumulative effects of sports concussion on motor cortex inhibition. *Neurosurgery*, *61*(2), 329–336.

Dunning, J., Daly, J. P., Lomas, J. P., Lecky, F., Batchelor, J., & Mackway-Jones, K. (2006). Derivation of the children's head injury algorithm for the prediction of important clinical events decision rule for head injury in children. *Archives of Disease in Childhood*, *91*(11), 885–891.

Durham, S. R., Liu, K. C., & Selden, N. R. (2006). Utility of serial computed tomography imaging in pediatric patients with head trauma. *Journal of Neurosurgery*, *105*(5, Suppl.), 365–369.

Falimirski, M. E., Gonzalez, R., Rodriguez, A., & Wilberger, J. (2003). The need for head computed tomography in patients sustaining loss of consciousness after mild head injury. *Journal of Trauma*, *55*(1), 1–6.

Farmer, M. Y., Singer, H. S., Mellits, E. D., Hall, D., & Charney, E. (1987). Neurobehavioral sequelae of minor head injuries in children. *Pediatric Neuroscience*, *13*(6), 304–308.

Fay, T. B., Yeates, K. O., Taylor, H. G., Bangert, B., Dietrich, A., Nuss, K. E., et al. (2010). Cognitive reserve as a moderator of postconcussive symptoms in children with complicated and uncomplicated mild traumatic brain injury. *Journal of the International Neuropsychology Society*, *16*(1), 94–105.

Galloway, N. R., Tong, K. A., Ashwal, S., Oyoyo, U., & Obenaus, A. (2008). Diffusion-weighted imaging improves outcome prediction in pediatric traumatic brain injury. *Journal of Neurotrauma*, *25*(10), 1153–1162.

Garnett, M. R., Blamire, A. M., Corkill, R. G., Cadoux-Hudson, T. A., Rajagopalan, B., & Styles, P. (2000). Early proton magnetic resonance spectroscopy in normal-appearing brain correlates with outcome in patients following traumatic brain injury. *Brain*, *123*(Pt. 10), 2046–2054.

Gasparovic, C., Yeo, R., Mannell, M., Ling, J., Elgie, R., Phillips, J., et al. (2009). Neurometabolite concentrations in gray and white matter in mild traumatic brain injury: An 1H-magnetic resonance spectroscopy study. *Journal of Neurotrauma*, *26*(10), 1635–1643.

Govindaraju, V., Gauger, G. E., Manley, G. T., Ebel, A., Meeker, M., & Maudsley, A. A. (2004). Volumetric proton spectroscopic imaging of mild traumatic brain injury. *American Journal of Neuroradiology*, *25*(5), 730–737.

Greenes, D. S., & Schutzman, S. A. (1997). Infants with isolated skull fracture: What are their clinical characteristics, and do they require hospitalization? *Annals of Emergency Medicine*, *30*(3), 253–259.

Greenes, D. S., & Schutzman, S. A. (1999). Clinical indicators of intracranial injury in head-injured infants. *Pediatrics, 104*(4 Pt 1): 861–867.

Greenes, D. S., & Schutzman, S. A. (2001). Clinical significance of scalp abnormalities in asymptomatic head-injured infants. *Pediatric Emergency Care, 17*(2), 88–92.

Haacke, E. M., Xu, Y., Cheng, Y. C., & Reichenbach, J. R. (2004). Susceptibility weighted imaging (SWI). *Magnetic Resonance in Medicine, 52*(3), 61–618.

Hattingen, E., Raab, P., Franz, K., Lanfermann, H., Setzer, M., Gerlach, R., et al. (2008). Prognostic value of choline and creatine in WHO grade II gliomas. *Neuroradiology, 50*(9), 759–767.

Haydel, M. J. (2005). Clinical decision instruments for CT scanning in minor head injury. *Journal of the American Medical Association, 294*(12), 1551–1553.

Haydel, M. J., & Shembekar, A. D. (2003). Prediction of intracranial injury in children aged five years and older with loss of consciousness after minor head injury due to nontrivial mechanisms. *Annals of Emergency Medicine, 42*(4), 507–514.

Henry, L. C., Tremblay, S., Boulanger, Y., Ellemberg, D., & Lassonde, M. (2010). Neuro-metabolic changes in the acute phase after sports concussions correlate with symptom severity. *Journal of Neurotrauma, 27*(1), 65–76.

Hergan, K., Oser, W., & Langle Jun, I. (2002). [Implementation of BIRADSTM together with an organization of percutaneous breast biopsies: experiences, reactions]. *Rofo, 174*(12), 1516–1521.

Hessen, E., & Nestvold, K. (2009). Indicators of complicated mild TBI predict MMPI-2 scores after 23 years. *Brain Injury, 23*(3), 234–242.

Hofman, P. A., Nelemans, P., Kemerink, G. J., & Wilmink, J. T. (2000). Value of radiological diagnosis of skull fracture in the management of mild head injury: Meta-analysis. *Journal of Neurology, Neurosurgery, and Psychiatry, 68*(4), 416–422.

Hollingworth, W., Vavilala, M. S., Jarvik, J. G., Chaudhry, S., Johnston, B. D., Layman, S., et al. (2007). The use of repeated head computed tomography in pediatric blunt head trauma: Factors predicting new and worsening brain injury. *Pediatric Critical Care Medicine, 8*(4), 348–356; CEU quiz, 357.

Holshouser, B. A., Ashwal, S., Luh, G. Y., Shu, S., Kahlon, S., Auld, K. L., et al. (1997). Proton MR spectroscopy after acute central nervous system injury: Outcome prediction in neonates, infants, and children. *Radiology, 202*(2), 487–496.

Holshouser, B. A., Ashwal, S., Shu, S., & Hinshaw, D. B., Jr. (2000). Proton MR spectroscopy in children with acute brain injury: Comparison of short and long echo time acquisitions. *Journal of Magnetic Resonance Imaging, 11*(1), 9–19.

Holshouser, B. A., Tong, K. A., & Ashwal, S. (2005). Proton MR spectroscopic imaging depicts diffuse axonal injury in children with traumatic brain injury. *American Journal of Neuroradiology, 26*(5), 1276–1285.

Hughes, D. G., Jackson, A., Mason, D. L., Berry, E., Hollis, S., & Yates, D. W. (2004). Abnormalities on magnetic resonance imaging seen acutely following mild traumatic brain injury: Correlation with neuropsychological tests and delayed recovery. *Neuroradiology, 46*(7), 550–558.

Huisman, T. A. (2003). Diffusion-weighted imaging: Basic concepts and application in cerebral stroke and head trauma. *European Radiology, 13*(10), 2283–2297.

Huisman, T. A., Sorensen, A. G., Hergan, K., Gonzalez, R. G., & Schaefer, P. W. (2003). Diffusion-weighted imaging for the evaluation of diffuse axonal injury in closed head injury. *Journal of Computer Assisted Tomography, 27*(1), 5–11.

Hunter, J. V., Thornton, R. J., Wang, Z. J., Levin, H. S., Roberson, G., Brooks, W. M., et al. (2005). Late proton MR spectroscopy in children after traumatic brain injury: Correlation with cognitive outcomes. *American Journal of Neuroradiology, 26*(3), 482–488.

Inglese, M., Li, B. S., Rusinek, H., Babb, J. S., Grossman, R. I., & Gonen, O. (2003). Diffusely elevated cerebral choline and creatine in relapsing–remitting multiple sclerosis. *Magnetic Resonance Medicine, 50*(1), 190–195.

Iverson, G. L. (2006). Complicated vs. uncomplicated mild traumatic brain injury: Acute neuropsychological outcome. *Brain Injury, 20*(13–14), 1335–1344.

Jones, K., Patrick, G., & Hickner, J. (2010). When is it safe to forego a CT in kids with head trauma? *Journal of Family Practice, 59*(3), 159–164.

Kashluba, S., Hanks, R. A., Casey, J. E., & Millis, S. R. (2008). Neuropsychologic and functional outcome after complicated mild traumatic brain injury. *Archives of Physical Medicine and Rehabilitation, 89*(5), 904–911.

Kennedy, R. E., Livingston, L., Marwitz, J. H., Gueck, S., Kreutzer, J. S., & Sander, A. M. (2006). Complicated mild traumatic brain injury on the inpatient rehabilitation unit: A multicenter analysis. *Journal of Head Trauma Rehabilitation, 21*(3), 260–271.

Klig, J. E., & Kaplan, C. P. (2010). Minor head injury in children. *Current Opinion in Pediatrics, 22*(3), 257–261.

Klingberg, T., Vaidya, C. J., Gabrieli, J. D., Moseley, M. E., & Hedehus, M. (1999). Myelination and organization of the frontal white matter in children: A diffusion tensor MRI study. *NeuroReport, 10*(13), 2817–2821.

Kuppermann, N. (2008). Pediatric head trauma: The evidence regarding indications for emergent neuroimaging. *Pediatric Radiology, 38*(Suppl. 4), S670–674.

Kuppermann, N., Holmes, J. F., Dayan, P. S., Hoyle, J. D., Jr., Atabaki, S. M., Holubkov, R., et al. (2009). Identification of children at very low risk of clinically-important brain injuries after head trauma: A prospective cohort study. *Lancet, 374*(9696), 1160–1170.

Lange, R. T., Iverson, G. L., & Franzen, M. D. (2009). Neuropsychological functioning following complicated vs. uncomplicated mild traumatic brain injury. *Brain Injury, 23*(2), 83–91.

Le Bihan, D., Mangin, J. F., Poupon, C., Clark, C. A., Pappata, S., Molko, N., et al. (2001). Diffusion tensor imaging: Concepts and applications. *Journal of Magnetic Resonance Imaging, 13*(4), 534–546.

Levin, H. S., Hanten, G., Roberson, G., Li, X., Ewing-Cobbs, L., Dennis, M., et al. (2008a). Prediction of cognitive sequelae based on abnormal computed tomography findings in children following mild traumatic brain injury. *Journal of Neurosurgery: Pediatrics, 1*(6), 461–470.

Levin, H. S., Wilde, E. A., Chu, Z., Yallampalli, R., Hanten, G. R., Li, X., et al. (2008b). Diffusion tensor imaging in relation to cognitive and functional outcome of traumatic brain injury in children. *Journal of Head Trauma Rehabilitation, 23*(4), 197–208.

Maguire, J. L., Boutis, K., Uleryk, E. M., Laupacis, A., & Parkin, P. C. (2009). Should a head-injured child receive a head CT scan?: A systematic review of clinical prediction rules. *Pediatrics, 124*(1), e145–e154.

Makoroff, K. L., Cecil, K. M., Care, M., & Ball, W. S., Jr. (2005). Elevated lactate as an early marker of brain injury in inflicted traumatic brain injury. *Pediatric Radiology, 35*(7), 668–676.

Malec, J. F., Brown, A. W., Leibson, C. L., Flaada, J. T., Mandrekar, J. N., Diehl, N. N., et al. (2007). The Mayo classification system for traumatic brain injury severity. *Journal of Neurotrauma, 24*(9), 1417–1424.

Melo, J. R., Reis, R. C., Lemos-Junior, L. P., Azevedo-Neto, A., Oliveira, D. W., Garcia, F. R., et al. (2008). Skull radiographs and computed tomography scans in children and adolescents with mild head trauma. *Arquivos de Neuro-Psiquiatria, 66*(3B), 708–710.

Moffett, J. R., Ross, B., Arun, P., Madhavarao, C. N., & Namboodiri, A. M. (2007). N-Acetylaspartate in the CNS: From neurodiagnostics to neurobiology. *Progress in Neurobiology, 81*(2), 89–131.

Niogi, S. N., & Mukherjee, P. (2010). Diffusion tensor imaging of mild traumatic brain injury. *Journal of Head Trauma Rehabilitation, 25*(4), 241–255.

Osmond, M. H., Klassen, T. P., Wells, G. A., Correll, R., Jarvis, A., Joubert, G., et al. (2010). CATCH: A clinical decision rule for the use of computed tomography in children with minor head injury. *Canadian Medical Association Journal, 182*(4), 341–348.

Palchak, M. J., Holmes, J. F., Vance, C. W., Gelber, R. E., Schauer, B. A., Harrison, M. J., et al. (2003). A decision rule for identifying children at low risk for brain injuries after blunt head trauma. *Annals of Emergency Medicine, 42*(4), 492–506.

Panigrahy, A., Nelson, M. D., Jr., & Bluml, S. (2010). Magnetic resonance spectroscopy in pediatric neuroradiology: Clinical and research applications. *Pediatric Radiology, 40*(1), 3–30.

Parizel, P. M., Ceulemans, B., Laridon, A., Ozsarlak, O., Van Goethem, J. W., & Jorens, P. G. (2003). Cortical hypoxic–ischemic brain damage in shaken-baby (shaken impact) syndrome: Value of diffusion-weighted MRI. *Pediatric Radiology, 33*(12), 868–871.

Parry, L., Shores, A., Rae, C., Kemp, A., Waugh, M. C., Chaseling, R., et al. (2004). An investigation of neuronal integrity in severe paediatric traumatic brain injury. *Child Neuropsychology, 10*(4), 248–261.

Ponsford, J., Willmott, C., Rothwell, A., Cameron, P., Ayton, G., Nelms, R., et al. (1999). Cognitive and behavioral outcome following mild traumatic head injury in children. *Journal of Head Trauma Rehabilitation, 14*(4), 360–372.

Povlishock, J. T., & Christman, C. W. (1995). The pathobiology of traumatically induced axonal injury in animals and humans: A review of current thoughts. *Journal of Neurotrauma, 12*(4), 555–564.

Prasad, M. R., Ewing-Cobbs, L., Swank, P. R., & Kramer, L. (2002). Predictors of outcome following traumatic brain injury in young children. *Pediatric Neurosurgery, 36*(2), 64–74.

Schaefer, P. W., Huisman, T. A., Sorensen, A. G., Gonzalez, R. G., & Schwamm, L. H. (2004). Diffusion-weighted MR imaging in closed head injury: High correlation with initial Glasgow Coma Scale score and score on modified Rankin scale at discharge. *Radiology, 233*(1), 58–66.

Schnellinger, M. G., Reid, S., & Louie, J. (2010). Are serial brain imaging scans required for children who have suffered acute intracranial injury secondary to blunt head trauma? *Clinical Pediatrics (Philadelphia), 49*(6), 569–573.

Schumann, M., Stiller, D., Thomas, B., Brinker, T., & Samii, M. (2000). 1H-MR spectroscopic monitoring of posttraumatic metabolism following controlled cortical impact injury: Pilot study. *Acta Neurochirurgica, 76*(Suppl.), 3–7.

Schutzman, S. A., Barnes, P., Duhaime, A. C., Greenes, D., Homer, C., Jaffe, D., et al. (2001). Evaluation and management of children younger than two years old with apparently minor head trauma: Proposed guidelines. *Pediatrics, 107*(5), 983–993.

Schutzman, S. A., & Greenes, D. S. (2001). Pediatric minor head trauma. *Annals of Emergency Medicine, 37*(1), 65–74.

Sehgal, V., Delproposto, Z., Haacke, E. M., Tong, K. A., Wycliffe, N., Kido, D. K., et al. (2005). Clinical applications of neuroimaging with susceptibility-weighted imaging. *Journal of Magnetic Resonance Imaging, 22*(4), 439–450.

Shane, S. A., & Fuchs, S. M. (1997). Skull fractures in infants and predictors of associated intracranial injury. *Pediatric Emergency Care, 13*(3), 198–203.

Sigmund, G. A., Tong, K. A., Nickerson, J. P., Wall, C. J., Oyoyo, U., & Ashwal, S. (2007). Multimodality comparison of neuroimaging in pediatric traumatic brain injury. *Pediatric Neurology, 36*(4), 217–226.

Simon, B., Letourneau, P., Vitorino, E., & McCall, J. (2001). Pediatric minor head trauma:

Indications for computed homographic scanning revisited. *Journal Trauma, 55*: 231–237.

Suh, D. Y., Davis, P. C., Hopkins, K. L., Fajman, N. N., & Mapstone, T. B. (2001). Nonaccidental pediatric head injury: Diffusion-weighted imaging findings. *Neurosurgery, 49*(2), 309–318; discussion, 318–320.

Thiessen, M. L., & Woolridge, D. P. (2006). Pediatric minor closed head injury. *Pediatric Clinics of North America, 53*(1), 1–26, v.

Tong, K. A., Ashwal, S., Holshouser, B. A., Nickerson, J. P., Wall, C. J., Shutter, L. A., et al. (2004). Diffuse axonal injury in children: Clinical correlation with hemorrhagic lesions. *Annals of Neurology, 56*(1), 36–50.

Tong, K. A., Ashwal, S., Holshouser, B. A., Shutter, L. A., Herigault, G., Haacke, E. M., et al. (2003). Hemorrhagic shearing lesions in children and adolescents with posttraumatic diffuse axonal injury: Improved detection and initial results. *Radiology, 227*(2), 332–339.

Tong, K. A., Ashwal, S., Obenaus, A., Nickerson, J. P., Kido, D., & Haacke, E. M. (2008). Susceptibility-weighted MR imaging: A review of clinical applications in children. *American Journal of Neuroradiology, 29*(1), 9–17.

Vagnozzi, R., Signoretti, S., Tavazzi, B., Floris, R., Ludovici, A., Marziali, S., et al. (2008). Temporal window of metabolic brain vulnerability to concussion: A pilot 1H-magnetic resonance spectroscopic study in concussed athletes—Part III. *Neurosurgery, 62*(6), 1286–1295.

Walz, N. C., Cccil, K. M., Wade, S. L., & Michaud, L. J. (2008). Late proton magnetic resonance spectroscopy following traumatic brain injury during early childhood: Relationship with neurobehavioral outcomes. *Journal of Neurotrauma, 25*(2), 94–103.

Wilde, E. A., Bigler, E. D., Haider, J. M., Chu, Z., Levin, H. S., Li, X., et al. (2006a). Vulnerability of the anterior commissure in moderate to severe pediatric traumatic brain injury. *Journal of Child Neurology, 21*(9), 769–776.

Wilde, E. A., Chu, Z., Bigler, E. D., Hunter, J. V., Fearing, M. A., Hanten, G., et al. (2006b). Diffusion tensor imaging in the corpus callosum in children after moderate to severe traumatic brain injury. *Journal of Neurotrauma, 23*(10), 1412–1426.

Wilde, E. A., McCauley, S. R., Hunter, J. V., Bigler, E. D., Chu, Z., Wang, Z. J., et al. (2008). Diffusion tensor imaging of acute mild traumatic brain injury in adolescents. *Neurology, 70*(12), 948–955.

Williams, D. H., Levin, H. S., & Eisenberg, H. M. (1990). Mild head injury classification. *Neurosurgery, 27*(3), 422–428.

Wozniak, J. R., Krach, L., Ward, E., Mueller, B. A., Muetzel, R., Schnoebelen, S., et al. (2007). Neurocognitive and neuroimaging correlates of pediatric traumatic brain injury: A diffusion tensor imaging (DTI) study. *Archives of Clinical Neuropsychology, 22*(5), 555–568.

Wu, T. C., Wilde, E. A., Bigler, E. D., Yallampalli, R., McCauley, S. R., Troyanskaya, M., et al. (2010). Evaluating the relationship between memory functioning and cingulum bundles in acute mild traumatic brain injury using diffusion tensor imaging. *Journal of Neurotrauma, 27*(2), 303–307.

Yeo, R. A., Phillips, J. P., Jung, R. E., Brown, A. J., Campbell, R. C., & Brooks, W. M. (2006). Magnetic resonance spectroscopy detects brain injury and predicts cognitive functioning in children with brain injuries. *Journal of Neurotrauma, 23*(10), 1427–1435.

CHAPTER 10

Physical and Neurological Exam

Joseph A. Grubenhoff and Aaron Provance

EPIDEMIOLOGY AND THE IMPORTANCE OF THE PHYSICAL AND NEUROLOGICAL EXAM

Traumatic brain injury (TBI) represents a major health burden for U.S. children. According to data collected from three national databases, TBI affects over 680,000 children annually in the United States (Faul, Xu, Wald, & Coronado, 2010; Langlois, Rutland-Brown, & Thomas, 2005). The vast majority of these patients are cared for in, and released from, emergency departments (EDs). However, these numbers likely underestimate the true burden of injury, as many patients are never evaluated in an ED or hospital (Setnik & Bazarian, 2007). There is considerable overlap in the initial clinical presentation of patients with mild TBI (mTBI) compared to those with moderate to severe injuries (Iverson, Lovell, Smith, & Franzen, 2000). This overlap challenges health care providers treating patients in the acute period following a head injury, as they must quickly determine which victims have suffered potentially lethal or permanently disabling insults. Although this book focuses on the pediatric victim of mTBI, an understanding of the spectrum of TBI, especially its more severe manifestations, is germane to the care of all patients with head injury.

Spectrum of Injury

At the most basic level, TBI severity is divided into mild, moderate, and severe categories. Classification most often occurs according to the Glasgow Coma Scale (GCS): mild = 13–15, moderate = 9–12, and severe ≤ 8. It is important to recognize that these divisions represent a continuum of injury, and the borders of these divisions are indistinct. For example, it is possible to have a GCS of 15 in the face of an epidural hematoma, a surgical emergency. In contrast, the metabolic derangements of mTBI can lead to severe compromise in cerebral function, potentially requiring intubation for protection of the airway even in the absence of acute findings on computed tomography (CT). This complexity requires the prudent clinician to be cognizant of the continuum so that potentially life-threatening injuries are identified.

Additionally, TBI does not always occur in isolation and the clinician must consider the possibility of associated injuries, particularly those of the neck and spine. Cervical spine injuries are rare among children but not insignificant. In two large trauma registries, cervical spine injuries were found in 1–2% of all pediatric trauma victims (Brown, Brunn, & Garcia, 2001; Platzer et al., 2007). The multicenter prospective National Emergency X-Radiography Utilization Study (NEXUS) reported similar findings (Viccellio et al., 2001). Motor vehicle collision accounts for the majority of spine injuries among all age groups, followed by falls for children ≤ 8 years and sports-related mechanisms in children > 8 years (Cirak et al., 2004; Patel, Tepas, Mollitt, & Pieper, 2001). These mechanisms are also the most commonly associated with TBI, thus highlighting the importance of careful attention to protection of the cervical spine during the initial evaluation of the head-injured patient.

Goals of the Physical and Neurological Exam

The physical and neurological exam serves to (1) identify life threatening injuries; (2) direct referral decisions in settings outside the ED (e.g., sideline, school); (3) provide direction in obtaining appropriate imaging studies; and (4) identify associated injuries. The exam is divided into two phases. The first phase is common to the care of any trauma victim and consists of a *primary survey* focusing on airway, breathing, circulation, neurological disability, and exposure of the patient (ABCDE). Once life-threatening conditions have been recognized and stabilized, the examination proceeds to a *secondary survey*, including a focused history and a thorough physical and neurological exam. A *tertiary survey* (laboratory and radiographic studies) may be indicated based on the findings in the primary and secondary surveys.

PRIMARY SURVEY

Airway and Cervical Spine

Acute care of the head trauma victim must aim to prevent any secondary injury. Paramount among these considerations is providing adequate oxygen delivery to the central nervous system. This begins by ensuring a patent airway. In a patient who is ambulating immediately following injury, speaking clearly, demonstrating no respiratory distress, and reporting no complaints of neck pain, the provider can be relatively reassured that the airway is patent and a cervical spine or spinal cord injury is unlikely.

When the mechanism of injury involves considerable biomechanical force (e.g., high-speed or rollover motor vehicle collision, axial loading of the spine during a football tackle) or the patient displays a significant depression in level of consciousness, then a more cautious approach is indicated. The airway should be cleared of any foreign material, blood, teeth, or vomitus. Because head trauma is frequently associated with cervical spine and/or spinal cord injury, manipulation of the neck in order to open the airway should be avoided and movement of the patient prior to the arrival of emergency medical personnel should be avoided, assuming this does not place the patient at risk for further injury. A jaw thrust performed by placing the fingers posterior to the angles of the mandible and moving the mandible anteriorly is the preferred method of opening the airway (Ralston, Hazinski, Zaritsky, Schexnayder, & Kleinman 2005; see Figure 10.1). If this maneuver is insufficient, placement of an oral airway—a plastic device inserted over the tongue with a rigid conduit for airflow and flange allowing the teeth to hold it in place—may facilitate opening the airway; this device should be used only in the unconscious patient as its use may induce vomiting in conscious victims. If a patent airway is not obtained after these measures, then the child is in need of care by providers with advanced airway management skills.

Concomitant with the interventions described above, the cervical spine should be immobilized. Until a rigid cervical collar can be fitted, manual immobilization with the hands placed on the sides of the head can be performed (Figure 10.2). Ideally, this is accomplished with a rigid cervical collar (Figure 10.3). If a cervical collar is not readily available, manual immobilization or securing the head to a spine board, using tape and towel rolls placed on either side of the head, is acceptable.

In the helmeted athlete (e.g., football, lacrosse, hockey) who has sustained a blow to head, the helmet and shoulder pads should remain in place unless the airway is compromised. The helmet should never be removed without removal of the shoulder pads because this could hyperextend the cervical spine, worsening a potential cord injury. In the case of an unconscious patient with airway compromise, the face mask should be removed. Specific tools should be used to remove the face mask (Figure 10.4). These tools include power drills to remove screws or specific clippers to cut the face mask fasteners. The face mask should also be removed prior to transportation to the ED via ambulance (Petrizzi, Reisman, & Cole, 2007). Face mask removal provides unobstructed access to the airway, allowing the health care professional to assess vital signs and initiate resuscitation as needed (Kleiner & Cantu, 1996).

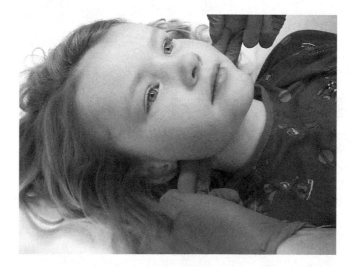

FIGURE 10.1. Jaw thrust maneuver: The fingers are place on the posterior aspect of the angle of the mandible and the jaw is pushed anteriorly.

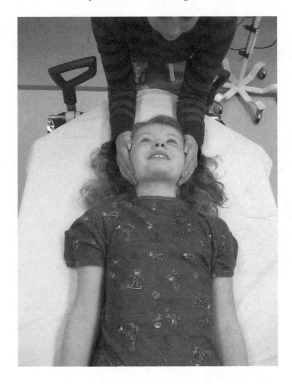

FIGURE 10.2. Manual in-line cervical immobilization.

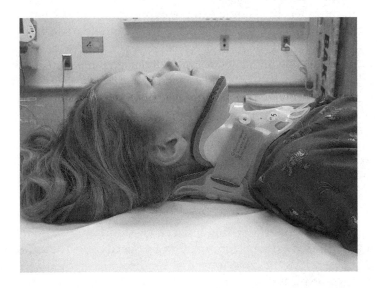

FIGURE 10.3. Appropriate placement of a cervical collar with neck in neutral position.

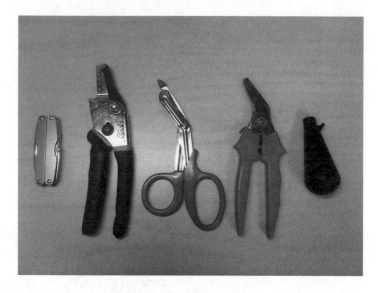

FIGURE 10.4. Tools for removal of helmet face mask: from left to right: pocket multi-tool, FMx-tractor2® face mask removal tool, trauma shears, heavy duty shears, Riddell Quick Release® Face Mask Installation Tool.

In rare instances, the injured athlete may need cardiopulmonary resuscitation on the field requiring the removal of helmet and shoulder pads. This requires two trained health professionals who are comfortable performing the maneuver. The jaw pads are removed and the air bladders are deflated prior to removal of the helmet shell. This can be accomplished by using a tongue depressor or reflex hammer to remove the jaw pads one at a time prior to helmet removal. One person pulls the ear holes apart and lifts the helmet off of the athlete's head while the second person maintains stabilization of the cervical spine. Prior to shoulder pad removal, jerseys and shirts are cut from the neck to the waist at the anterior midline. All straps and laces are cut from the front of the shoulder pads. Maintaining cervical stabilization, the shoulder pads are removed after the helmet has been removed. This technique is performed by pulling the back of the shoulder pads past the athlete's neck and head superiorly. Care must be taken to not change alignment of the trunk, neck, and head throughout these procedures (Waninger, 2004; see Figure 10.5).

Breathing

Victims of mTBI rarely require assisted breathing. A conscious patient who is verbal and shows no respiratory distress is breathing effectively. When the patient demonstrates a depressed level of consciousness, the provider should carefully evaluate the effectiveness of respirations. The depth and regularity of breathing need special attention. A slow rate or shallow or irregular respiratory pattern may herald Cushing's triad (hypertension, bradycardia, and irregular respirations), which is the result of tentorial herniation of the uncus of the temporal lobe leading to direct pressure on the brainstem. This finding requires immediate measures to decrease intracranial pressure.

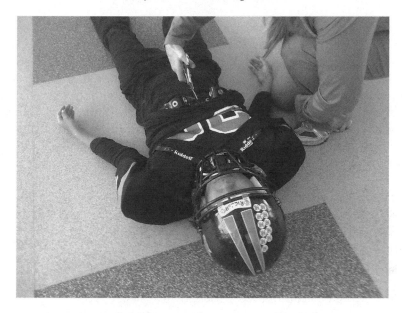

FIGURE 10.5. Shoulder pad removal.

Circulation

Circulatory disturbance is unusual in the setting of mTBI, whereas altered mental status—a potential sign of circulatory end organ dysfunction—is common. Depressed consciousness, nonetheless, should prompt the provider to consider more severe brain injury or cervical spinal cord injury. Elevation of intracranial pressure due to swelling or intracranial hemorrhage may produce hypertension as the autonomic nervous system attempts to maintain cerebral perfusion pressure.

Neurogenic (spinal) shock may be present. Neurogenic shock should be considered in the patient who displays hypotension in the absence of tachycardia or signs of peripheral vasoconstriction: mottled skin, cool extremities, and weak pulses.

Disability

During the primary survey, a truncated neurological exam is performed to rapidly identify signs of central nervous system dysfunction. The principal parts of this portion are an examination of pupil size and light reactivity and assignment of a GCS score. Any findings during this portion of the exam indicate the need for life-saving interventions, urgent imaging, and neurosurgical consultation.

A single dilated pupil (anisocoria) may indicate early tentorial herniation placing pressure on the ipsilateral third cranial nerve or diffuse cerebral edema (Greenes, 2006). Bilateral pupil dilation and loss of light reactivity results from progression of tentorial herniation, diffuse cerebral edema, or ischemic/anoxic brain injury. It is important to consider the use of illicit drugs during the pupil evaluation of the head-injured patient as well. Sympathomimetic agents (e.g., cocaine, amphetamines) and benzodiazepines are two commonly abused classes of drugs and may contribute to a patient's head trauma and cause pupil dilation.

The GCS deserves special attention in the discussion of the physical examination of the victim of TBI. Teasdale and Jennett (1974) first introduced the concept of a brief objective scale to classify the depth of coma found among victims of head trauma more than three decades ago. No other scale has been as widely adopted for triage, acute management, and prediction of outcomes after TBI (Marcin & Pollack, 2002). This simple scale is useful for initially assessing disability rapidly and monitoring early clinical changes, and it has been incorporated into many other trauma scales (Sternbach 2000). It allows for unambiguous discussion of a patient's condition across institutions. The GCS, particularly the motor component, is a reliable predictor of outcomes after moderate and severe TBI (Fabbri, Servadei, Marchesini, Stein, & Vandelli, 2008; Healey et al., 2003; Ting, Chen, Hsieh, & Chan, 2010). Haukoos, Gill, Rabon, Gravitz, and Green (2007) argued that a simplified motor score is equally reliable and easier to use. For a detailed discussion regarding the predictive utility of the GCS, the reader is referred to McNett (2007).

The GCS performs less well in the evaluation and management of mTBI victims. Convention suggests that a GCS of 13–15 indicates mTBI. Several authors have noted favorable outcomes for head-injured patients with higher GCS scores (Bishara, Partridge, Godfrey, & Knight, 1992; Pal, Brown, & Fleiszer, 1989; Young et al., 1981). However, the measures of favorable outcomes used in these studies focus on gross neurological functioning, such as the Glasgow Outcome Scale (GOS), rather than on specific assessments of cognitive functioning and persistent symptoms. For example, a top score of 5 on the GOS scale, which indicates good recovery, still allows the patient to have minor residual problems; these problems are not elucidated in the scale. Additionally, even a GCS score of 15 can be associated with significant mTBI symptoms among children (Grubenhoff, Kirkwood, Gao, Deakyne, & Wathen, 2010). That is, the GCS exhibits a ceiling effect when assessing mTBI.

Recognizing these limitations, the Glasgow Coma Score—Extended (GCS-E) was devised (Nell, Yates, & Kruger, 2000). The GCS-E includes an assessment of the duration of posttraumatic amnesia associated with mTBI (see Table 10.1). Nell and colleagues found rates of amnesia between 27 and 30% among head-injured patients with a GCS score of 13–15. In a study of adult patients, the GCS-E predicted the development of certain mTBI symptoms as well as poorer cognitive performance on the Standardized Assessment of Concussion (Drake, McDonald, Magnus, Gray, & Gottshall 2006). No studies have assessed the performance of the GCS-E among children. Despite these limitations, the GCS remains an important part of the immediate neurological assessment of children with head injuries because of its value in readily identifying more severe brain injury.

Exposure

Completely exposing the body of a victim of an isolated head injury with a GCS of 13–15 is not typically necessary. In contrast, any victim who is suspected of having multisystem injuries or who has significant alteration of consciousness requires removal of clothing to allow for rapid identification of other possible injuries. It is important to consider ambient conditions that may adversely affect the patient and delay this phase of the primary survey until the patient is evaluated in a climate-controlled environment (e.g., training room, ED).

TABLE 10.1. Glasgow Coma Scale and Glasgow Coma Scale—Extended

GCS	Score	GCS-E	Score
Eye Response		No amnesia	7
Spontaneous opening	4	Amnesia ≤ 30 minutes	
Open to verbal stimuli	3	Amnesia 30 minutes–	5
Open to painful stimuli	2	< 3 hours	4
No opening	1	Amnesia 3–< 24 hours	3
		Amnesia 1–7 days	
Verbal Response		Amnesia 8–30 days	2
Oriented speech	5	Amnesia 31–90 days	1
Confused or disoriented	4		
Inappropriate words	3		
Incomprehensible sounds	2		
No verbal response			
Motor Response			
Obeys commands	6		
Localizes pain	5		
Withdraws from pain	4		
Flexor posturing to pain	3		
Extensor posturing to pain	2		
No motor response	1		

INITIAL MANAGEMENT OF LIFE-THREATENING CONDITIONS

A detailed discussion of the care of the severely neurologically injured child is beyond the scope of this chapter. However, a brief discussion of the initial treatment of the patient with head trauma who may have life-threatening conditions is relevant. *Any time a life-threatening injury is suspected, activation of emergency medical services is indicated.* While awaiting the arrival of trained prehospital personnel, certain key interventions are appropriate.

Cervical Spine Immobilization/Airway Control

The reader is referred to the Airway and Cervical Spine section of the Primary Survey above.

Treatment of Elevated Intracranial Pressure

Although uncommon with mild or even moderate TBI, any patient with a head injury is at some risk of elevated intracranial pressure (ICP). If a patient has a GCS < 8, anisocoria, hypertension with bradycardia, irregular respirations, or complaints of severe headache, the head of the bed should be elevated to 30° to allow gravity to assist in venous drainage from the skull. However, maintaining appropriate spine immobilization is of paramount importance, so elevation of the head should be done only in patients who are not suspected of having cervical spine injury or who are appropriately immobilized. For patients requiring assisted ventilation, hyperventilation can acutely lower ICP via vasoconstriction. This effect is lost after approximately 30 minutes.

Seizures

The incidence of seizures among children with mTBI is not well established, although they do occur in a small minority of children (see Davis, Chapter 6, this volume). The surroundings of a patient experiencing a posttraumatic seizure should be cleared of any objects that may harm the patient. The patient should be laid in the rescue position: lying on the side with the downward leg straight and the upward leg hip and knee flexed, with the upward hand supporting the head. If a suction device is available, secretions and vomitus should be cleared from the mouth. With the exception of suction devices, no objects should be inserted into the mouth of the seizing patient. Doing so could induce vomiting or obstruct the airway further. Use of a finger sweep should be discouraged, as this could lead to injuries such as bite wounds. Administer supplemental oxygen if available; cerebral metabolic rates and, consequently, oxygen demand are increased during a seizure. Support of breathing is not usually necessary early in the course of a seizure. Although the patient may appear apneic, it is likely that he or she is only breathing more shallowly, and supplemental oxygen should be sufficient to maintain oxygen delivery to the brain. If cyanosis develops or the seizure persists for more than 2 minutes, ventilatory support may be required.

SECONDARY SURVEY

Although it is important to identify and address life-threatening injuries in victims of TBI, most patients will not require any significant resuscitative efforts. Attention can then be turned to a focused history and physical exam.

History

The history begins with obtaining the time of injury, mechanism involved, impact surface, and any modifying factors such as the use of protective equipment. Immediate postinjury events such as loss of consciousness, posttraumatic seizure, disorientation, and first aid measures should also be evaluated.

After inquiring about the injury itself, attention can turn to the symptoms that resulted from the injury. This is best accomplished using a concussion symptom inventory. Many concussion symptom inventories are available in the literature (e.g., Sports Concussion Assessment Tool, Standardized Assessment of Concussion, Acute Concussion Evaluation), though none has been proven to be superior. Chapter 12 of this volume, by Janusz, Sady, and Gioia, provides a comprehensive discussion of these instruments.

In addition to somatic complaints, victims of mTBI often display cognitive difficulties. Several studies of adults have found early cognitive impairment during evaluation in the ED (Naunheim, Matero, & Fucetola, 2008; Petersen, Stull, Collins, & Wang, 2009; Sheedy, Geffen, Donnelly, & Faux, 2006) and on the sideline (McCrea, 2001; McCrea et al., 1998). Assessing cognitive function of children in the ED is particularly difficult given their ongoing mental development and lack of population-level normative data for screening instruments. One should not rely exclusively on a brief screen of orientation to person, place, and time (e.g., "What is your last name?", "What state are we in?", "What day is it?") and general knowledge ("Who is the president?") to assess the degree of cognitive impairment. These questions do not address the major cognitive domains that tend to be primarily affected by mTBI (e.g., attention, concentration, and memory) and may lead to false reassurance that no cognitive deficits exist. The clinician must attempt to elicit from parents or other caregivers any signs of impaired cognition.

Many authors have questioned the validity of symptom inventories when evaluating and managing victims of mTBI due to multiple factors. Several studies have examined the frequency of mTBI symptoms in various populations that do not have a history of head injury. Adult patients with a history of depression, even in the absence of head injury, often report symptoms common to postconcussion syndrome (PCS; Iverson, 2006; Suhr & Gunstad, 2002). This trend has also been noted in healthy adult populations (Gouvier, Uddo-Crane, & Brown, 1988; Iverson & Lange, 2003; Machulda, Bergquist, Ito, & Chew, 1998). Confounders such as malingering, workers' compensation claims, and civil litigation proceedings have also been cited as reasons to suspect the validity of symptom reporting. These issues are much less likely to affect children. However, it is important to consider that children may exaggerate or feign symptoms following mTBI (Kirkwood & Kirk, 2010). Until the pathophysiological mechanisms for symptoms associated with mTBI are delineated clearly, there will likely be controversy surrounding the importance of symptom inventories.

Additional historical information relevant to the evaluation of the child with a suspected mTBI is shown in Table 10.2. A previous history of mTBI and participation in other activities at high risk for mTBI need to be considered. Important factors to delineate include the number of prior concussions, as well as their duration and proximity to the current injury.

TABLE 10.2. Historical Information to Obtain When Evaluating Children with Head Injury

Medical history	Surgical history	Social history

Prior mTBI(s)
  Number
  Severity of injury
  Duration of symptoms
  Most recent TBI
	Intracranial shunt
	Tumor resection
		Organized sports
		Recreational sports
		Recreational vehicle use
		Use of alcohol or controlled
		  substances

Seizure disorder		
Bleeding disorder or use of anti-coagulants		
History of headaches		

Psychiatric illness
  ADHD
  Depression
  Bipolar disorder
  Anxiety disorder		

Note. ADHD, attention-deficit/hyperactivity disorder.

Physical and Neurological Exam

The physical exam performed in the acute care setting is guided by the mechanism of injury and the patient's complaints and symptoms. When multisystem trauma is a concern, examination of the chest, abdomen, and pelvis is important. This section focuses on examination of the structures of the head, face, and neck and the central nervous system.

The scalp should be closely examined for bruising, hematomas (localized swelling), and lacerations. Although these findings are unlikely to be of significant consequence to the patient, they may alert the provider to more serious cranial or intracranial injuries. Bruising over the mastoid bone (Battle's sign) is suggestive of a skull base fracture, which, in turn, suggests that a high degree of force was applied to the skull. Skull base fractures carry a high risk of injury to the structures of the middle and inner ear. Complications include conductive hearing loss due to disruption of the ear bones, injury to the facial (VII) and vestibulocochlear (VIII) cranial nerves, and meningitis from translocation of middle ear or sinus bacteria. Hematomas, especially those that are large or exhibit a boggy quality on palpation, may suggest underlying skull fracture. Lacerations, although usually superficial, should be explored while maintaining appropriate aseptic precautions. A laceration at the site of a skull fracture defines an open skull fracture, which also carries a risk of meningitis.

Ear examination includes inspection for any fluid or blood draining from the ear canal; either may be suggestive of a temporal bone fracture. Hemotympanum (blood behind the ear drum) may also be noted with temporal bone fracture. This finding may evolve over time, and if there is strong suspicion, repeat examination can be useful. A bedside test for the presence of cerebrospinal fluid (CSF) in bloody ear drainage involves placing a drop of blood on tissue or filter paper; a ring of fluid extending outside the drop of blood ("halo" sign) has been considered to be suggestive of the presence of CSF. However, the sensitivity and specificity for an associated skull fracture have not been established, so the absence of a "halo" should not be construed as proof that no skull fracture exists.

Examination of the eyes should include not only the function of the cranial nerves as detailed below but also the orbits. Attention should be given to the presence of bruising around the eyes (raccoon eyes), which could signal a skull base fracture. Swelling around the eyes may indicate fracture of the facial bones.

The nose should be inspected for clear or bloody drainage, hematomas of the nasal septum, and deformity. Clear drainage from the nose may suggest skull base fracture. Nose bleeds are likely due to trauma to the veins just inside the nose. Hematomas of the septum require drainage to prevent bony erosion. Palpation may reveal deformity that is not appreciated on inspection due to swelling.

During the examination of the mouth, the patient's ability to open the mouth should be noted first. Limitation in range of motion or pain with movement at the temporomandibular joints (TMJ) should alert the provider to the possibility of fracture or dislocation. The jaw should be palpated for tenderness, especially at the TMJ. A simple bedside maneuver to assess for jaw fractures is performed by having the patient bite a wooden tongue depressor positioned between the molars. The patient is then instructed to break the tongue depressor by bending it with his or her hand. Inability to do so may suggest a fracture. Inspect the teeth for fractures, avulsions, inward or sideways displacement, and abnormal alignment of the biting surfaces. The upper central incisors are most frequently injured due to their prominence. If dental pain is reported, an assessment of tenderness and stability within the socket is indicated. Any lacerations of the tongue should be noted; however, most tongue lacerations do not require repair. In adolescents, the use of alcohol and other intoxicants must be considered in the setting of blunt head trauma, especially in the presence of altered mental status. Thus, any unusual odors from the mouth or clothing should be observed.

As noted previously, cervical spine injury is uncommon among pediatric trauma victims but the most common mechanisms are the same as for TBI. Consequently, a careful and thorough examination of the cervical spine is mandatory, especially in cases of high-velocity impacts or substantial axial loads applied to the cervical spine (e.g., motor vehicle crash, "spearing" injury in football, diving). The thoracolumbar spine should also be examined in the face of high-energy mechanisms. If a patient presents for care with a cervical collar in place, the collar should not be removed for the exam unless an assistant can maintain in-line immobilization during the exam. If the patient is ambulatory at the time of presentation, a cervical collar should be applied for any of the following findings: concerning mechanism, moderate to severe pain, weakness, numbness and tingling, loss of bowel or bladder control, sustained erection, focal neurological findings, altered mental status, or intoxication.

Careful palpation of each spinous process for tenderness, "step-off (a loss of normal alignment of vertebral spinous processes)," and crepitus (crackling or grating feeling or sound under the skin) should be performed. The paraspinal muscles need to be palpated for tenderness, as cervical strain can be associated with muscle spasm and torticollis. In the immobilized patient and after examination of distal motor function and reflexes, the patient should be "log-rolled" and the thoracic and lumbar spine examined in similar fashion (Figure 10.6).

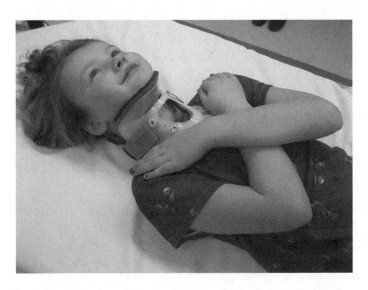

FIGURE 10.6. Preparation of patient for log roll.

Criteria exist for the removal of a rigid cervical collar without obtaining radiographs, often referred to as "clinical clearance" (Hoffman, Wolfson, Todd, & Mower, 1998). Patients must meet all of the following criteria: normal level of alertness, no focal neurological deficit, no evidence of intoxication, no posterior midline neck tenderness, and no painful distracting injury. When these criteria were specifically examined in a pediatric cohort, they performed similarly as in adults (Viccellio et al., 2001). However, the authors noted that there were few young children (< 8 years old) in the study. More recently, a multicenter retrospective study of children < 16 years old with blunt trauma found that a different set of criteria may be more appropriate in this setting (Leonard et al., 2010). Having any one of the factors (altered mental status, focal neurological findings, neck pain, torticollis, substantial torso injury, conditions predisposing to cervical spine injury, diving, and high-risk motor vehicle crash) was 98% sensitive (95% confidence interval [CI]: 96–99%), though not specific, for identifying cervical spine injury. As altered mental status is a hallmark of mTBI, great caution should be exercised when considering removal of a rigid cervical collar based on clinical features alone. Options include allowing return to a normal level of alertness prior to attempting clinical clearance or performing cervical spine imaging. Discontinuation of a cervical collar should be carried out only by a physician skilled in the evaluation of cervical spine injury (e.g., emergency, orthopedist, trauma surgeon, or neurosurgeon).

Cranial Nerves and Papilledema

Cranial nerves should be evaluated with the resources that are available at the site of care. Most of the cranial nerves can be easily assessed. Papilledema (swelling of the optic nerve) is not commonly assessed on the sideline due to the need of an ophthalmoscope and dark environment. Many physicians find it difficult to perform this examination in the clinic setting without dilation of the pupils, which may be contraindicated in patients with altered mental status. Papilledema may indicate elevated ICP; however, there is a lack of evidence regarding the sensitivity and specificity of this exam finding in the face of head trauma. If identified, papilledema may indicate the need for neuroimaging, but its absence does not exclude the possibility of intracranial injury.

Station and Gait

Gait should be evaluated when mTBI is suspected. Thirty percent of patients report symptoms of impaired balance and altered coordination after mTBI (Basford et al., 2003). Serial neurological testing every 5–10 minutes on the sideline includes continued monitoring of gait and station. In the ED, ataxia that is not resolving should prompt the provider to consider a period of observation in the hospital.

Cerebellar Function

The Romberg test and assessment of rapid alternating movements are commonly used to assess posterior column and cerebellar function. The Romberg test evaluates proprioception and balance by asking the patient to stand with the feet together and eyes closed for 20 seconds. The arms are extended with the palms up. Any significant swaying or movement of the feet is a positive test. Inability to coordinate rapid alternating movements, such as flipping the palms back and forth on the lap, also suggests cerebellar dysfunction.

Strength and Sensation

Strength and sensation of the extremities should be assessed after head injury. Alterations of strength or sensation, especially if unilateral or restricted to a single limb, should be considered indicative of a significant spinal cord or intracranial injury until proven otherwise. Serial testing should include repeat evaluation of strength and sensation. Specific dermatome and motor function of nerves should be ascertained by health care professionals to expedite the determination of the level of injury.

Reflexes

Reflexes in the upper and lower extremities should be assessed immediately after and in the clinic following a head injury. Hyperactive reflexes should alert the clinician to a possible upper motor neuron lesion such as an intracranial hemorrhage or cord compression. Reflexes are graded on a 0–4 scale (0–no response, 1–hypoactive, 2–normal, 3–more reactive, 4–hyperactive). The reflexes typically assessed are those of the brachioradialis, biceps, triceps, patellar, and Achilles tendons.

Mini-Mental Status Examination

The mini-mental status examination is also felt by some neurologists to be one of the more sensitive tests when evaluating for loss of cognitive function. This test offers a quick and simple way to quantify cognitive function difficulties. The mini-mental status examination assesses orientation, attention, immediate and delayed recall, language, and motor skills; it poses particular challenges when used to assess young children and has not been validated in this age group. The clinician needs to clarify the child's use of words to describe mood, thought, content, or perceptions. A preliminary study analyzed the mini-mental status examination in children to assess the relationship between scores and children's mental age and intelligence (Rubial-Alvarez et al., 2007). The mini-mental state exam scores correlated significantly with children's chronological and mental ages.

EMERGENT IMAGING

Ashwal, Tong, Bartnik-Olson, and Holshouser (Chapter 9, this volume) include an extensive review of various brain imaging modalities and their roles in the evaluation of children with mTBI. This section reviews indications for imaging in the first hours after injury. Providers caring for children with acute mTBI should recognize that the goals of imaging shortly after injury are different from those of children who have persistent, severe, or unusual symptoms days to weeks or longer after the acute injury.

Computed Tomography

In the last three decades, the frequency of computed tomography (CT) scanning for myriad indications has increased. Brenner and Hall (2007) showed that between 1980 and 2005, the number of CT scans performed annually in the United States increased from approximately 5 million to about 60 million. This trend has also been noted specifically for children evaluated emergently after suffering head trauma. One study showed the rate of head CT nearly doubling between 1995 and 2003 (Blackwell, Gorelick, Holmes, Bandyopadhyay, & Kuppermann, 2007). Yet, visible pathology is uncommon (~ 5% of children who undergo head CT scan), and less than 1% of these children require neurosurgical intervention (Kuppermann, 2008). Additionally, one must consider the risk of malignancy due to exposure to ionizing radiation. Estimates place the risk at one lethal malignancy for every 2,000–5,000 head CT scans (Brenner, 2002; Brenner & Hall, 2007; Hall, 2002).

Providers evaluating patients in the hours following a blunt head injury must weigh the benefit of finding an injury that requires emergent intervention (neurosurgery, intubation for airway protection) against the risks of obtaining a CT scan (ionizing radiation, sedation, resource utilization). The goal in this immediate time frame is to identify injuries that are potentially life-threatening or debilitating and prevent or ameliorate mortality and morbidity. Several studies have attempted to identify risk factors for brain injuries that are visible on CT scan (Palchak et al., 2003; Quayle et al., 1997; Sun, Hoffman, & Mower, 2007; Warden, Brownstein, & Del Beccaro, 1997). These studies were limited by relatively small sample sizes, retrospective designs, or data collection from only one center.

In 2009, Kuppermann et al. published the results of a multicenter trial that included over 42,000 children with nontrivial head trauma in the prior 24 hours and who had a GCS of 14 or 15. The specific aim was to define criteria to identify those children who are at very low risk of TBI that may result in death, the need for neurosurgery, intubation > 24 hours, or admission to the hospital for ≥ 2 nights. Their prediction rule was devised based on the findings of approximately three-quarters of the study sample and then validated in the remaining quarter. Six factors were identified among children 2 years and older that, if absent, had a negative predictive value of 99.95% (95% CI, 99.81–99.99%) for TBIs requiring intervention (see Table 10.3). Given the rarity of serious TBI in this study, most patients presenting for emergent evaluation after blunt head trauma will not require emergent imaging.

TABLE 10.3. Factors Indicating That a Patient Is Not at Very Low Risk of a TBI Requiring Intervention

- Altered mental status[a]
- Signs of basilar skull fracture[a]
- Loss of consciousness > 5 seconds
- Any history of vomiting
- Severe headache
- Severe mechanism

[a]Either of these findings carried ~ 4% risk, whereas the others carried ~ 1% risk.

Beyond 24 hours, the utility of a head CT scan decreases significantly and continues to decline in the following weeks. The indications for CT scans more than 24 hours after injury are much less clear, and there is a lack of evidence to guide clinical decision making. Conservatively, in the week following injury, progressively worsening symptoms, new severe symptoms not present in the first 24 hours after injury, or new neurological deficits should prompt the provider to consider a head CT scan. However, if the patient's condition warrants imaging, other modalities (e.g., MRI) provide more detailed structural or functional information; the provider should consider whether such studies can be obtained in lieu of a CT scan, while not placing the patient at risk for a catastrophic outcome.

Magnetic Resonance Imaging

During the emergent evaluation of children with blunt head trauma when more severe intracranial injury or skull fracture is suspected, there is little value in obtaining a magnetic resonance image (MRI) of the brain rather than a CT scan. CT is superior for identifying fractures and acute bleeding when compared to MRI. Additionally, CT is very rapid with newer-generation scanners able to perform a head CT in 30–60 seconds. This obviates the need for sedation and its associated risks and provides information in a timely fashion when making decisions regarding the need for operative intervention. MRI may take 45 minutes or longer, depending on use of contrast, patient cooperation, and availability of personnel and a scanner. Patients requiring brain imaging may display variable levels of cooperation or depressed mental status. MRI often requires procedural sedation in order to obtain high-quality images in young children or those with altered mental status. However, there is a relative contraindication to sedation because it complicates subsequent evaluation for changes in mental or neurological status. These factors render MRI an inappropriate acute imaging modality in the vast majority of blunt head trauma. Concerns for ischemia due to a cerebrovascular accident (stroke) or severe edema are exceptions and may warrant MRI.

DIFFERENTIAL DIAGNOSIS

Unfortunately, the signs and symptoms of mTBI are relatively nonspecific; they can be seen in other conditions that also affect children who have suffered blunt head trauma. After completing a thorough history, physical, and neurological exam, the practitioner should generate a differential diagnosis to ensure that alternate or comorbid conditions are considered and addressed. For example, headache is a common feature of mTBI but is also frequently experienced by patients with dehydration, heat exhaustion/stroke, exertional headaches, or migraines.

Exertional Headache

Benign exertional headache occurs in many sporting events, with the most common being running and weight lifting. The prevalence of exertional headache in adolescents has been reported to be as high as 30% in students between 13 and 15 years of age (Chen, Fuh, Lu, & Wang, 2009). It is defined by bilateral throbbing at onset, which may develop into a migraine-type headache. The headache is exacerbated by physical exercise and activities and may last between several minutes to 24 hours. Weightlifting with maximal lifts significantly elevates systolic and diastolic blood pressures and should be avoided in athletes with a previous diagnosis of exertional headache. Valsalva maneuvers with strenuous exercise are known to induce exertional headaches (McCrory, 2010). Avoiding excessive exertion during physical activities may prevent exertional headaches. Exertional headache is not associated with any intracranial or systemic disorders.

Heat Exhaustion/Stroke

Heat exhaustion is defined as the inability to continue physical activity because of fatigue often associated with increased core body temperature, which frequently occurs with exercise in a hot and humid environment (Coyle, 2000). Dehydration due to increased sweating and decreased fluid intake compounds heat exhaustion. The core body temperature is increased above normal, but is below 40° C (104° F). The athlete may experience syncope during the sporting event. Symptoms such as headaches, nausea, and vomiting can occur with heat exhaustion and can be confused with symptoms of mTBI.

Heat stroke is a medical emergency defined by core body temperature ≥ 40° C and central nervous system dysfunction such as delirium and seizures. Heat stroke can also lead to cerebral damage or internal organ damage if not treated immediately (Coyle, 2000). Mental status changes with heat stroke can be confused with a head injury if the athletic activity is not being observed continuously. This can occur in mass participation events such as mountain bike races, marathons, or other outside events. It is important to note that the effects of heat-related illness fall along a continuum.

Footballer's Migraine

Footballer's migraine, also known as trauma-triggered migraine, occurs routinely during sporting events. A study evaluating the prevalence of headaches in elite professional Australian footballers found 80% of subjects reporting headaches during competition. Of the headaches reported, 34% met the diagnosis of footballer's migraine (McCrory, Heywood, & Coffey, 2005a). Trauma-triggered migraine has been reported mainly by men in contact sports (Williams & Nukada, 1994). Even mild trauma can sometimes induce a posttraumatic migraine headache. Footballer's migraine presents as a classic migraine, which may include visual field deficits. This most commonly presents in young men immediately after suffering a blow to the head while playing football. In some cases, young football players may need to give up the sport if the condition is too severe or does not respond to pharmaceutical agents. McCrory, Heywood, and Ugoni (2005b) showed that 86% of migraines with aura and 100% of migraines without aura responded to sumatriptan nasal spray. Complete relief of the headaches at 2 hours was reported by 71% of players with migraines with aura and 90% of those without aura. The authors concluded that sumatriptan nasal spray may be a valuable, effective, and convenient treatment of footballer's headache.

Transient Cortical Blindness

One specific entity that has been recognized after minor trauma to the head is transient cortical blindness. Although very frightening for the athlete, this symptom is usually benign and resolves within a 1- to 2-hour period after the head injury.

REFERRAL DECISIONS

Immediate Referral to an ED

Any deterioration in mental status, including a loss of consciousness, focal neurological deficit, or suspected cervical spine injury, should prompt immediate transfer to an ED via emergency medical services. Most physicians would also send the athlete with prolonged loss of consciousness or active vomiting to the ED for observation and potential neuroimaging.

Primary Care Physician's Office

Most concussions can be evaluated in the primary care physician's office within 1–3 days after the injury. The majority of concussion symptoms will resolve within a 7- to 10-day period and return-to-play decisions are usually made by the athlete's primary care physician at that time. Continuing medical education and continued review of current literature in this field are vital to appropriate decision making regarding return to play for the athlete. Once again, return-to-play decisions should be made on an individual basis. History of previous concussions, severity of previous concussions, nature of the injury, burden to the athlete, and duration of symptoms should all be factored into these decisions.

Sports Medicine Clinic

Referral to a sports medicine clinic should be made when the primary care physician is uncomfortable treating the concussed athlete. Sports medicine physicians are required to be up to date on current concussion management and return-to-play decisions. Sports medicine clinics will most likely have a network of communication set up between the parents, teachers and school officials, certified athletic trainers, and the health care provider. Academic relief while the patient is symptomatic will usually be required. The sports medicine physician will make the decision, when it is appropriate, to refer to the more specialized concussion clinic.

Specialized Concussion Clinic

Specialized concussion clinics are designed to evaluate and treat the most complicated and severe concussions. Neuropsychologists and physicians who are comfortable and knowledgeable at treating complex or multiple concussions usually staff these clinics. Prolonged PCS and other complications are more appropriately treated in these specialized concussion clinics. Health care providers in these clinics can make referrals for cognitive rehabilitation therapy.

SUMMARY

The immediate postinjury physical and neurological exam is likely to reveal few if any significant findings in the victim of mTBI. However, this portion of evaluation is an indispensible component of the care of all victims of blunt head trauma. It allows the athletic trainer, team physician, or school nursing personnel to activate emergency medical services or refer a patient to the ED or primary care provider's office. It allows the emergency care provider to identify potentially life-threatening injuries and decide when imaging studies are indicated. Furthermore, the physical and neurological exam allows for generation of a differential diagnosis and pursuit of alternate diagnoses.

Future research should focus on methods to quantify the severity of mTBI with regard to the expected duration of sequelae as well as identify treatments that may alter the course of recovery, starting in the acute period. The former may include graded symptom inventories, quantification of biomarkers specific to TBI, and identification of preinjury factors and comorbidities that are likely to influence the recovery process. The latter should include study of cognitive and physical rest periods and medications to treat or prevent PCS.

REFERENCES

Basford, J. R., Chou, L. S., Kaufman, K. R., Brey, R. H., Walker, A., Malec, J. F., et al. (2003). An assessment of gait and balance deficits after traumatic brain injury. *Archives of Physical Medicine and Rehabilitation, 84,* 343–349.

Bishara, S. N., Partridge, F. M., Godfrey, H. P., & Knight, R. G. (1992). Post-traumatic amnesia and Glasgow Coma Scale related to outcome in survivors in a consecutive series of patients with severe closed-head injury. *Brain Injury, 6,* 373–380.

Blackwell, C. D., Gorelick, M., Holmes, J. F., Bandyopadhyay, S., & Kuppermann, M. (2007). Pediatric head trauma: Changes in use of computed tomography in emergency departments in the United States over time. *Annals of Emergency Medicine, 49,* 320–324.

Brenner, D. J. (2002). Estimating cancer risks from pediatric CT: Going from the qualitative to the quantitative. *Pediatric Radiology, 32,* 228–300.

Brenner, D. J., & Hall, E. J. (2007). Computed tomography: An increasing source of radiation exposure. *New England Journal of Medicine, 357,* 2277–2284.

Brown, R. L., Brunn, M. A., & Garcia, V. F. (2001). Cervical spine injuries in children: A review of 103 patients treated consecutively at a level 1 pediatric trauma center. *Journal of Pediatric Surgery, 36,* 1107–1114.

Chen, S. P., Fuh, J. L., Lu, S. R., & Wang, S. J. (2009). Exertional headache: A survey of 1,963 adolescents. *Cephalagia, 29,* 401–407.

Cirak, B., Ziegfeld, S., Knight, V. M., Chang, D., Avellino, A. M., & Paidas, C. M. (2004). Spinal injuries in children. *Journal of Pediatric Surgery, 39,* 607–612.

Coyle, J. F. (2000). Thermoregulation. In J. A. Sullivan & S. J. Anderson (Eds.), *Care of the young athlete* (1st ed., pp. 70–71). Oklahoma City, OK: American Academy of Pediatrics and American Academy of Orthopedic Surgeons.

Drake, A. I., McDonald, E. C., Magnus, N. E., Gray, N., & Gottshall, K. (2006). Utility of Glasgow Coma Scale—Extended in symptom prediction following mild traumatic brain injury. *Brain Injury, 20,* 469–475.

Fabbri, A., Servadei, F., Marchesini, G., Stein, S. C., & Vandelli, A. (2008). Early predictors of unfavorable outcome in subjects with moderate head injury in the emergency department. *Journal of Neurology, Neurosurgery, and Psychiatry, 79*, 567–573.

Faul, M., Xu, L., Wald, M. M., & Coronado, V. G. (2010). *Traumatic brain injury in the United States: Emergency department visits, hospitalizations, and deaths.* Atlanta, GA: Centers for Disease Control and Prevention, National Center for Injury Prevention and Control.

Gouvier, W. D., Uddo-Crane, M., & Brown, L. M. (1988). Base rates of post-concussional symptoms. *Archives of Clinical Neuropsychology, 3*, 273–278.

Greenes, D. S. (2006). Neurotrauma. In G. R. Fleisher, S. Ludwig, & F. M. Henretig (Eds.), *Textbook of pediatric emergency medicine* (5th ed., pp. 1363–1364). Philadelphia: Lippincott, Williams & Wilkins.

Grubenhoff, J. A., Kirkwood, M., Gao, D., Deakyne, S., & Wathen, J. (2010). Evaluation of the Standardized Assessment of Concussion in a pediatric emergency department. *Pediatrics, 126*, 688–695.

Hall, E. J. (2002). Lessons we have learned from our children: Cancer risks from diagnostic radiology. *Pediatric Radiology, 32*, 700–706.

Haukoos, J. S., Gill, M. R., Rabon, R. E., Gravitz, C. S., & Green, S. M. (2007). Validation of the Simplified Motor Score for the prediction of brain injury outcomes after trauma. *Annals of Emergency Medicine, 50*, 18–24.

Healey, C., Osler, T. M., Rogers, F. B., Healey, M. A., Glance, L. G., Kilgo, P. D., et al. (2003). Improving the Glasgow Coma Scale score: Motor score alone is a better predictor. *Journal of Trauma, 54*, 671–678.

Hoffman, J. R., Wolfson, A. B., Todd, K., & Mower, W. R. (1998). Selective cervical spine radiography in blunt trauma: Methodology of the National Emergency X-Radiography Utilization Study (NEXUS). *Annals of Emergency Medicine, 32*, 461–469.

Iverson, G. L. (2006). Misdiagnosis of the persistent postconcussion syndrome in patients with depression. *Archives of Clinical Neuropsychology, 21*, 303–310.

Iverson, G. L., & Lange, R. T. (2003). Examination of "postconcussion-like" symptoms in a healthy sample. *Applied Neuropsychology, 10*, 137–144.

Iverson, G. L., Lovell, M. R., Smith, S., & Franzen, M. D. (2000). Presence of abnormal CT scans following mild head injury. *Brain Injury, 14*, 1057–1061.

Kirkwood, M. W., & Kirk, J. W. (2010). The base rate of suboptimal effort in a pediatric mild TBI sample: Performance on the Medical Symptom Validity Test. *The Clinical Neuropsychologist, 24*, 860–872.

Kleiner, D. M., & Cantu, R. C. (1996). *A current comment: Football helmet removal.* Indianapolis, IN: American College of Sports Medicine.

Kuppermann, N. (2008). Pediatric head trauma: The evidence regarding indications for emergent neuroimaging. *Pediatric Radiology, 38*(Suppl. 4), S670–S674.

Kuppermann, N., Holmes, J. F., Dayan, P. S., Hoyle, J. D., Jr., Atabaki, S. M., Holubkov, R., et al. (2009). Identification of children at very low risk of clinically-important brain injuries after head trauma: A prospective cohort study. *Lancet, 374*, 1160–1170.

Langlois, J. A., Rutland-Brown, W., & Thomas, K. E. (2005). The incidence of traumatic brain injury among children in the United States: Differences by race. *Journal of Head Trauma Rehabilitation, 20*, 229–238.

Leonard, J. C., Kuppermann, N., Olsen, C., Babcock-Cimpello, L., Brown, K., Mahajan, P., et al. (2010). Factors associated with cervical spine injury in children after blunt trauma. *Annals of Emergency Medicine, 58*(2), 145–155.

Machulda, M. M., Bergquist, T. F., Ito, V., & Chew, S. (1998). Relationship between stress, coping, and postconcussion symptoms in a healthy adult population. *Archives of Clinical Neuropsychology, 13*, 415–424.

Marcin, J. P., & Pollack, M. M. (2002). Triage scoring systems, severity of illness measures, and mortality prediction models in pediatric trauma. *Critical Care Medicine, 30*(Suppl. 11), S457–S467.

McCrea, M. (2001). Standardized mental status testing on the sideline after sport-related concussion. *Journal of Athletic Training, 36,* 274–279.

McCrea, M., Kelly, J. P., Randolph, C., Kluge, J., Bartolic, E., Finn, G., et al. (1998). Standardized assessment of concussion (SAC): On-site mental status evaluation of the athlete. *Journal of Head Trauma Rehabilitation, 13,* 27–35.

McCrory, P. (2010). Sports Concussion. In P. Brukner & K. Khan (Eds.), *Clinical sports medicine* (3rd ed., pp. 200–206). New York: McGraw-Hill.

McCrory, P., Heywood, J., & Coffey, C. (2005a). Prevalence of headache in Australian footballers. *British Journal of Sports Medicine, 39,* e10.

McCrory, P., Heywood, J., & Ugoni, A. (2005b). Open label study of intranasal sumatriptan (Imigran) for footballer's headache. *British Journal of Sports Medicine, 39,* 552–554.

McNett, M. (2007). A review of the predictive ability of Glasgow Coma Scale scores in head-injured patients. *Journal of Neuroscience Nursing, 39,* 68–75.

Naunheim, R. S., Matero, D., & Fucetola, R. (2008). Assessment of patients with mild concussion in the emergency department. *Journal of Head Trauma Rehabilitation, 23,* 116–122.

Nell, V., Yates, D. S., & Kruger, J. (2000). An extended Glasgow Coma Scale (GCS-E) with enhanced sensitivity to mild brain injury. *Archives of Physical Medicine and Rehabilitation, 81,* 614–617.

Pal, J., Brown, R., & Fleiszer, D. (1989). The value of the Glasgow Coma Scale and Injury Severity Score: Predicting outcome in multiple trauma patients with head injury. *Journal of Trauma, 29,* 746–748.

Palchak, M. J., Holmes, J. F., Vance, C. W., Gelber, R. E., Schauer, B. A., Harrison, M. J., et al. (2003). A decision rule for identifying children at low risk for brain injuries after blunt head trauma. *Annals of Emergency Medicine, 42,* 492–506.

Patel, J. C., Tepas, J. J., 3rd, Mollitt, D. L., & Pieper, P. (2001). Pediatric cervical spine injuries: Defining the disease. *Journal of Pediatric Surgery, 36,* 373–376.

Peterson, S. E., Stull, M. J., Collins, M. W., & Wang, H. E. (2009). Neurocognitive function of emergency department patients with mild traumatic brain injury. *Annals of Emergency Medicine, 53,* 796–803.

Petrizzi, M., Reisman, A., & Cole, S. (2007, April). *Sideline management assessment response techniques.* Workshop presented at the American Medical Society for Sports Medicine annual meeting, Albuquerque, NM.

Platzer, P., Jaindl, M., Thalhammer, G., Dittrich, S., Kutscha-Lissberg, F., Vecsei, V., et al. (2007). Cervical spine injuries in pediatric patients. *Journal of Trauma, 62,* 389–396.

Quayle, K. S., Jaffe, D. M., Kuppermann, N., Kaufman, B. A., Lee, B. C., Park, T. S., et al. (1997). Diagnostic testing for acute head injury in children: When are head computed tomography and skull radiographs indicated? *Pediatrics, 99,* E11.

Ralston, M., Hazinski, M. F., Zaritsky, A. L., Schexnayder, S. M., & Kleinman, M. E. (Eds.). (2006). *PALS provider manual.* Dallas, TX: American Heart Association.

Rubial-Alvarez, S., Machado, M. C., Sintas, E., de Sola, S., Böhm, P., & Peña-Casanova, J. (2007). A preliminary study of the mini-mental state examination in a Spanish child population. *Journal of Child Neurology, 22*(11), 1269–1273.

Setnik, L., & Bazarian, J. J. (2007). The characteristics of patients who do not seek medical treatment for traumatic brain injury. *Brain Injury, 21,* 1–9.

Sheedy, J., Geffen, G., Donnelly, J., & Faux, S. (2006). Emergency department assessment of mild traumatic brain injury and prediction of post-concussion symptoms at one month post injury. *Journal of Clinical and Experimental Neuropsychology, 28,* 755–772.

Sternbach, G. L. (2000). The Glasgow Coma Scale. *Journal of Emergency Medicine, 19,* 67–71.

Suhr, J. A., & Gunstad, J. (2002). Postconcussive symptom report: The relative influence of head injury and depression. *Journal of Clinical and Experimental Neuropsychology, 24,* 981–993.

Sun, B. C., Hoffman, J. R., & Mower, W. R. (2007). Evaluation of a modified prediction instrument to identify significant pediatric intracranial injury after blunt head trauma. *Annals of Emergency Medicine, 49,* 325–332.

Teasdale, G., & Jennett, B. (1974). Assessment of coma and impaired consciousness: A practical scale. *Lancet, 2,* 81–84.

Ting, H. W., Chen, M. S., Hsieh, Y. C., & Chan, C. L. (2010). Good mortality prediction by Glasgow Coma Scale for neurosurgical patients. *Journal of the Chinese Medical Association, 73,* 139–143.

Viccellio, P., Simon, H., Pressman, B. D., Shah, M. N., Mower, W. R., & Hoffman, J. R. (2001). A prospective multicenter study of cervical spine injury in children. *Pediatrics, 108,* E20.

Waninger, K. N. (2004). Management of the helmeted athlete with suspected cervical spine injury. *American Journal of Sports Medicine, 32,* 1331–1350.

Warden, C. R., Brownstein, D. R., & Del Beccaro, M. A. (1997). Predictors of abnormal findings of computed tomography of the head in pediatric patients presenting with seizures. *Annals of Emergency Medicine, 29,* 518–523.

Williams, S. J., & Nukada, H. (1994). Sport and exercise headache: Part 2. Diagnosis and classification. *British Journal of Sports Medicine, 28*(2), 96–100.

Young, B., Rapp, R. P., Norton, J. A., Haack, D., Tibbs, P. A., & Bean, J. R. (1981). Early prediction in outcome of head-injured patients. *Journal of Neurosurgery, 54,* 300–303.

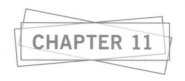

CHAPTER 11

Balance Testing

Tamara C. Valovich McLeod and Kevin M. Guskiewicz

CENTRAL NERVOUS SYSTEM CONTRIBUTIONS TO BALANCE

The assessment of balance following mild traumatic brain injury (mTBI) can play an important part in determining impairments, as the maintenance of postural equilibrium requires an intact and integrated central nervous system (CNS). *Balance*, defined as the process of maintaining one's center of gravity within the base of support, is controlled through a hierarchy that includes the cerebral cortex, cerebellum, basal ganglia, brainstem, and spinal cord (Guyton, 1986; Vander, Sherman, & Luciano, 1990). The cerebral cortex is the highest level of the hierarchy and involves the brain areas responsible for attention, concentration, emotion, and the association cortex for integrating input from other brain structures. The middle levels of the hierarchy include the sensorimotor complex, cerebellum, parts of the basal ganglia, and some brainstem nuclei, with the cerebellum important in balance coordination and interpreting information coming from numerous sources (e.g., muscles, joints, ears, eyes, skin) within the body (Guyton, 1986; Vander et al., 1990). The brainstem and spinal cord (where the motor neurons exit) make up the lowest level of the hierarchy and receive input from the middle level via the descending pathways.

The maintenance of postural equilibrium or balance requires the functioning of both sensory and motor processes. Sensory organization requires the CNS to process and integrate information from the sensory systems (visual, vestibular, and somatosensory), including timing, direction, and amplitude of postural responses from those inputs (Guskiewicz, 2011). Although three sensory inputs are available, the CNS tends to utilize information from one input at a time when determining the body's orientation. In healthy adults, the use of information from the somatosensory system is preferred. In contrast, young children tend to rely more on visual cues (Assaiante & Amblard, 1995; Nashner, 1982; Riach & Hayes, 1987). Vestibular cues become important sources of sensory information in patients with vestibular deficits, especially when visual or somatosensory cues are impaired or are sending inaccurate information (Nashner, Black, & Wall, 1982). The motor process involves muscle coordination, which determines the sequencing and distribution of the motor responses required to maintain balance. Motor processes include reflexes, automatic and adaptive postural responses, and voluntary movements of the ankle, thigh, and trunk muscles.

IDENTIFIED BALANCE DEFICITS FOLLOWING mTBI

Deficits in balance ability have been reported in patients with mTBI (Gagnon, Forget, Sullivan, & Friedman, 1998; Gagnon, Swaine, Friedman, & Forget, 2004; Guskie-wicz, Perrin, & Gansneder, 1996; Riemann & Guskiewicz, 2000), as well as in those with moderate–severe TBI (Geurts, Ribbers, Knoop, & van Limbeek, 1996; Inger-soll & Armstrong, 1992; Katz-Leurer, Rotem, Keren, & Meyer, 2009a; Katz-Leurer, Rotem, Lewitus, Keren, & Meyer, 2008b). Brain injury has been shown to lead to changes in the normal weighing and integration of sensory cues, resulting in pos-tural instabilities. Therefore, these patients must reorganize their pattern of remain-ing sensory cues that establish postural control (Rubin, Woolley, Dailey, & Goebel, 1995). Additionally, self-reported symptoms such as dizziness, tinnitus, lighthead-edness, blurred vision, and/or photophobia often accompany mTBI. The symptoms often relate to one of the three sensory systems (visual, vestibular, somatosensory) and may affect the patient's perception of sensory cues (Campbell & Parry, 2005; Geurts et al., 1996; Greenwald et al., 2001; Guskiewicz, Ross, & Marshall, 2001; Ingersoll & Armstrong, 1992). Ingersoll and Armstrong (1992) used postural stabil-ity assessments to investigate the effects of closed-head injuries of different degrees of severity on postural sway in adults. Assessments took place 7–9 years following the closed-head injury. Those who had suffered severe head injuries (loss of consciousness [LOC] > 6 hours) displayed more anterior–posterior and medial–lateral sway than mildly head-injured or normal subjects, although total sway did not differ between groups. The researchers also reported that individuals who suffered a severe head injury tended to maintain their center of balance at a greater distance from their base of support (Ingersoll & Armstrong, 1992).

In athletic populations, deficits in postural control have been investigated pri-marily in collegiate athletes, with transient impairments in balance lasting between 3 and 10 days postinjury (Cavanaugh et al., 2005; Guskiewicz et al., 1996, 2001; McCrea et al., 2003; Riemann & Guskiewicz, 2000). In a meta-analysis of sport con-cussion studies, Broglio and Puetz (2008) identified six investigations that assessed postural control, in high school and collegiate athletes, that used either instrumented or clinical assessment methods. A large effect of concussion on postural control was noted immediately following the concussion (effect size = –2.56) and within the 2 weeks following the initial assessment (effect size = –1.16), indicating that balance impairments can exist up to 2 weeks postinjury.

Guskiewicz et al. (1996) evaluated the postural stability of high school and collegiate athletes acutely following concussion and reported impaired postural sta-bility 1–3 days following injury, with recovery occurring between days 3 and 5. The difference between the control and concussion groups was more evident when

sensory input was altered with a foam or moving surface. In addition, the participants with concussion tended to maintain their center of balance further from their
base of support on day 1 following injury. A follow-up investigation using only collegiate athletes confirmed the earlier results by demonstrating decreased postural
stability until 3 days following the concussion, with recovery occurring between
days 3 and 5 (Guskiewicz, Riemann, Perrin, & Nashner, 1997). Additionally, the
use of the NeuroCom Sensory Organization Test (SOT) during the follow-up study
allowed for the isolation of visual, vestibular, and somatosensory contributions to
balance. Evaluation of the sensory ratios indicated a significantly lower visual ratio
in the concussion group on day 1 postinjury, with no differences between groups on
the vestibular and somatosensory ratios (Guskiewicz et al., 1997). More recently,
an investigation using the SOT and a clinical balance assessment, the Balance Error
Scoring System (BESS), reported impairments in postural stability with decreases in
the composite equilibrium score (see Figure 11.1), visual and vestibular ratios (Figure
11.2), and increases in BESS errors (Figure 11.3) at day 1 postinjury, compared to
a preseason baseline score (Guskiewicz et al., 2001). Concussed collegiate athletes
also had impaired postural stability at days 1, 3, and 5 postinjury, compared to the
healthy control group on the total BESS score, SOT composite score, and visual
and vestibular ratios, supporting the findings that concussed athletes have problems
under balance conditions involving sensory conflict (unstable surface and absent or
inaccurate visual cues).

   Although the majority of sport-concussion studies have assessed collegiate athletes, there have been some investigations into the effect of TBI on balance in children
(Gagnon et al., 1998, 2004; Katz-Leurer et al., 2009a; Katz-Leurer, Rotem, Keren, &
Meyer, 2009b; Katz-Leurer, Rotem, Lewitus, Keren, & Meyer, 2008a, 2008b; Kuhtz-
Buschbeck et al., 2003). One study (Gagnon et al., 2004) evaluated children at 1, 4,
and 12 weeks following mTBI (Glasgow Coma Scale [GCS] 13–15), with an otherwise unremarkable neurological exam. Balance assessments included the Bruininks–

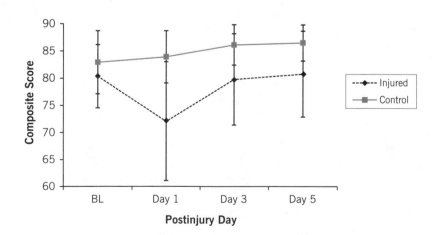

FIGURE 11.1. Composite score means (±SD) on the Sensory Organization Test for 36 concussed
and 36 control college-age subjects across test sessions. Higher scores represent better performance. From Guskiewicz, Ross, and Marshall (2001). Copyright 2001 by the National Athletic
Trainers' Association. Reprinted by permission. Reprinted with permission from *The Journal of
Athletic Training*.

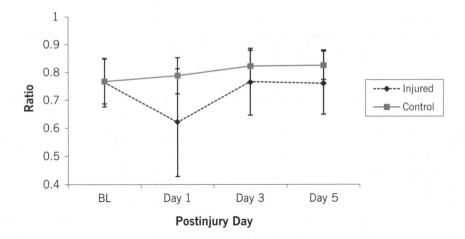

FIGURE 11.2. Vestibular ratio means (±SD) on the Sensory Organization Test for 36 concussed and 36 control college-age subjects across test sessions. Higher scores represent better performance. From Guskiewicz, Ross, and Marshall (2001). Copyright 2001 by the National Athletic Trainers' Association. Reprinted by permission.

Oseretsky Test of Motor Proficiency (BOTMP), the Pediatric Clinical Test of Sensory Interaction on Balance (P-CTSIB), and the Postural Stress Test (PST). Children with mTBI demonstrated worse balance than healthy children at all time points and across all tasks of the BOTMP. Deficits in balance among those with mTBI were also noted on the P-CTSIB in the eyes-closed conditions of the tandem stance on both firm and foam surfaces (Gagnon et al., 2004). More recent investigations of dynamic balance and gait following severe TBI (GCS ≤ 8 for 6 hours) have reported decreased functional reach, slower timed up and go (TUG), smaller step length, increased step time, slower gait velocity, and increased gait variability compared to typically developing

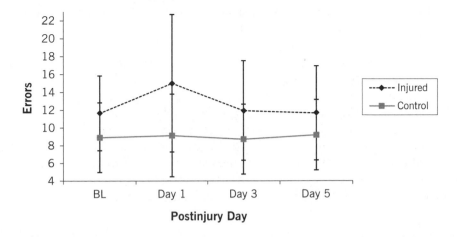

FIGURE 11.3. Balance Error Scoring System total score means (±SD) for 36 concussed and 36 control college-age subjects across test sessions. Lower scores represent better performance. From Guskiewicz, Ross, and Marshall (2001). Copyright 2001 by the National Athletic Trainers' Association. Reprinted by permission.

children (Katz-Leurer et al., 2009a, 2008b). Although the majority of balance deficits following mTBI are temporary and resolve in a sequential manner, these deficits are important to recognize and assess during the individual's recovery.

BALANCE ASSESSMENT APPROACHES, STRATEGIES, AND TOOLS

The assessment of balance can be accomplished using a variety of assessment techniques and tools capable of evaluating different characteristics of balance. Balance can be assessed under static conditions, dynamic conditions (e.g., unstable surface, moving platform), or during more functional tasks. Furthermore, some assessments require sophisticated equipment, whereas others are more clinical and "low-tech" in nature. Table 11.1 summarizes several of the balance assessments that may be appropriate for the evaluation of balance in the pediatric population post TBI.

Sensory Organization Test

The SOT is an instrumented balance assessment performed on a specialized force plate system aimed at altering sensory cues available to the somatosensory or visual inputs while measuring the patient's ability to maintain a quiet stance. The SOT uses six different conditions, with the patient completing three trials of each condition to assess balance (see Figure 11.4). The test protocol consists of three 20-second trials under three different visual conditions (eyes open, eyes closed, sway-referenced) and two different surface conditions (fixed, sway-referenced). Sway referencing causes the orientation of the support surface or surround to remain constant relative to body position. Patients are asked to stand as motionless as possible for each of the 20-second trials in a bilateral stance with the feet shoulder width apart. During sway-referenced support surface conditions (Conditions 4, 5, 6), the force plate tilts synchronously with the patient's anterior-posterior center of gravity (A-P COG) sway. Similarly, during sway-referenced visual surround conditions (Conditions 3 and 6), the visual surround tilts synchronously with anterior-posterior center of gravity (A-P COG) sway. The SOT can assess patients' ability to ignore the inaccurate information from the sway-referenced senses.

An overall composite equilibrium score, indicating a person's level of performance during all of the trials in the SOT, is calculated, with higher scores representing better balance performance. The composite score is the average of the following 14 scores: the condition 1 average score, the condition 2 average score, and the three equilibrium scores from each of the trials in conditions 3–6. The relative differences between the equilibrium scores of various conditions are calculated using ratios to reveal specific information about each of the sensory systems involved with maintaining balance (see Table 11.2). The SOT has been studied in children, and normative data are available for children age 3 years and older (see Table 11.3).

Clinical Test of Sensory Interaction on Balance

A technique described by Shumway-Cook and Horak (1986), called the Clinical Test of Sensory Interaction and Balance (CTSIB), has been used to assess balance and

TABLE 11.1. Summary of Assessments for the Evaluation of Balance Following Childhood mTBI

Assessment	Characteristics	Format	Advantages	Disadvantages	TBI populations studied
Balance Error Scoring System (BESS)	Clinical—static	Six 20-second balance assessments on firm and foam surfaces; eyes closed; score the number of errors	Easy to administer; minimal equipment; low cost; validated against SOT	Scores can be affected by fatigue and learning effects	College and high school athletes
Clinical Test of Sensory Interaction on Balance (CTSIB)	Clinical—static	6–12 sensory conditions; firm and foam surfaces; eyes open, eyes closed, visual conflict dome; measures time in stance and sway	Easy to administer; minimal equipment needs; low cost	Sway measure is often subjective	College and high school athletes (CTSIB); children and adolescents (P-CTSIB)
Modified Functional Reach Test (MFRT)	Clinical—dynamic	Limits of stability assessment in three directions; measured in distance leaned from a starting point	Easy to administer; low cost; minimal equipment needs	Limited reports in the literature	Children and adolescents; mild to severe TBI
Timed Up and Go (TUG)	Clinical—dynamic	Timed walk from a seated position to a marked point, returning to the seated position	Easy to administer; moderate to good association with P-CTSIB		Children and adolescents; mild to severe TBI
Gait	Instrumented—dynamic	Normal walking in a laboratory setting; measured by typical gait parameters	Functional activity; easy instructions for patients	Require gait analysis instrumentation	Children and adolescents; college athletes; mild to severe TBI
Sensory Organization Test (SOT)	Instrumented—dynamic	Six 20-second balance tests; firm and moving surfaces; eyes open, eyes closed, sway-referenced vision; measures equilibrium score, sensory ratios	Ability to isolate sensory information; established norms for children; published literature in concussed athletes	Cost of device	College and high school athletes

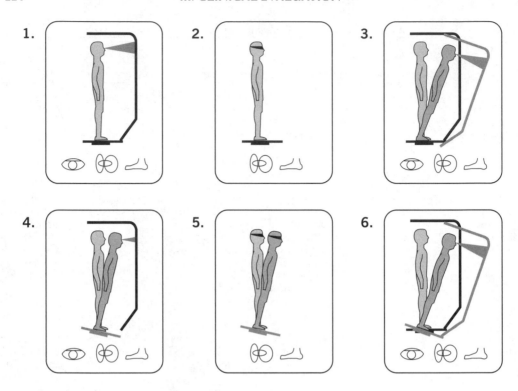

FIGURE 11.4. Sensory Organization Test conditions. Reprinted with permission from Neurocom, a Division of Natus Medical Incorporated.

systematically remove or provide inaccurate sensory input from one or more of the three sensory systems. The balance test uses combinations of three visual and two support surface conditions during static balance trials. The visual conditions include (1) eyes open, (2) eyes closed (absent vision), and (3) a visual conflict dome for producing inaccurate visual input. The surface conditions include (1) a firm surface (stable) and (2) a medium-density foam surface (unstable). Table 11.2 describes the conditions and primary sensory system targeted for the CTSIB. The CTSIB can be scored by quantifying sway through several techniques, including (1) subjective sway assessment using a numeric rating (1 = minimal sway, 2 = mild sway, 3 = moderate sway, 4 = fall); (2) measurement of the time in seconds that the patient can remain erect for each condition; or (3) evaluation of body displacement through the use of posture grids or plumb lines (Shumway-Cook & Horak, 1986). The balance tasks can also be performed on a standard force plate allowing an instrumented measure of postural sway to be obtained (Guskiewicz et al., 1996).

   A pediatric version of the CTISIB, the Pediatric Clinical Test of Sensory Interaction for Balance (P-CTSIB), has been developed and uses the same surfaces and visual conditions (Crowe, Deitz, Richardson, & Atwater, 1990; Dietz, Richardson, Atwater, Crowe, & Odiorne, 1991; Gagnon, Swaine, & Forget, 2006; Westcott, Crowe, Deitz, & Richardson, 1994). In addition to the double-leg stance commonly used in the CTSIB, a tandem stance condition (see Figure 11.5) is added to the pediatric version, resulting in 12 balance conditions. During the test the patient is asked to stand

TABLE 11.2. Sensory Conditions of the Sensory Organization Test, Clinical Test of Sensory Interaction on Balance, and Pediatric CTSIB

Condition	Targeted sensory system	CTSIB/P-CTSIB		SOT	
		Vision	Surface	Vision	Surface
1	All available	Eyes open	Stable	Eyes open	Stable
2	Somatosensory and vestibular	Eyes closed	Stable	Eyes closed	Stable
3	Somatosensory and vestibular	Visual-conflict dome	Stable	Sway-referenced surround	Stable
4	Visual and vestibular	Eyes open	Foam	Eyes open	Sway-referenced platform
5	Vestibular	Eyes closed	Foam	Eyes closed	Sway-referenced platform
6	Vestibular	Visual-conflict dome	Foam	Sway-referenced surround	Sway-referenced platform

quietly and attempt to remain stable for up to 30 seconds while being tested on all six sensory conditions in both bilateral and tandem stance conditions. For each trial the time (seconds) the patient was able to remain balanced without needing to make postural adjustments is measured, along anterior-posterior and medial-lateral sway. Sway can be scored subjectively, as noted above with the CTSIB, or objectively using grid systems or plumb lines. A balance summary score, ranging from 0 to 5, is also given. This summary score takes into account the sway amplitude and the time in balance. Westcott et al. (1994) found test–retest reliability coefficients for combined sensory condition scores ranging from .45 to .69 with the feet together and from .44 to .83 in the tandem stance for children between 4 and 9 years of age on the P-CTSB.

TABLE 11.3. NeuroCom Sensory Organization Test Age-Appropriate Normative Values for the Equilibrium Score

Age	Stable eyes open	Stable eyes closed	Stable sway-referenced	Unstable eyes open	Unstable eyes closed	Unstable sway-referenced	Composite score
3–4	62.9	65.3	42.1	15.6	2.8	1.4	31.7
5–6	69.2	61.6	58.2	34.5	8.8	6.1	39.8
7–8	80.4	71.62	73.4	43.9	8.4	11.1	48.1
9–10	81.6	77.5	76.5	47.9	25.4	6.8	52.6
11–13	86.6	85.7	82.2	52.2	21.8	23.3	58.6
14–15	87.2	86.8	83.3	67.5	28.7	29.9	63.9
16–59	90	85	86	70	52	48	70

Based on Nashner (1993) and Hirabayashi and Iwasake (1995).

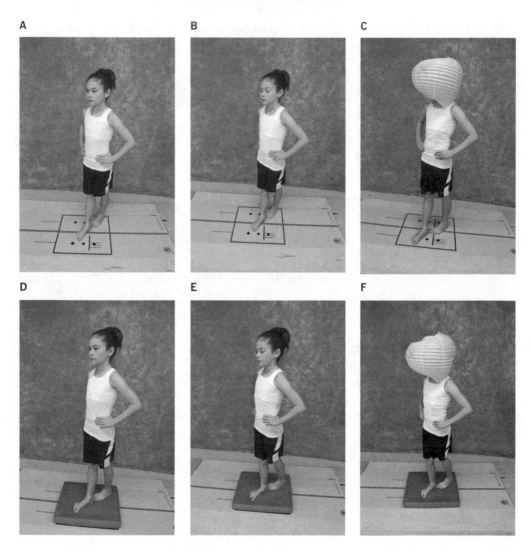

FIGURE 11.5. The Pediatric Clinical Test of Sensory Integration on Balance (P-CTSIB). Shown are the tandem stance conditions. The test can also be done with feet together.

Balance Error Scoring System

Prior to the use of computerized force platform systems, the Romberg test was commonly used to evaluate postural stability following injury. The original Romberg test has been criticized as being too subjective and insensitive to changes in postural stability (Jansen, Larsen, & Mogens, 1982). A clinical field assessment for postural stability, the BESS, has been shown to be a reliable measure of postural stability and correlates well with computerized posturography measures (Guskiewicz et al., 2001; Riemann, Guskiewicz, & Shields, 1999). The BESS comprises a series of clinical balance tests that progressively challenge the sensory systems through variations in stance (double-leg, single-leg, tandem) and surface (firm, foam) (see Figure 11.6). The double-leg stance (A and D) is performed with the feet touching at the arches, creating a small base of support. During the single-leg stance (B and E), the patient is asked to maintain the on-stance leg in 20–30 degrees of hip flexion and 40–50 degrees of knee flexion. The tandem stance (C and F) is performed with the patient standing with one foot in front of the other so that the heel of the front foot and the toes of the rear foot are in contact. Many studies have standardized the test leg and used the nondominant leg as the stance leg for the single-leg conditions and the back leg for the tandem stance. Patients are asked to stand quietly in the required test position with their hands on their hips. Once the eyes are closed, the 20-second trial begins. During each condition, patients are told that upon losing their balance they should return to the starting position as quickly as possible and continue balancing until asked to stop.

As opposed to other clinical measures of postural stability that assess either time until touching down or number of touchdowns in a specified amount of time

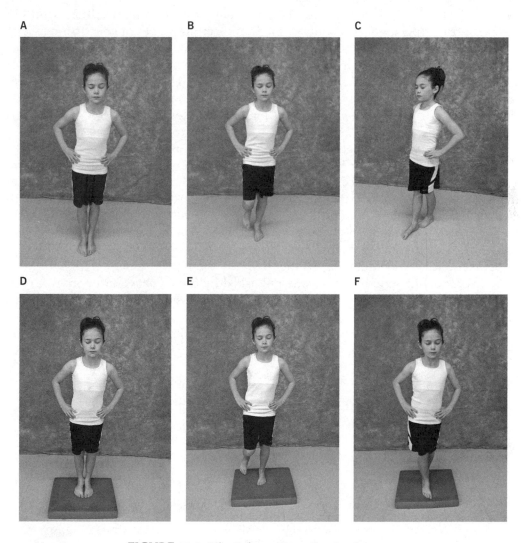

FIGURE 11.6. The Balance Error Scoring System.

(Ekdahl, Jarnlo, & Andersson, 1989), the scoring of errors allows the clinician to be more stringent and specific regarding the subject's ability to maintain postural stability (Riemann et al., 1999). Table 11.4 presents the scored BESS errors. The errors scored during each condition are summed, resulting in a total BESS score. If a patient is unable to remain in the proper stance for at least 5 seconds during a trial, the trial is considered to be incomplete and a standard error score of 10 is assigned. The BESS requires minimal equipment, is portable, and has been demonstrated as a useful and cost-effective sideline technique to evaluate postural stability following concussion. The BESS has been found sensitive in detecting acute postural stability alterations up to day 3 postconcussion and can be used to assist clinicians in evaluating concussion when laboratory force platforms are unavailable or impractical (Guskiewicz et al., 2001; McCrea et al., 2003). Several investigators have reported the inter- and intra-rater reliabilities of the BESS, which have been found to range between .57 and .96 and .58 and .98, respectively (see Table 11.5).

Unlike the SOT, there is not a substantial database of normative BESS scores in the pediatric population. In a study of measurement properties of concussion assessment tools, Valovich McLeod, Barr, McCrea, and Guskiewicz (2006) provided normative values on the BESS in a small sample of children between 9 and 14 years of age. The total BESS score across the entire sample was 15.5 ± 5.8 errors, with scores for males (17.4 ± 5.2 errors) slightly higher than females (13.5 ± 5.6 errors). Younger (9–11 years) athletes had a significantly higher BESS total score (18.5 ± 4.7 errors) compared to older (12–14 years) athletes (13.0 ± 5.3 errors).

Attempts have been made to modify the BESS to improve reliability and make the test easier to administer for clinicians at all levels. Hunt, Ferrara, Bornstein, and Baumgartner (2009) assessed the reliability of the BESS, as originally described (Riemann et al., 1999) and in a modified format. The researchers found that the reliability of the BESS could be increased from $r = .60$ to $r = .88$ by having subjects perform three trials of a modified BESS that consisted of four conditions (single-firm, tandem-firm, single-foam, tandem-foam). However, this modified version has yet to be used in pediatric studies or following mTBI.

A second BESS modification was published by the Concussion in Sport Group following the 3rd International Conference on Concussion in Sport. The consensus group acknowledged that balance deficits exist postconcussion and advocated for the use of postural stability assessments as a component of a comprehensive concussion assessment (McCrory et al., 2009). The group included a coordination and balance

---

TABLE 11.4. Types of Errors for the Balance Error Scoring System

- Lifting hand off iliac crest(s)
- Opening eyes
- Step, stumble, or fall
- Moving hip into more than 30° of flexion or abduction
- Lifting the forefoot or heel
- Remaining out of the test position for greater than 5 seconds

The BESS score is calculated by adding 1 error point for each error committed during each of the six 20-second trials.

TABLE 11.5. Reliability of the Balance Error Scoring System in Pediatric Samples

Author	Sample	Reliability measure	Reliability scores	Comment
Valovich McLeod et al. (2004)	Adolescents (9–14 years)	Intratester	Total BESS ICC(2,1) = 0.98; SEM = 1.01	Individual condition reliabilities ranged from .87 to .95.
Valovich McLeod et al. (2006)	Adolescents (9–14 years)	Test–retest	ICC (2,1) = 0.70; SEM = 3.3	60-day test–retest interval
Hunt et al. (2009)	Adolescents (13–19 years)	Intraclass reliability coefficient	Total BESS r = .60; single and tandem stances only (four conditions) r = .71 Modified BESS r = .88 (three trials), r = .84 (two trials)	The Modified BESS (mBESS) included three trials of four conditions (single-firm, tandem-firm, single-foam, tandem-foam).

testing section in the Sport Concussion Assessment Tool–2 (SCAT2) using a modification of the BESS. In this modification, the three stances on the firm condition are used. The modified BESS score is calculated by adding one error point for each error during the three 20-second tests. The maximum total number of errors for any single condition is 10. The error scores for the three conditions are then summed and subtracted from 30. It is important to note that with this modified scoring system, lower scores indicate worse performance or impaired balance.

Functional Assessments

Other researchers have studied the use of more functional assessments for the evaluation of balance following mTBI. Select tests that have been investigated for their use in patients with TBI are discussed below.

The functional reach test (FRT) has been used in the evaluation of children with mild–severe TBI and cerebral palsy, as well as with typically developing children (Katz-Leurer et al., 2008a, 2008b, 2009a). The FRT measures functional reaching ability by requiring the patient to reach as far as he or she can while staying within the limits of his or her stability. The patient is tested in three positions: (1) standing with the preferred hand near a wall and leaning forward, (2) standing with the back to the wall and leaning to the preferred side, and (3) standing with the back to the wall and leaning to the nonpreferred side. All tasks are performed in front of a grid consisting of 5 cm × 5 cm squares hanging on the wall. Each task is measured in terms of the distance (cm) moved while leaning. The FRT has demonstrated excellent within-session reliability (ICC = 0.92–0.97) in children with TBI (Katz-Leurer et al., 2008a); however, it has not yet been used serially to track recovery during the acute time frame after mTBI.

The TUG is another functional test of balance that has been studied in children with TBI (Katz-Leurer et al., 2008a, 2008b, 2009a). To start the test, the patient is seated in a chair with hips flexed to 90 degrees and feet flat on the floor. When cued to start, the patient stands, walks a distance of 3 meters, turns at a marked point, walks back to the chair, and sits down. The test measures the amount of time (seconds) taken to perform the task from "go" until the patient is seated. The within-session reliability of the TUG in children with TBI has been reported to be good (ICC = 0.96; Katz-Leurer et al., 2008a), but there has yet to be published studies investigating its sensitivity to detect mTBI-related deficits in a serial manner to track recovery after injury.

Measures of gait can also be used to assess balance following mTBI (Katz-Leurer et al., 2009a, 2009b; Parker, Osternig, van Donkelaar, & Chou, 2007, 2008). Gait parameters, including step length, step time, step width, and step variability, have been assessed using the GaitRite System (GAITRite, CIR Systems Inc., Clifton, NJ) in children with differing severities of TBI and have shown increased variability in step time and step length and decreased gait speed (Katz-Leurer et al., 2008b, 2009b). Investigations of collegiate athletes with mTBI have used more sophisticated motion analysis systems to assess center of mass displacement, peak velocity in the medial–lateral direction, average gait velocity, and maximum separation between center of mass and the center of pressure of the stance foot (Catena, van Donkelaar, & Chou, 2009; Parker et al., 2007, 2008).

METHODOLOGICAL AND CONCEPTUAL ISSUES OF BALANCE ASSESSMENT

Age-Related Changes

Postural stability, as with other motor skills, varies with the developmental stage of the child and will impact the interpretation of balance assessments following mTBI. The development of postural stability and control strategies results from complex interactions between the neural and muscular–skeletal systems (Shumway-Cook & Woollacott, 1995). Neural contributions include the motor and sensory processing of information, higher-level mapping, and processes for adapting to alterations of posture; muscular–skeletal contributions include joint range of motion, biomechanical properties of the body segments, and muscle properties (Shumway-Cook & Woollacott, 1995).

The development of postural control has been identified and studied according to various models, including the reflex hierarchical theory (Shumway-Cook & Woollacott, 1995), the systems perspective (Shumway-Cook & Woollacott, 1995), Williams's theoretical model (see Table 11.6; Williams, Fisher, & Tritschler, 1983), and Assaiante and Amblard's (1995) periods of ontogenesis. Although these models differ to some degree, all seem to define stages or periods of transition through which the child must go before developing adult-like postural control and stability. The stage-like pattern of postural stability development described by these models is likely an extension of the stages of motor development described by Kugler, Kelso, and Turvey (1982), which demonstrate stepwise qualitative changes in the organization of movement. The characteristic patterns of movement organization are described by short periods of time that are spent in transition phases in which the child is considered unstable, followed by stable organization plateaus that are maintained for longer periods of time (Kugler et al., 1982). Progression of this stepwise development occurs until the child reaches adult-like qualities of the motor skill, or in this case, adult-like postural stability.

TABLE 11.6. Williams's Theoretical Model of Balance Abilities

Level	Balance tasks	Characteristics	Nature of underlying somatosensory, vestibular, and visual patterns
I	Sit, stand	• Static position • Stable base • Vision used	Somatosensory and vestibular patterns established in visual framework
II A	Walk, run	• Dynamic position • Stable base • Vision used	Visual framework maintained; somatosensory–vestibular patterns varied
B	Two-foot stand, eyes closed	• Static position • Stable base • Vision eliminated	Established somatosensory–vestibular patterns maintained; visual framework removed
C	One-foot stand, eyes open	• Static position • Unstable base • Vision used	Visual framework maintained; established proprioceptive–vestibular patterns varied
III A	Beam walk	• Dynamic position • Unstable base • Vision used	Visual framework maintained; somatosensory–vestibular patterns of II-A varied
B	One-foot stand, eyes closed	• Static position • Unstable base • Vision eliminated	Somatosensory–vestibular patterns of II-A maintained; visual framework removed
IV	Beam walk, eyes closed	• Dynamic position • Unstable base • Vision eliminated	Somatosensory–vestibular patterns of III-A maintained; visual framework removed

Note. Data from Williams, Fisher, and Tritschler (1983).

Since the development of postural control and stability is bound by the complex interactions between several body systems, differences exist between the postural control of healthy children and adults (Shumway-Cook & Woollacott, 1995). These developmental differences occur in both the sensory and motor processes controlling balance and include (1) development of the individual sensory systems, (2) development of sensory strategies for organizing multiple inputs, (3) development of muscle strength and changes in the relative mass of body segments, (4) development of motor coordination or neuromuscular response synergies, and (5) development of adaptive and anticipatory mechanisms to modify postural control.

The development of the visual, vestibular, and somatosensory systems occurs independently, but all contribute to the maturation of postural control and stability. The *visual system* is the dominant sensory system regulating postural control in infants and young children (Assaiante & Amblard, 1995; Forssberg & Nashner, 1982), especially in static conditions. In one study, children less than 4 years of age were unable to complete the eyes-closed conditions of one investigation, demonstrating a high reliance on vision (Riach & Hayes, 1987). This same investigation found that as development continues, the extent to which vision is used to maintain balance decreases, as measured by the Romberg quotient (RQ = eyes closed/eyes open). Younger children (4–5 years) swayed more with eyes open than eyes closed, giving them a low RQ value, a finding that is not abnormal in younger children. RQ values reach adult values by 9–11 years of age (Riach & Hayes, 1987).

Development of the *vestibular system* occurs shortly after birth (Forssberg & Nashner, 1982) but does not seem to play a crucial role in postural stability until the age of 7. At this time, the vestibular system is predominantly used to maintain head stabilization in space as the child gains the ability to separate head and trunk stabilization, as noted in period three of the ontogenic model (Assaiante & Amblard, 1995). Following the child's transition into this period of development, the vestibular contribution closely resembles that of an adult, but seems to be insensitive to fine movements (Lee & Aronson, 1974).

Finally, *somatosensory system* development occurs later in the emergence of postural stability and as the last stage prior to adult-like postural stability (Shumway-Cook & Woollacott, 1985, 1995). Research has demonstrated an increased reliance on somatosensory information in children from 4 to 6 years of age (Shumway-Cook & Woollacott, 1985), with the contribution to postural stability at this age most often apparent after practicing a task (Lee & Aronson, 1974).

Although each of the three sensory systems develops independently over the course of childhood, successful adult-like postural control strategies cannot be developed until the child is able to resolve conflicts involving these three sensory systems. Utilizing balance tasks such as the P-CTSIB and moving platforms, alterations to one or more of the sensory systems and the resulting balance strategies have been investigated. Children of all ages tend to be able to use cues from each of the three sensory systems (Deitz et al., 1991); however, the extent to which they utilize each and their ability to successfully integrate the systems varies with age. Age 7 appears to be a critical age, after which children are able to utilize integration strategies successfully in response to conflicts of information. Forssberg and Nashner (1982) found that children under the age of 7 were unable to balance when somatosensory and visual cues were eliminated. In fact, the performance of these younger children during tasks involving altered support and visual conditions resembled the performance of patients with vestibular deficits (Forssberg & Nashner, 1982). An evaluation of SOT composite equilibrium and vestibular equilibrium scores in children of varying ages showed a progressive linear increase in balance as a function of age, whereas visual equilibrium scores were significantly associated with the subject's height (Cumberworth, Patel, Rogers, & Kenyon, 2007). There were no age-related associations with the somatosensory equilibrium score. These findings suggest that visual and vestibular functions mature in an age-dependent manner through 16 years of age, whereas somatosensory function develops at a younger age.

Shumway-Cook and Woollacott (1985) summarized the development of sensory interaction based on their investigation of young (≤ 3 years), middle (4–6 years), and older (7–10 years) children in response to a balance task on a moving platform. Children less than 3 years of age tended to use only visual and vestibular information as their primary means of control. These children found it difficult to suppress inaccurate visual inputs and were unable to correct for altered somatosensory inputs (Shumway-Cook & Woollacott, 1985). Children in the middle group seemed to shift away from their reliance on vision and increased their awareness of somatosensory inputs. During this age period, the children demonstrated adult-like sensory integration strategies, but had some difficulties in suppressing inaccurate information and resolving conflicts. However, they were able to achieve and maintain balance following practice of the task (Shumway-Cook & Woollacott, 1985). In contrast, the children in the older group displayed response patterns to altered conditions that were comparable to results demonstrating a mature process of sensory organization.

Fatigue

Balance ability can be affected by a number of factors, including fatigue. A decrease in postural stability following fatigue or exertion has been found in previous studies utilizing both whole-body (Fox, Mihalik, Blackburn, Battaglini, & Guskiewicz, 2008; Lepers, Bigard, Diard, Gouteyron, & Guezennec, 1997; Nardone, Tarantola, Galante, & Schieppati, 1998; Susco, Valovich McLeod, Gansneder, & Shultz, 2004) and isolated muscle fatigue (Fox et al., 2008; Vuillerme, Nougier, & Prieur, 2001) and has been reported using varying methods of assessing balance. Studies utilizing the BESS, in young adults, have demonstrated a decrease in postural stability, resulting in an increase in total BESS errors, following an exertion or fatigue protocol (Fox et al., 2008; Susco et al., 2004; Wilkins, Valovich McLeod, Perrin, & Gansneder, 2004). Scores on the BESS tend to recover to prefatigued levels following 13–20 minutes of rest or recovery (Fox et al., 2008; Susco et al., 2004). Several investigations have also found decreases in postural stability as measured by instrumented posturography with significant increases in sway path more prominent under conditions that involve eye closure (Nardone et al., 1998). Similarly, utilizing the SOT to measure postural stability following a 25-km run, Lepers et al. (1997) found a significant decrease in postural stability during the posttest in all of the conditions except the fixed-support/eyes-open condition. Balance performance had decreased the most during the sway-referenced/eyes-closed condition (Condition 5) and the sway-referenced/ sway-referenced condition (Condition 6) when the subjects needed to rely on vestibular input as their only accurate sensory input. In addition, the sensory isolation ratios for vision (4:1) and vestibular inputs (5:1) decreased following the exercise protocol, indicating that the subjects did not make effective use of either of these inputs following fatigue (Lepers et al., 1997).

Learning Effects

Another factor that can influence the interpretation of balance assessment scores is practice or learning effects. This factor may be even more important to understand when assessing balance in children and adolescents with respect to their continued motor development and ability to learn tasks. Learning effects can be influenced by both the nature of the balance task and the time intervals between the test sessions. The nature of the balance assessment is an important factor in determining whether learning will take place and the time course of the learning. Learning effects have been demonstrated in static force platform (Hamman, Longridge, Mekjavic, & Dickinson, 1995; Nordahl, Aasen, Dyrkorn, Eiksvik, & Molavaer, 2000; Riemann et al., 1999) and clinical assessments (Valovich, Perrin, & Gansneder, 2003). In addition, tasks that require novel or unusual activities tend to demonstrate a greater learning effect. These tasks may include impaired visual feedback, unstable or moving surfaces, or dynamic movement patterns.

In an investigation of repeated stabilometric testing in adults, Nordahl et al. (2000) found that the largest amount of learning occurred on a foam surface with eyes closed and with the least amount of time between test sessions. The researchers found no learning effects for any stance in which the eyes were open, but noted high learning potential with loss of visual reference or changed proprioceptive input. These findings were substantiated using the BESS in both high school (Valovich, Perrin, & Gansneder, 2003) and youth athletes (Valovich McLeod et al., 2004). High school athletes were given repeated administrations of the BESS every other day for four test sessions. Total BESS score decreased with each administration and was significantly lower than baseline on days 5 and 7. Although the total BESS score showed a learning effect, not all BESS conditions contributed equally to the learning. The largest learning effects were apparent on the conditions involving the foam surfaces and single-leg stances, which were significantly different than baseline on day 7 (Valovich et al., 2003).

The interval between test sessions has also been shown to be an important factor in postural stability learning effects. Using the BESS, Valovich et al. (2003) found that the number of errors decreased over each test session and were significantly different than the baseline by day 5. During this time, subjects were tested with a very short interval between test sessions (1 day). Another investigation of the influences of time intervals between repeated test sessions with stabilometric testing found that subjects with the shortest time interval between test sessions (11 days) had significantly greater learning on various postural sway parameters compared to groups who had test–retest time intervals of 17, 31, and 115 days (Nordahl et al., 2000). However, other investigations have found learning with substantially longer periods between test sessions (Hamman et al., 1995; Strange Hansen, Dieckmann, Jensen, & Jakobsen, 2000).

Although the majority of postural stability research on learning effects has been conducted with adult populations, pediatric populations are equally susceptible to learning effects and maturation with repeated testing. Previous work investigating the reliability of tiltboard balance assessments in young children has demonstrated practice or learning effects during the retest session (Atwater, Crowe, Deitz, & Richardson, 1991; Broadstone, Westcott, & Deitz, 1993) that are most prominent in the eyes-closed condition (Atwater et al., 1991). A follow up study also demonstrated a clear practice effect (Broadstone et al., 1993), especially with a novel task. Additionally, learning effects were found with the heel-to-toe stances of the P-CTSIB (Westcott et al., 1994). Children performed better on the retest for all six conditions, although significant learning effects were found only on the absent vision, inaccurate vision, and accurate somatosensory conditions (Westcott et al., 1994).

SUMMARY AND FUTURE RESEARCH DIRECTIONS

Consensus conferences have established that the assessment and management of sport-related mTBI or "sport concussion" should involve a multisystem approach, whereby the clinician assesses a variety of cerebral functions. The most basic, yet important, component includes monitoring symptoms that manifest at the time of injury and that may increase or decrease in severity during subsequent evaluations. The subjectivity involved with using only a *symptom assessment*, however, can leave the clinician without a clear picture of the athlete's true mental status. *Neuropsychological testing* has become a mainstay in the sports medicine community for assessing the cognitive domain of neurological functioning.

Because selected areas of the brain responsible for the maintenance of postural stability can also be affected by mTBI, postural stability testing has gained credence for assessing the motor domain of neurological functioning after injury. As outlined in our review, multiple studies using sophisticated force plate technology and/or less technical clinical balance tests have identified postural stability deficits lasting several days following sport-related mTBI. These studies suggest that *postural stability (balance) testing*, along with assessment of symptom severity and cognitive function, should be considered reliable and valid tools in the management of patients suffering from mTBI. Studies investigating the relationship between these three clinical measures following mTBI have been inconclusive; at best they appear to be only mildly correlated in athletes suffering mild to moderate concussions. Thus, it is strongly recommended that all three components be assessed following concussion, especially in the pediatric population where the consequences of misdiagnosing a concussion run a higher risk of a catastrophic outcome.

More recently, researchers have begun investigating the efficacy of *dual-task rehabilitation strategies* (combined postural stability and cognitive tasks) for treating athletes with lingering postconcussion symptoms. Although little research currently exists involving this rehabilitation strategy, training both the cognitive and postural control systems concurrently might be helpful in retraining executive attentional networks that are typically disrupted following TBI. Studies involving dual-task postural control and the effects of cognitive demand in conjunction with focus of attention have identified that secondary cognitive activities improve postural performance by shifting the focus of overt attention away from a highly automatized activity (Huxhold, Li, Schmiedek, & Lindenberger, 2006; Wulf, Shea, & Park, 2001b). Postural stability improves under these dual-task conditions, which is consistent with the hypothesis of *constrained action* (Wulf, McNevin, & Shea, 2001a). Instead of the dual task interfering with postural control, the external focus of attention, which is provided by the secondary perceptual task, enables the postural control system to self-organize automatically. Therefore, in many of these studies, postural stability (and other motor tasks) improves when a perceptual task of low cognitive demand is added. It is important to recognize, however, that a secondary task with a given level of cognitive demand may have different functional effects on individuals who differ in their amount of attentional resources, such as with older individuals or individuals recovering from neurological impairment. For example, because older adults are more limited in attentional capacity, memory tasks that are more cognitively demanding may result in attentional resource competition between cognition and postural control performance, and consequently negatively affect postural control. In contrast, due to their relatively higher level of cognitive capacity, younger adults do not experience increasing resource competition with the same nominal level of cognitive demands, and their postural performance may not demonstrate those same impairments under the dual-task conditions (Huxhold et al., 2006). This theory needs to be tested in the pediatric population to determine its application to rehabilitation following TBI. New game technologies such as the Nintendo Wii Balance Board have provided the medical community with options for training pediatric patients or athletes on dual-task activities. Current research suggests that this approach may have utility in rehabilitation settings whereby concussed athletes can train neural networks responsible for performing divided attention tasks (Clark et al., 2010).

A major consideration for future research should be aimed at understanding the effect of variable priority instructions (randomly shifting attention between tasks) versus fixed-priority instructions (placing equal amounts of attention on both tasks). This combination has the greatest potential to simulate sport-related activities that require both motor and cognitive functions to work concurrently. Most of the studies to date utilized fixed-priority instructions; however, one provided three different sets of instructions to see how healthy subjects would respond. In most studies, subjects were able to focus more on the cognitive tasks and improve cognitive performance when given the instructions to do so but were not able to do this with balance performance (Rankin, Woollacott, Shumway-Cook, & Brown, 2000; Shumway-Cook & Horak, 1986; Silsupadol et al., 2009; Silsupadol, Siu, Shumway-Cook, & Woollacott, 2006; Siu & Woollacott, 2007). Balance performance did not change under any of the conditions, indicating the prioritization of balance (postural control) over the cognitive task in normal healthy individuals. Balance is an attentionally demanding task; therefore, in order to train an individual's balance/postural control, a certain amount of allocated attention is necessary. However, more research is needed to assess the validity and reliability of these dual-task measures, specifically in an active pediatric population. Future studies should identify tasks that combine balance and cognitive attention, perhaps using virtual reality or computer games that will task both motor and cognitive functions. These tasks should be age-appropriate and developed specifically for use with the pediatric patient with TBI.

REFERENCES

Assaiante, C., & Amblard, B. (1995). An ontogenetic model for the sensorimotor organization of balance control in humans. *Human Movement Science, 14*, 13–43.

Atwater, S. W., Crowe, T. K., Deitz, J. C., & Richardson, P. K. (1991). Interrater and test–retest reliability of two pediatric balance tests. *Physical Therapy, 70*, 79–87.

Broadstone, B. J., Westcott, S. L., & Deitz, J. C. (1993). Test–retest reliability of two tiltboard tests in children. *Physical Therapy, 73*, 618–625.

Broglio, S. P., & Puetz, T. W. (2008). The effect of sport concussion on neurocognitive function, self-report symptoms and postural control: A meta-analysis. *Sports Medicine, 38*(1), 53–67.

Campbell, M., & Parry, A. (2005). Balance disorder and traumatic brain injury: Preliminary findings of a multi-factorial observational study. *Brain Injury, 19*(13), 1095–1104.

Catena, R. D., van Donkelaar, P., & Chou, L. S. (2009). Different gait tasks distinguish immediate vs. long-term effects of concussion on balance control. *Journal of NeuroEngineering and Rehabilitation, 6*, 25.

Cavanaugh, J. T., Guskiewicz, K. M., Giuliani, C., Marshall, S., Mercer, V., & Stergiou, N. (2005). Detecting altered postural control after cerebral concussion in athletes with normal postural stability. *British Journal of Sports Medicine, 39*(11), 805–811.

Clark, R. A., Bryant, A. L., Pua, Y., McCrory, P., Bennell, K., & Hunt, M. (2010). Validity and reliability of the Nintendo Wii Balance Board for assessment of standing balance. *Gait Posture, 31*(3), 307–310.

Crowe, T. K., Deitz, J. C., Richardson, P. K., & Atwater, S. W. (1990). Interrater reliability of the Pediatric Clinical Test of Sensory Interaction for Balance. *Physical and Occupational Therapy in Pediatrics, 10*(4), 1–27.

Cumberworth, V. L., Patel, N. N., Rogers, W., & Kenyon, G. S. (2007). The maturation of balance in children. *Journal of Laryngology and Otology, 121*(5), 449–454.

Deitz, J. C., Richardson, P. K., Atwater, S. W., Crowe, T. K., & Odiorne, M. (1991). Performance of normal children on the Pediatric Clinical Test of Sensory Interaction for Balance. *Occupational Therapy Journal of Research, 11*(6), 336–356.

Ekdahl, C., Jarnlo, G. B., & Andersson, S. I. (1989). Standing balance in healthy subjects: Evaluation of a quantitative test battery on a force platform. *Scandinavian Journal of Rehabilitation Medicine, 21*(4), 187–195.

Forssberg, H., & Nashner, L. M. (1982). Ontogenetic development of postural control in man: Adaptation to altered support and visual conditions during stance. *Journal of Neuroscience, 2*(5), 545–552.

Fox, Z. G., Mihalik, J. P., Blackburn, J. T., Battaglini, C. L., & Guskiewicz, K. M. (2008). Return of postural control to baseline after anaerobic and aerobic exercise protocols. *Journal of Athletic Training, 43*(5), 456–463.

Gagnon, I., Forget, R., Sullivan, S. J., & Friedman, D. (1998). Motor performance following a mild traumatic brain injury in children: An exploratory study. *Brain Injury, 12*(10), 843–853.

Gagnon, I., Swaine, B., & Forget, R. (2006). Exploring the comparability of the Sensory Organization Test and the Pediatric Clinical Test of Sensory Interaction for Balance in children. *Physical and Occupational Therapy: Pediatrics, 26*(1–2), 23–41.

Gagnon, I., Swaine, B., Friedman, D., & Forget, R. (2004). Children show decreased dynamic balance after mild traumatic brain injury. *Archives of Physical Medicine and Rehabilitation, 85*(3), 444–452.

Geurts, A. C., Ribbers, G. M., Knoop, J. A., & van Limbeek, J. (1996). Identification of static and dynamic postural instability following traumatic brain injury. *Archives of Physical Medicine and Rehabilitation, 77*(7), 639–644.

Greenwald, B. D., Cifu, D. X., Marwitz, J. H., Enders, L. J., Brown, A. W., Englander, J. S., et al. (2001). Factors associated with balance deficits on admission to rehabilitation after traumatic brain injury: A multicenter analysis. *Journal of Head Trauma Rehabilitation, 16*(3), 238–252.

Guskiewicz, K. M. (2011). Balance assessment in the management of sport-related concussion. *Clinical Sports Medicine, 30*(1), 89–102, ix.

Guskiewicz, K. M., Perrin, D. H., & Gansneder, B. M. (1996). Effect of mild head injury on postural stability in athletes. *Journal of Athletic Training, 31*(4), 300–306.

Guskiewicz, K. M., Riemann, B. L., Perrin, D. H., & Nashner, L. M. (1997). Alternative approaches to the assessment of mild head injury in athletes. *Medical Science and Sports and Exercise, 29*(7, Suppl.), S213–S221.

Guskiewicz, K. M., Ross, S. E., & Marshall, S. W. (2001). Postural stability and neuropsychological deficits after concussion in collegiate athletes. *Journal of Athletic Training, 36*(3), 263–273.

Guyton, A. (1986). *Textbook of medical physiology.* Philadelphia: Saunders.

Hamman, R., Longridge, N. S., Mekjavic, I., & Dickinson, J. (1995). Effect of age and training schedules on balance improvement exercises using visual biofeedback. *Journal of Otolaryngology, 24*(4), 221–229.

Hirabayashi, S., & Iwasake, Y. (1995). Developmental perspective of sensory organization on postural control. *Brain and Development, 17*, 111–113.

Hunt, T. N., Ferrara, M. S., Bornstein, R. A., & Baumgartner, T. A. (2009). The reliability of the modified Balance Error Scoring System. *Clinical Journal of Sports Medicine, 19*(6), 471–475.

Huxhold, O., Li, S. C., Schmiedek, F., & Lindenberger, U. (2006). Dual-tasking postural control: Aging and the effects of cognitive demand in conjunction with focus of attention. *Brain Research Bulletin, 69*(3), 294–305.

Ingersoll, C. D., & Armstrong, C. W. (1992). The effects of closed-head injury on postural sway. *Medical Science and Sports and Exercise, 24*(7), 739–743.

Iwasake, Y. (1995). Developmental perspective of sensory organization on postural control. *Brain and Development, 17*, 111–113.

Jansen, E., Larsen, R., & Mogens, B. (1982). Quantitative Romberg's test: Measurement and computer calculations of postural stability. *Acta Neurologica Scandinavica, 66*, 93–99.

Katz-Leurer, M., Rotem, H., Keren, O., & Meyer, S. (2009a). Balance abilities and gait characteristics in post-traumatic brain injury, cerebral palsy and typically developed children. *Developmental Neurorehabilitation, 12*(2), 100–105.

Katz-Leurer, M., Rotem, H., Keren, O., & Meyer, S. (2009b). The relationship between step variability, muscle strength and functional walking performance in children with post-traumatic brain injury. *Gait Posture, 29*(1), 154–157.

Katz-Leurer, M., Rotem, H., Lewitus, H., Keren, O., & Meyer, S. (2008a). Functional balance tests for children with traumatic brain injury: Within-session reliability. *Pediatric Physical Therapy, 20*(3), 254–258.

Katz-Leurer, M., Rotem, H., Lewitus, H., Keren, O., & Meyer, S. (2008b). Relationship between balance abilities and gait characteristics in children with post-traumatic brain injury. *Brain Injury, 22*(2), 153–159.

Kugler, P. N., Kelso, J. A. S., & Turvey, M. T. (1982). On the control and co-ordination of naturally developing systems. In J. A. S. Kelso & J. E. Clark (Eds.), *The development of movement control and co-ordination* (pp. 5–78). Chichester, UK: Wiley.

Kuhtz-Buschbeck, J. P., Hoppe, B., Golge, M., Dreesmann, M., Damm-Stunitz, U., & Ritz, A. (2003). Sensorimotor recovery in children after traumatic brain injury: Analyses of gait, gross motor, and fine motor skills. *Developmental Medicine and Child Neurology, 45*(12), 821–828.

Lee, D. N., & Aronson, E. (1974). Visual proprioceptive control of standing infant humans. *Perception and Psychophysics, 15*(3), 529–532.

Lepers, R., Bigard, A. X., Diard, J. P., Gouteyron, J. F., & Guezennec, C. Y. (1997). Posture control after prolonged exercise. *European Journal of Applied Physiology, 76*, 55–61.

McCrea, M., Guskiewicz, K. M., Marshall, S. W., Barr, W., Randolph, C., Cantu, R. C., et al. (2003). Acute effects and recovery time following concussion in collegiate football players: The NCAA Concussion Study. *Journal of the American Medical Association, 290*(19), 2556–2563.

McCrory, P., Meeuwisse, W., Johnston, K., Dvorak, J., Aubry, M., Molloy, M., et al. (2009). Consensus statement on Concussion in Sport 3rd International Conference on Concussion in Sport held in Zurich, November 2008. *Clinical Journal of Sports Medicine, 19*(3), 185–200.

Nardone, A., Tarantola, J., Galante, M., & Schieppati, M. (1998). Time course of stabilometric changes after a strenuous treadmill exercise. *Archives of Physical Medicine and Rehabilitation, 79*, 920–924.

Nashner, L. M. (1982). Adaptation of human movement to altered environments. *Trends in Neuroscience, 5*, 358–361.

Nashner, L. M. (1993). Practical biomechanics and physiology of balance. In B. P. Jacobson, C. W. Newman, & J. M. Kartush (Eds.), *Handbook of balance function testing* (pp. 261–275). St. Louis, MO: Mosby Year Book.

Nashner, L. M., Black, F. O., & Wall, C., 3rd. (1982). Adaptation to altered support and visual conditions during stance: Patients with vestibular deficits. *Journal of Neuroscience, 2*(5), 536–544.

Nordahl, S. H., Aasen, T., Dyrkorn, B. M., Eiksvik, S., & Molavaer, O. I. (2000). Static stabilometry and repeated testing in a normal population. *Aviation Space and Environmental Medicine, 71*(9), 889–893.

Parker, T. M., Osternig, L. R., van Donkelaar, P., & Chou, L. S. (2007). Recovery of cognitive and dynamic motor function following concussion. *British Journal of Sports Medicine, 41*(12), 868–873; discussion, 873.

Parker, T. M., Osternig, L. R., van Donkelaar, P., & Chou, L. S. (2008). Balance control during gait in athletes and non-athletes following concussion. *Medical Engineering and Physics, 30*(8), 959–967.

Rankin, J. K., Woollacott, M. H., Shumway-Cook, A., & Brown, L. A. (2000). Cognitive influence on postural stability: A neuromuscular analysis in young and older adults. *Journal of Gerontolology: A Biological Science: Medical Science, 55*(3), M112–M119.

Riach, C. L., & Hayes, K. C. (1987). Maturation of postural sway in young children. *Developmental Medicine and Child Neurology, 29*, 651–658.

Riemann, B. L., & Guskiewicz, K. M. (2000). Effects of mild head injury on postural stability as measured through clinical balance testing. *Journal of Athletic Training, 35*(1), 19–25.

Riemann, B. L., Guskiewicz, K. M., & Shields, E. W. (1999). Relationship between clinical and forceplate measure of postural stability. *Journal of Sport Rehabilitation, 8*, 71–82.

Rubin, A. M., Woolley, S. M., Dailey, V. M., & Goebel, J. A. (1995). Postural stability following mild head or whiplash injuries. *American Journal of Otology, 16*(2), 216–221.

Shumway-Cook, A., & Horak, F. B. (1986). Assessing the influence of sensory interaction on balance. *Physical Therapy, 66*(10), 1548–1550.

Shumway-Cook, A., & Woollacott, M. H. (1985). The growth of stability: Postural control from a developmental perspective. *Journal of Motor Behavior, 17*(2), 131–147.

Shumway-Cook, A., & Woollacott, M. H. (1995). *Motor control: Theory and practical applications.* Baltimore: Williams & Wilkins.

Silsupadol, P., Shumway-Cook, A., Lugade, V., van Donkelaar, P., Chou, L. S., Mayr, U., et al. (2009). Effects of single-task versus dual-task training on balance performance in older adults: A double-blind, randomized controlled trial. *Archives of Physical Medicine and Rehabilitation, 90*(3), 381–387.

Silsupadol, P., Siu, K. C., Shumway-Cook, A., & Woollacott, M. H. (2006). Training of balance under single- and dual-task conditions in older adults with balance impairment. *Physical Therapy, 86*(2), 269–281.

Siu, K. C., & Woollacott, M. H. (2007). Attentional demands of postural control: The ability to selectively allocate information-processing resources. *Gait Posture, 25*(1), 121–126.

Strange Hansen, M., Dieckmann, B., Jensen, K., & Jakobsen, B. W. (2000). The reliabiliy of balance tests performed on the kinesthetic ability trainer (KAT). *Knee Surgery, Sports Traumatology, Arthroscopy, 8*, 180–185.

Susco, T. M., Valovich McLeod, T. C., Gansneder, B. M., & Shultz, S. J. (2004). Balance recovers within 20 minutes after exertion as measured by the Balance Error Scoring System. *Journal of Athletic Training, 39*(3), 241–246.

Valovich, T. C., Perrin, D. H., & Gansneder, B. M. (2003). Repeat administration elicits a practice effect with the Balance Error Scoring System but not with the Standardized Assessment of Concussion in high school athletes. *Journal of Athletic Training, 38*(1), 51–56.

Valovich McLeod, T. C., Barr, W. B., McCrea, M., & Guskiewicz, K. M. (2006). Psychometric and measurement properties of concussion assessment tools in youth sports. *Journal of Athletic Training, 41*(4), 399–408.

Valovich McLeod, T. C., Perrin, D. H., Guskiewicz, K. M., Shultz, S. J., Diamond, R., & Gansneder, B. M. (2004). Serial administration of clinical concussion assessments and learning effects in healthy young athletes. *Clinical Journal of Sports Medicine, 14*(5), 287–295.

Vander, A., Sherman, J., & Luciano, D. (1990). Human physiology: *The mechanisms of body function* (5th ed.). New York: McGraw-Hill.

Vuillerme, N., Nougier, V., & Prieur, J. M. (2001). Can vision compensate for a lower limb muscular fatigue for controlling posture in humans? *Neuroscience Letters, 308,* 106–106.

Westcott, S. L., Crowe, T. K., Deitz, J. C., & Richardson, P. (1994). Test–retest reliability of the Pediatric Clinical Test of Sensory Interaction for Balance. *Physical and Occupational Therapy in Pediatrics, 14*(1), 1–22.

Wilkins, J. C., Valovich McLeod, T. C., Perrin, D. H., & Gansneder, B. M. (2004). Performance on the Balance Error Scoring System decreases after fatigue. *Journal of Athletic Training, 39*(2), 156–161.

Williams, H. G., Fisher, J. M., & Tritschler, K. A. (1983). Descriptive analysis of static postural control in 4, 6, and 8 year old normal and motorically awkward children. *American Journal of Physical Medicine, 62*(1), 12–26.

Wulf, G., McNevin, N., & Shea, C. H. (2001a). The automaticity of complex motor skill learning as a function of attentional focus. *Quarterly Journal of Experimental Psychology A, 54*(4), 1143–1154.

Wulf, G., Shea, C., & Park, J. H. (2001b). Attention and motor performance: Preferences for and advantages of an external focus. *Research Quarterly for Exercise and Sport, 72*(4), 335–344.

CHAPTER 12

Postconcussion Symptom Assessment

Jennifer A. Janusz, Maegan D. Sady, and Gerard A. Gioia

In recent years, the focus of concussion assessment and management has shifted away from severity grading systems (Eckner & Kutcher, 2010). Concussion assessment is now widely considered to require an individualized, multifaceted approach. Evaluation of a patient's or athlete's symptoms is considered a key component of any postinjury assessment. To this end, research has focused on developing methods to assess and monitor postconcussion symptoms. In both athlete and nonathlete populations, evidence suggests that symptom report is apt to be at least as sensitive to the effects of concussion as neurocognitive or balance testing (Broglio & Puetz, 2008; Yeates, 2010). Furthermore, because many return-to-play guidelines state that an athlete should be symptom-free before returning to play, the careful use of such measures becomes an important part of the clinical decision-making process.

Self-report symptom scales typically assess somatic (e.g., headache, fatigue), cognitive (e.g., forgetfulness, inattention), and emotional/behavioral (e.g., irritability, disinhibition) symptoms commonly seen after a concussion. These scales are a practical method for evaluating and tracking postconcussion symptoms, and research is actively exploring their use, feasibility, reliability, and validity in capturing such symptomatology. Among adult athletes, the sensitivity of scales to concussive symptoms has consistently been shown (Randolph et al., 2009). However, research is just beginning to explore the use of these measures with youth athletes (Gioia, Schneider, Vaughan, & Isquith, 2009).

In 2004, the 2nd International Conference on Concussion in Sport Group recognized the specialized needs of the pediatric athlete in managing postconcussive symptoms (McCrory et al., 2005). Vast differences exist between younger and older athletes not only with respect to their neurological maturation and pathophysiological responses to injury, but also in regard to the expectations of their day-to-day activities (Kirkwood, Yeates, & Wilson, 2006). Because children need to be understood differently than adults, developmentally appropriate guidelines for concussion management, as well as associated clinical tools, are essential.

In the creation of postconcussion symptom measures, age has been recognized as an important consideration. As in other areas of child assessment, specific measures for children require the use of age-appropriate wording and response formats. The appropriate measurement of symptoms in children versus adults requires a number of questions to be answered. For example, how young can children accurately report symptoms? Can young children understand traditional, rank-order ratings, or do they require simpler binary ratings? Can young children understand and accurately report symptoms such as dizziness? When should the symptom vocabulary change to adult usage? Furthermore, given the potential importance of monitoring symptoms serially from preinjury baseline to postinjury assessment, normal maturation that might occur during that time frame also needs to be considered in the development of symptom measures (McCrory, Collie, Anderson, & Davis, 2004).

As compared to assessment with adults, the inclusion of key adults in monitoring and managing a child's symptoms is also essential. Parents are obviously important informants regarding the functioning of their children, but teachers and coaches can provide additional information not easily observed by parents (Gioia et al., 2009). The inclusion of these informed adults in symptom assessment is a common practice in many aspects of the behavioral assessment of children, with measures such as the Child Behavior Checklist (CBCL; Achenbach & Rescorla, 2001), Behavior Rating Inventory of Executive Function (BRIEF; Gioia, Isquith, Guy, & Kenworthy, 2000), and the Pediatric Quality of Life Inventory (PedsQL; Varni, Seid, & Rode, 1999) frequently used to obtain information regarding a child's behavioral, emotional, and cognitive functioning. The relationship between parent and child ratings needs to be considered in pediatric assessment to appreciate the relative contribution of both to an understanding of the child's status.

Finally, regardless of whether instruments are used with children or adults, the measures must demonstrate appropriate psychometric properties, including evidence of appropriate reliability and validity, examined through well-designed studies with appropriate sample sizes. As these measures are frequently used in monitoring symptom change over time, the inclusion of reliable change metrics is an important feature.

This chapter provides an overview of the current literature regarding postconcussion symptom scales for children and adolescents, reviewing the development, use with children and adolescents, and available psychometric evidence for each. Regarding the psychometric evidence, we report the various lines of evidence for reliability and validity available for each instrument. As a brief review, *reliability* refers to the internal consistency and stability over time of an instrument, whereas *validity* refers to the accuracy with which the instrument's scores can be interpreted to reflect a particular construct (e.g., somatic symptoms) or criterion (e.g., presence of concussion, improved recovery). Validity is not measured by a single indicator. Instead, evidence supporting the valid interpretation of a measure's scores is evaluated based on multiple sources (Campbell & Fiske, 1959), including (1) the content of the measure; (2) the presence of expected developmental changes in the scores; (3) the convergence and divergence of scores with those of other measures; (4) the clarity, coherence, and consistency of the measure's internal structure (typically by factor analysis); (5)

TABLE 12.1. Description of Symptom Assessment Measures

Measure	No. of items	Response format	Age range	Self-report	Parent-report
GSC/GSS	16–20	7-point Guttman scale	Middle/high school	Yes	No
CSI	12	7-point Guttman scale	High school	Yes	No
RPCSQ	16	5-point Guttman scale	8–18 years	Yes	No
ACE	22	2-point Guttman scale	3–18 years	No	Yes
HBI					
—Child report	50	4-point Guttman scale	8–15 years	Yes	
—Parent report	50	4-point Guttman scale	8–15 years		Yes
PCS—Interview	15	2-point Guttman scale	8–15 years	Yes	Yes
PCSI					
—Parent report	20	7-point Guttman scale	5–18 years		Yes
—Child self-report (5–7)	13	3-point Guttman scale	5–7 years	Yes	
—Child self-report (8–12)	17	3-point Guttman scale	8–12 years	Yes	
—Adolescent self-report (13–18)	20	7-point Guttman scale	13–18 years	Yes	
PCS	22	7-point Guttman scale	11–18 years	Yes	No

Note. GSC/GSS, Graded Symptom Checklist/Scale; CSI, Concussion Symptom Inventory; RPCSQ, Rivermead Post-Concussion Symptoms Questionnaire; ACE, Acute Concussion Evaluation;
HBI, Health and Behavior Inventory; PCS—Interview, Post-Concussion Symptom Interview; PCSI, Post-Concussion Symptom Inventory; PCS, Post-Concussion Scale.

discriminating profiles of scores within and between various groups of children with varying clinical conditions (e.g., concussion, attention-deficit/hyperactivity disorder [ADHD], depression); (6) sensitivity to expected changes in symptoms over the course of recovery following a concussion; and (7) sensitivity and specificity of scores for detecting the presence or absence of a concussion. Finally, this review reports whether reliable change score metrics are available for each measure. Reliable change metrics employ a statistical method for determining when clinical change over time is beyond that expected by chance, regression to the mean, or practice effects. Table 12.1 describes the characteristics of each measure.

INSTRUMENTS

Graded Symptom Checklist/Scale

Description

The Graded Symptom Scale (GSS) and the Graded Symptom Checklist (GSC) are both derived from the Head Injury Scale (HIS; Piland, Motl, Ferrara, & Peterson, 2003), a theoretically derived, self-report measure that has predominantly been used with adult athletes. The GSS consists of 16 items that are rated on Guttman-type scaling[1] in terms of severity (0 = not having the symptom to 6 = severe symptom) and duration (number of days present during the week; Mailer, Valovich-McLeod, & Bay, 2008). From the severity scale, a total symptom score (TSS) and the total number of symptoms endorsed (TSE) are calculated. On the GSC, symptoms are assessed through 20 items. Raters endorse whether they are experiencing the symptom that day and rate its severity on a 7-point Guttman scale, from "no symptom" to "severe symptom" (Piland, Motl, Guskiewicz, McCrea, & Ferrara, 2006). The TSS and the TSE can be calculated (Register-Mihalik, Guskiewicz, Mann, & Shields, 2007).

Use with Children and Adolescents

Mailer and colleagues (2008) report use of the GSS in 126 nonconcussed middle school students, with a mean age of 13.1 years. The GSC was used with a large sample of male high school athletes (N = 1,089), with a mean age of 16 years, as well as with a sample of male high school and collegiate athletes, also with a mean age of 16 years (Register-Mihalik, Guskiewicz, Mann, & Shields, 2007).

Psychometric Studies

Mailer et al. (2008) found excellent test–retest reliability for TSS (intraclass correlation coefficient [ICC] = .93) and TSE (ICC = .88) scales of the GSS. Marginal to excellent test–retest reliability was also found on the individual symptoms for the severity (ICC = .65–.89) and duration (ICC = .56–.96) scales.

Piland and colleagues (2006) used 16 of the 20 GCS items that were on the original HIS scale to examine the measure's factor structure. They explored a three-factor structure for both a 16-item version and a 9-item version. Although adequate support was found for the 16-item version, the 9-item version resulted in the strongest indices. The three factors included somatic symptoms (headache, nausea, and balance problems), neurobehavioral symptoms (sleeping more than usual, drowsiness, and fatigue), and cognitive symptoms (feeling slowed down, feeling in a fog, and difficulty concentrating).

In a study assessing the relationship between headache and postconcussion symptoms, those reporting headache at baseline assessment had more symptoms postinjury than those without headache at baseline. Across headache and nonheadache groups, both the TSE and the TSS increased at days 1 and 3 postinjury, with symptom resolution by day 7 (Register-Mihalik et al., 2007).

Summary

The GSS and GCS are derived from the HIS, a theoretically driven measure. Items on the HIS, and subsequently the GSS/GCS, were chosen to be representative of concussive symptoms reported in the literature and consistent with other postconcussion

---

[1] Note: As a point of clarification, technically a Guttman-type scale consists of a unidimensional-ordered response scale with items that are ranked in order from the least extreme to most extreme position. In contrast, a Likert scale (Likert, 1932) is a bipolar scale running from one extreme (e.g., Strongly Disagree) through a neutral point (No Opinion) to the opposite extreme (Strongly Agree).

symptoms scales for adults. As such, there is less developmental basis for the item selection of this measure than those that were created specifically for children. The GSS/GCS is a self-report measure, with no parent version available. Test–retest reliability has been reported to be adequate for the GSS. Convergent validity (relationship to other factors), internal structure (factor analysis), and criterion validity (group differences) have all been explored with the GCS, and indicate that the measure is sensitive to postconcussion symptoms. While the GCS was used serially, a reliable change index (RCI) was not calculated. Given that the study samples have consisted of mostly older male teens, the findings may not generalize to younger children or females.

Concussion Symptom Inventory

Description

The Concussion Symptom Inventory (CSI; Randolph et al., 2009) consists of 12 items rated on a 7-point Guttman scale (0 = absent; 6 = severe). The rating form also includes an area for written text to describe symptoms not rated on the scale.

Use with Children and Adolescents

The only identified study using the CSI describes its development with a large sample of 16,000 high school and college athletes. The data were combined from several data sets. A mean age or age range for the combined sample was not provided.

Psychometric Evidence

This is the first empirically derived postconcussion symptom scale and uses one of the largest samples to date. Randolph and colleagues (2009) combined data sets on symptom scales from three separate projects: the Concussion Prevention Initiative, the NCAA Concussion Study, and Project Sideline. The project included baseline symptom scores for over 16,000 high school and college athletes and over 600 postconcussion symptom scores. For postinjury assessments, five data points were common to all studies: immediately postinjury, postgame, day 1, day 3, and day 5. Although the symptoms assessed varied slightly between studies, all were rated on a 7-point Guttman scale.

In developing the scale, the authors first eliminated items that were considered insensitive to concussion in the acute phase of the injury. To be retained, an item needed an effect size of at least 0.3 on at least two of the five postinjury assessments. This analysis resulted in the elimination of 13 items. Three other items were also eliminated: sensitivity to noise and sensitivity to light, as these were combined in the NCAA data set, and neck pain that was considered attributable to cervical strain and not directly related to concussion. This left a total of 12 symptoms. Receiver-operating characteristic (ROC) analyses were then conducted to ensure that scale sensitivity was not diminished by the loss of items. ROC curves on day 1 for both the CSI and the original 27-item version were nearly identical, suggesting that both were equally effective in detecting concussion symptoms. The authors present minimum, maximum, and mean scores on the scale across the assessment points, with scores significantly elevated immediately postinjury through day 3 and returning to baseline levels by day 5.

Summary

This is the only postconcussion symptom scale with an empirical basis for item selection, and its strengths include the use of stringent psychometric techniques in its development and its derivation from data from an impressively large number of concussed and nonconcussed athletes. The authors also demonstrate its sensitivity to postconcussion symptoms and short-term serial use, although no RCI metrics are reported. Only one article has been published thus far on the CSI, focusing on its scale development. Future research is needed to explore its reliability and validity. Because the CSI was developed on a sample of high school and college athletes, developmental factors may not have been taken into consideration in its creation. A parent-report version is not available. The exact number of participants at specific ages is difficult to determine, but in reviewing the sample description, at least a quarter of the baseline data was obtained from college football players through the NCAA Concussion Study. As such, validation of the CSI is recommended specifically with younger adolescent athletes and other nonconcussed pediatric patient groups. Females appear to be underrepresented in the sample, necessitating exploration of the scale's validity with female athletes.

Rivermead Post Concussion Symptoms Questionnaire

Description

The Rivermead Post Concussion Symptoms Questionnaire (RPCSQ; King, Crawford, Wenden, Moss, & Wade, 1995; Wrightson & Gronwall, 1999) is a 16-item self-report measure first used with adults. Items on the RPCSQ were generated by reviewing commonly reported postconcussive symptoms in the literature (King et al., 1995). Symptoms are rated as compared to "usual levels" to account for presence of preinjury symptoms. The severity of symptoms are rated on a 5-point Guttman scale, ranging from 0 (absence of symptom) to 4 (a severe problem). A total score is calculated, as well as three subscales: cognitive, emotional, and somatic (Gagnon, Swaine, Friedman, & Forget, 2005; Wilde et al., 2008).

Use with Children and Adolescents

The RPCSQ has been used with children ages 8–18 (Gagnon et al., 2005; Iverson & Goetz, 2004; Wilde et al., 2008).

Psychometric Evidence

Iverson and Goetz (2004) report on the reliability of the RPCSQ in a sample of 15- to 20-year-old hockey players. They indicate high internal consistency reliability (Cronbach alpha = 0.89) and split-half reliability ($r = .88$). Test–retest reliability over a 1-year interval was, however, low (Pearson $r = .24$; Spearman $r = .23$).

Two studies report evidence for the validity of the RPCSQ. Gagnon and colleagues (2005) used the RPSCQ in a study evaluating children's self-efficacy in relation to their practice of physical activities before and after concussion. Differences on the RPCSQ were found between children who had sustained a concussion and matched controls at 1, 4, and 12 weeks postinjury. Through serial use of the RPCSQ, the authors found a decrease in symptoms across the three visits, suggesting sensitivity to recovery of symptoms. However, reliable change metrics were not calculated.

Wilde et al. (2008) used the RPCSQ to examine the relationship between concussion symptoms and neuroimaging techniques, specifically diffusion tensor imaging tractography. As with Gagnon's study, the RPCSQ discriminated between groups of concussed and nonconcussed children, with higher postconcussion symptom scores reported by the concussed group for the total symptom raw score (Cohen's d = 1.57), as well as the three symptom subscales (Cohen's d for Cognitive = 1.35; Affective = 1.12; Somatic = 1.58).

Summary

Although the RPCSQ has been used with children as young as age 8, it has some limitations in its broader application to child and adolescent populations. The measure was not developed specifically for children, and no parent-report version is available. Iverson and Goetz (2004) report appropriate internal consistency and split-half reliability, but the low test–retest reliability suggests limitations regarding its stability over time. Although the Gagnon et al. (2005) and Wilde (2008) studies include boys and girls in their samples, no gender differences in symptom reports were explored. Furthermore, the sample size for the Wilde (2008) study was quite small, consisting of only 10 children with mild traumatic brain injury (mTBI) and 10 controls, rendering these group findings preliminary evidence of validity at best. Although studies provide evidence of criterion validity through group differences, no other validity studies have been conducted. The authors suggest using three subscales in interpreting scores; however, factor analysis has not been provided to support these domains. No reliable change metrics have been calculated.

Acute Concussion Evaluation

Description

The Acute Concussion Evaluation (ACE; Gioia, Collins, & Isquith, 2008a) is a clinical interview administered to the child's caretaker as part of a clinical examination or over the phone as a triage measure. The ACE was developed with two primary goals: (1) to create an evidence-based protocol for use in assessing mTBI in the medical setting, and (2) to link assessment information with direct postinjury recommendations for families. To this end, the mTBI literature was reviewed to determine what information is considered important when diagnosing mTBI. The ACE protocol is organized into three subsections: (1) information regarding injury characteristics, including details of the blow to the head (e.g., direct vs. indirect, location), presence of retrograde and anterograde amnesia and/or loss of consciousness; (2) ratings of 22 postconcussion symptoms on a binary yes (symptom present)–no (symptom not present) scale, endorsement of whether symptoms change with physical and cognitive activity, and a general rating of how "different" the child is from his or her usual self; and (3) identification of risk factors that may prolong recovery, including premorbid history of headaches, learning disabilities, and/or attention-deficit/hyperactivity disorder. The ACE also includes "red flags" for neurological deterioration that requires acute management, including seizures, focal neurological signs, and/or slurred speech. Guidance and recommendations for management are provided via the ACE Care Plan, which gives suggestions for the child at home and school, as well as guidelines for return to sports (Gioia & Collins, 2006). The ACE and ACE Care Plan are part of the Centers for Disease Control and Prevention (CDC) "Heads Up to Clinicians: Brain Injury in Your Practice" toolkit (CDC, 2007).

Use with Children and Adolescents

In the study conducted by Gioia and colleagues (2008a), the ACE was completed via telephone with 354 parents of children ages 3–18 years (M = 13.4 years; SD = 3.3 years) who had sustained concussion.

Psychometric Evidence

Examination of the item-scale membership of the ACE by calculation of item–total correlations indicates moderate correlations of most of the scale's symptoms with the total score. The symptoms most highly correlated were fatigue (.50), feeling slowed down (.49), and feeling more emotional (.52). Those with the least correlation were vomiting (.13), sleeping less often than usual (.16), and numbness/tingling (.19); the authors point out that these are also the least endorsed items. The ACE also demonstrated high internal consistency, with an alpha coefficient of .82. Interrater reliability was explored by comparing overall scores for four raters who completed 35 or more ACE ratings with parents. No differences between the raters were apparent after controlling for injury characteristics and demographics. The ACE symptom checklist and parent-report Post-Concussion Symptom Inventory (PCSI) scores were also found to correlate significantly (Gioia et al., 2008a).

With respect to evidence for the validity of the ACE, several lines are presented. The ACE total symptom score significantly predicted parent- and self-ratings on the PCSI administered 1 week later in the clinic (r = .68; r = .59, respectively), but was less related to preconcussion baseline ratings. There were also strong relationships between the frequency of symptoms reported on the ACE and the frequency of symptoms reported in other comparison samples of concussed athletes. Factor analysis provided evidence of construct validity, revealing a four-factor model (Somatic, Emotional, Cognitive, and Sleep), generally consistent with factors identified in the concussion literature (Gioia et al., 2008a).

Summary

The ACE is a unique measure, in that it was developed to provide a systematic, evidence-based protocol for use by clinicians in diagnosing mTBI in the clinic setting.

Furthermore, the ACE is the only symptom assessment measure linked to management suggestions through the ACE Care Plan. The ACE is also a relatively quick way to assess symptoms, as the authors report a mean administration time of 5.5 minutes (*SD* = 2.1). However, because it was developed to be administered by a clinician, it requires the time of a clinician to do so and, as such, is less easily administered than a self-completed questionnaire.

The ACE was specifically developed to be used with parents as reporters of their child's symptom presentation, and developmental factors were thus taken into consideration. Questions focus on issues relevant to children and adolescents. For example, an assessment of "risk factors" specific to the pediatric population is included. Given its developmental nature, the ACE can be used with parents of children as young as 3 years of age. Unlike other measures, the ACE includes questions assessing key clinical information beyond symptoms, including injury characteristics and risk factors for recovery, which may help the clinician with interpretation and understanding expectations for recovery. Although no self-report version is available, the ACE showed a strong relationship with self-report versions of the PCSI; Gioia et al., 2008a, 2009).

Another strength of the ACE is its psychometric properties; it has adequate internal consistency and interrater reliability. Validity of the ACE has been established through the examination of its factor structure, and it has demonstrated sensitivity to postconcussion symptoms through its significant relationship to other postconcussion measures. The ACE has not yet been studied serially, and therefore no reliable change metrics are reported. The ACE was explored in an adequate sample size, with a majority of male participants (65%); male–female gender differences have not been examined.

Health and Behavior Inventory

Description

The Health and Behavior Inventory (HBI) was originally developed for use with children who have moderate to severe TBI (Barry, Taylor, Klein, & Yeates, 1996). Items on the HBI were selected based on previous research of symptoms following moderate to severe TBI, as well as review of similar symptom questionnaires (Yeates et al., 1999). Item content overlapped with other concussion rating scales, resulting in a 62-item version of the HBI used by Yeates and colleagues (1999) in a study of postconcussive symptoms in children with and without mTBI.

The current version of the HBI consists of 20 items assessing cognitive and somatic symptoms. The frequency of the symptom over the past week is rated on a 4-point scale, from "never" to "often." Parent and child versions include the same symptoms, although the items of the child version are worded in the first person to be developmentally appropriate. For example, for the parent item, "has difficulty showing emotions," the child item is "I have problems showing how I feel" (Ayr, Yeates, Taylor, & Brown, 2009). In addition to a total score, factor analysis has supported the use of scales for somatic, cognitive, and emotional symptoms for the parent version, and somatic and cognitive symptoms for the child version (Ayr et al., 2009).

Use with Children and Adolescents

The HBI has been used with children ages 8–15 and their parents (Ayr et al., 2009; Ganesalingam et al., 2008; Taylor et al., 2010; Yeates et al., 1999).

Psychometric Evidence

Factor analysis of the parent version yielded three consistent scales (i.e., Somatic, Cognitive, and Emotional), with internal reliabilities (IRs) ranging from .89 to .95. Although a fourth behavioral factor was identified on baseline, it did not emerge from analyses of the 3-month assessment. Analysis of the child ratings yielded two consistent factors, Somatic (IR = .86) and Cognitive (IR = .89). The symptoms loading on the Somatic and Cognitive factors were very similar for the parent and child versions. However, despite similarities between scale items, only moderate correlations between parent and child report were seen for the Cognitive (r = .27) and Somatic (r = .39) domains. For 3-month postinjury ratings, only a moderate correlation remained for the Cognitive scale (r = .31; Ayr et al., 2009).

Studies have shown the HBI to be sensitive to differences between children with mTBI and those with other injuries (Taylor et al., 2010; Yeates et al., 1999), as well as to recovery over time. Taylor and colleagues assessed symptoms with the HBI across several time points (baseline, 1-month, 3-month, and 12-month postinjury assessment). Although group differences between parent-reported somatic symptoms were initially apparent, symptoms resolved by the 12-month assessment, with no group differences at that point. However, for cognitive symptoms, group differences were greatest at the 3-month assessment and remained throughout the follow-up period. Regarding self-report ratings, group differences were not seen for cognitive symptoms, but children with mTBI reported more somatic symptoms than orthopedic injury controls initially, with no differences seen by the 3-month assessment. Reliable change methodology has been applied to the HBI, with children with mTBI being more likely to demonstrate reliable increases in somatic and cognitive symptom scores, with cognitive symptoms persisting to 12 months in some children (Yeates et al., in press). Recently, Moran et al. (2011) examined the sensitivity and specificity of the parent-report HBI in classifying group membership (mTBI vs. orthopedic injury) and severity (mTBI with/without loss of consciousness [LOC]). Classification rates were higher for group membership (75%/71.6% sensitivity, 82.5%/68.2% specificity at 11 days/3 months) than for severity (mTBI with LOC, sensitivity 43.1%/35.6%; mTBI without LOC, 51.9%/61.3%).

Relationships between the HBI and other outcome measures have been studied. High parent ratings of cognitive and somatic symptoms have been associated with more perceived family burden and parental distress (Ganesalingam et al., 2008). The relationship between injury characteristics and postconcussive symptoms on the HBI has also been demonstrated, with LOC associated with significantly higher ratings of cognitive symptoms on the parent scale. Marginal relationships were also found between hospitalization and elevated ratings of cognitive symptoms, whereas motor-vehicle-related trauma was associated with parent-rated emotional symptoms (Taylor et al., 2010).

Hajek et al. (2011) considered item-level correlation between parent and child versions of the HBI in both mTBI and orthopedic injury groups. In both groups, correlations were generally significant but moderate. In the mTBI group, general agreement between parent and child report was seen for cognitive symptoms, but children endorsed higher levels of somatic symptoms at all four assessment intervals.

Summary

The HBI has the advantage of including both parent- and child-report versions for use with children as young as 8 years old. The authors were sensitive to age in the scale's development, and items are worded to be understandable for children. Studies exploring the HBI have adequate sample sizes, with generally equivalent percentages of boys and girls; however, gender differences have not been explored. The HBI exhibits good internal consistency and reliability. Several studies have demonstrated the scale's validity, including its underlying factor structure, relationship to other variables, and sensitivity to group differences. Classification rates have also been examined. Serial assessment shows decreasing scores over time, suggesting sensitivity to recovery. Reliable change metrics have been applied to the HBI. Given the psychometric strength of the HBI and its demonstrated utility with pediatric mTBI, it is listed as a core measure in the NINDS Common Data Elements for pediatric TBI outcomes (McCauley et al., 2011).

Post-Concussion Symptom Interview

Description

The Post-Concussion Symptom Interview (PCS-Interview; Mittenberg, Wittner, & Miller, 1997) asks parents and children to indicate the presence or absence of 15 symptoms over the preceding week. Items include cognitive, somatic, and emotional symptoms and were chosen for their similarities to those listed for post-concussion syndrome in the International Classification of Diseases (ICD-10; World Health Organization, 1992) and research criteria for post-concussional disorder in the *Diagnostic and Statistical Manual of Mental Disorders* (DSM-IV; American Psychiatric Association, 1994).

Use with Children and Adolescents

Recent studies have used the PCS-Interview with children ages 8–15 years (Ganesalingam et al., 2008; Hajek et al., 2011; Taylor et al., 2010; Yeates et al., 2009). Mittenberg et al.'s (1997) original study used the measure with children as young as age 5.

Psychometric Evidence

Ganesalingam et al. (2008) completed PCS-Interviews with 181 children with mTBI and 97 children with orthopedic injuries and their parents. The parent PCS-Interview exhibited adequate interitem reliability, with .71 for the total sample, .60 for the concussion group, and .82 for the orthopedic group. The child interview exhibited similar reliabilities, with .70 for the total sample, .71 for the concussion group, and .68 for the orthopedic group.

Differences between an orthopedic group and a group with diagnosed mTBI were found on both the parent and child versions of the PCS-Interview. Parents of children with mTBI reported more symptoms at baseline and 1-month follow-up, but not at 3 or 12 months. Children with mTBI reported more symptoms at all assessment intervals. On the parent-report version, the number of symptoms reported increased from baseline to 1 month, and from 1 month to 3 months, with a significant decrease from 3 months to 12 months. A somewhat different pattern was seen on the child-report version, with symptom counts increasing from baseline through the 3-month assessment, but then not changing significantly from 3 to 12 months.

Four different recovery trajectories for postconcussion symptoms were identified with the PCS-Interview: no symptoms, moderate persistent symptoms, high acute/resolved symptoms, and high acute/persistent symptoms (Yeates et al., 2009). Variables such as LOC, posttraumatic amnesia, Glasgow Coma Scale score < 15, disorientation, and other mental status changes were associated with higher levels of acute symptoms. Group differences were found, with children with mTBI more likely to be in the high acute/resolved and high/acute persistent groups than children with orthopedic injuries.

The PCS-Interview has shown a positive relationship with other variables as well. In the Ganesalingam et al. (2008) study, higher symptom reports on both parent and child PCS-Interviews were associated with greater perceived family burden and parental distress.

Low to moderate agreement was seen between overall parent and child ratings across serial assessment (Total Sample r = .31–.38; Hajek et al., 2011; Taylor et al., 2010). At an item level, correlations between parent and child report were significant but modest (Hajek et al., 2011). Children endorsed more symptoms than their parents, with the difference becoming larger over time (Hajek et al., 2011).

The PCS-Interview has shown good correlation with the HBI, a well-validated measure previously described. The total number of symptoms endorsed on the parent PCS-Interview was moderately correlated with parent ratings of somatic (r = .42), cognitive (r = .55), and emotional (r = .56) symptoms on the HBI. Correlations were even stronger between the child PCS-Interview and the child HBI (r = .66–.71; Taylor et al., 2010).

Summary

The PCS-Interview is a theoretically based measure specifically developed for use with the pediatric population, with both parent- and self-report versions. Unlike other measures that rate symptoms on a more differentiated Guttman scale, the PCS-Interview provides, in essence, a symptom count and may be a quick way to obtain information regarding the basic presence or absence of symptoms. Although its interview format may have benefits, one disadvantage is that it is less easily administered than a self-completed questionnaire.

Although one study of the PCS-Interview used this measure down to age 5, more recent studies have demonstrated its utility in children age 8 years and older. Studies using the PCS-Interview have adequate sample sizes and generally equal numbers of boys and girls, although differences between gender symptom presentations have not been explored. Reasonable evidence of the scale's internal consistency, reliability, and validity has been presented. The PCS-Interview is sensitive to concussion, with decreases in symptoms seen over time and a demonstrated relationship to injury-related variables. Despite its serial use, RCI has not been explored.

Post-Concussion Symptom Inventory

Description

The PCSI (Gioia, Janusz, Isquith, & Vincent, 2008b; Gioia et al., 2009) is a set of scales for parent-, teacher-, and self-report of symptoms. Self-report forms were designed to be developmentally appropriate in terms of item content, wording, and response format. As such, three self-report versions are available for different age groups: 5–7 years (13 items, 3-point Guttman scale), 8–12 years (17 items, 3-point Guttman scale), and 13–18 years (20 items, 7-point Guttman scale). The parent and teacher versions consist of 20 items rated on a 7-point Guttman scale. Physical, cognitive, emotional, and fatigue symptoms are rated.

Use with Children and Adolescents

Studies have used parent-, teacher-, and self-report versions with children ages 5–18 years (Diver, Gioia, & Anderson, 2007; Gioia et al., 2008b; Schneider & Gioia, 2007; Vaughan, Gioia, & Vincent, 2008).

Psychometric Evidence

Several types of reliability of the PCSI have been examined. All three versions demonstrate strong internal consistency with varying samples:

- Parent 5–12 normative sample (n = 705), alpha = .81; concussion sample (n = 268), alpha = .95
- Parent 13–18 normative sample (n = 311), alpha = .75; concussion sample (n = 201), alpha = .95
- Child ages 5–7 normative sample (n = 103), alpha = .82; concussion sample (n = 47), alpha = .83
- Child ages 8–12 normative sample (n = 407), alpha = .91; concussion sample (n = 206), alpha = .91
- Child ages 13–18 normative sample (n = 318), alpha = .91; concussion sample (n = 198), alpha = .94 (Gioia, Vaughan, & Isquith, 2011).

Test–retest reliability of the PCSI is also good for the child measures (ages 5–7 r = .79; ages 8–12 r = .89; Gioia et al., 2011) but was not available for the 13- to 18-year-old scale. Interrater reliability was examined via correlations between parent and child ratings. The relationships are consistently higher in clinical samples than normative, likely due to the range restriction in the latter:

- Child ages 5–7 normative sample (n = 148), r = .14; concussion sample (n = 34), r = .36
- Child ages 8–12 normative sample (n = 543), r = .15; concussion sample (n = 169), r = .55
- Child ages 13–18 normative sample (n = 313), r = .13; concussion sample (n = 217), r = .65 (Gioia et al., 2011).

The scale structure of the PCSI is supported by factor analysis conducted via a combined confirmatory–exploratory factor analysis method for the three age groups (Gioia et al., 2011). The resulting factor solutions were then submitted to confirmatory analysis on PCSI data from samples of uninjured control children. Exploratory and confirmatory factor analyses of the PCSI supported a three-factor model (Physical, Cognitive, and Emotional) with 13 items for 5- to 7-year-olds, four factors (Physical, Cognitive, Emotional, Fatigue) with 17 items for 8- to 12-year-olds, and four factors using 20 items for the 13- to 18-year-old adolescents and for the parent PCSI for the 5- to 18-year age range. The PCSI structure is generally consistent with factors from other concussion symptom scales described in the literature.

Studies of children, adolescent, and parent normative samples find low symptom base rates across the versions of the PCSI (Gioia et al., 2008b; Schneider & Gioia, 2007). The PCSI has been shown to differentiate children with concussion from noninjured controls. Additional longitudinal analyses of symptom manifestation using growth curve modeling in 5- to 12-year-olds with concussion demonstrated significant improvement in symptom ratings over the recovery period (Gioia et al., 2011). Group membership was predicted using discriminant function analysis. To establish the relative predictive utility of the parent versus child reports of the PCSI, discriminant function analyses were conducted and found that parent reports are most predictive in children ages 5–7. When used in combination with neurocognitive measures of response speed, self-rated symptoms were most predictive of concussion group membership, particularly in 8- to 12-year-olds (Gioia et al., 2011); predictive validity needs to be explored in adolescents. Reliable change metrics have been developed for the various forms of the PCSI. Symptom validity has also been examined, with cutoff scores provided for unusual symptom reports both for noninjured baseline reports and for postinjury symptom reports.

Gender differences have been explored with the PCSI (Gioia et al., 2011; Schneider & Gioia, 2007). No differences were found in the noninjured control sample. In children with concussion, the youngest age group exhibited few differences between boys and girls for their symptom reports. Differences, however, were found in the 8- to 12-year and 13- to 18-year groups, with girls endorsing more symptoms than boys.

Summary

The PCSI is a relatively new symptom assessment measure. Three different self-report versions of the PCSI are available, based on the child's age, with differences in wording and response format. A parent-report version has also been developed. The initial studies have appropriate sample sizes and include children as young as 5 years. Appropriate reliability is demonstrated for each of the scales, which were developed based on factor analyses. Gender differences have been explored, although only for the self-report version for ages 5–12. Prospective, longitudinal studies have shown evidence for the measure's sensitivity to injury. Reliable change metrics have been developed to assist with serial assessments. The utility of the PCSI has yet to be used in independent studies to further establish its validity. Given the emerging psychometric strength of the PCSI with pediatric mTBI, it is listed as a supplementary measure in the NINDS Common Data Elements for pediatric TBI outcomes (McCauley et al., 2011).

Post-Concussion Scale

Description

The Post-Concussion Scale (PCS; Lovell & Collins, 1998) is a 22-item self-report measure. Symptom items were chosen based on the authors' experience with both professional and amateur athletes, with items worded to reflect the language of the players rather than medical terminology. Symptoms are rated on a 7-point Guttman severity scale, from 0, "no symptom," to 6, "severe symptom." The scale was developed to be used along with neuropsychological testing, and it is administered as part of the Immediate Post-Concussion Assessment and Cognitive Testing (ImPACT) computerized assessment, although a paper version is also available (Lovell et al., 2006).

Use with Children and Adolescents

The majority of pediatric studies have used the PCS with high school athletes (Collins et al., 2003; Field, Collins, Lovell, & Maroon, 2003; Iverson, Lovell, & Collins, 2003; Lau, Collins, & Lovell, 2011; Lovell et al., 2006; McClincy, Lovell, Pardini, Collins, & Spore, 2006; Schatz, Pardini, Lovell, Collins, & Podell, 2006; Van Kampen, Lovell, Pardini, Collins, & Fu, 2006), although one study used the PCS with a sample of children down to 11 years of age (Blinman, Houseknecht, Snyder, Wiebe, & Nance, 2009).

Psychometric Evidence

The PCS has been shown to have high internal consistency in both normal samples (Cronbach alpha = .89–.94) and concussed samples (alpha = .92–.93; Lovell et al., 2006), as well as marginal test–retest reliability (r = .65; Iverson & Goetz, 2004). Construct validity of the PCS has been examined, with a four-factor structure reported (Pardini et al., 2004), identifying Somatic, Cognitive, Emotional, and Sleep dimensions. Several studies have demonstrated differences between concussed and nonconcussed samples, with the concussed group reporting more symptoms (Field et al., 2003; Iverson et al., 2003; Lovell et al., 2006; Schatz et al., 2006; Van Kampen et al., 2006). Following concussion, an increase in symptom report is seen from baseline to first postinjury assessment (within 24–72 hours), with gradual decline in symptom report over time and return to baseline levels typically by 7–14 days postinjury (Field et al., 2003; Lovell et al., 2006; McClincy et al., 2006). A similar pattern of recovery was demonstrated by Blinman et al. (2009) in their sample of younger children, with marked improvement seen for most subjects 2–3 weeks after injury. Collins and colleagues (2003) classified subjects as having good postinjury presentation or poor postinjury presentation and found that symptom scores resulted in similar classification as ImPACT neurocognitive testing. McClincy (2006) also found similar recovery patterns on both neurocognitive testing and symptom report.

In assessing change over time, several studies applied RCI metrics. Van Kampen and colleagues (2006) found that 64% of the concussed sample at day 2 postinjury demonstrated an increase in symptom scores that exceeded reliable change expectations, compared to only 9% of the control sample. Iverson et al. (2003) provide reliable change estimates for the PCS, with a decline or improvement of 10 points considered significant.

Schatz et al. (2006) explored the sensitivity and specificity of the PCS. When used in conjunction with ImPACT scores, sensitivity was 81.9% and specificity was 89.4%. Using the PCS score, Processing Speed Composite, Visual Memory Composite, and Impulse Control Composite, in combination, correctly classified 85.5% of the cases as concussed or nonconcussed. More recently, Lau et al. (2011) found increased sensitivity and specificity when using the PCS in conjunction with neurocognitive testing. When used alone, the PCS had a sensitivity of 40.8% and specificity of 79.3% in predicting recovery, defined as taking greater than 14 days to recover. When combined with ImPACT variables, sensitivity increased to 65.2%, whereas specificity remained essentially unchanged.

Many PCS studies combine both high school and college athletes. When these groups are considered independently, the results reflect possible differences in reported recovery rates. Whereas Lovell and colleagues (2006) did not see a difference in symptom reporting between high school and college athletes, Field et al. (2003) found that high school athletes reported more symptoms than controls up to 7 days postinjury while no differences were seen between college athletes and controls by 3 days after injury.

For most studies using high school and college samples, the participants are predominantly male. Only one study (Lovell et al., 2006) considered males and females separately, and differences were seen, with high school women reporting more symptoms than men; as such, normative data are presented by gender. In their study of younger children, Blinman et al. (2009) found that girls had higher mean symptom scores at initial testing, but not at follow-up.

Summary

The PCS is a theoretically derived scale. Like many of the other symptom assessment measures, it was developed for use with adults and has primarily been used with high school and college athletes, with only one study reporting use in children down to age 11. No parent-report version is available. For studies that compared high school and college athletes, differences were found possibly on developmental grounds. Therefore, more research is needed to fully understand its use in the younger high school population. Gender differences have been explored, resulting in different norms for males and females. Available literature reports appropriate reliability (internal consistency; test–retest reliability) and several lines of evidence for its validity (factor structure, sensitivity to injury and recovery, relationship to other measures, classification based on injury presentation). Unlike other measures, RCI metrics have been calculated with suggestions provided for consideration of significant score change.

METHODOLOGICAL AND CONCEPTUAL ISSUES

Several key issues are highlighted by this review. First, the developmental appropriateness of the symptom assessment instruments is an essential aspect of a child measure (Gioia et al., 2009). Only four measures (HBI, PCS-Interview, PCSI, and ACE) were developed for specific use with children and their parents. With the exception of the ACE, each of these four measures has both parent-report and child-report versions. Two of the child-report measures, the HBI and the PCSI, made developmentally appropriate changes to item wording and response format for younger age groups. Additional research with younger populations is needed with the other child-report measures not specifically developed for children to determine their appropriateness. Furthermore, they are limited by their lack of associated parent versions.

Obtaining parent-report measures in addition to child-report ones has also shown value in the assessment of children's status. Correlations are generally low to moderate between parent and child raters, despite similar items on the scales (Gioia et al., 2009; Hajek et al., 2011). At least one study suggested differences between parent and child reports of cognitive versus somatic symptoms (Hajek et al., 2011). The PCSI parent-report measure also demonstrated a stronger relationship to the younger child's injury status than the child's symptom report (Gioia et al., 2011). These findings suggest that parents and children have different perspectives in assessing postconcussion symptoms. Certain symptoms may be less easily observed and rated by parents, whereas others may be less defined for the child to reliably identify. As such, both parent and child ratings are needed to completely assess symptoms, and one cannot be substituted for the other (Hajek et al., 2011).

Another methodological issue revealed by this review is the limited age range that has been studied to date, and the lack of attention to the possible age-related differences in symptom manifestation. Most of the published studies examined combined high school and college samples. Yet Field and colleagues (2003) found modest differences between high school and college athletes in their symptom recovery, suggesting that there may indeed be clinical differences between these two age groups. Combining these large age spans in studies can limit the ability to generalize their findings, and future research will need to explore the reliability and validity of measures in each group independently.

A related issue is the predominance of males in the study samples, particularly at the high school level. Although this may not be entirely unexpected given the higher overall incidence of concussion among males, it is clinically important to understand the nature of concussion symptoms and their recovery in females specifically. Several studies have found differences between high school females and males, with females reporting more symptoms (Lovell et al., 2006; Schneider & Gioia, 2007). Increased postinjury symptom report has also been noted among female college athletes (Broshek et al., 2005; Frommer et al., 2011). Normative data are presented separately by gender for the PCS for this reason (Lovell et al., 2006). Differences between males' and females' symptom reports were found in younger children, ages 5–12 years, with the PCSI (Gioia et al., 2011). Further exploration of gender differences among younger age groups is warranted.

A consideration not yet explored in the pediatric literature is the impact of the assessment instrument's format on symptom report. In research with adult samples, differences have been found between symptom rating methods and open-ended interviews. Villemure, Nolin, and LeSage (2011) found that participants reported more symptoms when they completed a checklist than when they were asked to freely identify their symptoms. Participants also reported slightly different symptoms with each method. Similar findings were seen in a study conducted by Iverson, Brooks, Ashton, and Lange (2010), in that more symptoms were endorsed on a paper-and-pencil symptom rating scale than during an open-ended interview. Furthermore, the symptoms that were endorsed on the rating scale were of a greater severity than that reported during the interview. Although the two measures reviewed, the ACE and the PCS-Interview, are completed in an interview format, neither is an open-ended interview. Rather, both ask about the presence of specific symptoms. Because these findings suggest that adults may either overreport symptoms on questionnaire measures or underreport on interviews, comparisons between checklist and interview methods should be explored in the pediatric population as well.

SUMMARY AND FUTURE DIRECTIONS

This review finds adequate though variable psychometric support for eight post-concussion symptom assessment measures. As summarized in Table 12.2, seven of eight measures report some type of reliability examination, with six providing multiple lines of evidence. Seven measures report internal consistency reliabilities (GSC, RPCSQ, ACE, HBI, PCS-Interview, PCSI, PCS), four report test–retest reliabilities (GSC, RPCSQ, PCSI, PCS), and three provide interrater reliability (ACE, HBI, PCSI). Three of the measures have translated their stability coefficients into reliable change metrics (HBI, PCSI, PCS). With respect to the seven types of validity described above, all eight measures provide at least four lines of evidence. All provide adequate evidence of general content validity, in that the instruments include commonly accepted symptoms, although only one of the measures used empirically derived item selection and scaling (CSI). Only four instruments provide some indication of developmentally oriented content (ACE, HBI, PCS-Interview, PCSI), and none examined the developmental sensitivity of scores. Seven studies explored the convergence of the symptoms with other measures (all but the CSI). Factor structure is reported for four measures (HBI, ACE, PCSI, and PCS). Because postconcussion symptoms are not considered a unitary construct, but rather composed of symptom clusters, clarifying the factor structure of measures is important (Gioia et al., 2009). All symptom scales provide evidence of their ability to discriminate between concussed and nonconcussed groups. Six of the measures report serial use and sensitivity to change across recovery (CSI, RPCSQ, HBI, PCS-Interview, PCSI, PCS). Given that a primary purpose for the use of these measures is to monitor symptom change over time, fully understanding scales' abilities to detect such change reliably is important for their clinical use. Sensitivity and specificity analyses were provided for four of the measures (CSI, HBI, PCSI, and PCS).

TABLE 12.2. Psychometric Evidence Summary of Symptom Assessment Measures

Measure	Reliability	Validity	Reliable change	Total no. of psychometric indicators
GSC/GSS	1, 2	1, 3, 4, 5		6
CSI	—	1, 5, 6, 7		4
RPCSQ	1, 2	1, 3, 5, 6		6
ACE	2, 3	1, 3, 5, 6		6
HBI: Child	1, 3	1, 3, 4, 5, 6, 7		8
HBI: Parent	1, 3	1, 3, 4, 5, 6, 7		8
PCS-Interview	2	1, 3, 4, 5, 6		6
PCSI: Child 5–7	1, 2, 3	1, 3, 4, 5, 6, 7	Yes	9
PCSI: Child 8–12	1, 2, 3	1, 3, 4, 5, 6, 7	Yes	9
PCSI: Adolescent	1, 2, 3	1, 3, 4, 5, 6, 7	Yes	9
PCSI: Parent	1, 3	1, 3, 4, 5, 6, 7		8
PCS	1, 2	1, 3, 4, 5, 6, 7	Yes	8

Note. Measures: GSC/GSS, Graded Symptom Checklist/Scale; CSI, Concussion Symptom Inventory; RPCSQ, Rivermead Post-Concussion Symptoms Questionnaire; ACE, Acute Concussion Evaluation; HBI, Health and Behavior Inventory; PCS-Interview, Post-Concussion Symptom Interview; PCSI, Post-Concussion Symptom Inventory; PCS, Post-Concussion Scale. *Reliability:* 1 = internal consistency, 2 = test–retest, 3 = interrater. *Validity:* 1 = content, 2 = developmental adaptation, 3 = relationship to other measures, 4 = internal structure, 5 = group discrimination, 6 = sensitivity to recovery, 7 = sensitivity/specificity for group membership.

The development and use of postconcussion symptom measures with children and adolescents has gained increasing attention over the past 10 years. An adequate body of evidence of reliability and validity is growing, although more research needs to be conducted. The progression of instrument development has proceeded from young adult to adolescent, with a small literature now available for children as young as 5 years. Despite the development of measures specific to pediatric populations, the focus has been largely on school-age children, age 8 and older, and adolescents, with only three measures used with children age 7 and younger. As such, exploring ways of assessing postconcussion symptoms in the preschool population will be important for future research.

Furthermore, many of the studies reviewed use student athletes in their samples. Given the wide-reaching nature of concussion, exploration of symptoms and their assessment in the general population will be important as well. Although many studies use these measures for serial assessments, few document reliable change metrics. Given that these measures will primarily be used clinically to determine recovery over time, having an understanding of "clinically meaningful" change is essential, as is quantifying the risks associated with elevated scores. Many studies document validity, but more work is needed regarding the reliability of measures. Also, although studies document sensitivity of the scale to concussion, in that more symptoms are reported in concussed than nonconcussed samples, normative expectations have not been developed. Although current guidelines suggest comparing postinjury assessment to preinjury baseline levels, understanding the general incidence of "symptoms" in the noninjured population is also important for normative comparison. Despite the need for future investigation, current findings suggest that these measures can be used effectively in clinical settings.

REFERENCES

Achenbach, T. M., & Rescorla, L. A. (2001). *Manual for the ASEBA School-Age Forms and Profiles*. Burlington, VT: University of Vermont, Research Center for Children, Youth, and Families.

American Psychiatric Association. (1994). *Diagnostic and statistical manual of mental disorders* (4th ed.). Washington, DC: Author.

Ayr, L. K., Yeates, K. O., Taylor, H. G., & Brown, M. (2009). Dimensions of post-concussive symptoms in children with mild traumatic brain injuries. *Journal of the International Neuropsychological Society, 15*, 19–30.

Barry, C. T., Taylor, H. G., Klein, S., & Yeates, K. O. (1996). Validity of neurobehavioral symptoms reported in children with traumatic brain injury. *Child Neuropsychology, 2*, 213–226.

Blinman, T. A., Houseknecht, E., Snyder, C., Wiebe, D. J., & Nance, M. L. (2009). Postconcussive symptoms in hospitalized pediatric patients after mild traumatic brain injury. *Journal of Pediatric Surgery, 44*, 1223–1228.

Broglio, S. P., & Puetz, T. W. (2008). The effect of sport concussion on neurocognitive function, self-report symptoms, and postural control: A meta-analysis. *Sports Medicine, 38*, 53–67.

Broshek, D. K., Kaushik, T., Freeman, J. R., Erlanger, D., Webbe, F., & Barth, J. T. (2005). Sex differences in outcome following sports-related concussion. *Journal of Neurosurgery, 102*, 856–863.

Campbell, D. T., & Fiske, D. W. (1959). Convergent and discriminant validation by the multitrait–multimethod matrix. *Psychological Bulletin, 56*, 81–105.

Centers for Disease Control and Prevention. (2007). *Heads up: Brain injury in your practice*. Atlanta, GA: Centers for Disease Control. Retrieved May 1, 2011 from *www.cdc.gov/concussion/headsup/physicians_tool_kit.html*.

Collins, M. W., Iverson, G. L., Lovell, M. R., McKeag, D. B., Norwig, J., & Maroon, J. (2003). On-field predictors of neuropsychological and symptom deficit following sports-related concussion. *Clinical Journal of Sports Medicine, 13*, 222–229.

Diver, T., Gioia, G., & Anderson, S. (2007). Discordance of symptom report across clinical and control groups with respect to parent and child. *Journal of the International Neuropsychological Society, 13*(Suppl. 1), 63.

Eckner, J. T., & Kutcher, J. S. (2010). Concussion symptom scales and sideline assessment tools: A critical literature update. *Current Sports Medicine Report, 9*, 8–15.

Field, M., Collins, M. W., Lovell, M. R., & Maroon, J. (2003). Does age play a role in recovery from sports-related concussion?: A comparison of high school and collegiate athletes. *Journal of Pediatrics, 142*, 546–543.

Frommer, L. J., Gurka, K. K., Cross, K. M., Ingersoll, C. D., Comstock, R. D., & Saliba, S. A. (2011). Sex differences in concussion symptoms of high school athletes. *Journal of Athletic Training, 46*, 76–84.

Gagnon, I., Swaine, B., Friedman, D., & Forget, R. (2005). Exploring children's self-efficacy related to physical activity performance after mild traumatic brain injury. *Journal of Head Trauma Rehabilitation, 20*, 436–439.

Ganesalingam, K., Yeates, K. O., Ginn, M. S., Taylor, H. G., Dietrich, A., Nuss, K., et al. (2008). Family burden and parental distress following mild traumatic brain injury in children and its relationship to post-concussive symptoms. *Journal of Pediatric Psychology, 33,* 621–629.

Gioia, G. A., & Collins, M. (2006). *Acute concussion evaluation (ACE): Physician/clinician version.* Available at *www.cdc.gov/ncipc/tbi/PhysiciansTool_Kit.htm.*

Gioia, G. A., Collins, M., & Isquith, P. K. (2008a). Improving identification and diagnosis of mild traumatic brain injury with evidence: Psychometric support for the acute concussion evaluation. *Journal of Head Trauma Rehabilitation, 23,* 230–242.

Gioia, G. A., Isquith, P. K., Guy, S. C., & Kenworthy, L. (2000). *Manual for the Behavior Rating Inventory of Executive Function.* Lutz, FL: Psychological Assessment Resources.

Gioia, G. A., Janusz, J., Isquith, P., & Vincent, D. (2008b). Psychometric properties of the parent and teacher Post-Concussion Symptom Inventory (PCSI) for children and adolescents. *Journal of the International Neuropsychological Society, 14*(Suppl. 1), 204.

Gioia, G. A., Schneider, J. C., Vaughan, C. G., & Isquith, P. K. (2009). Which symptom assessments and approaches are uniquely appropriate for paediatric concussion? *British Journal of Sports Medicine, 43*(S1), i13–i22.

Gioia, G. A., Vaughan, C. G., & Isquith, P. K. (2011). *Manual for pediatric Immediate Post-Concussion Assessment and Cognitive Testing.* Pittsburgh, PA: ImPACT Applications.

Hajek, C. A., Yeates, K. O., Taylor, H. G., Bangert, B., Dietrich, A., Nuss, K. E., et al. (2011). Agreement between parents and children on ratings of post-concussive symptoms following mild traumatic brain injury. *Child Neuropsychology, 17,* 17–33.

Iverson, G. L., Brooks, B. L., Ashton, V. L., & Lange, R. T. (2010). Interview versus questionnaire symptom reporting in people with the postconcussion syndrome. *Journal of Head Trauma Rehabilitation, 25,* 23–30.

Iverson, G. L., & Goetz, M. (2004). Practical consideration for interpreting change following brain injury. In M. R. Lovell, R. J. Echemendia, J. T. Barth, & M. W. Collin (Eds.), *Traumatic brain injury in sports: An international neuropsychological perspective* (pp. 323–356). Exton, PA: Swets & Zeitlinger.

Iverson, G. L., Lovell, M. R., & Collins, M. W. (2003). Interpreting change on ImPACT following sport concussion. *The Clinical Neuropsychologist, 7,* 460–467.

King, N. S., Crawford, S., Wenden, F. J., Moss, N. E., & Wade, D. T. (1995). The Rivermead Post Concussion Symptoms Questionnaire: A measure of symptoms commonly experienced after head injury and its reliability. *Journal of Neurology, 242,* 587–592.

Kirkwood, M. W., Yeates, K. O., & Wilson, P. E. (2006). Pediatric sport-related concussion: A review of the clinical management of an oft-neglected population. *Pediatrics, 117,* 1359–1371.

Lau, B. C., Collins, M. W., & Lovell, M. R. (2011). Sensitivity and specificity of subacute computerized neurocognitive testing and symptom evaluation in predicting outcomes after sports-related concussion. *American Journal of Sports Medicine, 39,* 1209–1216.

Likert, R. (1932). A technique for the measurement of attitudes. *Archives of Psychology, 140*(52), 5–55.

Lovell, M. R., & Collins, M. W. (1998). Neuropsychological assessment of the college football player. *Journal of Head Trauma Rehabilitation, 13,* 9–26.

Lovell, M. R., Iverson, G. L., Collins, M. W., Podell, K., Johnston, K. M., Pardini, D., et al. (2006). Measurement of symptoms following sports-related concussion: Reliability and normative data for the Post-Concussion Scale. *Applied Neuropsychology, 13,* 166–174.

Mailer, B. J., Valovich-McLeod, T. C., & Bay, R. C. (2008). Healthy youth are reliable in reporting symptoms on a graded symptom scale. *Journal of Sports Rehabilitation, 17,* 11–20.

McCauley, S., Wilde, E., Anderson, V., Bedell, G., Beers, S., Campbell, T., et al. (2011) Recommendations for the use of common outcome measures in pediatric traumatic brain injury research. *Journal of Neurotrauma*. Advance online publication. doi: 10.1089/neu.2011.1838.

McClincy, M. P., Lovell, M. R., Pardini, J., Collins, M. W., & Spore, M. K. (2006). Recovery from sports concussion in high school and collegiate athletes. *Brain Injury, 20*, 33–39.

McCrory, P., Collie, A., Anderson, V., & Davis, G. (2004). Can we manage sport related concussion in children the same as in adults? *British Journal of Sports Medicine, 38,* 516–519.

McCrory, P., Johnston, K., Meeuwise, W., Aubry, M., Cantu, R., Dvorak, J., et al. (2005). Summary and agreement statement of the second International Conference on Concussion in Sport. *British Journal of Sports Medicine, 39*, 196–204.

Mittenberg, W., Wittner, M. S., & Miller, L. J. (1997). Postconcussion syndrome occurs in children. *Neuropsychology, 11*, 447–452.

Moran, L. M., Taylor, G., Rusin, J., Bangert, B., Dietrich, A., Nuss, K. E., et al. (2011). Do postconcussive symptoms discriminate injury severity in pediatric mild traumatic brain injury? *Journal of Head Trauma Rehabilitation, 26*, 348–354.

Pardini, D., Stump, J., Lovell, M., Collins, M., Moritz, K., & Fu, F. (2004). The Post-Concussion Symptom Scale (PCSS): A factor analysis. *British Journal of Sports Medicine, 38*, 661–662.

Piland, S. G., Motl, R. W., Ferrara, M. S., & Peterson, C. L. (2003). Evidence for the factorial and construct validity of a self-report concussion symptoms scale. *Journal of Athletic Training, 38*, 104–112.

Piland, S. G., Motl, R. W., Guskiewicz, K. M., McCrea, M., & Ferrara, M. S. (2006). Structural validity of a self-report concussion-related symptom scale. *Medicine and Science in Sports and Exercise, 38*, 27–32.

Randolph, C., Millis, S., Barr, W. B., McCrea, M., Guskiewicz, K. M., Hammeke, T. A., et al. (2009). Concussion Symptom Inventory: An empirically derived scale for monitoring resolution of symptoms following sports-related concussion. *Archives of Clinical Neuropsychology, 24*, 219–229.

Register-Mihalik, J., Guskiewicz, K. M., Mann, J. D., & Shields, E. W. (2007). The effects of headache on clinical measures of neurocognitive function. *Clinical Journal of Sports Medicine, 17*, 282–288.

Schatz, P., Pardini, J. E., Lovell, M. R., Collins, M. W., & Podell, K. (2006). Sensitivity and specificity of the ImPACT test battery for concussion in athletes. *Archives of Clinical Neuropsychology, 21*, 91–99.

Schneider, J., & Gioia, G. (2007). Psychometric properties of the Post-Concussion Symptom Inventory (PCSI) in school age children. *Developmental Neuropsychology, 10*, 282.

Taylor, H. G., Dietrich, A., Nuss, K., Wright, M., Rusin, J., Bangert, B., et al. (2010). Postconcussive symptoms in children with mild traumatic brain injury. *Neuropsychology, 24*, 148–159.

Van Kampen, D. A., Lovell, M. R., Pardini, J., Collins, M. W., & Fu, F. H. (2006). The "value added" of neurocognitive testing after sport-related concussion. *American Journal of Sports Medicine, 34*, 1630–1635.

Varni, J. W., Seid, M., & Rode, C. A. (1999). The PedsQL: Measurement model for the Pediatric Quality of Life inventory. *Medical Care, 37*, 126–139.

Vaughan, C. G., Gioia, G., & Vincent, D. (2008). Initial examination of self-reported postconcussion symptoms in normal and mTBI children ages 5 to 12. *Journal of the International Neuropsychological Society, 14*(Suppl. 1), 207.

Villemure, R., Nolin, R., & LeSage, N. (2011). Self-reported symptoms during post-mild traumatic brain injury in acute phase: Influence of interviewing method. *Brain Injury, 25*, 53–64.

Wilde, E. A., McCauley, S. R., Hunter, J. V., Bigler, E. D., Chu, Z., Wang, Z. J., et al. (2008).

Diffusion tensor imaging of acute mild traumatic brain injury in adolescents. *Neurology, 70*, 948–955.

World Health Organization. (1992). *ICD-10 Classifications of Mental and Behavioural Disorder: Clinical Descriptions and Diagnostic Guidelines.* Geneva: Author.

Wrightson, P., & Gronwall, D. (1999). *Mild head injury: A guide to management.* New York: Oxford University Press.

Yeates, K. O. (2010). Mild traumatic brain injury and post-concussive symptoms in children and adolescents. *Journal of the International Neuropsychological Society, 16,* 953–960.

Yeates, K. O., Kaizar, E., Rusin, J., Bangert, B., Dietrich, A., Nuss, K., et al. (2012). Reliable change in post-concussive symptoms and its functional consequences among children with mild traumatic brain injury. *Archives of Pediatrics and Adolescent Medicine.* Epub ahead of print. Retrieved March 15, 2012, doi:10.1001/archpediatrics.2011.1082.

Yeates, K. O., Luria, J., Bartkowski, H., Rusin, J., Martin, L., & Bigler, E. D. (1999). Postconcussive symptoms in children with mild closed head injuries. *Journal of Head Trauma Rehabilitation, 14,* 337–350.

Yeates, K. O., Taylor, H. G., Rusin, J., Bangert, B., Dietrich, A., Nuss, K., et al. (2009). Longitudinal trajectories of postconcussive symptoms in children with mild traumatic brain injuries and their relationship to acute clinical status. *Pediatrics, 123,* 735–743.

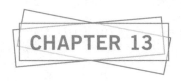

CHAPTER 13

Cognitive Screening
and Neuropsychological Assessment

Doug Bodin and Nicole Shay

Traumatic brain injury (TBI) is a leading cause of hospitalization and death among children and adolescents and therefore represents a major public health problem (Langlois, Rutland-Brown, & Thomas, 2006). Most studies of TBI prevalence and incidence only include injuries associated with hospitalization, resulting in fewer documented cases of TBI that are on the milder end of the injury spectrum, such as mild TBI (mTBI) and concussion (Yeates, 2010). The term *concussion* has been used most prevalently in the sports medicine field to describe head injuries that result in transient neurological changes (see Tator, 2009). No formal consensus exists within the neuropsychological and medical community regarding the difference, if any, between mTBI and concussion (Bodin, Yeates, & Klamar, 2012).

THE ROLE OF COGNITIVE SCREENING
AND NEUROPSYCHOLOGICAL ASSESSMENT

The role of neuropsychological assessment in pediatric mTBI initially arose out of concerns that mTBI may lead to significant cognitive, psychosocial, and academic dysfunction (Beers, 1992; Boll, 1983). These early reviews engendered the notion that mTBI represents a "silent epidemic" (Satz, 2001), which brought increased attention from clinicians and researchers alike. More recent studies have suggested that mTBI does not, *in most cases*, result in persisting cognitive, psychosocial, or academic deficits (Carroll et al., 2004; Ponsford et al., 1999; Satz, 2001; Thompson & Irby, 2003; Yeates & Taylor, 2005). Nevertheless, comprehensive neuropsychological assessment is recommended in cases of multiple concussions or when recovery is not progressing as expected (Halstead & Walter, 2010; Kirkwood, Yeates, & Wilson, 2006).

Over the past decade, increased attention has been paid to sports-related concussions, leading to an emphasis on the role of neuropsychology in the cognitive screening of concussed athletes. The National Athletic Trainers' Association (NATA) has supported the use of symptom checklists, neuropsychological testing, and postural stability testing in the assessment and treatment of concussion (Guskiewicz et al., 2004). NATA's recommendations also include the use of baseline screening of neuropsychological functioning in all athletes. In other words, they recommend that all athletes be screened prior to participating in high-risk competitive sports. Moreover, NATA recommends that follow-up testing, including neuropsychological testing, be conducted to assist in determining when athletes can safely return to play. Nonetheless, most athletic trainers do not follow through on their own organization's recommendations. In a study of 927 athletic trainers, only 3% of those surveyed report following through with an assessment of all areas recommended in NATA's guidelines, and only 18% pursue neuropsychological testing (Notebaert & Guskiewicz, 2005).

The Vienna summary statement (Aubry et al., 2002) of the 1st International Conference on Concussion in Sport established two important principles (1) No single concussion grading system exists with sufficient evidence to make decisions regarding return to play, so decisions should be made on a case-by-case basis; and (2) neuropsychological testing is one of the cornerstones of the process in making decisions for appropriate medical management. This conference established the importance of the neuropsychological evaluation in the assessment and treatment of concussion for all patients. The Prague summary statement of the Second International Conference on Concussion in Sport provided continued support for the use of neuropsychological testing in concussion evaluation (McCrory et al., 2005). The Prague work group classified concussions as "simple" (resolution of symptoms within 7–10 days) or "complex" (persistent symptoms, concussive convulsions, prolonged loss of consciousness, or prolonged cognitive impairment). Critics voiced concern that patients diagnosed with simple concussions would not receive neuropsychological evaluation because the guidelines no longer placed an emphasis on neuropsychological assessment for all patients, but instead focused on assessment for those patients with complex concussions (Shuttleworth-Edwards, 2008). The Zurich summary statement (McCrory et al., 2009) of the Third International Conference on Concussion in Sport also emphasized the role of neuropsychological assessment in the management of concussed athletes and abandoned the use of the *simple* versus *complex* classification system. The American Academy of Pediatrics has also supported the use of neuropsychological assessment in sports-related concussions, although they acknowledge several limitations in the use of cognitive screening and neuropsychological assessment (Halstead & Walter, 2010).

NEUROPSYCHOLOGICAL TOOLS OF THE TRADE

Before discussing specific tools used in mTBI/concussion assessment, a brief mention of relevant psychometric properties is essential (see Table 13.1). In concussion assessment the tests utilized must have high test–retest reliability and validity to set the stage for high sensitivity, specificity, and positive predictive power. In addition, establishing

TABLE 13.1. Definition of Relevant Psychometric Terms

Psychometric term	Definition
Test–retest reliability	Whether scores on a specific measure/battery are stable across multiple administrations
Test validity	Whether the test/battery measures what it is supposed to measure
Sensitivity	Probability of a positive test result, given a particular diagnosis/deficit
Specificity	Probability of a negative test result, given the absence of a particular diagnosis/deficit
Positive predictive power	Probability that a diagnosis/deficit exists, given a positive test result
Reliable change index	Method of determining that a change in test performance is not due to error or normal variation
Practice effects	Improvement in test performance as a result of previous exposure to the test

"reliable change" is important in determining if a change in scores on a specific test or battery represents a significant improvement or decline in test performance. An in-depth review of these concepts is beyond the scope of this chapter; several related reviews are available (Broglio, Ferrara, Macciocchi, Baumgartner, & Elliott, 2007a; Collie et al., 2004; Randolph, McCrea, & Barr, 2005; Strauss, Sherman, Spreen, & Slick, 2006; Valovich McLeod, Barr, McCrea, & Guskiewicz, 2006).

The assessment of a child's or adolescent's cognitive status is an important component of the interdisciplinary clinical management of mTBI. Kirkwood et al. (2008) present a useful model for the role of neuropsychology in the assessment and management of pediatric mTBI across different recovery stages. This model defines the acute stage as time of injury through 3 days postinjury, the postacute stage as between 4 days and 3 months postinjury, and the long-term stage as 4 months postinjury through recovery (Kirkwood et al., 2008). This review of the approaches, strategies, and tools used in the cognitive screening and neuropsychological assessment of mTBI follows the model used by Kirkwood et al. (2008), although we acknowledge that considerable overlap exists between certain recovery stages and assessment strategies used therein. Clinicians must keep in mind the time elapsed since the injury occurred, as well as the age of the person being assessed. Recovery from concussion is a dynamic process that changes rapidly. Within the first 3 days of the injury, during the acute phase, the goal should be identification of medical emergencies, recognition of the concussion, stabilization of the patient, and education of parents and teachers (Gioia, Isquith, Schneider, & Vaughan, 2009a; Kirkwood et al., 2008). During the postacute phase, from 3 days to 3 months following the concussion, the goal of the neuropsychological evaluation should be the identification of lingering physical and cognitive symptoms to aid in treatment planning (Kirkwood et al., 2008). Beyond 3 months, any lingering symptoms from concussion would warrant a complete neuropsychological assessment.

Acute Phase

Several measures have been developed to assess recovery from pediatric TBI during the acute and postacute phases and to assist with assigning injury severity labels (see Table 13.2). The Children's Orientation and Amnesia Test (COAT; Ewing-Cobbs, Levin, Fletcher, Miner, & Eisenberg, 1990) was developed to measure orientation and memory recovery during the acute phase of TBI recovery. Scores on the COAT have been found to predict postinjury memory function up to 12 months after TBI (Ewing-Cobbs et al., 1990). The Westmead Post-Traumatic Amnesia Scale (WPTAS; Shores, Marosszeky, Sandanam, & Batchelor, 1986) was designed to be administered at hourly intervals and has been used in children as young as 7 years of age. A relatively recent version of the WPTAS has been developed for preschool-age children (Rocca, Wallen, & Batchelor, 2008), although validation studies in clinical populations are forthcoming. The COAT and WPTAS were not developed specifically for the mTBI/concussion population, but have been used across the severity spectrum.

The Standardized Assessment of Concussion (SAC; McCrea, Kelly, & Randolph, 2000) is a 10-minute screening test that has been shown to be reliable and valid in adult patients with concussion (McCrea, Kelly, Kluge, Ackley, & Randolph, 1997). Studies have supported the use of the SAC in an adult emergency department population (Naunheim, Matero, & Fucetola, 2008) and in high school and college athlete populations (McCrea, 2001). The Sport Concussion Assessment Tool (SCAT) was developed as part of the 2nd International Conference on Concussion in Sport (McCrory et al., 2005) to provide both patient education and physician assessment. The cognitive screening portion of the SCAT essentially includes items from the SAC and the Maddocks questions for sideline concussion assessment (Maddocks, Dicker, & Saling, 1995). The SCAT2 was developed as part of the 3rd International Conference on Concussion in Sport (McCrory et al., 2009), which concluded that validation studies were needed. At the present time, the SAC and SCAT have been used predominately in adolescent and adult populations, with a relative scarcity of screening batteries for school-age children.

A study of the SAC in a pediatric population revealed that the overall SAC score may not be sensitive to concussion in children presenting to an emergency department (Grubenhoff, Kirkwood, Gao, Deakyne, & Wathen, 2010). Instead, the graded-symptom checklist included in the SAC element appeared to discriminate best between concussed and nonconcussed children. The graded-symptom checklist questions that demonstrated the best discriminability were dizziness, photophobia, and memory disturbance. An additional pediatric study found that the SAC appears to measure different areas of cognitive functioning than traditional paper-and-pencil tests, suggesting that the SAC should be used in combination with more traditional neuropsychological assessment (Valovich McLeod et al., 2006).

Postacute Phase

Relatively recently, neuropsychologists have been called upon to develop and administer measures of cognitive screening during the initial days to weeks following mTBI. These activities have occurred, for the most part, in the context of sports concussions in adolescents and young adults, with a more limited focus on school-age children.

TABLE 13.2. Commonly Used Neuropsychological Instruments for Pediatric Concussion Assessment

Test	Stage of recovery	Brief description	Strengths/weaknesses
Children's Orientation and Amnesia Test (COAT; Ewing-Cobbs et al., 1990)	Acute	• Orally administered • Measures posttraumatic amnesia • Age range: 3–15 years • 5- to 10-minute administration time	• Used serially in rehab settings with moderate to severe TBI • Norms for 3–15 years • Adequate reliability and validity
Westmead Post-Traumatic Amnesia Scale (WPTAS; Shores et al., 1986)	Acute	• Orally administered • Measures posttraumatic amnesia • School-age and preschool-age versions • 5- to 10-minute administration time	• Used serially in rehab settings with moderate to severe TBI • Separate preschool and school-age norms • Reliability and validity data in pediatric populations needed
Standardized Assessment of Concussion (SAC; McCrea, Kelly, & Randolph, 2000)	Acute and subacute	• Orally administered • Brief mental status and neurological screener • Adolescent to adult • 5- to 10-minute screening test	• Developed for sideline use but has been used in medical settings • Published adult/adolescent norms • Emerging pediatric reliability/validity data
Sport Concussion Assessment Tool–2 (SCAT2; McCrory et al., 2009)	Acute and subacute	• Orally administered • SAC plus additional sideline assessment items • Adolescent to adult • 5- to 10-minute administration time	• Normative data forthcoming • Psychometric support for individual components (e.g., SAC), but no peer-reviewed studies of entire instrument
Trail Making Test	Subacute and long-term	• Paper and pencil • Measures processing speed and cognitive flexibility • 8 years and up • 5- to 10-minute administration time	• Norms for ages 8 and up • Adequate sensitivity but susceptible to practice effects
Digit Span Test	Subacute and long-term	• Orally administered • Measure of auditory attention and working memory • Norms available for 5 years and above • 5-minute administration time	• Multiple versions available • Norms for ages 5 age up • Low sensitivity
Symbol Digit Modalities Test	Subacute and long-term	• Paper and pencil • Measures processing speed • 8 years and up • 5-minute administration time	• Norms for 8 years and up • Adequate sensitivity but questionable reliability
ImPACT (University of Pittsburgh)	Acute and subacute	• Computerized battery • Measures memory, reaction time, impulse control, and visual motor speed • Developed for high school, college, and professional athletes; pediatric version is forthcoming • 20- to 25-minute administration time	• Baseline model • Adolescent and adult norms • Limited peer-reviewed data to support reliability, validity, and clinical utility

(cont.)

TABLE 13.2. *(cont.)*

Test	Stage of recovery	Brief description	Strengths/weaknesses
AxonSport (formerly CogSport)	Acute and subacute	• Computerized battery • Measures speed, accuracy, and response consistency • Adolescent to adult • 15- to 20-minute administration time	• Baseline model • Adolescent and adult norms • Limited peer-reviewed support for reliability, validity, and clinical utility
Headminder Concussion Resolution Index (Headminder Inc.)	Acute and subacute	• Computerized battery • Measures processing speed, simple reaction time, and complex reaction time • High school age and older • 20- to 25-minute administration time	• Web-based administration • Adolescent and adult norms • Some support for adequate reliability and reliable change index scores • Limited peer-reviewed support for sensitivity and validity.

Following is a critical review of traditional paper-and-pencil measures and computerized programs that are commonly used to screen cognitive functioning during the postacute phase of mTBI.

Paper-and-Pencil Cognitive Screening

Currently, many neuropsychologists use traditional paper-and-pencil screens of concussion that typically include brief neuropsychological testing. Generally, relatively few areas of cognition are screened because concussion is seen to affect particular functions disproportionately, including attention, reaction time, working memory, and processing speed (Dikmen, Machamer, Winn, & Temkin, 1995). Because few areas of cognition are evaluated, difficulties arise with the reliability of brief neuropsychological screens (Ellemberg, Henry, Macciocchi, Guskiewicz, & Broglio, 2009; Randolph et al., 2005). A number of neuropsychological tests, which are used as screeners, possess some of the psychometric properties required for a good concussion assessment instrument, but often do not possess all of the requirements and have primarily been validated in adolescent and adult populations. Some of the tests that have been found to have high sensitivity to concussion include the Trail Making Test (Macciocchi, Barth, Alves, Rimel, & Jane, 1996) and the Symbol Digit Modalities Test (Broglio, Macciocchi, & Ferrara, 2007b). Although the Trail Making Test does have high sensitivity for concussion, it is susceptible to practice effects (Macciocchi et al., 1996), thereby reducing positive predictive power. The Digit Span Test has also often been utilized as a measure of focused attention and working memory, but has been found to have low sensitivity (Ellemberg et al., 2009).

Macciocchi and colleagues (1996) argue, however, that regardless of which neuropsychological screening tests are utilized, practice effects will always occur when measures are given over brief periods of time. Thus, the use of change scores over time should be the main outcome measure used to assess improvement in neuropsychological functioning (Randolph et al., 2005). On the other hand, other methods of assessment have been employed to account for practice effects. In a study by Hinton-

Bayre, Geffen, Geffen, McFarland, and Friis (1999), the authors used multiple baseline assessments in order to *create* practice effects. By adopting this strategy, the athletes in their study should have reached peak performance prior to any injury and could then subsequently be followed to assess decrements should an injury occur. Although this strategy is novel and has promise, it is unrealistic for clinical purposes because of the time and expense involved in completing multiple assessments.

Computerized Cognitive Screening

Although paper-and-pencil tests are generally quick and simple to administer, a number of problems are associated with them (Collie, Darby, & Maruff, 2001; Gioia et al., 2009a). When neuropsychological tests are used for repeated assessment, the measures must be extremely sensitive to identify declines and improvement over time. In addition, practice effects must be controlled for by administering equivalent, alternate forms of a test. Few paper-and-pencil tests have alternate forms, and this poses problems for repeat administrations. In addition, traditional paper-and-pencil tests can be susceptible to interrater biases and can show significant practice effects (Collie et al., 2001). Yet another problem is that paper-and-pencil measures may be insensitive to the subtle changes in reaction time that are often a symptom of concussion (Maroon et al., 2000). Paper-and-pencil neuropsychological tests typically require trained neuropsychologists to both administer and interpret the result, which often is difficult when assessment occurs on the athletic field, in the emergency department, or in physicians' offices.

With these problems in mind, a number of computerized cognitive screening programs have been developed for concussion assessment and monitoring in both acute and postacute phases. Although several computerized batteries are available, the majority of these programs were designed for adults. The three most commonly used computerized batteries for high school athletes are the ImPACT (University of Pittsburgh, Pittsburgh, PA), CogSport (CogState Ltd., Victoria, Australia), and Headminder Concussion Resolution Index (Headminder Inc., New York, NY). The computerized tests are quick to administer and can be administered to multiple patients at once without requiring a neuropsychologist. Moreover, to avoid practice effects, several alternate forms of the tests are available. The computerized batteries have been widely used by high schools, colleges, professional sports teams, and sports medicine clinics as part of a baseline model of concussion assessment. One problem associated with computerized batteries is that neuropsychologists are often not accessible by physicians' offices, schools, or sports medicine clinics to assist in interpreting the results. Because of the limited scope of computerized programs, interpretation of the results may be difficult for the untrained professional (Maerlender et al., 2010). Computerized batteries typically involve serial assessments; thus, sensitivity of the measures and test–retest reliability are very important. Overall, the sensitivity of computerized neuropsychological assessments has been found to be in the moderate range. In a study of high school athletes with concussion, the athletes were evaluated using ImPACT within 3 days of their concussion (Schatz, Pardini, Lovell, Collins, & Podell, 2006). Using symptom report and cognitive performance, the ImPACT program was able to correctly identify 81.9% of concussed athletes as evidencing either cognitive impairment or elevated symptoms related to the concussion. Another study of college-age athletes who sustained concussions during play reported a lower sensitivity on the ImPACT, with only 62.5% sensitivity, and a slightly higher sensitivity of the Headminder Concussion Resolution Index (78.6%; Broglio et al., 2007b).

Test–retest reliability of computerized batteries has often been assessed over short time periods, which does not provide sufficient evidence for stability over longer time periods. Unpublished data by the University of Georgia Department of Sports Medicine (as cited in Broglio et al., 2007a) suggested that the mean time between initial baseline assessment and time of concussion was 45 days, much longer than the test–retest time periods of days or a few weeks reported by the publishers (e.g., Erlanger et al., 2001). Broglio and colleagues (Broglio et al., 2007a) assessed the test–retest reliability of ImPACT, Headminder Concussion Resolution Index, and Concussion Sentinel (the previous version of CogSport) at 45 and 50 days postbaseline. The authors found that the test–retest reliabilities of all of the programs over 45 days were lower than had been shown in previous publications (Collie et al., 2003; Erlanger et al., 2001). Test–retest reliabilities of several indices were in the minimally acceptable range for clinical purposes (i.e., around .60). None of the tests reached levels typically considered acceptable for test–retest reliability (i.e., > .75).

Although the test–retest reliability of computerized batteries has been questioned, multiple studies have demonstrated the sensitivity of computerized batteries. In a study by Lovell and colleagues (2007), athletes who sustained a concussion during a sporting event were evaluated on the ImPACT test battery within a mean of 6 days following their concussion and then again at about 35 days postinjury. The athletes were compared to a control group on the battery. Athletes who sustained a concussion performed worse on ImPACT than nonconcussed controls at the assessment immediately following the injury, but not by 35 days postinjury. Another study of the ImPACT test battery in concussed athletes revealed neurocognitive deficits 2, 7, and 14 days following concussion (McClincy, Lovell, Pardini, Collins, & Spore, 2006). Thus, computerized batteries, such as ImPACT, have provided both clinicians and researchers with information regarding the period of time during which neurocognitive deficits typically exist after concussion. These batteries also provide clinicians with concrete data on the recovery process for individual athletes. As the number of computerized programs continues to grow, these measures will require careful evaluation to determine whether they are appropriate tools for use with clinical populations.

Overall, cognitive screening of mTBI has grown rapidly over the past decade. However, significant concerns have been noted regarding the psychometric properties of both traditional and computerized cognitive screening, leading some authors to question the use of these tools in clinical applications (see Randolph et al., 2005; also see Macciocchi, 2005). Unfortunately for the pediatric clinician, the majority of the paper-and-pencil and computerized cognitive screening batteries have only been evaluated in the older adolescent and young-adult populations. A pediatric version of the ImPACT is currently under development (Gioia et al., 2006, 2009b), but published data regarding reliability and validity in clinical populations are not yet available.

Long-Term Phase

During the long-term recovery phase following mTBI (i.e., beyond 4 months postinjury), formal neuropsychological evaluation is occasionally needed. Although mTBI typically does not result in lasting deficits, especially for the mildest forms such as concussion, a formal neuropsychological evaluation is needed in cases of either repeat concussion and/or persisting injury-related symptoms (Halstead & Walter, 2010; Kirkwood, Yeates, & Wilson, 2006). Formal pediatric neuropsychological evaluations typically involve a review of medical records, interviews with parents and/or teacher, and the assessment of a wide variety of cognitive domains, including overall cognitive ability, language, visual–spatial/visual–perceptual functions, memory, attention, executive functions, sensory–motor functions, academic achievement, and adaptive and behavioral functioning. Pediatric neuropsychological evaluations should be conducted within a framework of understanding the multiple and reciprocal developmental and environmental contexts in which the child/adolescent operates (see Baron, 2010; Bernstein, 2000). During the long-term phase of recovery from mTBI, formal neuropsychological evaluations can be used to document persisting deficits, determine noninjury factors that are influencing outcome, and assist with clinical and academic planning (Kirkwood et al., 2008).

METHODOLOGICAL AND CONCEPTUAL ISSUES

Clinicians and researchers who conduct cognitive screening or neuropsychological assessment of pediatric mTBI need to be aware of multiple and potentially controversial methodological and conceptual issues. First, a myriad of factors can influence outcomes from pediatric mTBI, including injury severity, age at time of injury, premorbid cognitive and behavioral functioning, genetic vulnerability, previous injuries, family functioning, comorbid conditions, motivational factors, and issues surrounding postinjury clinical management (Kirkwood et al., 2008). Several of these factors that are thought to be most important in clinical contexts are discussed below.

Age Effects

The age at which a child or adolescent sustains an mTBI may play an important role in potential outcomes. In the past, younger brains were often held to be more likely to recover from injury than older brains because of the greater potential for plasticity. However, recent research has suggested that immature brains are not likely to respond well to diffuse injuries (e.g., Kolb & Gibb, 2007), as can be the case in TBI. The immature brain's response to TBI is a complex process involving multiple biomechanical and pathophysiological processes (Kirkwood et al., 2006). In addition, mTBI sustained at a young age may affect the later development of cognitive functions that have not yet emerged (e.g., certain executive functions), such that deficits may not be evident until the child reaches a later age. In the case of mTBI, studies have shown that high school athletes may demonstrate more protracted rates of recovery following concussion than older athletes (Field, Collins, Lovell, & Maroon, 2003; Pellman, Lovell, Viano, & Casson, 2006). Age effects have also been found for rates of postconcussion symptoms in children following mTBI (Taylor et al., 2010). There is also an emerging literature on the effects of mTBI in preschool children (Anderson et al., 2006; Anderson, Catroppa, Morse, Haritou, & Rosenfeld, 2001; Gronwall, Wrightson, & McGinn, 1997).

Assessment of Effort and Motivation

The assessment of effort and motivation in pediatric mTBI is essential, given the role of subjective symptom complaints and cognitive test performance in the clinical decision-making process. Clinically, substantial attention is paid to the formal assessment of effort and motivation in cases involving litigation with adult patients, but comparatively little notice is given to these issues in pediatric neuropsychology. Many adults with mTBI have been shown to display suboptimal effort on neuropsychological testing (Larrabee, 2003). In addition, performance on measures of effort has been shown to be related to both symptom report and neuropsychological test performance (Lange, Iverson, Brooks, & Ashton Rennison, 2010). Unfortunately, relatively few pediatric clinicians and researchers routinely use measures of effort in their evaluations and investigations. Kirkwood and Kirk (2010) examined the rate of suboptimal effort in a pediatric mTBI sample and found a high (17%) rate of suboptimal effort. These results, although in need of replication, suggest that the assessment of effort and motivation should be considered in the cognitive screening or neuropsychological assessment of pediatric mTBI.

Non-Injury-Related Factors

A challenging issue in the context of pediatric mTBI is determining whether neuropsychological deficits are secondary to noninjury factors, such as premorbid status, comorbid conditions, or family functioning. The estimation of a child's or adolescent's premorbid level of cognitive functioning is often based on information such as preinjury school performance, parent report of preinjury performance, parental education and socioeconomic status, and performance on measures of word reading (Yeates & Taylor, 1997). The estimation of premorbid cognitive ability, although imprecise, is potentially important, given that studies have suggested that preinjury cognitive ability may moderate mTBI outcomes (Fay et al., 2010). In addition to premorbid cognitive ability, weaknesses in specific cognitive skills prior to mTBI, such as attention span, can also influence injury outcomes (Yeates et al., 2005). Family environment can, as well, be a predictor of outcomes following pediatric TBI (Yeates et al., 1997).

Baseline Model

The use of the "baseline model" of cognitive screening following concussions has become increasingly popular. In clinical practice, the baseline model involves administering a battery of neuropsychological tests (typically, computerized batteries) to athletes prior to the beginning of the season to obtain a measure of preinjury cognitive functioning. If an injury occurs, the cognitive battery is repeated, and scores are compared to baseline performance to determine when the athlete is no longer displaying injury-related cognitive deficits (i.e., when the athlete's score returns to the level obtained prior to the season). As mentioned earlier, this model has enjoyed much popularity and has been endorsed as part of multiple sports medicine and athletic training organizations guidelines. Despite the popularity of the baseline model, its utility in guiding return-to-play decisions has been criticized on both statistical and theoretical grounds (Kirkwood, Randolph, & Yeates, 2009; Randolph, 2011). More specifically, questions have arisen as to whether neuropsychological tests have the psychometric properties needed to reliably detect concussion-related effects. In addition, the use of neuropsychological testing within the baseline model may not add incremental value beyond subjective reports of postconcussion symptoms (Kirkwood et al., 2009). The use of procedures such as calculating a reliable change index is becoming a "gold standard" in measuring recovery and is essential in using the baseline model to make clinical decisions.

SUMMARY AND FUTURE RESEARCH DIRECTIONS

Cognitive screening and neuropsychological assessment following pediatric mTBI should be part of an interdisciplinary approach to clinical management. During the acute and postacute phases of mTBI recovery, brief cognitive screening can be used to track recovery of commonly affected neuropsychological functions, such as attention, memory, and processing speed. Traditional paper-and-pencil measures of cognitive functioning have been used to evaluate postacute functioning; however, concerns have arisen regarding the psychometric properties of these instruments, especially in children and when used in repeat administrations. In the past decade, computerized batteries have been developed and widely used in the area of sports concussion management. These computerized batteries have also been criticized on psychometric and empirical grounds. If postconcussive symptoms continue past the typical recovery period (i.e., beyond 3–4 months), a more formal neuropsychological evaluation is indicated to document persisting deficits, rule out non-injury-related factors that may contribute to persistent symptoms, and assist with ongoing clinical management.

Clinicians should bear in mind that no gold-standard tool is available for cognitive screening and neuropsychological assessment of children with mTBI. All measures have pros and cons that must be weighed when deciding which measure or measures will best suit a specific patient population. Practitioners should also recognize that concerns continue to be raised about the value of the "baseline model" in improving clinical decision making following a concussion. Research must continue in this area to determine whether cognitive testing in the baseline model provides any incremental value to the assessment of concussion, above and beyond traditional symptom-based assessment. Additional research also is needed to develop measures to assess cognitive recovery during the acute phase for preschool and school-age children. Finally, more research is needed to understand the role of noninjury factors, such as genetic vulnerability and motivation/effort, in influencing outcomes from mTBI.

REFERENCES

Anderson, V., Catroppa, C., Dudgeon, P., Morse, S. A., Haritou, F., & Rosenfeld, J. V. (2006). Understanding predictors of functional recovery and outcome 30 months following early childhood head injury. *Neuropsychology, 20,* 42–57.

Anderson, V., Catroppa, C., Morse, S. A., Haritou, F., & Rosenfeld, J. V. (2001). Outcome from mild head injury in young children: A prospective study. *Journal of Clinical and Experimental Neuropsychology, 23,* 705–717.

Aubry, M., Cantu, R., Dvorak, J., Graf-Baumann, T., Johnston, K., Kelly, J., et al. (2002). Summary and agreement statement of the First International Conference on Concussion in Sport, Vienna 2001: Recommendations for the improvement of safety and health of athletes who may suffer concussive injuries. *British Journal of Sports Medicine*, *36*, 6–10.

Baron, I. S. (2010). Maxims and a model for the practice of pediatric neuropsychology. In K. O. Yeates, M. D. Ris, H. G. Taylor, & B. F. Pennington (Eds.), *Pediatric neuropsychology: Research, theory, and practice* (2nd ed., pp. 473–498). New York: Guilford Press.

Beers, S. (1992). Cognitive effects of mild head injury in children and adolescents. *Neuropsychology Review*, *3*, 281–320.

Bernstein, J. H. (2000). Developmental neuropsychological assessment. In K. O. Yeates, M. D. Ris, & H. G. Taylor (Eds.), *Pediatric neuropsychology: Research, theory, and practice* (pp. 405–438). New York: Guilford Press.

Bodin, D., Yeates, K. O., & Klamar, K. (2012). Definition and classification of concussion. In J. N. Apps & K. Walter (Eds.), *Pediatric and adolescent concussion: Diagnosis, management, and outcome* (pp. 9–20). New York: Springer.

Boll, T. J. (1983). Minor head injury in children: Out of sight but not out of mind. *Journal of Clinical Child Psychology*, *12*, 74–80.

Broglio, S. P., Ferrara, M. S., Macciocchi, S. N., Baumgartner, T. A., & Elliot, R. (2007a). Test–retest reliability of computerized concussion assessment programs. *Journal of Athletic Training*, *42*, 509–514.

Broglio, S. P., Macciocchi, S. N., & Ferrara, M. S. (2007b). Sensitivity of the concussion assessment battery. *Neurosurgery*, *60*, 1050–1058.

Carroll, L. J., Cassidy, J. D., Peloso, P. M., Borg, J., von Holst, H., Holm, L., et al. (2004). Prognosis for mild traumatic brain injury: Results of the WHO Collaborating Centre Task Force on Mild Traumatic Brain Injury. *Journal of Rehabilitation Medicine*, *43*(Suppl.), 84–105.

CogSport. Retrieved January 2011, from *www.cogsport.com*.

Collie, A., Darby, D., & Maruff, P. (2001). Computerized cognitive assessment of athletes with sports related head injury. *British Journal of Sports Medicine*, *35*, 297–302.

Collie, A., Maruff, P., Makdissi, M., McCrory, P., McStephen, M., & Darby, D. (2003). CogSport: Reliability and correlation with conventional cognitive test used in postconcussion medical evaluations. *Clinical Journal of Sport Medicine*, *13*, 28–32.

Collie, A., Maruff, P., Makdissi, M., McStephen, M., Darby, D. G., & McCrory, P. (2004). Statistical procedures for determining the extent of cognitive change following concussion. *British Journal of Sports Medicine*, *38*, 273–278.

Concussion Resolution Index. (1999). New York: Headminder.

Dikmen, S. S., Machamer, J. E., Winn, H. R., & Temkin, N. R. (1995). Neuropsychological outcome at 1-year post head injury. *Neuropsychology*, *59*, 80–90.

Ellemberg, D., Henry, L. C., Macciocchi, S. N., Guskiewicz, K. M., & Broglio, S. P. (2009). Advances in sport concussion assessment: From behavioral to brain imaging measures. *Journal of Neurotrauma*, *26*, 2365–2382.

Erlanger, D. M., Saliba, E., Barth, J. T., Almquist, J., Webright, W., & Freeman, J. (2001). Monitoring resolution of postconcussion symptoms in athletes: Preliminary results of a web-based neuropsychological test protocol. *Journal of Athletic Training*, *36*, 280–287.

Ewing-Cobbs, L., Levin, H. S., Fletcher, J. M., Miner, M. E., & Eisenberg, H. M. (1990). The Children's Orientation and Amnesia Test: Relationship to severity of acute head injury and to recovery of memory. *Neurosurgery*, *27*, 683–691.

Fay, T. B., Yeates, K. O., Taylor, H. G., Bangert, B., Dietrich, A., Nuss, K. E., et al. (2010). Cognitive reserve as a moderator of postconcussive symptoms in children with complicated and uncomplicated mild traumatic brain injury. *Journal of the International Neuropsychological Society*, 16, 94–105.

Field, M., Collins, M. W., Lovell, M. R., & Maroon, J. (2003). Does age play a role in recovery from sports-related concussion?: A comparison of high school and collegiate athletes. *Journal of Pediatrics*, 142, 546–553.

Gioia, G. A., Isquith, P. K., Schneider, J. C., & Vaughan, C. G. (2009a). New approaches to assessment and monitoring of concussion in children. *Topics in Language Disorders*, 29, 266–281.

Gioia, G. A., Isquith, P. K., Schneider, J. C., Vaughan, C. G., Vincent, D. T., Leaffer, E., et al. (2009b). Initial validation of a pediatric version of the Immediate Post-Concussion Assessment and Cognitive Testing (ImPACT) Battery [Abstract]. *British Journal of Sports Medicine*, 43(Suppl. 1), i92.

Gioia, G. A., Janusz, J., Diver, T., Natale, M., Anderson, S., Dipinto, M., et al. (2006). Initial development of the pediatric version of the Immediate Post-Concussion Assessment and Cognitive Testing (ImPACT) battery [Abstract]. *Journal of the International Neuropsychological Society*, 12(Suppl. 1), i39.

Gronwall, D., Wrightson, P., & McGinn, V. (1997). Effect of mild head injury during the preschool years. *Journal of the International Neuropsychological Society*, 3, 592–597.

Grubenhoff, J. A., Kirkwood, M., Gao, D., Deakyne, S., & Wathen, J. (2010). Evaluation of the Standardized Assessment of Concussion in a pediatric emergency department. *Pediatrics*, 126, 688–695.

Guskiewicz, K. M., Bruce, S. L., Cantu, R. C., Ferrara, M. S., Kelly, J. P., McCrea, M., et al. (2004). National Athletic Trainers' Association position statement: Management of sport-related concussion. *Journal of Athletic Training*, 39, 280–297.

Halstead, M. E., & Walter, K. D. (2010). Clinical report: Sport-related concussion in children and adolescents. *Pediatrics*, 126, 597–615.

Hinton-Bayre, A. D., Geffen, G. M., Geffen, L. B., McFarland, K. A., & Friis, P. (1999). Concussion in contact sports: Reliable change indices of impairment and recovery. *Journal of Clinical Experimental Neuropsychology*, 21, 70–86.

ImPACT. Retrieved January 2011, from *www.impacttest.com*.

Kirkwood, M. W., & Kirk, J. W. (2010). The base rate of suboptimal effort in a pediatric mild TBI sample: Performance on the medical symptom validity test. *The Clinical Neuropsychologist*, 24, 860–872.

Kirkwood, M. W., Randolph, C., & Yeates, K. O. (2009). Returning pediatric athletes to play after concussion: The evidence (or lack thereof) behind baseline neuropsychological testing. *Acta Pædiatrica*, 98, 1409–1411.

Kirkwood, M. W., Yeates, K. O., Taylor, H. G., Randolph, C. R., McCrea, M., & Anderson, V. A. (2008). Management of pediatric mild traumatic brain injury: A neuropsychological review from injury through recovery. *The Clinical Neuropsychologist*, 22, 769–800.

Kirkwood, M. W., Yeates, K. O., & Wilson, P. E. (2006). Pediatric sport-related concussion: A review of the clinical management of an oft-neglected population. *Pediatrics*, 117, 1359–1371.

Kolb, B., & Gibb, R. (2007). Brain plasticity and recovery from early cortical injury. *Developmental Psychobiology*, 49, 107–118.

Lange, R. T., Iverson, G. L., Brooks, B. L., & Ashton Rennison, V. L. (2010). Influence of poor effort on self-reported symptoms and neurocognitive test performance following mild traumatic brain injury. *Journal of Clinical and Experimental Neuropsychology*, 32, 961–972.

Langlois, J. A., Rutland-Brown, W., & Thomas, K. E. (2006). *Traumatic brain injury in the United States: Emergency department visits, hospitalizations, and deaths*. Atlanta, GA:

Centers for Disease Control and Prevention, National Center for Injury Prevention and Control.

Larrabee, C. J. (2003). Detection of malingering using atypical performance patterns on standard neuropsychological tests. *The Clinical Neuropsychologist, 17,* 410–425.

Lovell, M. R., Pardini, J. E., Welling, J., Collins, M. W., Bakal, J., Lazar, N., et al. (2007). Functional brain abnormalities are related to clinical recovery and time to return-to-play in athletes. *Neurosurgery, 61,* 352–360.

Macciocchi, S. N. (2005). Commentary. *Journal of Athletic Training, 40,* 152–153.

Macciocchi, S. N., Barth, J. T., Alves, W., Rimel, R. W., & Jane, J. A. (1996). Neuropsychological functioning and recovery after mild head injury in collegiate athletes. *Neurosurgery, 39,* 510–514.

Maddocks, D. L., Dicker, G. D., & Saling, M. M. (1995). The assessment of orientation following concussion in athletes. *Clinical Journal of Sports Medicine, 5,* 32–33.

Maerlender, A., Flashman, L., Kessler, A., Kumbhani, S., Greenwald, R., Tosteson, T., et al. (2010). Examination of the construct validity of ImPACT computerized test, traditional, and experimental neuropsychological measures. *The Clinical Neuropsychologist, 24,* 1309–1325.

Maroon, J. C., Lovell, M. R., Norwig, J., Podell, K., Powell, J. W., & Hartl, R. (2000). Cerebral concussion in athletes: Evaluation and neuropsychological testing. *Neurosurery, 47,* 659–669.

McClincy, M. P., Lovell, M. R., Pardini, J., Collins, M. W., & Spore, M. K. (2006). Recovery from sports concussion in high school and collegiate athletes. *Brain Injury, 20,* 33–39.

McCrea, M. (2001). Standardized mental status testing on the sideline after sport-related concussion. *Journal of Athletic Training, 36,* 274–279.

McCrea, M., Kelly, J. P., Kluge, J., Ackley, B., & Randolph, C. (1997). Standardized assessment of concussion in football players. *Neurology, 48,* 586–588.

McCrea, M., Kelly, J. P., & Randolph, C. (2000). *Standardized Assessment of Concussion (SAC): Manual for administration, scoring, and interpretation* (2nd ed.). Waukesha, WI: CNS Inc.

McCrory, P., Johnston, K., Meeuwise, W., Aubry, M., Cantu, R., Dvorak, J., et al. (2005). Summary and agreement statement of the 2nd International Conference on Concussion in Sport, Prague 2004. *Clinical Journal of Sport Medicine, 15,* 48–55.

McCrory, P., Meeuwisse, W., Johnston, K., Dvorak, J., Aubry, M., Molloy, M., et al. (2009). Consensus statement on concussion in sport: 3rd International Conference on Concussion in Sport, Zurich, November 2008. *Clinical Journal of Sports Medicine, 19,* 185–195.

Naunheim, R. S., Matero, D., & Fucetola, R. (2008). Assessment of patients with mild concussion in the emergency department. *Journal of Head Trauma Rehabilitation, 23,* 116–122.

Notebaert, A. J., & Guskiewicz, K. M. (2005). Current trends in athletic training practice for concussion assessment and management. *Journal of Athletic Training, 40,* 320–325.

Pellman, E. J., Lovell, M. R., Viano, D. C., & Casson, I. R. (2006). Concussion in professional football: Recovery of NFL and high school athletes assessed by computerized neuropsychological testing: Part 12. *Neurosurgery, 58,* 263–274.

Ponsford, J., Willmott, C., Rothwell, A., Cameron, P., Ayton, G., Nelms, R., et al. (1999). Cognitive and behavioral outcome following mild traumatic head injury in children. *Journal of Head Trauma Rehabilitation, 12,* 360–372.

Randolph, C. (2011). Baseline neuropsychological testing in managing sport-related concussion: Does it modify risk? *Current Sports Medicine Reports, 10,* 21–26.

Randolph, C., McCrea, M., & Barr, W. B. (2005). Is neuropsychological testing useful in the management of sport-related concussion? *Journal of Athletic Training, 40,* 139–152.

Rocca, A., Wallen, M., & Batchelor, J. (2008). The Westmead Post-Traumatic Amnesia Scale for Children (WPTAS-C) aged 4 and 5 years old. *Brain Impairment*, 9, 14–21.

Satz, P. (2001). Mild head injury in children and adolescents. *Current Directions in Psychological Science*, 10, 106–109.

Schatz, P., Pardini, J. E., Lovell, M. R., Collins, M. W., & Podell, K. (2006). Sensitivity and specificity of the ImPACT Test Battery for concussion in athletes. *Archives of Clinical Neuropsychology*, 21, 91–99.

Shores, E. A., Marosszeky, J. E., Sandanam, J., & Batchelor, J. (1986). Preliminary validation of a scale for measuring the duration of post-traumatic amnesia. *Medical Journal of Australia*, 144, 569–572.

Shuttleworth-Edwards, A. B. (2008). Central or peripheral?: A positional stance in reaction to the Prague statement on the role of neuropsychological assessment in sports concussion management. *Archives of Clinical Neuropsychology*, 23, 479–485.

Strauss, E., Sherman, E. M., Spreen, O., & Slick, D. J. (2006). Psychometrics in neuropsychological assessment. In E. Strauss, E. M. Sherman, & O. Spreen (Eds.), *A compendium of neuropsychological tests: Administration, norms, and commentary* (pp. 3–43). New York: Oxford University Press.

Tator, C. H. (2009). Let's standardize the definition of concussion and get reliable incidence data. *Canadian Journal of Neurological Sciences*, 36, 429–435.

Taylor, H. G., Dietrich, A., Nuss, K., Wright, M., Rusin, J., Bangert, B., et al. (2010). Postconcussive symptoms in children with mild traumatic brain injury. *Neuropsychology*, 24, 148–159.

Thompson, M. D., & Irby, J. W. (2003). Recovery from mild head injury in pediatric populations. *Seminars in Pediatric Neurology*, 10, 130–139.

Valovich McLeod, T. C., Barr, W. B., McCrea, M., & Guskiewicz, K. M. (2006). Psychometric and measurement properties of concussion assessment tools in youth sports. *Journal of Athletic Training*, 41, 399–408.

Yeates, K. O. (2010). Traumatic brain injury. In K. O. Yeates, M. D. Ris, H. G. Taylor, & B. F. Pennington (Eds.), *Pediatric neuropsychology: Research, theory, and practice* (2nd ed., pp.112–146). New York: Guilford Press.

Yeates, K. O., Armstrong, K., Janusz, J., Taylor, H. G., Wade, S., Stancin, T., et al. (2005). Long term attention problems in children with traumatic brain injury. *Journal of the American Academy of Child and Adolescent Psychiatry*, 44, 574–584.

Yeates, K. O., & Taylor, H. G. (1997). Predicting premorbid neuropsychological functioning following pediatric traumatic brain injury. *Journal of Clinical and Experimental Neuropsychology*, 19, 825–837.

Yeates, K. O., & Taylor, H. G. (2005). Neurobehavioral outcomes of mild head injury in children and adolescents. *Pediatric Rehabilitation*, 8, 5–16.

Yeates, K. O., Taylor, H. G., Drotar, D., Wade, S., Kein, S., & Stancin, T. (1997). Premorbid family environment as a predictor of neurobehavioral outcomes following pediatric TBI. *Journal of the International Neuropsychological Society*, 3, 617–630.

PART IV

CLINICAL INTERVENTION

CHAPTER 14

Active Rehabilitation
for Slow-to-Recover Children

Grant L. Iverson, Isabelle Gagnon, and Grace S. Griesbach

No evidence-based guidelines exist for treatment and rehabilitation services for children and adolescents who are slow to recover following a mild traumatic brain injury (mTBI). While children are acutely injured, we believe that it is prudent to provide them and their families with early education and reassurance as well as to strongly encourage (1) rest, (2) taking time off from sports (including noncontact activities such as physical education classes in school and extracurricular dance), and (3) avoiding vigorous play. During this time period children might also benefit from substantial reductions in mental activity and stimulation, such as attending school, writing exams, or playing video games. Mental and physical rest following injury has been strongly encouraged for sport-related concussion in agreement and consensus statements (McCrory et al., 2005, 2009).

From a practical perspective, enforcement of complete rest, especially for active children and adolescents involved in many sports, is very difficult, and determinations of how much school is reasonable to miss are not easy to make. Basically, parents are expected to monitor injured children's symptoms and to work with a physician and other health care professionals who have expertise in concussion management (if available) on a plan for returning to school, extracurricular activities, and sports. As we wait for scientific evidence to accumulate regarding the best strategies for managing the acute recovery period and for returning to activities, common sense and clinical judgment prevail.

Fortunately, most children who sustain mTBIs appear to recover, functionally, within the first few weeks postinjury. Some children, however, report persisting symptoms. For children with persisting symptoms, four options are available for ongoing management: (1) encourage continued rest and avoid vigorous activity; (2) allow the child to engage in limited activities under parental supervision; (3) provide symptomatic treatment (e.g., analgesics and antimigraine medications for headaches, or psychological treatment for behavioral issues); or (4) implement active rehabilitation. The first two options rely on "watchful waiting."

The purpose of this chapter is to encourage an active approach to treatment and rehabilitation for children who are slow to recover after an mTBI, in order to reduce symptoms and improve functioning in a more timely manner. Children who are slow to recover are at risk for secondary problems and consequences if their normal activities are curtailed for extended periods of time—while they wait for complete resolution of symptoms. These problems include, but are not limited to, physical deconditioning, anxiety and stress, mild depression, irritability, and acting-out behavior at home and at school. Moreover, as time passes, the strength of the association between the neurobiology of the original injury and the ongoing symptoms likely diminishes, whereas the importance of preexisting factors (e.g., mental health problems, attention-deficit/hyperactivity disorder [ADHD], social–emotional adjustment issues) and current noninjury factors (e.g., dispositional, mental health, situational, and environmental issues) increases. Eventually, for most cases, determining what is causing, maintaining, or exacerbating symptoms becomes nearly impossible. Thus, prolonged activity restrictions might actually be iatrogenic in some cases.

There is a dearth of direct scientific evidence that active rehabilitation with children who are slow to recover after mTBI is time-effective, cost-effective, or clinically efficacious. There simply has been very little clinical research in this area. However, considerable indirect evidence, in multiple areas, supports an active rehabilitation approach. In the first section of this chapter, we provide the rationale for encouraging rest and providing education and reassurance while acutely injured—prior to initiating active rehabilitation. In the second section, we review diverse lines of indirect evidence that support an active rehabilitation approach. In the third section, we discuss education and reassurance as an early intervention strategy. In the fourth section, we describe an active rehabilitation program based at Montreal Children's Hospital. The chapter concludes with a summary and directions for future research.

RATIONALE FOR REST DURING THE "TEMPORAL WINDOW"

The rationale for rest following concussion comes from four lines of evidence. First, based on neuroscience literature, concussions are assumed to cause complex, interwoven cellular and vascular changes characterized by ionic shifts, abnormal energy metabolism, diminished cerebral blood flow, and impaired neurotransmission (Giza & Hovda, 2001, 2004). The stretching of axons results in an indiscriminate release of neurotransmitters and uncontrolled ionic fluxes. Mechanoporation, the development of transient membrane pores due to mechanical force, allows calcium (Ca^{2+}) influx and potassium (K^+) efflux, contributing to rapid and widespread depolarization. Cells respond by activating ion pumps in an attempt to restore the normal membrane potential, increasing glucose utilization (i.e., accelerated glycolysis). There also appears to be impaired oxidative metabolism. These factors contribute to a state of hypermetabolism, which occurs in tandem with decreased cerebral blood flow. During the early postinjury period, cerebral metabolism is likely dedicated to restoring cerebral function. Thus, placing an energy demand on the system, through exercise, could compromise restorative events.

Second, concussions can have an enormously adverse effect on physical and cognitive functioning in the first few days postinjury. In a meta-analysis of 39 studies, the acute adverse effect of sport-related concussion on objectively measured cognition was shown to be large (Hedge's $g = -.81$), and the adverse effect on balance ($g = -2.56$) and subjective symptoms ($g = -3.31$) was very large (Broglio & Puetz, 2008). As seen in Figure 14.1, the "average" acute effect of concussion on cognition is comparable to the effect of early dementia. Notably, if the "average" deviation from normal is approximately one standard deviation, then some people will have no appreciable cognitive deficits, and some will have extremely low cognitive test scores (e.g., > 2 SDs from the mean). As seen in Figure 14.2, the acute effect of concussion on balance and subjectively experienced symptoms is enormous. In addition to

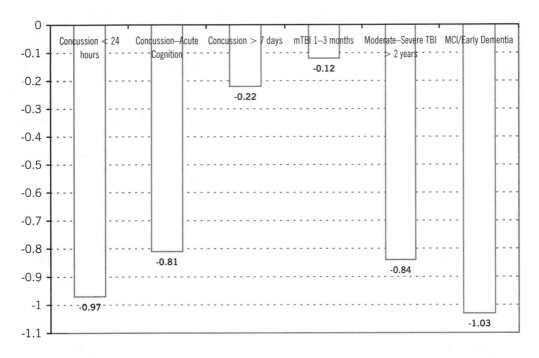

FIGURE 14.1. Meta-analytic effect sizes: Adverse effects on neuropsychological functioning. As a rule, the studies in the meta-analyses do not involve children, but some involve high school athletes. Effect sizes typically are expressed in pooled, weighted standard deviation units. However, across studies, there are some minor variations in the methods of calculation. By convention, effect sizes of 0.2 are considered small, 0.5 medium, and 0.8 large. This is from a statistical, not necessarily clinical, perspective. For this figure, the overall effect on cognitive or neuropsychological functioning is reported. Effect sizes less than 0.3 should be considered very small and difficult to detect in individual patients because the patients and control groups largely overlap. Sport-related concussion < 24 hours and > 7 days from Belanger and Vanderploeg (2005); concussion–acute from Broglio and Puetz (2008); mTBI 1–3 months and moderate-severe > 24 months in Schretlen and Shapiro (2003); and mild cognitive impairment (MCI) or early dementia based on memory testing (Bäckman, Jones, Berger, Laukka, & Small, 2005).

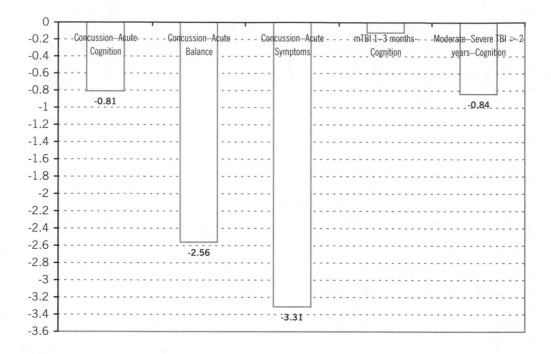

FIGURE 14.2. Meta-analytic effect sizes: Adverse effects of mTBI on functioning. As a rule, the studies in the meta-analyses do not involve children, but some involve high school athletes. Effect sizes typically are expressed in pooled, weighted standard deviation units. However, across studies, there are some minor variations in the methods of calculation. Sport-related concussion–acute from Broglio and Puetz (2008); mTBI 1–3 months and moderate–severe > 24 months in Schretlen and Shapiro (2003).

objective evidence of cognitive and balance impairments, concussions are associated with widespread physical (e.g., headaches, dizziness, nausea, light and noise sensitivity, fatigue, hypersomnia/insomnia) and neurobehavioral (e.g., irritability, emotional dysregulation) symptoms in the acute postinjury period.

Third, evidence is emerging in the animal literature that there is a "temporal window" of vulnerability during which a second injury results in magnified cognitive and behavioral deficits and greater levels of traumatic axonal injury (Laurer et al., 2001; Longhi et al., 2005; Vagnozzi et al., 2007). That is, mice that are reinjured during this temporal window have worse behavioral and neurobiological outcomes than mice who are reinjured after the temporal window. Taken together, human studies illustrate that concussions can have an enormously adverse effect on subjective symptoms, balance, and cognition in the first 48 hours postinjury—and animal studies show that reinjury during the temporal window can lead to worse outcome. Thus, from a clinical management perspective, promoting rest during the acute recovery period prevents possible magnified pathophysiology attributable to overlapping injuries.

Finally, as described later in this chapter, when animals are allowed to exercise too soon after an injury, they do not show exercise-induced increases in molecular markers of neuroplasticity. Disruptions in cellular function due to metabolic alterations might interfere with the positive effects of exercise on neurobiology. Brain injuries result in alterations such as mitochondrial dysfunction, decreases in blood flow, and changes in glucose metabolism that compromise neuronal functioning and signaling. Theoretically, increasing energy demand during the period of restoration and recovery could compound the hypermetabolism and slow the recovery process. These lines of evidence support the recommendation for rest during the acute recovery period. However, the optimal duration of this rest period following very mild injuries is unknown, but is likely to be days (rather than weeks to months).

EDUCATION AND REASSURANCE
AS AN EARLY INTERVENTION STRATEGY

Most research relating to education and reassurance as a treatment intervention following mTBI has been done with adults. In general, adults who participate in these early intervention programs, consisting of educational materials plus various additional treatments and/or assessments (e.g., neuropsychological testing, meeting with a therapist, reassurance, access to a multidisciplinary team), report fewer postconcussion symptoms at 3 months postinjury (Ponsford et al., 2001, 2002) and at 6 months postinjury (Minderhoud, Boelens, Huizenga, & Saan, 1980; Mittenberg, Tremont, Zielinski, Fichera, & Rayls, 1996; Wade, King, Wenden, Crawford, & Caldwell, 1998) compared to adults who receive standard hospital treatment. The educational brochures or sessions typically provide information regarding common symptoms, likely time course of recovery, reassurance of recovery, and suggested coping strategies following mTBI (e.g., Mittenberg et al., 1996; Paniak, Toller-Lobe, Reynolds, Melnyk, & Nagy, 2000; Ponsford et al., 2002; Wade et al., 1998).

Ponsford and colleagues (2001) conducted the only study involving early education and reassurance intervention for children who have sustained mTBIs. One group of children with mTBIs was assessed at 1 week and 3 months postinjury, and a second group was assessed at 3 months only. The first group received an information brochure describing symptoms and coping strategies, and those seen only at 3 months did not receive this booklet. The symptoms resolved for most children by 3 months postinjury. Children with a previous brain injury or a history of learning or behavior problems were more likely to report ongoing symptoms. The group that received the information booklet reported fewer symptoms at 3 months postinjury than the group that did not receive this booklet.

There are a number of recommendations for managing mTBI in children. First, children should rest during the acute stage of recovery; they should reduce physical and cognitive activities. Second, in collaboration with their parents, children should monitor their symptoms and discuss them with their doctor. Third, some students, after returning to school, might benefit from (a) taking rest breaks as needed, (b) spending fewer hours at school, (c) being given more time to take tests or complete assignments, (d) receiving help with schoolwork, and/or (e) reducing time spent on the computer, reading, or writing (*www.cdc.gov/concussion/pdf/TBI_factsheet_ TEACHERS-508-a.pdf*). Finally, returning to sports or vigorous physical activity should be a gradual and stepwise process. These strategies are effective for most children, most of the time. For those who have poor outcome after following these recommendations, however, alternative and innovative management strategies are needed.

RATIONALE FOR EXERCISE AS TREATMENT

Converging lines of evidence suggest that exercise should be included as a core component of treatment for children and adults who have poor long-term outcome following mTBI. The evidence presented in this section converges to illustrate some of the benefits of exercise, and particularly of aerobic endurance exercise, on brain health and functioning. This evidence comes from both animal and human studies—the human studies are mostly with adults and older adults.

Neuroplasticity

Exercise facilitates molecular markers of neuroplasticity and promotes neurogenesis (Michelini & Stern, 2009; Neeper, Gomez-Pinilla, Choi, & Cotman, 1995; van Praag, 2008). One of the key molecules that exercise increases is brain-derived neurotrophic factor (BDNF; see glossary of neuroscience terms in Table 14.1). BDNF is well known for increasing neuronal survival and facilitating long-term potentiation (LTP; Kang, Welcher, Shelton, & Schuman, 1997; Suen et al., 1997). LTP is one of the key mechanisms underlying synaptic plasticity and is thought to have a vital role in the formation of memories. BDNF expression is, in large part, activity dependent (Thoenen, 1995). Exercise-induced BDNF increases are prevalent in the hippocampus, a region of the brain that is involved with long-term memory (Neeper et al., 1995). Because of its beneficial effects, delivery of BDNF to the traumatically injured brain has been pursued. However, because BDNF does not freely cross the blood–brain barrier, exogenous delivery of BDNF to the brain has been challenging. The fact that exercise increases BDNF in an endogenous manner makes it particularly relevant for TBI treatment and rehabilitation. Other growth factors that are increased with exercise are vascular endothelial growth factor (VEGF; Fabel et al., 2003) and insulin-like growth factor 1 (IGF 1; Carro, Trejo, Busiguina, & Torres-Aleman, 2001). Both VEGF and IGF are known to increase vascularization and neuronal proliferation.

In addition to growth factors, exercise increases other proteins that enhance neural function and cognitive performance. Proteins such as synapsin I, calcium/calmodulin-dependent protein kinase II (CaMKII), and cyclic-AMP response-element-binding protein (CREB) have been found to increase with exercise. These exercise-induced increases in synapsin I, CaMKII and CREB are also observed after experimental brain injury, as they are typically seen in the uninjured brain (see Table 14.1; Griesbach, Hovda, Molteni, Wu, & Gomez-Pinilla, 2004b). Multiple other effects of exercise have an influence on synaptic plasticity and neural protection. For example, exercise has been shown to increase angiogenic factors (Ding et al., 2004), reduce oxidative stress (Navarro, Gomez, Lopez-Cepero, & Boveris, 2004; Pan et

TABLE 14.1. Glossary of Neuroscience Terms

Term	Function	Effects of exercise
Angiogenesis	It is the growth of new blood vessels, also known as *vascularization*.	It is found to occur with exercise.
Brain-derived neurotrophic factor (BDNF)	It is a protein in the neurotrophin family of growth factors. This protein can facilitate the growth and differentiation of new neurons and synapses. BDNF helps with neuronal survival after injury and facilitates synaptic function.	It increases with exercise (Cotman & Berchtold, 2002; Neeper et al., 1995).
Calcium/calmodulin-dependent protein kinase II (CaMKII)	It facilitates synaptic plasticity through the regulation of glutamate receptors.	It increases with exercise (Vaynman, Ying, & Gomez-Pinilla, 2003).
Cytokines	These are intercellular messengers with pro- or anti-inflammatory properties.	Some cytokines that are involved in neurodegenerative diseases decrease with exercise (Ang, Wong, Moochhala, & Ng, 2004; Ding, Vaynman, Souda, Whitelegge, & Gomez-Pinilla, 2006).
Growth factors	Proteins (and other substances) that can stimulate cell growth, differentiation, and proliferation.	These are increased with exercise (Neeper, Gomez-Pinilla, Choi, & Cotman, 1996).
Insulin-like growth factor 1 (IGF1)	Hormone involved in growth and tissue remodeling that has been found to be involved in neurogenesis and neuroprotection.	It increases with exercise (Carro et al., 2001).
Long-term potentiation (LTP)	Increase in neuronal signal transmission that is believed to underlie learning and memory.	It is facilitated with exercise (Farmer et al., 2004).
Neurotrophins	A family of proteins that facilitates the development, growth, function, and survival of neurons.	Some neurotrophins, such as BDNF, are increased with exercise.
Neuronal proliferation	Also known as neurogenesis or the formation of new neuronal cells.	It is facilitated with exercise (van Praag et al., 1999).
Oxidative stress	Results in the production of free radicals that can compromise cell function and lead to cell death.	Exercise decreases oxidized proteins (Griesbach et al., 2008; Navarro et al., 2004).
Synaptogenesis	It is the formation of synapses and results in the increase of intracellular signaling.	It is increased with exercise.
Vascular endothelial growth factor (VEGF)	Family of cytokines that stimulate blood vessel growth.	It is increased with exercise (Fabel et al., 2003).

al., 2007; Wu, Ying, & Gomez-Pinilla, 2004), and increase hippocampal cerebral blood flow. It has also been shown to increase hippocampal neurogenesis (van Praag, Christie, Sejnowski, & Gage, 1999; van Praag, Shubert, Zhao, & Gage, 2005) and increase an array of genes involved in synaptic plasticity (Tong, Shen, Perreau, Balazs, & Cotman, 2001).

Neurotransmitter Systems and Mental Health

Exercise is associated with changes in the neurotransmitter systems of the brain. The glutamatergic, dopaminergic, noradrenergic, and serotonergic systems demonstrate particular benefits (Chaouloff, 1989; Molteni, Ying, & Gomez-Pinilla, 2002), which in turn contribute to improved mood and to a general sense of well-being (Callaghan, 2004; Conn, 2010; Duman, 2005). In adults, exercise can be an effective treatment for mild and even more severe depression (Babyak et al., 2000; Daley, 2008; Dunn, Trivedi, Kampert, Clark, & Chambliss, 2005; Lawlor & Hopker, 2001; Mead et al., 2008, 2009; Penninx et al., 2002; Rethorst, Wipfli, & Landers, 2009), but its use in clinical practice remains limited, especially as an adjunct to established treatment approaches such as psychotherapy or pharmacotherapy (Strohle, 2009).

The effect of exercise on anxiety has been examined in many studies with adults (Barbour, Edenfield, & Blumenthal, 2007; Greenwood & Fleshner, 2008; Herring, O'Connor, & Dishman, 2010; Wang et al., 2010). Broman-Fulks and Storey (2008) reported that brief aerobic exercise is associated with reduction in anxiety sensitivity (i.e., the tendency to fear and dwell upon anxiety-related symptoms). Smits and colleagues (2008) randomly assigned participants with elevated anxiety sensitivity to a 2-week exercise intervention, exercise plus cognitive therapy, and wait-list control. Both exercise conditions resulted in a large beneficial change in anxiety sensitivity. Merom and colleagues randomized clinical patients with anxiety disorders to group cognitive behavior therapy with either exercise or educational information as an adjunct. Patients in the exercise groups reported greater improvement in anxiety and stress (Merom et al., 2008). In a meta-analysis of the effects of exercise on anxiety, Wipfli, Rethorst, and Landers (2008) reported an overall effect size of −0.48. This medium effect size represents a substantial reduction in anxiety among exercise groups compared to no-treatment control groups.

Cognitive Functioning

Most research relating to exercise and cognitive functioning has been conducted with adults and older adults. In a meta-analysis of 29 studies, people who were randomly assigned to receive aerobic exercise training had small improvements in attention, processing speed, memory, and executive functioning (Smith et al., 2010). The mechanisms by which exercise and level of fitness are associated with improved cognition are not well understood. In fact, another meta-analysis of the literature concluded that the cardiovascular–aerobic fitness hypothesis, as the primary mechanism or mediator for the relation between exercise and improved cognition, is not supported. These authors encouraged additional research on other physiological and psychological variables that might influence the relation between exercise and cognition (Etnier, Nowell, Landers, & Sibley, 2006).

The direct and indirect effects of exercise, and overall fitness, on brain functioning, cognition, and academic performance in children have been a topic of considerable interest. In a study of 259 public school children, aerobic capacity was positively associated, and body mass was negatively associated, with academic achievement. Greater aerobic fitness was associated with better performance in reading and mathematics (Castelli, Hillman, Buck, & Erwin, 2007). Davis and colleagues randomized sedentary overweight children to low-dose exercise, high-dose exercise, or a control condition. The exercise sessions were 5 days per week for 15 weeks. Those in the high-dose exercise group performed better on a test of executive functioning than children in the control group (Davis et al., 2007). Groups of children with varying levels of fitness have also been studied on specific cognitive tasks. For example, children have been classified as having higher fitness levels versus lower fitness levels and then compared on cognitive testing, such as memory and executive functioning. In some studies, children with high fitness levels perform better on cognitive testing (Buck, Hillman, & Castelli, 2008; Chaddock, Hillman, Buck, & Cohen, 2011). Researchers have designed experiments in which children complete cognitive tasks before and after an aerobic exercise session, in comparison to before and after rest or sedentary activities. Children tend to perform better on tests of attention and executive functioning after the exercise session (Hillman et al., 2009). In a study of adolescents, an exercise session was not associated with improved electrophysiological indices of cognitive control—but level of fitness was (Stroth et al., 2009).

Fitness and Brain Morphology

Recently, researchers have investigated the association between fitness and brain morphology in children. Chaddock and colleagues (2010a) reported that children with greater fitness levels showed greater bilateral hippocampal volumes and better performance on a memory test than children with lower fitness levels. This research team also examined the relation between level of fitness and basal ganglia morphology in children. Children with greater fitness levels showed greater volumes of the dorsal (but not ventral) striatum relative to children with lesser fitness levels. The children with greater fitness also performed better on a test of attentional control (Chaddock et al., 2010b).

Self-Esteem

Exercise is associated with higher ratings of self-esteem (Ekeland, Heian, Hagen, Abbott, & Nordheim, 2004). When examining if exercise alone or exercise as part of a comprehensive intervention could improve self-esteem among children and young adolescents, Ekeland et al. (2004) reported that exercise has positive short-term effects on self-esteem in children and young people while having positive effects on general physical health.

Sleep, Pain, and Headaches

Exercise is associated with improved sleep quality (Youngstedt, 2005). Furthermore, evidence indicates that exercise is associated with reduced pain and disability in patients with chronic low back pain (Bell & Burnett, 2009; Henchoz & Kai-Lik So, 2008), and it has been studied for its beneficial effects on the treatment of migraines and other types of headaches. Headaches are one of the hallmark symptoms of mTBI in children, and it is a symptom that they complain about when they fail to recover swiftly after their injury. Researchers have reported that regular long-term aerobic exercise reduces migraine frequency, severity, and duration (Koseoglu, Akboyraz, Soyuer, & Ersoy, 2003; Lockett & Campbell, 1992), possibly due to increased nitric oxide production (Narin, Pinar, Erbas, Ozturk, & Idiman, 2003); however, methodological limitations with research in this area may limit confidence in these findings (Busch & Gaul, 2008). In many studies, investigators use submaximal aerobic exercise, with intensities varying between 50 and 85% of maximal heart rate, to explore the impact of exercises on migraines.

Exercise as Treatment for Brain Injury in Animals

Both clinical and animal studies have indicated that exercise has neuroprotective qualities and is beneficial for physical and mental health. What remains uncertain is if and when it should be implemented after brain injury, and more specifically after an mTBI. In other words, it is not clear whether the beneficial effects of exercise are dependent on a specific time window, and we do not know if recovery can be hampered if exercise is implemented too early. Several studies relating to exercise following brain injuries in animals have been conducted by Griesbach and colleagues. These rodent exercise studies indicate that a therapeutic window should be taken into consideration when utilizing voluntary exercise to enhance neural function following the concussive injury model of fluid percussion brain injury (FPI; an experimental method for inducing mild–moderate brain injuries; Griesbach et al., 2004b). Rats underwent an FPI and were housed with or without access to a voluntary running wheel. Exercise began either the day of the injury or 2 weeks afterward. The beneficial effects of exercise were found only if exercise was delayed. The animals that were given access to a running wheel from 14 to 21 days postinjury did show an increase in BDNF and other molecular markers of plasticity. Injured rats with the delayed exercise also performed better on a hippocampal-dependent learning and memory task when compared to sedentary FPI rats with the same postinjury delay. A later study showed that the exercise-induced increase in BDNF was associated with better performance on a learning and memory task, in that BDNF blockade reversed the cognitive effects of exercise (Griesbach, Sutton, Hovda, Ying, & Gomez-Pinilla, 2009). However, rats that were allowed to exercise during the first week postinjury failed to show an increase in BDNF and other target proteins, such as synapsin I and CREB. In addition, the acutely exercised FPI rats also performed worse in the behavioral task when compared to injured rats that were not exercised and were tested at the same postinjury time (Griesbach et al., 2004b). Moreover, molecular markers of plasticity that increased in sedentary counterparts were reduced when rats were acutely exercised (in the first week postinjury; Griesbach, Gomez-Pinilla, & Hovda, 2004a). These findings suggest that premature exercise compromises compensatory responses to the injury. In these studies, early physiological stimulation through voluntary exercise reduced the capacity for neuroplasticity.

Animal studies also suggest that the time window is dependent on the particular characteristics or severity of the injury, such that the necessary delay for exercise to be effective after an FPI is severity dependent (Griesbach, Gomez-Pinilla, & Hovda, 2007). Along these lines, variations in the biomechanical forces and region of damage might influence the outcome of exercise. When rats were allowed to exercise acutely following a controlled cortical impact injury, an increase in BDNF was observed (Griesbach, Hovda, Gomez-Pinilla, & Sutton, 2008). In contrast to the FPI model that was used in the previously mentioned studies, the controlled cortical impact injury results in an area of pronounced focal cell death with less diffusivity. In the cortical impact study, notably, the injured rats chose not to exercise as much in the first 3 days after the injury compared to rats that underwent an FPI.

The reasons for the lack of exercise-induced increases in BDNF during a "temporal window" are unknown. Disruptions in cellular function due to postinjury metabolic alterations might interfere with the effects of exercise. TBI results in alterations such as mitochondrial dysfunction, decreases in blood flow, and changes in glucose metabolism that compromise neuronal functioning and signaling. During the early postinjury period, cerebral metabolism is likely to be dedicated to restoring cerebral function. Thus, placing an energy demand on the system, through exercise, can compromise restorative events. In addition TBI disrupts the regulation of stress hormones, such as corticosteroids, which are known to influence BDNF expression. A recent study in rats indicated that the stress response is heightened for the first week postinjury after a mild FPI (Griesbach, Hovda, Tio, & Taylor, 2011). This finding raises the possibility that elevations in glucocorticoids, which are known to suppress levels of BDNF and CREB, contribute to the undesired effects (i.e., poor performance in the water maze and suppression of molecular markers of plasticity) of early exercise that have been observed after FPI.

The translation of findings in animal studies to humans is not straightforward. As indicated above, the response to exercise appears to be dependent on the injury characteristics (e.g., more severe injuries require longer rest periods prior to exercise). In contrast to animal studies that control for subject and injury homogeneity, studying the effects of exercise in injured human subjects is challenging due to the diversity of the subjects and injury characteristics, as well as lack of consistency within and between studies in regard to postinjury assessment intervals.

HUMAN STUDIES INVOLVING EXERCISE AND ACTIVITY LEVEL FOLLOWING mTBI

Guidelines for returning children to physical activity following injury are typically derived from adult recommendations, which in turn are usually based on expert consensus rather than empirical data. Generally, the consensus-based standard of care requires that symptomatic children be restricted from participating in physical activity (McCrory et al., 2009; Purcell, 2009). While symptoms are present, both cognitive and physical rest are advocated to allow the restoration of normal brain metabolism and resolution of disrupted physiological activity (Giza & Hovda, 2001). Due to obvious methodological and ethical issues, very little human research is available on the relationship between activity levels in the acute postinjury period, or on the duration of a rest period in relation to the resolution or persistence of symptoms.

Majerske and colleagues (2008) studied 86 high school student athletes who were retrospectively assigned to one of the following five groups, based on their self-reported postconcussion activity level at the time of their follow-up visits to a concussion clinic: (1) no school or exercise activity (n = 35); (2) school activity only (n = 77); (3) school activity and light activity at home (e.g., slow jogging, mowing the lawn; n = 57); (4) school activity and sports practice (n = 26); (5) school activity and participation in a sports game (n = 9) (Majerske et al., 2008). The group that seemed to function the best cognitively was #3 (school and light activity at home), and the group that functioned the worst cognitively was #5 (school and return to competition). This quasi-experimental retrospective cohort study is interesting and provocative, but does not allow causal inferences. It suggests a relationship, however, between activity level and cognitive functioning acutely and postacutely following injury. The lack of clear information about the time lapse between injury and complete symptom recovery, as well as activity level in relation to the acuteness of the injury, makes it difficult to interpret the results when trying to determine the optimal duration of a recommended rest period following injury.

Using a different approach, McCrea et al. (2009) explored the impact of a symptom-free waiting period on clinical outcome and risk of reinjury after sport-related concussions in high school and college athletes. In their prospective, nonrandomized study, 635 athletes with concussion were grouped based on the presence and duration of a symptom-free waiting period before they returned to sports participation after their injury. The majority of athletes (60.3%) observed a symptom-free waiting period that lasted from 1 day to 7 days or more. The other athletes returned to play immediately after symptom resolution or, for some, prior to complete recovery from the concussion. No differences in outcome 45 or 90 days postinjury could be found between the two groups. With regard to risks of sustaining a second concussion during the same playing season, the researchers reported that although the overall incidence of repeat concussions was low (3.78%), the overwhelming majority of them occurred within 10 days of the initial injury, whether the athlete had observed a symptom-free waiting period or not. This finding was presented as supporting the hypothesis of a time-sensitive window of cerebral vulnerability postconcussion.

Both of these studies are worthy of note in that they are among the first to challenge a common consensus-based guideline recommendation (McCrory et al., 2009) supporting the application of a symptom-free waiting period with all concussed athletes, and an even longer one in younger children. The nonrandomized nature of the designs precludes definitive conclusions, but they are a first step in trying to determine the optimal duration of a symptom-free waiting period or even if the need for this waiting period is supported by empirical evidence. The methodology used in these studies relies on retrospective or secondary analyses of data collected clinically as part of routine care, or from other ongoing studies, illustrating the inherent ethical difficulties in manipulating level of activity participation following concussion in human subjects. Although most experts agree that initial rest is beneficial, at least until symptom resolution, when children are slow to recover following an mTBI, the literature does not provide specific recommendations regarding rehabilitation strategies. Rather, in sports at least, the recommendation is simply to rest and limit activities. With no mention of a time limit, clinicians are left with little information regarding treatment strategies to promote recovery in more complex cases.

Exercise as Treatment for mTBI in Humans

In a retrospective survey study of adults who had sustained TBIs of all severities, Gordon and colleagues (1998) reported that those individuals who engaged in exercise reported fewer symptoms of depression and better general health status than those who did not exercise. In a series of experimental treatment studies with adults who had sustained moderate–severe TBIs, Driver and colleagues showed that aquatic exercise is associated with improved self-esteem, health-promoting behaviors, and improved psychological functioning (Driver & Ede, 2009; Driver, O'Connor, Lox, & Rees, 2004; Driver, Rees, O'Connor, & Lox, 2006). Gemmell and Leathem (2006) provided a 6-week course of tai chi to a small sample of individuals with TBIs. Compared to a wait-list control group, they reported significant improvements in psychological functioning and mental health. Blake and Batson (2009) also reported that participation in tai chi was associated with improvements in self-esteem and psychological functioning in adults with TBIs.

In terms of mTBI, Iverson and colleagues developed the British Columbia Concussion Rehabilitation Program (BC-CRP), based on mental and physical circuit training, for injured adults with workers' compensation claims who were slow to recover (Iverson, Brooks, Azevedo, & Gaetz, 2006). A "circuit" consists of 14 minutes of sustained mental activity (i.e., Connors Continuous Performance Test—Second Edition), followed by sustained physical activity (i.e., exercise bike for 15 minutes), then a 15-minute rest period. A "session" consists of three circuits, lasting 2.5 hours. Sessions are done daily, 3–5 days per week. Pre- and postsession concussion symptom ratings are obtained for each session, using an abbreviated version of the Post-Concussion Scale. A person progresses, in stages, after completing *three consecutive sessions without significant symptom elevation*. Each stage has an increasingly intense physical component (increasing bike tension and increasing revolutions per minute—tailored to the individual needs and physical conditioning of the injured worker), but maintains the same cognitive and rest components. Outside the circuit training, we reinforce the importance of maintaining daily activity, such as 15- to 30-minute walks with family or friends and cognitive activities such as reading, sudoko, and crosswords. Counseling regarding good sleep hygiene is provided. The BC-CRP is well suited for injured workers with protracted recovery from an mTBI. It provides active rehabilitation, physical and mental conditioning, and is easily provided in conjunction with education, psychotherapy, counseling, and/or work-specific rehabilitation. This program, however, has not been studied in clinical research or clinical trials to evaluate its efficacy.

Similarly, Leddy et al. (2010) set out to test the safety and effectiveness of subsymptom threshold exercise training for the treatment of postconcussion syndrome in adults. In their study, individuals who had been experiencing postconcussion symptoms at rest for more than 6 weeks (mean duration of 19 weeks) were enrolled in an intervention consisting of aerobic exercises of a duration and intensity determined with the administration of a graded treadmill test. Individuals reported no adverse events during the intervention, experienced resolution of their postconcussion symptoms, and had a successful return to activities (sports or work).

THE MONTREAL CHILDREN'S HOSPITAL ACTIVE REHABILITATION PROGRAM FOR SLOW-TO-RECOVER CHILDREN AND ADOLESCENTS

Children who fail to recover in the expected time from an mTBI pose a challenge to practitioners involved in their care, whether in the context of sports teams, school involvement, or within the health care system. For these slow-to-recover children who fail to return to preinjury status after the expected initial recovery period, guidelines are broad, unclear with regard to interventions, and unhelpful to the professionals who are faced with determining the best approach to management. The Montreal Children's Hospital (MCH) is a tertiary care pediatric university teaching hospital, and as part of the trauma programs within the institution, an mTBI (or concussion) clinic serves two specific groups of children. First, children who have been asymptomatic at rest for 5–7 days undergo a physical and cognitive exertion test as part of their gradual return-to-activities protocol. Children in this group thus benefit from an opportunity to become increasingly active in a supervised environment, to ensure that they remain asymptomatic under cognitive and cardiovascular stress. The second group of children is composed of those who remain symptomatic at rest 4 weeks after their mTBI, for whom the term *slow to recover* has been used. As stated previously, current consensus-based recommendations focus on a period of physical and cognitive rest until symptom resolution, with a gradual return to activity once symptoms subside. If those symptoms persist, children and teens are faced with a prolonged period of inactivity and a "wait-and-see" approach that may itself contribute to the persistence of symptoms, as it can with any athletic injury. A rehabilitation intervention that aims at facilitating recovery, therefore, appeared as an appropriate step. Faced with the mission of returning children who were slow to recover to activities (academic and physical) after their mTBI, clinicians in the MCH trauma programs designed an innovative active rehabilitation program that is described in Gagnon, Galli, Friedman, Grilli, and Iverson (2009).

The approach used at the MCH is based on a theoretical model anchored in current neuroscience evidence, as well as on the clinical expertise of professionals involved in the care of children with mTBI. Before children enter the intervention, a screening of general neurological status, balance, coordination, cognitive functioning, and postconcussion symptoms is performed to document preintervention status as well as to determine if there are any contraindications to exercise. Before beginning the active rehabilitation protocol, children are also assessed by a neuropsychologist who conducts a clinical interview aimed at establishing preinjury cognitive, psychosocial, and emotional functioning—and exploring possible personal factors contributing to the persistence of symptoms.

The graded rehabilitation is comprised of four components. First, submaximal (60% maximal capacity) aerobic training is provided for up to 15 minutes. Second, light coordination exercises, up to 10 minutes, are tailored to the child's favorite activity or main sport. Third, visualization and imagery techniques are introduced. Finally, a home program allows continued training outside the clinic, thus facilitating school attendance and minimizing disruptions to the child's daily life. The program is summarized in Figure 14.3.

All program activities are based on principles derived from a variety of the studies discussed in this chapter and also summarized in Gagnon et al. (2009). For the *aerobic* component, children are asked to choose between fast-paced walking/light jogging on a treadmill or peddling a stationary bicycle, both of which can be used in conjunction with an interactive gaming system (e.g., Nintendo Wii) to provide distraction and further enjoyment of the activity. Using a portable heart rate monitor (e.g., Polar monitor and chest strap), children are instructed to exercise at a maximal heart rate corresponding to 60% of their maximal capacity for no more than 15 minutes. *Coordination* exercises are tailored to the child's favorite sport or physical activity and last a maximum of 10 minutes. Heart rate continues to be monitored throughout this phase of the program. If at any point during the physical exertion (aerobic activities and coordination exercises), any of the symptoms found on the Post-Concussion Scale—Revised appear or increase, the activity is terminated and the duration recorded. *Visualization* and imagery techniques are introduced as a third component to reinitiate positive experiences in relation to participation in physical activity. The child is asked to choose a motor component of his or her sport or favorite activity at which he or she is usually successful and that is finite in duration (e.g., a particular football drill). The physical therapist discusses the technique of positive visualization and proceeds to practice with the child in the clinic to achieve realistic timing and motor imagery of the chosen activity. Throughout the components of the intervention, children and their families are provided reassurance and engaged in a

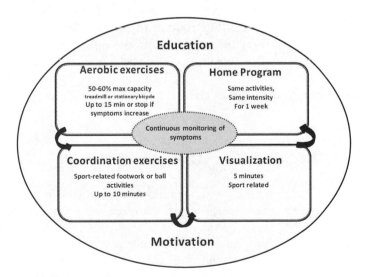

FIGURE 14.3. Montreal Children's Hospital rehabilitation after concussion program. From Gagnon, Galli, Friedman, Grilli, and Iverson (2009). Copyright 2009 by Taylor & Francis Ltd. Reprinted by permission.

discussion that reviews information regarding the likely time course of recovery and general coping strategies that they were given during the acute period postinjury. This component helps to determine the personal meaning and impact of the mTBI on the child and parents, and its consequences on their daily lives. Clinicians also watch for, and address, the impact of other life stressors on children's symptoms. Strong emotional reactions to having symptoms or overpathologizing the symptoms can also be addressed. These discussions are a segue for teaching coping skills to the child and parent to reduce their stress and anxiety.

The final component is a home program that includes all parts of the intervention. The home program lasts approximately 20 minutes daily (monitored with the use of a log) and is continued until the next planned weekly visit to the clinic for reassessment. The child and parents are also instructed to interrupt the home session and contact the Neurotrauma Program if any worsening of symptoms occurs. Finally, the child is followed weekly until symptom-free at rest for 1 week. At that time, the standard return-to-activity protocol, including exertion testing and graded return to activities, is initiated.

Outcome from participation in this intervention has been positive, although results remain anecdotal without the inclusion of a proper control group to gather empirical data. In Gagnon et al. (2009), a case series of 16 individuals who successfully returned to their activities following the active rehabilitation protocol is presented. Satisfaction with the intervention was reported as high and qualitative comments suggested greater empowerment for both children and parents when compared to their state prior to entering the program. Further testing of the intervention is underway to identify a subgroup of individuals who may benefit the most from such an approach.

Both this pediatric rehabilitation approach and the adult examples presented previously have advanced the concept that supervised and controlled aerobic exercise may be beneficial for individuals who fail to recover readily after an mTBI. Although these strategies appear promising, they remain in exploratory stages. To date, little emphasis has been placed on trying to determine the optimal "dosage" or protocol to use with clinical patients. Moreover, none of the reported studies used a control group of equivalent slow-to-recover individuals randomized to different intervention strategies, thus making it difficult to attribute recovery solely to the proposed rehabilitation programs.

CONCLUSIONS AND FUTURE DIRECTIONS

Fortunately, most children who experience mild brain injuries in sports or daily life recover swiftly. A minority, however, do not. Children who are slow to recover present a challenge to the health care system. At present, no evidence-based guidelines exist for how to manage children who experience atypical recovery. In the initial days following injury, both mental and physical rest have been strongly encouraged (McCrory et al., 2005, 2009). The optimal time period for rest, however, is unknown. From a practical perspective, children need to, and naturally will, transition back into an active lifestyle. Clinicians must decide when to transition from activity restrictions and watchful waiting to more active treatment and rehabilitation.

There is evolving interest in using exercise as an adjunctive treatment for people who have sustained TBIs (Devine & Zafonte, 2009; Lojovich, 2010; Mossberg, Amonette, & Masel, 2010). Converging lines of diverse medical and scientific evidence support the use of exercise as a core component of treatment for children and adults who have poor outcome from mTBI. However, some important questions remain unanswered. The optimal period of rest following injury is unknown, and it might differ across the lifespan. Similarly, we do not know when it is most clinically efficacious to begin increasing a child's activity levels. We do not know the most beneficial types of exercise, or the best frequency, intensity, and duration of training sessions. We do not know the dispositional and/or clinical characteristics of injured children that might facilitate or hinder the beneficial treatment effects of exercise. A tremendous amount of research will be necessary to answer these questions. With time, we are confident that clinical researchers will make important advances that will facilitate evidence-based recommendations for treatment and rehabilitation of children who are slow to recover after mTBI.

REFERENCES

Ang, E. T., Wong, P. T., Moochhala, S., & Ng, Y. K. (2004). Cytokine changes in the horizontal diagonal band of Broca in the septum after running and stroke: A correlation to glial activation. *Neuroscience, 129*(2), 337–347.

Babyak, M., Blumenthal, J. A., Herman, S., Khatri, P., Doraiswamy, M., Moore, K., et al. (2000). Exercise treatment for major depression: Maintenance of therapeutic benefit at 10 months. *Psychosomatic Medicine, 62*, 633–638.

Bäckman, L., Jones, S., Berger, A. K., Laukka, E. J., & Small, B. J. (2005). Cognitive impairment in preclinical Alzheimer's disease: A meta-analysis. *Neuropsychology, 19*(4), 520–531.

Barbour, K. A., Edenfield, T. M., & Blumenthal, J. A. (2007). Exercise as a treatment for depression and other psychiatric disorders: A review. *Journal of Cardiopulmonary Rehabilitation and Prevention, 27*(6), 359–367.

Belanger, H. G., & Vanderploeg, R. D. (2005). The neuropsychological impact of sports-related concussion: A meta-analysis. *Journal of the International Neuropsychological Society, 11*(4), 345–357.

Bell, J. A., & Burnett, A. (2009). Exercise for the primary, secondary and tertiary prevention of low back pain in the workplace: A systematic review. *Journal of Occupational Rehabilitation, 19*(1), 8–24.

Blake, H., & Batson, M. (2009). Exercise intervention in brain injury: A pilot randomized study of tai chi qigong. *Clinical Rehabilitation, 23*(7), 589–598.

Broglio, S. P., & Puetz, T. W. (2008). The effect of sport concussion on neurocognitive function, self-report symptoms, and postural control: A meta-analysis. *Sports Medicine, 38*(1), 53–67.

Broman-Fulks, J. J., & Storey, K. M. (2008). Evaluation of a brief aerobic exercise intervention for high anxiety sensitivity. *Anxiety, Stress, and Coping, 21*(2), 117–128.

Buck, S. M., Hillman, C. H., & Castelli, D. M. (2008). The relation of aerobic fitness to Stroop task performance in preadolescent children. *Medicine and Science in Sports and Exercise, 40*(1), 166–172.

Busch, V., & Gaul, C. (2008). Exercise in migraine therapy: Is there any evidence for efficacy? A critical review. *Headache, 48*(6), 890–899.

Callaghan, P. (2004). Exercise: A neglected intervention in mental health care? *Journal of Psychiatry and Mental Health Nursing*, *11*(4), 476–483.

Carro, E., Trejo, J. L., Busiguina, S., & Torres-Aleman, I. (2001). Circulating insulin-like growth factor I mediates the protective effects of physical exercise against brain insults of different etiology and anatomy. *Journal of Neuroscience*, *21*(15), 5678–5684.

Castelli, D. M., Hillman, C. H., Buck, S. M., & Erwin, H. E. (2007). Physical fitness and academic achievement in third- and fifth-grade students. *Journal of Sport and Exercise Psychology*, *29*(2), 239–252.

Chaddock, L., Erickson, K. I., Prakash, R. S., Kim, J. S., Voss, M. W., Vanpatter, M., et al. (2010a). A neuroimaging investigation of the association between aerobic fitness, hippocampal volume, and memory performance in preadolescent children. *Brain Research*, *1358*, 172–183.

Chaddock, L., Erickson, K. I., Prakash, R. S., VanPatter, M., Voss, M. W., Pontifex, M. B., et al. (2010b). Basal ganglia volume is associated with aerobic fitness in preadolescent children. *Developmental Neuroscience*, *32*(3), 249–256.

Chaddock, L., Hillman, C. H., Buck, S. M., & Cohen, N. J. (2011). Aerobic fitness and executive control of relational memory in preadolescent children. *Medicine and Science in Sports and Exercise*, *43*(2), 344–349.

Chaouloff, F. (1989). Physical exercise and brain monoamines: A review. *Acta Physiologica Scandinavia*, *137*, 1–13.

Conn, V. S. (2010). Depressive symptom outcomes of physical activity interventions: Meta-analysis findings. *Annals of Behavioral Medicine*, *39*(2), 128–138.

Cotman, C. W., & Berchtold, N. C. (2002). Exercise: A behavioral intervention to enhance brain health and plasticity. *Trends in Neurosciences*, *25*(6), 295–301.

Daley, A. (2008). Exercise and depression: A review of reviews. *Journal of Clinical Psychology in Medical Settings*, *15*(2), 140–147.

Davis, C. L., Tomporowski, P. D., Boyle, C. A., Waller, J. L., Miller, P. H., Naglieri, J. A., et al. (2007). Effects of aerobic exercise on overweight children's cognitive functioning: A randomized controlled trial. *Research Quarterly for Exercise and Sport*, *78*(5), 510–519.

Devine, J. M., & Zafonte, R. D. (2009). Physical exercise and cognitive recovery in acquired brain injury: A review of the literature. *PM & R: The Journal of Injury, Function, and Rehabilitation*, *1*(6), 560–575.

Ding, Q., Vaynman, S., Souda, P., Whitelegge, J. P., & Gomez-Pinilla, F. (2006). Exercise affects energy metabolism and neural plasticity-related proteins in the hippocampus as revealed by proteomic analysis. *European Journal of Neuroscience*, *24*(5), 1265–1276.

Ding, Y. H., Luan, X. D., Li, J., Rafols, J. A., Guthinkonda, M., Diaz, F. G., et al. (2004). Exercise-induced overexpression of angiogenic factors and reduction of ischemia/reperfusion injury in stroke. *Current Neurovascular Research*, *1*(5), 411–420.

Driver, S., & Ede, A. (2009). Impact of physical activity on mood after TBI. *Brain Injury*, *23*(3), 203–212.

Driver, S., O'Connor, J., Lox, C., & Rees, K. (2004). Evaluation of an aquatics programme on fitness parameters of individuals with a brain injury. *Brain Injury*, *18*(9), 847–859.

Driver, S., Rees, K., O'Connor, J., & Lox, C. (2006). Aquatics, health-promoting self-care behaviours and adults with brain injuries. *Brain Injury*, *20*(2), 133–141.

Duman, R. S. (2005). Neurotrophic factors and regulation of mood: Role of exercise, diet and metabolism. *Neurobiology of Aging*, *26*(Suppl. 1), 88–93.

Dunn, A. L., Trivedi, M. H., Kampert, J. B., Clark, C. G., & Chambliss, H. O. (2005). Exercise treatment for depression: Efficacy and dose response. *American Journal of Preventative Medicine*, *28*(1), 1–8.

Ekeland, E., Heian, F., Hagen, K. B., Abbott, J., & Nordheim, L. (2004). Exercise to improve self-esteem in children and young people. *Cochrane Database of Systematic Reviews* (1), CD003683.

Etnier, J. L., Nowell, P. M., Landers, D. M., & Sibley, B. A. (2006). A meta-regression to examine the relationship between aerobic fitness and cognitive performance. *Brain Research Reviews*, *52*(1), 119–130.

Fabel, K., Tam, B., Kaufer, D., Baiker, A., Simmons, N., Kuo, C. J., et al. (2003). VEGF is necessary for exercise-induced adult hippocampal neurogenesis. *European Journal of Neuroscience*, *18*(10), 2803–2812.

Farmer, J., Zhao, X., van Praag, H., Wodtke, K., Gage, F. H., & Christie, B. R. (2004). Effects of voluntary exercise on synaptic plasticity and gene expression in the dentate gyrus of adult male Sprague–Dawley rats *in vivo*. *Neuroscience*, *124*(1), 71–79.

Gagnon, I., Galli, C., Friedman, D., Grilli, L., & Iverson, G. L. (2009). Active rehabilitation for children who are slow to recover following sport-related concussion. *Brain Injury*, *23*(12), 956–964.

Gemmell, C., & Leathem, J. M. (2006). A study investigating the effects of tai chi chuan: Individuals with traumatic brain injury compared to controls. *Brain Injury*, *20*(2), 151–156.

Giza, C. C., & Hovda, D. A. (2001). The neurometabolic cascade of concussion. *Journal of Athletic Training*, *36*(3), 228–235.

Giza, C. C., & Hovda, D. A. (2004). The pathophysiology of traumatic brain injury. In M. R. Lovell, R. J. Echemendia, J. T. Barth, & M. W. Collins (Eds.), *Traumatic brain injury in sports* (pp. 45–70). Lisse, Switzerland: Swets & Zeitlinger.

Gordon, W. A., Sliwinski, M., Echo, J., McLoughlin, M., Sheerer, M. S., & Meili, T. E. (1998). The benefits of exercise in individuals with traumatic brain injury: A retrospective study. *Journal of Head Trauma Rehabilitation*, *13*(4), 58–67.

Greenwood, B. N., & Fleshner, M. (2008). Exercise, learned helplessness, and the stress-resistant brain. *Neuromolecular Medicine*, *10*(2), 81–98.

Griesbach, G. S., Gomez-Pinilla, F., & Hovda, D. A. (2004a). The upregulation of plasticity-related proteins following TBI is disrupted with acute voluntary exercise. *Brain Research*, *1016*(2), 154–162.

Griesbach, G. S., Gomez-Pinilla, F., & Hovda, D. A. (2007). Time window for voluntary exercise-induced increases in hippocampal neuroplasticity molecules after traumatic brain injury is severity dependent. *Journal of Neurotrauma*, *24*(7), 1161–1171.

Griesbach, G. S., Hovda, D. A., Gomez-Pinilla, F., & Sutton, R. L. (2008). Voluntary exercise or amphetamine treatment, but not the combination, increases hippocampal brain-derived neurotrophic factor and synapsin I following cortical contusion injury in rats. *Neuroscience*, *154*(2), 530–540.

Griesbach, G. S., Hovda, D. A., Molteni, R., Wu, A., & Gomez-Pinilla, F. (2004b). Voluntary exercise following traumatic brain injury: Brain-derived neurotrophic factor upregulation and recovery of function. *Neuroscience*, *125*(1), 129–139.

Griesbach, G. S., Hovda, D. A., Tio, D., & Taylor, A. N. (2011). Heightening of the stress response during the first weeks after a mild traumatic brain injury. *Neuroscience*, *178*, 147–158.

Griesbach, G. S., Sutton, R. L., Hovda, D. A., Ying, Z., & Gomez-Pinilla, F. (2009). Controlled contusion injury alters molecular systems associated with cognitive performance. *Journal of Neuroscience Research*, *87*(3), 795–805.

Henchoz, Y., & Kai-Lik So, A. (2008). Exercise and nonspecific low back pain: A literature review. *Joint Bone Spine*, *75*(5), 533–539.

Herring, M. P., O'Connor, P. J., & Dishman, R. K. (2010). The effect of exercise training on anxiety symptoms among patients: A systematic review. *Archives of Internal Medicine*, *170*(4), 321–331.

Hillman, C. H., Pontifex, M. B., Raine, L. B., Castelli, D. M., Hall, E. E., & Kramer, A. F. (2009). The effect of acute treadmill walking on cognitive control and academic achievement in preadolescent children. *Neuroscience, 159*(3), 1044–1054.

Iverson, G. L., Brooks, B. L., Azevedo, A., & Gaetz, M. (2006, September). *Modifying the British Columbia Concussion Recovery Program for use with injured adults with post-concussion syndrome.* Poster presented at the Brain Injury of the Americas Conference (North American Brain Injury Society—NABIS), Maimi, FL.

Kang, H., Welcher, A. A., Shelton, D., & Schuman, E. M. (1997). Neurotrophins and time: Different roles for TrkB signaling in hippocampal long-term potentiation. *Neuron, 19*(3), 653–664.

Koseoglu, E., Akboyraz, A., Soyuer, A., & Ersoy, A. O. (2003). Aerobic exercise and plasma beta endorphin levels in patients with migrainous headache without aura. *Cephalalgia, 23,* 972–976.

Laurer, H. L., Bareyre, F. M., Lee, V. M., Trojanowski, J. Q., Longhi, L., Hoover, R., et al. (2001). Mild head injury increasing the brain's vulnerability to a second concussive impact. *Journal of Neurosurgery, 95*(5), 859–870.

Lawlor, D. A., & Hopker, S. W. (2001). The effectiveness of exercise as an intervention in the management of depression: Systematic review and meta-regression analysis of randomised controlled trials. *British Medical Journal, 322*(7289), 763–767.

Leddy, J. J., Kozlowski, K., Donnelly, J. P., Pendergast, D. R., Epstein, L. H., & Willer, B. (2010). A preliminary study of subsymptom threshold exercise training for refractory post-concussion syndrome. *Clinical Journal of Sport Medicine, 20*(1), 21–27.

Lockett, D. M., & Campbell, J. F. (1992). The effects of aerobic exercise on migraine. *Headache, 32,* 50–54.

Lojovich, J. M. (2010). The relationship between aerobic exercise and cognition: Is movement medicinal? *Journal of Head Trauma Rehabilitation, 25*(3), 184–192.

Longhi, L., Saatman, K. E., Fujimoto, S., Raghupathi, R., Meaney, D. F., Davis, J., et al. (2005). Temporal window of vulnerability to repetitive experimental concussive brain injury. *Neurosurgery, 56*(2), 364–374.

Majerske, C. W., Mihalik, J. P., Ren, D., Collins, M. W., Reddy, C. C., Lovell, M. R., et al. (2008). Concussion in sports: Postconcussive activity levels, symptoms, and neurocognitive performance. *Journal of Athletic Training, 43*(3), 265–274.

McCrea, M., Guskiewicz, K., Randolph, C., Barr, W. B., Hammeke, T. A., Marshall, S. W., et al. (2009). Effects of a symptom-free waiting period on clinical outcome and risk of reinjury after sport-related concussion. *Neurosurgery, 65*(5), 876–882; discussion, 882–883.

McCrory, P., Johnston, K., Aubry, M., Cantu, R., Dvorak, J., Graf-Baumann, T., et al. (2005). Summary of the Second International Conference on Concussion in Sport, Prague, Czech Republic. *Clinical Journal of Sport Medicine, 15*(2), 48–55.

McCrory, P., Meeuwisse, W., Johnston, K., Dvorak, J., Aubry, M., Molloy, M., et al. (2009). Consensus statement on concussion in sport: The 3rd International Conference on Concussion in Sport held in Zurich, November 2008. *British Journal of Sports Medicine, 43*(Suppl. 1), i76–i90.

Mead, G. E., Morley, W., Campbell, P., Greig, C. A., McMurdo, M., & Lawlor, D. A. (2008). Exercise for depression. *Cochrane Database of Systematic Reviews* (4), CD004366.

Mead, G. E., Morley, W., Campbell, P., Greig, C. A., McMurdo, M., & Lawlor, D. A. (2009). Exercise for depression. *Cochrane Database of Systematic Reviews* (3), CD004366.

Merom, D., Phongsavan, P., Wagner, R., Chey, T., Marnane, C., Steel, Z., et al. (2008). Promoting walking as an adjunct intervention to group cognitive behavioral therapy for anxiety disorders: A pilot group randomized trial. *Journal of Anxiety Disorders, 22*(6), 959–968.

Michelini, L. C., & Stern, J. E. (2009). Exercise-induced neuronal plasticity in central auto-nomic networks: Role in cardiovascular control. *Experimental Physiology, 94*(9), 947–960.

Minderhoud, J. M., Boelens, M. E., Huizenga, J., & Saan, R. J. (1980). Treatment of minor head injuries. *Clinical Neurology and Neurosurgery, 82*(2), 127–140.

Mittenberg, W., Tremont, G., Zielinski, R. E., Fichera, S., & Rayls, K. R. (1996). Cognitive-behavioral prevention of postconcussion syndrome. *Archives of Clinical Neuropsychol-ogy, 11*(2), 139–145.

Molteni, R., Ying, Z., & Gomez-Pinilla, F. (2002). Differential effects of acute and chronic exercise on plasticity-related genes in the rat hippocampus revealed by microarray. *European Journal of Neuroscience, 16*(6), 1107–1116.

Mossberg, K. A., Amonette, W. E., & Masel, B. E. (2010). Endurance training and cardio-respiratory conditioning after traumatic brain injury. *Journal of Head Trauma Rehabili-tation, 25*(3), 173–183.

Narin, S. O., Pinar, L., Erbas, D., Ozturk, V., & Idiman, F. (2003). The effects of exercise and exercise-related changes in blood nitric oxide level on migraine headache. *Clinical Rehabilitation, 17*(6), 624–630.

Navarro, A., Gomez, C., Lopez-Cepero, J. M., & Boveris, A. (2004). Beneficial effects of moderate exercise on mice aging: Survival, behavior, oxidative stress, and mitochondrial electron transfer. *American Journal of Physiology: Regulatory, Integrative and Com-parative Physiology, 286*(3), R505–R511.

Neeper, S. A., Gomez-Pinilla, F., Choi, J., & Cotman, C. (1995). Exercise and brain neurotro-phins. *Nature, 373*(6510), 109.

Neeper, S. A., Gomez-Pinilla, F., Choi, J., & Cotman, C. W. (1996). Physical activity increases mRNA for brain-derived neurotrophic factor and nerve growth factor in rat brain. *Brain Research, 726*(1–2), 49–56.

Pan, Y. X., Gao, L., Wang, W. Z., Zheng, H., Liu, D., Patel, K. P., et al. (2007). Exercise training prevents arterial baroreflex dysfunction in rats treated with central angiotensin II. *Hypertension, 49*(3), 519–527.

Paniak, C., Toller-Lobe, G., Reynolds, S., Melnyk, A., & Nagy, J. (2000). A randomized trial of two treatments for mild traumatic brain injury: 1 year follow-up. *Brain Injury, 14*(3), 219–226.

Penninx, B. W., Rejeski, W. J., Pandya, J., Miller, M. E., Di Bari, M., Applegate, W. B., et al. (2002). Exercise and depressive symptoms: A comparison of aerobic and resistance exercise effects on emotional and physical function in older persons with high and low depressive symptomatology. *Journals of Gerontology: Series B, Psychological Sciences and Social Sciences, 57*(2), P124–P132.

Ponsford, J., Willmott, C., Rothwell, A., Cameron, P., Ayton, G., Nelms, R., et al. (2001). Impact of early intervention on outcome after mild traumatic brain injury in children. *Pediatrics, 108*(6), 1297–1303.

Ponsford, J., Willmott, C., Rothwell, A., Cameron, P., Kelly, A. M., Nelms, R., et al. (2002). Impact of early intervention on outcome following mild head injury in adults. *Journal of Neurology, Neurosurgery, and Psychiatry, 73*(3), 330–332.

Purcell, L. (2009). What are the most appropriate return-to-play guidelines for concussed child athletes? *British Journal of Sports Medicine, 43*(Suppl. 1), i51–i55.

Rethorst, C. D., Wipfli, B. M., & Landers, D. M. (2009). The antidepressive effects of exer-cise: A meta-analysis of randomized trials. *Sports Medicine, 39*(6), 491–511.

Schretlen, D. J., & Shapiro, A. M. (2003). A quantitative review of the effects of traumatic brain injury on cognitive functioning. *International Review of Psychiatry, 15*(4), 341–349.

Smith, P. J., Blumenthal, J. A., Hoffman, B. M., Cooper, H., Strauman, T. A., Welsh-Bohmer,

K., et al. (2010). Aerobic exercise and neurocognitive performance: A meta-analytic review of randomized controlled trials. *Psychosomatic Medicine, 72*(3), 239–252.

Smits, J. A., Berry, A. C., Rosenfield, D., Powers, M. B., Behar, E., & Otto, M. W. (2008). Reducing anxiety sensitivity with exercise. *Depression and Anxiety, 25*(8), 689–699.

Strohle, A. (2009). Physical activity, exercise, depression, and anxiety disorders. *Journal of Neural Transmission, 116*(6), 777–784.

Stroth, S., Kubesch, S., Dieterle, K., Ruchsow, M., Heim, R., & Kiefer, M. (2009). Physical fitness, but not acute exercise modulates event-related potential indices for executive control in healthy adolescents. *Brain Research, 1269,* 114–124.

Suen, P. C., Wu, K., Levine, E. S., Mount, H. T., Xu, J. L., Lin, S. Y., et al. (1997). Brain-derived neurotrophic factor rapidly enhances phosphorylation of the postsynaptic N-methyl-D-aspartate receptor subunit 1. *Proceedings of the National Academy of Sciences of the United States of America, 94*(15), 8191–8195.

Thoenen, H. (1995). Neurotrophins and neuronal plasticity. *Science, 270*(5236), 593–598.

Tong, L., Shen, H., Perreau, V. M., Balazs, R., & Cotman, C. W. (2001). Effects of exercise on gene-expression profile in the rat hippocampus. *Neurobiology of Disease, 8*(6), 1046–1056.

Vagnozzi, R., Tavazzi, B., Signoretti, S., Amorini, A. M., Belli, A., Cimatti, M., et al. (2007). Temporal window of metabolic brain vulnerability to concussions: Mitochondrial-related impairment—Part I. *Neurosurgery, 61*(2), 379–388; discussion, 388–389.

van Praag, H. (2008). Neurogenesis and exercise: Past and future directions. *Neuromolecular Medicine, 10*(2), 128–140.

van Praag, H., Christie, B. R., Sejnowski, T. J., & Gage, F. H. (1999). Running enhances neurogenesis, learning, and long-term potentiation in mice. *Proceedings of the National Academy of Sciences of the United States of America, 96*(23), 13427–13431.

van Praag, H., Shubert, T., Zhao, C., & Gage, F. H. (2005). Exercise enhances learning and hippocampal neurogenesis in aged mice. *Journal of Neuroscience, 25*(38), 8680–8685.

Vaynman, S., Ying, Z., & Gomez-Pinilla, F. (2003). Interplay between brain-derived neurotrophic factor and signal transduction modulators in the regulation of the effects of exercise on synaptic-plasticity. *Neuroscience, 122*(3), 647–657.

Wade, D. T., King, N. S., Wenden, F. J., Crawford, S., & Caldwell, F. E. (1998). Routine follow up after head injury: A second randomised controlled trial. *Journal of Neurology, Neurosurgery, and Psychiatry, 65*(2), 177–183.

Wang, C., Bannuru, R., Ramel, J., Kupelnick, B., Scott, T., & Schmid, C. H. (2010). Tai chi on psychological well-being: Systematic review and meta-analysis. *BMC Complementary and Alternative Medicine, 10,* 23.

Wipfli, B. M., Rethorst, C. D., & Landers, D. M. (2008). The anxiolytic effects of exercise: A meta-analysis of randomized trials and dose–response analysis. *Journal of Sport and Exercise Psychology, 30*(4), 392–410.

Wu, A., Ying, Z., & Gomez-Pinilla, F. (2004). The interplay between oxidative stress and brain-derived neurotrophic factor modulates the outcome of a saturated fat diet on synaptic plasticity and cognition. *European Journal of Neuroscience, 19*(7), 1699–1707.

Youngstedt, S. D. (2005). Effects of exercise on sleep. *Clinical Sports Medicine, 24*(2), 355–365, xi.

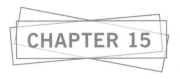

CHAPTER 15

Medical and Pain Management

Pamela E. Wilson and Gerald H. Clayton

Symptoms from mild traumatic brain injury (mTBI) will generally resolve within a short time frame. A small percentage of children and adolescents develops persistent postconcussive symptoms and require therapeutic intervention. The pathophysiological consequences of mTBI are myriad (see Babikian, DiFiori, & Giza, Chapter 5, this volume) and present as very complex phenomena that have physical and psychological implications. These phenomena are, in general, not well understood and limited empirical data are available, certainly in the pediatric and adolescent population. Therefore, much of the information on treatment that follows is extrapolated from the adult literature; pediatric-specific studies are noted where relevant.

The acute and subacute sequelae of mTBI result in part from changes in the homeostatic mechanisms of the brain. These include trauma-induced molecular cascades causing alterations in the neurochemical and ionic environment. The ability to respond to injury and return to normal cellular homeostasis affects behavior and symptomatology associated with mTBI. In addition, neuromuscular injuries may present in a manner similar to symptoms of central nervous system (CNS) origin. A number of techniques are now available to identify postinjury molecular, physiological, and structural alterations that can serve to document postconcussive changes and allow for potential associations to be discerned between symptoms and physiological mechanism. These tools provide the means to document injury severity and subsequent recovery beyond behavioral observation, and they provide guidance and direction for treatment. Several of these methods are currently in use clinically, whereas others are in the research phase but are approaching practical clinical use. It is important to note that other, non-neurological, factors can play a role in symptom complaints following mTBI.

Children and adolescents with mTBI present to a variety of health care providers, including those in primary care offices or emergency departments. These patients will have unique symptoms that need to be characterized and a treatment plan implemented. Works by several authors over the last decade have demonstrated that the symptoms associated with these injuries can, and should, be categorized into clusters (e.g., somatic, cognitive, emotional, and behavioral) (Ayr, Yeates, Taylor, & Browne, 2009; International Headache Society [IHS], 2004; Meares et al., 2006). A thorough review of treatment for each cluster of symptoms is beyond the scope of this chapter; however, we present a brief review of possible treatments for some of the most common somatic symptoms including *postconcussion headaches*; *dizziness, vertigo, and tinnitus*; *sleep problems and fatigue*; and *visual disturbances*.

POSTCONCUSSION HEADACHES

The most cited symptom after a concussion is headache. One should, however, take care in defining postconcussion headaches. As opined by Lane and Arcinegas (2002), the "true post-concussion headache" presumes that there is no premorbid definable headache disorder. The incidence of posttraumatic headaches (PTHAs) has been quoted as anywhere from 5 to 90% for both adults and children (Faux & Sheedy, 2008; Kraus, Fife, Cox, Ramstein, & Conroy, 1986; Lanser, Jennekens-Schinkel, & Peters, 1988; Uomoto & Esselman, 1993). Faux followed a population of adults with mTBI and found that 15% still had headaches at 3 months (Faux & Sheedy, 2008). In a study by Korinthenberg et al., 23 of 98 children still had a variety of somatic symptoms at 4–6 weeks postinjury, and 16.3% suffered from headaches (Korinthenberg, Schreck, Weser, & Lehmkuhl, 2004). Kirk et al., in their observational study of 117 children with mild head injuries, reported that 7.5% had headaches within 14 days of the injury, and these symptoms were still in evidence 8 weeks later (Kirk, Nagiub, & Abu-Arafeh, 2008). Other small studies have reported varying frequency of unresolved PTHA in children (Satz et al., 1997). Clearly, variations in study design and definition complicate the ability to draw a conclusion related to the incidence of PTHA.

Defining the type of headaches after mTBI is imperative for developing treatment strategies (Kirk et al., 2008). Kirk has commented that, based on symptoms, post-concussion headaches have features of both tension type and migraine. A study by Callaghan in 2001 characterized PTHA specifically in children and adolescents and demonstrated that chronic and episodic tension types were the most common, followed by migraine without aura and then mixed pattern (Callaghan & Abu-Arafeh, 2001). Studies in adults have found that chronic tension type headaches alone or in combination with migraine symptoms are very common (Baandrup & Jensen, 2005; Lew et al., 2006).

Headaches can be classified using standardized diagnostic criteria such as those contained in the International Classification of Headache Disorders–2 (ICHDs-2; IHS, 2004). Two broad categories for headaches currently exist: "primary," which has no organic or structural etiology, and "secondary," which can be related to an underlying etiology. This paradigm categorizes the four primary types of headache:as migraine, tension, trigeminal autonomic cephalalgia (including cluster), and other (thunderclap, hemicranium continua, new daily persistent, and hypnic). There are nine secondary headache classifications, including "headaches attributed to head and/or neck trauma." Posttraumatic and whiplash headaches fall within this category.

According to the ICHD-2, to classify a patient as having PTHA, the headaches must start within 7 days of the traumatic event and resolve within 3 months. Headaches that persist beyond that time interval are reclassified as chronic PTHA. An increase in baseline headache intensity does not fall into this classification. Adherence to these classification guidelines greatly facilitates direction of care.

Headache has been characterized globally as a manifestation of brain dysfunction (Gladstone, 2009). However, muscular–skeletal abnormalities and psychopathology also need to be factored into this clinical schema. Such a complex "differential diagnosis" often makes planning treatment difficult. As indicated above, correct classification is the definitive first step.

Migraine Headaches

By definition, migraine headaches are usually unilateral, pulsating, and of moderate intensity. Exercise may increase symptoms, and it is not uncommon to have nausea and light or noise sensitivity (IHS, 2004; Sjaastad, Fredriksen, & Pfaffenrath, 1998a; Sjaastad, Salvesen, Jansen, & Fredriksen, 1998b). Prevalence has been documented in a range of 8–23% in children up to age 15 years of age (Lipton, Silberstein, & Stewart, 1994). Genetically predisposed individuals often have a history of motion sickness or nonspecific gastrointestinal symptomatology (Solomon, 1998). Migraines are also known to have a comorbidity with underlying psychiatric diagnoses (Pakalnis, Gibson, & Colvin, 2005). Two popular theories on the origins and pathophysiology of migraine predominate: (1) *vascular theory* suggests that acute vasoconstriction results in brief ischemia, causing aura, whereas headache pain results from rebound vasodilation, causing activation of perivascular trigeminal nerve endings; (2) *central neuronal theory* suggests that circuits in the brain involved in sensory integration and filtering can be viewed as migraine generating (e.g., trigeminal ganglia and nucleus, areas within the pons and medulla, periaqueductal gray matter, hypothalamus and thalamus). To quote Ho et al., "Migraine triggers are likely to reflect a disturbance in overall balance of the circuits involved in the modulation of sensory activity, particularly those with relevance to the head" (Ho, Edvinsson, & Goadsby, 2010, p. 573). Recent work suggests that pharmacological agents such as calcitonin gene-related peptide (CGRP), triptans, and serotonin modulators may function not by modulating vasodilatory responses but by influencing the overall balance of interactive circuits focused on integrating sensory input, such as the trigeminal–cervical complex and the thalamus (Edvinsson & Ho, 2010; Ho et al., 2010; Hoskin, Kaube, & Goadsby, 1996; Olesen et al., 2004; Shields & Goadsby, 2006; Sprenger & Goadsby, 2009).

Treatment of posttraumatic migraine headaches follows the same principles employed in routine migraine management. Interventions can incorporate both traditional therapeutics and complementary strategies. Contemporary treatment will vary based on whether one is aiming for a symptomatic (i.e., abortive) or prophylactic therapy (see Tables 15.1 and 15.2 for common medications). Although some advocate for the use of first-line medications, nonpharmacological/complementary options are a reasonable adjunctive approach. A holistic approach often incorporates exercise, sleep management, stress reduction, and nutritional supplements (John, Sharma, Sharma, & Kankane, 2007; Sun-Edelstein & Mauskop, 2011). Behavioral interventions, including biofeedback and relaxation, are effective in pediatric migraine

TABLE 15.1. Pharmacological Prophylaxis of Headache

Category	Commonly used medication
Antiepileptics (AEDs)	Topiramate Valproic acid Gabapentine Levetiracetam Carbamazepine
Antidepressants	Tricyclics (TCAs) Amitriptyline Nortriptyline Trazodone
Antihypertensives	Beta blockers Propranolol
Serotonin (5-HT$_2$) antagonists	Methysergide Pizotifen

treatment (Nestoriuc, Martin, Rief, & Andrasik, 2008a; Nestoriuc, Rief, & Martin, 2008b; Sun-Edelstein & Mauskop, 2011). A multitude of medications has been used over the years, and most have at least some supporting data for efficacy. Traditional medications used for prevention include the antiepileptics (AEDs), antidepressants, antihypertensives, and serotonin receptor agonists (e.g., triptans) (Jokeit & Reed, 2011; Lewis, 2010). Recent data on onabotulinum toxin has also shown some promise in prevention of these headaches (Aurora et al., 2010; Delstanche & Schoenen, 2010; Diener et al., 2010; Dodick et al., 2010). Basilar type migraine or vestibular migraine in children is often resistant to treatment acutely; however, one study with children documented the effective use of topiramate in prevention, even though the mechanism of action remains unclear (Lewis & Paradiso, 2007).

Cervicogenic Headache

Cervicogenic headache (CEH) is a unique syndrome with the pathology originating in the cervical spine (Vincent, 2010). The diagnostic criteria for CEH have been debated

TABLE 15.2. Pharmacological Abortive Therapy (Typically Combination Therapy) for Headache

Category	Commonly used medication
Analgesics	Acetaminophen NSAIDs (e.g., naproxen sodium) Opioids (e.g., oxycodone, morphine)
Vasoconstrictors	Serotonin (5-HT$_1$) agonists Triptans (e.g., sumatriptan) Ergot alkaloids (alpha agonists) ergotamine, dihydroergotamine
Dopamine receptor hypersensitivity antagonists	Dopamine antagonists Metoclopramide and prochlorperazine

for years. Sjaastad et al. developed a diagnostic paradigm consisting of unilaterality, symptoms of neck involvement, and confirmation by diagnostic block (Sjaastad, Fredriksen, & Pfaffenrath, 1998a; Sjaastad, Salvesen, Jansen, & Fredriksen, 1998b). These criteria were developed in the adult population, and current practice does not differentiate their use with adults versus children. Unfortunately, few data exist specific to the diagnosis and treatment of children with CEH (Ormos, 2003). Clinical guidance stems from application of lessons learned from adults. The mechanisms and pathology of CEH are complex and still not completely understood. The trigeminal–cervical nucleus in the upper cervical spine receives sensory information from the trigeminal nerve and cervical roots (Biondi, 2005). Bogduk (2001) describes the mechanism as convergence of two separate afferent neurons on the same second-order neuron. When one of the neurons is carrying nociceptive information during the convergence process, it can influence the other neuron to sense pain. Therefore, CEHs can refer to any area in the head. The upper three cervical segments are most commonly involved in CEHs. A classic headache study done by Cyriax (1938) showed that injecting saline into the suboccipital muscles causes headaches (Cyriax, 1938). Relevant structures include not only muscles of the neck but also the facet joints and discs. See summary of structural relationships in Table 15.3.

Treatment of CEHs often includes rehabilitative therapy, manual medicine techniques, medication, injections, and surgical interventions. Grimshaw (2001) states that the entire neuromuscular system, which is dynamic, interactive, and functional, must be treated. Manual therapy for CEH (e.g., spinal manipulation) has been suggested to be efficacious for adults in a systematic review of randomized controlled trials in England, although several other publications suggest otherwise (Alcantara, 2011; Borusiak, Biedermann, Bosserhoff, & Opp, 2010; Bronfort, Haas, Evans, Leininger, & Triano, 2010). Medications prescribed are typically the same class as those used in primary headache syndromes. The use of the tricyclic antidepressants (TCAs), selective serotonin reuptake inhibitors (SSRIs), AEDs, and nonsteroidal anti-inflammatory drugs (NSAIDs) are all considered reasonable options (Feng & Schofferman, 2003). Injection techniques that infuse local anesthetics and corticosteroids are also used for both diagnosis and treatment (Fernandez-De-Las-Penas, 2010).

TABLE 15.3. Structural Relationships for Posttraumatic Cervical Pain

Structure	Referral pattern
Atlanto-occipital joint	Occipital region
C_2 neuralgia	Occipital referring to other cranial areas; eye watering and redness may occur ipsilaterally
C_{2-3} zygapophyseal joint	Base of skull and occipital region with referral to frontotemporal and periorbital; tenderness to direct palpation
Occipital neuralgia	Constant burning with some paroxysmal pain, numbness in scalp
Regional myofascial pain syndrome	Specific muscles have pain with referral pain, trigger points

Tension-Type Headache

Tension-type headache (TTH) is considered to be the most common type of headache in children following mTBI (Callaghan & Abu-Arafeh, 2001; Kirk et al., 2008). TTH tends to be bilateral and typically is described as a pressure or a squeezing sensation. These TTHs are moderate in intensity, and exercise does not increase symptoms. Generally there is no associated nausea or light and noise sensitivity (IHS, 2004; Sjaastad et al., 1998a, 1998b). In individuals with PTHA, 80% of the time these can be categorized as TTH (Schoenen & Jensen, 2006). TTHs have a complex pathophysiology that combines elements of genetic predisposition, muscle contraction, stress, and centralized pain. Treatment approaches are similar to those previously discussed for migraine and CEH. Nonpharmacological treatment incorporating relaxation and biofeedback is known to be effective (Sun-Edelstein & Mauskop, 2011). A synthesis of two meta-analyses and other data offered an unequivocal high rating for the evidence supporting efficacy and specificity of biofeedback for TTH (Nestoriuc et al., 2008a, 2008b; Sun-Edelstein & Mauskop, 2011). Acupuncture has also been shown to have mild beneficial effects when compared to sham treatment (Linde et al., 2009). Pharmacological treatment may include use of simple analgesics and NSAIDs. In addition, muscle relaxants and onabotulinum toxin injections may play a role in the treatment of TTH. However, a number of experts only recommend the use of onabotulinum toxin in migraines (Aurora et al., 2010; Blumenfeld et al., 2010; Delstanche & Schoenen, 2010; Diener et al., 2010; Dodick et al., 2010). Medication overuse may complicate recovery, leading to increased frequency of headaches, and should be kept in mind as a possible confounder (Lauwerier, Paemeleire, Van Damme, Goubert, & Crombez, 2011). In treating resistant TTH, practitioners should be mindful of recent data associating it with vitamin D deficiency and consider checking vitamin D levels and adding it to the treatment plan, as indicated (Prakash et al., 2010; Prakash & Shah, 2009).

Complementary and Alternative Medicine Approaches

The use of complementary and alternative medicine (CAM) in the treatment of headache is often the result of a lack of satisfaction with traditional medical approaches or frustration in dealing with pharmaceutical side effects. Numerous nutraceutical, behavioral, and physical modalities exist with varying levels of evidence for their efficacy. In the face of poor results with traditional care, these treatments may prove to be useful.

The most prevalent alternative pharmacological approaches to the treatment of headache include the use of electrolytes, vitamins, nutritional supplements, and herbs. Magnesium is associated with a number of physiological processes, although the most relevant to PTHA treatments are likely vasoconstriction and neurotransmitter release (Altura & Turlapaty, 1982; Coan & Collingridge, 1985). Low magnesium ion (Mg^{2+}) levels are suggested to be associated with migraine, based upon small population studies (Sun-Edelstein & Mauskop, 2011). Several studies and randomized controlled trials have also shown that returning Mg^{2+} levels to normal is associated with a decrease in the number of days with headache (Sun-Edelstein & Mauskop, 2011). Facchinetti et al. also showed that, when used for menstrual migraine prophylaxis, Mg^{2+} supplementation caused a significant decline in the number of days with headache and total pain scores (Facchinetti, Sances, Borella, Genazzani, & Nappi, 1991). Other studies of migraine prophylaxis have shown as much as a 42% decrease in attack frequency (Peikert, Wilimzig, & Kohne-Volland, 1996; Pfaffenrath et al., 1996). In contrast, certain studies have shown equivocal or negative results, which have been thought to be due at least in part to poor absorption associated with oral dosing (Pfaffenrath et al., 1996; Sun-Edelstein & Mauskop, 2011; Taylor et al., 2010).

Vitamin B2, or riboflavin, is an essential precursor to two flavin coenzymes necessary for electron transport, oxidation and/or reduction reactions, and the production of adenosine triphosphate (ATP). As such, it functions to stabilize membranes and, from an energy standpoint, is essential for cellular homeostasis. The discovery of metabolic abnormalities within the brains of patients with migraine suggests functional mitochondrial deficits (Sas, Pardutz, Toldi, & Vecsei, 2010). The role of riboflavin, in part, is to increase the activity of the respiratory chain, thereby increasing phosphorylation levels. Clinically, a randomized controlled trial of adults with migraine has shown that 400 mg B2 daily for 3 months resulted in a 50% reduction in attacks in over half of the patients, as compared to 15% in the placebo group (Schoenen, Jacquy, & Lenaerts, 1998). This research suggests that utilizing B2 in migraine prophylaxis may be beneficial. Coenzyme Q10 (CoQ10) also plays a role in electron transport within the mitochondria, and thus is important in energy generation within the cell. It has the capability to function as an antioxidant. In one randomized controlled trial, 100 mg CoQ10 three times a day significantly lessened frequency of attacks and headache days (Sandor et al., 2005). In a retrospective study of 1,550 pediatric patients with recurring headaches, Hershey et al. (2007) demonstrated low levels of CoQ10 in one-third of the population. CoQ10 supplementation led to a normalization of levels and statistically significant lessening of headache frequency.

Alpha lipoic acid (or thioctic acid or ALA) is a very strong nonenzymatic antioxidant that is both fat and water soluble. This property facilitates penetration into the CNS. In addition, it also plays a role in ATP production, making it an excellent compound for addressing mitochondrial compromise and improving glucose utilization. ALA has been tested in a variety of clinical disorders, including diabetic peripheral neuropathy, heart disease, and migraine (Magis et al., 2007). Magis et al. (2007) showed a trend toward statistical significance in decreasing migraines. Further studies are required to test these hypotheses and validate anecdotal reports of efficacy.

Two common herbal formulations have received attention in the treatment of headache: butterbur (*petasites hybridus* root extract) and feverfew (*Tanacetum parthenium*). Petadolex, a commercial preparation of butterbur extract, has been evaluated in several randomized controlled trials of adults and children, collectively showing a significant reduction in attack frequency and migraine days per month (Diener, Rahlfs, & Danesch, 2004; Grossmann & Schmidramsl, 2000; Lipton, Gobel, Einhaupl, Wilks, & Mauskop, 2004; Pothmann & Danesch, 2005). Butterbur's mechanism of action has been suggested to be due to its calcium channel interactions and inhibition of leukotriene synthesis, thereby altering the inflammatory processes often associated with migraine pathophysiology. Feverfew, often touted as useful in migraine prophylaxis, has been used for centuries in the treatment of headache. Its mechanisms of action are proposed to involve inhibition of platelet aggregation and subsequent serotonin release as well as an anti-inflammatory function related to prostaglandin synthesis (Heptinstall, Groenewegen, Spangenberg, &

Loesche, 1987; Heptinstall, White, Williamson, & Mitchell, 1985; Losche et al., 1987; Pugh & Sambo, 1988). A Cochrane review of safety and efficacy studies conducted in 2004 indicated that there was not enough evidence to state that feverfew was more successful at migraine prophylaxis than placebo. However, stabler formulations have been developed and tested in one small study (Diener, Pfaffenrath, Schnitker, Friede, & Henneicke-von Zepelin, 2005), which demonstrated a statistically significant reduction in migraine frequency.

Finally, acupuncture has been suggested as efficacious in the treatment of headache for many years and until recently recommendations have been unclear. A recent Cochrane review of migraine in 2009 concluded that acupuncture provided more benefit than routine care (Linde et al., 2009).

DIZZINESS, VERTIGO, AND TINNITUS

Balance is a complex process and relies on input from the visual, vestibular, and proprioceptive systems. The development of balance begins in infancy with an early emphasis on integration of information from the vestibular and visual systems. Integration of somatosensory data occurs at a later age. Children develop a vestibular–ocular reflex (VOR) by 10 months and by 5 years visual tracking is similar to an adult. The integration of all these systems does not mature until 12–14 years (Peterson, Christou, & Rosengren, 2006).

Dizziness is a nonspecific term and includes descriptions of light-headedness, an unstable feeling, or clumsiness. *Vertigo*, on the other hand, is a well-defined medical diagnosis. Vertigo is the sensation that the individual (subjective vertigo) or the environment (objective vertigo) is moving.

Dizziness and balance problems are a frequent complaint after mTBI. Niemensivu and colleagues studied the under-15-year-old population in Helsinki and found a prevalence rate of 8–15% (Niemensivu, Pyykko, Wiener-Vacher, & Kentala, 2006). Register-Mihalik et al. found that college athletes with PTHAs had an increased rate of balance problems as compared to those without headache (Register-Mihalik, Mihalik, & Guskiewicz, 2008).

Tinnitus, also known as ringing in the ears, frequently occurs after trauma. As stated by Shulman and Strashun (2009), "Normal function of the brain and ear is a reflection of a normal state of homeostasis between the fluid compartments in the brain, of cerebrospinal fluid and perilymph–endolymph in the labyrinth of the ear" (p. 119). As reviewed by Rauschecker et al., the tinnitus signal is normally cancelled out in the thalamus as part of an auditory–thalamic–limbic pathway (Rauschecker, Leaver, & Muhlau, 2010). Disruption or overrepresentation of frequencies due to injury may result in tinnitus. Therefore, damage to areas within this pathway could be suspect in persistent tinnitus.

Types of Disorders Causing Dizziness/Vertigo/Tinnitus

Temporal bone fractures, especially those classified as transverse, can extend into the labyrinth and cause damage to the vestibular system. In addition to vestibular symptoms there may be an associated hearing loss.

Benign positional paroxysmal vertigo (BPPV) is the most common etiology for dizziness and vertigo, although no epidemiological studies have been conducted to understand how often this may explain reported dizziness following pediatric mTBI. In general, the etiology of BPPV seems to be associated with debris collection of the otoconia that originates in the utricle and migrates to the semicircular canals. Classically, individuals will describe dizziness and vertigo with positional changes. The episodes are usually short lived but can occur several times per day. Tests for nystagmus are typically positive. BPPV is generally self-limiting and resolves spontaneously. Maneuvers designed to reposition debris can be effective in resolving symptoms (Oh, Kim, Han, & Lim, 2007; Post & Dickerson, 2010). Children with associated nausea may respond to an antiemetic (Hain & Yacovino, 2005).

Perilymphatic fistula is an abnormal opening between the middle and inner ear caused by an injury, usually to the round or oval window. Symptoms include not only dizziness and vertigo but also hearing loss. Valsalva-like maneuvers may increase symptoms. This condition may be difficult to diagnose and referral to a specialist should be made, if suspected. Treatment is conservative, with a short duration of simple bedrest and avoidance of strenuous activity (Prisman, Ramsden, Blaser, & Papsin, 2011). If this fails, then surgical intervention may be used to repair the leak.

Treatment

When treating vertigo and dizziness with pharmacological interventions, anticholinergics and H1 antihistamines may be the most effective (Sprenger & Goadsby, 2009). However, benzodiazepines, calcium channel antagonists, and dopamine receptor antagonists are also suggested treatment approaches (Sprenger & Goadsby, 2009). Anticholinergics, such as Meclazine and Dramamine, appear to have some effect on central receptors that increase motion tolerance (Sprenger & Goadsby, 2009). Antihistamines may act centrally, and benzodiazepines work by modulating gamma-aminobutyric acid (GABA) and act centrally to alter VOR activity.

Vestibular rehabilitation is a frequent treatment modality used in individuals with dizziness/vertigo. The basic program utilizes movement-based therapy to retrain the injured vestibular system. These programs incorporate desensitization techniques, eye exercises, head movements, and balance retraining. The Cochrane library recently reviewed 27 adult-based studies and reported moderate to strong evidence in support of these vestibular interventions for various etiologies (Hillier & McDonnell, 2011).

Tinnitus, on the other hand, is historically more difficult to treat. Treatments range from surgical cochlear implant to treatment with antiseizure medications (e.g., diazepam) that affect GABA transmission within the auditory–thalamic–limbic pathways (Fioretti, Eibenstein, & Fusetti, 2011; Rauschecker et al., 2010). TCAs (e.g., amitriptyline) have been tried but with varied results; further research is needed to identify therapeutic doses (Bayar, Boke, Turan, & Belgin, 2001; Langguth, Landgrebe, Wittmann, Kleinjung, & Hajak, 2010). At least one report has suggested that biofeedback may be more efficacious than amitriptyline (Podoshin, Ben-David, Fradis, Malatskey, & Hafner, 1995). Other nonpharmacological treatments are currently being tested, such as low-level laser therapy, phase-out sound cancellation treatment, cognitive-behavioral therapy, and tinnitus retraining therapy (Fioretti et al., 2011).

These all have met with some success, but larger focused trials are needed to confirm their efficacy.

SLEEP PROBLEMS AND FATIGUE

Disturbances in sleep and fatigue are noted sequelae of mTBI and appear to be common in adults as well as children (Orff, Ayalon, & Drummond, 2009). In a study of 122 individuals ages 15–65 years, sleep disturbance and fatigue were reported as the most common symptoms (Lundin, de Boussard, Edman, & Borg, 2006). Milroy found that parent report of sleep disturbance in children 7–12 years with mTBI was higher than in orthopedic controls (Milroy, Dorris, & McMillan, 2008). Blinman et al. followed 116 children, mean age of 14, with mTBI and reported that the most common initial symptoms were fatigue and headache, whereas at follow-up sleep disturbance was the most commonly reported symptom (Blinman, Houseknecht, Snyder, Wiebe, & Nance, 2009).

In general populations, various types of sleep disorders exist, including difficulties in falling and staying asleep (insomnia), problems staying awake (hypersomnia), problems adhering to a normal sleep–wake cycle, and sleep disruptive behaviors. Schreiber et al. (2008) did a study on adults with mTBI and found abnormal stage 2 sleep and excessive daytime episodes of falling asleep. Ayalon et al. studied 42 patients with mTBI and a diagnosis of insomnia (Ayalon, Borodkin, Dishon, Kanety, & Dagan, 2007). They found a circadian rhythm sleep disorder in 36% of this group, higher than the general sleep-clinic population.

Treatment interventions for sleep disturbances should always begin with an assessment of sleep hygiene, as poor sleep hygiene is a frequent cause of sleep disruption in pediatric populations (Thiedke, 2001). Medications are frequently prescribed and may help with sleep induction and maintenance (Orff et al., 2009; Sanchez-Barcelo, Mediavilla, & Reiter, 2011). Melatonin is a naturally occurring hormone produced in the pineal gland that may help with sleep induction. In addition, some individuals find other natural agents such as valerian (*Valeriana officinalis*) helpful for falling asleep. Schmitz and Jackel (1998) report that a mixture of hops and valerian was equal to benzodiazepines in treating nonchronic and nonpsychiatric sleep disorders. In 2007, Taibi et al. published a thorough review of 29 controlled trials that concluded that the safety profile of valerian was good, although evidence for efficacy was lacking (Taibi, Landis, Petry, & Vitiello, 2007). Medications such as trazadone or melatonin agonists have been suggested as appropriate treatment for those with brain injuries, including mTBI (Larson & Zollman, 2010).

VISUAL DISTURBANCES

Vision abnormalities are often associated acutely with mTBI. Frequently, the first visual symptom reported is blurred vision. After more severe mTBI, persistent visual abnormalities can be associated with cranial nerve injuries, especially the trochlear and abducens nerves. Such injuries are unusual after mTBI, although the trochlear nerve structure and length make it susceptible to trauma. Meienberg found 39 adult cases of trochlear nerve palsy after frontal or occipital blows to the head (Meienberg & Muri, 1992). Direct empirical studies of these injuries are lacking in children, and at this point, consist primarily of the occasional case report (Stiller-Ostrowski, 2010). Clinically, individuals with these types of injuries may have a head tilt to correct for a vertical diplopia. The injury causes the superior oblique muscle to weaken, precluding the ability to look up and out. Abducens nerve injuries cause the eye to have horizontal diplopia, preventing abduction of the eye. Some preliminary evidence indicates that visual tracking may be a method of evaluating recovery from a concussion. Maruta et al. used a visual tracking technique in adult patients with mTBI and controls and reported that gaze error variability during tracking may be a useful screening technique (Maruta, Lee, Jacobs, & Ghajar, 2010a; Maruta, Suh, Niogi, Mukherjee, & Ghajar, 2010b).

Photophobia, a common complaint with migraine and often associated with concussion, may be amenable to treatment with photochromic lenses, such as under conditions of excessive light exposure found outside on a bright day. A study of 169 Norwegian adults with migraine showed that attack frequency was increased during the artic summer when light is extremely bright, and those with migraine aura reported significantly more frequent use of sunglasses to alleviate symptoms (Alstadhaug, 2009). We are reminded by Solomon that treatment of PTHA and associated symptoms should follow the same principles as treatment of primary headache; however, care is recommended in that there can be nonorganic exaggeration of visual symptoms (Bengtzen, Woodward, Lynn, Newman, & Biousse, 2008; Solomon, 2009). Novel treatment paradigms such as targeting CGRP and its link to vasodilation as well as glutamate receptors are proposed as potential adjuncts (Asghar et al., 2010; Recober et al., 2009; Sprenger & Goadsby, 2009).

AUTONOMIC DYSFUNCTION

The autonomic nervous system regulates sympathetic and parasympathetic function. Limited studies in children have associated autonomic instability with concussion. Autonomic dysregulation is known to occur in severe brain injuries and should be considered after mTBI, even though the exact incidence is currently unknown (Blackman, Patrick, Buck, & Rust, 2004). Middleton presented a case of an athlete who had "white-out" episodes after a concussion (Middleton, Krabak, & Coppel, 2010). Autonomic testing suggested altered vascular tone and an abnormal heart rate response. Gall et al. examined 14 concussed athletes, age 18, with an acute concussion and found a lower "R-to-R interval," a rare associated change on electrocardiogram with subthreshold exercise (Gall, Parkhouse, & Goodman, 2004). They postulated an uncoupling between the autonomic and cardiovascular systems acutely. Recent research by Kanjwal et al. studied eight patients who developed postural orthostatic tachycardia syndrome (POTS) after a brain injury. They all developed orthostatic dizziness, fatigue, palpitations, and near syncope. Treatment interventions were successful in all but two (Kanjwal, Karabin, Kanjwal, & Grubb, 2010). An excellent recent review by Raj (2006) documents the variety of mechanisms that may result in POTS. Treatments reflect the varying pathophysiology involved and may include exercise, adrenergic blockade, methods to decrease sympathetic tone (e.g., clonidine), or vascular volume expanders such as erythropoietin or intravascular saline. The overall goal, in all cases, is to deal with autonomic dysregulation causing tachycardia. Raj also notes that no medications are specifically approved by the Food and Drug Administration (FDA) for this indication.

SOMATOFORM AND MALINGERING DISORDERS

At times clinicians may encounter individuals who have symptoms that seem out of proportion or inconsistent with the severity of the initial injury. Somatoform disorders and malingering need to be considered in this population. Conversion disorder is a specific type of somatoform disorder in which the medical diagnosis does not account for the physical complaints. By definition, these symptoms have a psychological explanation (e.g., response to environmental stressors) and are not under voluntary control. Malingering, on the other hand, is an intentional reporting of symptoms or an exaggeration of physical findings that occurs for external gain. In the pediatric population, the avoidance of school or schoolwork is one possible reason for intentionally produced exaggeration. A recent study by Kirkwood and Kirk (2010) found that a significant percentage (17%) of school-age children exerted suboptimal effort on neuropsychological testing following mTBI. No evidence-based treatment for children who exaggerate symptomology exists, although the first step to appropriate care is to attempt to identify the nonconcussive factors that may be contributing to the symptoms so that each factor can be addressed (Kirkwood, Kirk, Blaha, & Wilson, 2010).

CONCLUSION

In order to define appropriate treatment options, an understanding of the epidemiology of postconcussive signs and symptoms is critical, as is the recognition that they may be associated with underlying pathophysiology or any of a variety of nonneurological factors. To date, studies validating treatment interventions in children are limited and pediatric approaches are often defined by adult research and experience. Growing evidence in the literature focusing on the evaluation of treatments in children will continue to allow us to refine therapies and improve their efficacy and specificity.

REFERENCES

Alcantara, J. (2011). A critical appraisal of the clinical trial on spinal manipulative therapy (SMT) and pediatric cervicogenic headache. *Headache, 51*(1), 167–168.

Alstadhaug, K. B. (2009). Migraine and the hypothalamus. *Cephalalgia: An International Journal of Headache, 29*(8), 809–817.

Altura, B. M., & Turlapaty, P. D. (1982). Withdrawal of magnesium enhances coronary arterial spasms produced by vasoactive agents. *British Journal of Pharmacology, 77*(4), 649–659.

Asghar, M. S., Hansen, A. E., Kapijimpanga, T., van der Geest, R. J., van der Koning, P.,

Larsson, H. B., et al. (2010). Dilation by CGRP of middle meningeal artery and reversal by sumatriptan in normal volunteers. *Neurology*, 75(17), 1520–1526.

Aurora, S. K., Dodick, D. W., Turkel, C. C., DeGryse, R. E., Silberstein, S. D., Lipton, R. B., et al. (2010). Onabotulinumtoxin: A for treatment of chronic migraine: Results from the double-blind, randomized, placebo-controlled phase of the PREEMPT 1 trial. *Cephalalgia: An International Journal of Headache*, 30(7), 793–803.

Ayalon, L., Borodkin, K., Dishon, L., Kanety, H., & Dagan, Y. (2007). Circadian rhythm sleep disorders following mild traumatic brain injury. *Neurology*, 68(14), 1136–1140.

Ayr, L. K., Yeates, K. O., Taylor, H. G., & Browne, M. (2009). Dimensions of postconcussive symptoms in children with mild traumatic brain injuries. *Journal of International Neuropsychology Society*, 15(1), 19–30.

Baandrup, L., & Jensen, R. (2005). Chronic post-traumatic headache: A clinical analysis in relation to the International Headache Classification 2nd Edition. *Cephalalgia: An International Journal of Headache*, 25(2), 132–138.

Bayar, N., Boke, B., Turan, E., & Belgin, E. (2001). Efficacy of amitriptyline in the treatment of subjective tinnitus. *Journal of Otolaryngology*, 30(5), 300–303.

Bengtzen, R., Woodward, M., Lynn, M. J., Newman, N. J., & Biousse, V. (2008). The "sunglasses sign" predicts nonorganic visual loss in neuro-ophthalmologic practice. *Neurology*, 70(3), 218–221.

Biondi, D. M. (2005). Cervicogenic headache: A review of diagnostic and treatment strategies. *Journal of the American Osteopath Association*, 105(4, Suppl. 2), 16S–22S.

Blackman, J. A., Patrick, P. D., Buck, M. L., & Rust, R. S., Jr. (2004). Paroxysmal autonomic instability with dystonia after brain injury. *Archives of Neurology*, 61(3), 321–328.

Blinman, T. A., Houseknecht, E., Snyder, C., Wiebe, D. J., & Nance, M. L. (2009). Postconcussive symptoms in hospitalized pediatric patients after mild traumatic brain injury. *Journal of Pediatric Surgery*, 44(6), 1223–1228.

Blumenfeld, A., Silberstein, S. D., Dodick, D. W., Aurora, S. K., Turkel, C. C., & Binder, W. J. (2010). Method of injection of onabotulinumtoxin A for chronic migraine: A safe, well-tolerated, and effective treatment paradigm based on the PREEMPT clinical program. *Headache*, 50(9), 1406–1418.

Bogduk, N. (2001). Cervicogenic headache: Anatomic basis and pathophysiologic mechanisms. *Current Pain and Headache Reports*, 5(4), 382–386.

Borusiak, P., Biedermann, H., Bosserhoff, S., & Opp, J. (2010). Lack of efficacy of manual therapy in children and adolescents with suspected cervicogenic headache: Results of a prospective, randomized, placebo-controlled, and blinded trial. *Headache*, 50(2), 224–230.

Bronfort, G., Haas, M., Evans, R., Leininger, B., & Triano, J. (2010). Effectiveness of manual therapies: The UK evidence report. *Chiropractic and Osteopathy*, 18(3), 1–33.

Callaghan, M., & Abu-Arafeh, I. (2001). Chronic posttraumatic headache in children and adolescents. *Developmental Medicine and Child Neurology*, 43(12), 819–822.

Coan, E. J., & Collingridge, G. L. (1985). Magnesium ions block an N-methyl-D-aspartate receptor-mediated component of synaptic transmission in rat hippocampus. *Neuroscience Letters*, 53(1), 21–26.

Cyriax, J. (1938). Rheumatic headache. *British Medical Journal*, 2(4069), 1367–1368.

Delstanche, S., & Schoenen, J. (2010). Botulinum toxin for the treatment of headache: A promising path on a "dead end road"? *Acta Neurologica Belgica*, 110(3), 221–229.

Diener, H. C., Dodick, D. W., Aurora, S. K., Turkel, C. C., DeGryse, R. E., Lipton, R. B., et al. (2010). Onabotulinumtoxin A for treatment of chronic migraine: Results from the double-blind, placebo-controlled phase of the PREEMPT 2 trial. *Cephalalgia: An International Journal of Headache*, 30(7), 804–814.

Diener, H. C., Pfaffenrath, V., Schnitker, J., Friede, M., & Henneicke-von Zepelin, H. H.

(2005). Efficacy and safety of 6.25 mg t.i.d. feverfew CO_2-extract (MIG-99) in migraine prevention: A randomized, double-blind, multicentre, placebo-controlled study. *Cephalalgia: An International Journal of Headache, 25*(11), 1031–1041.

Diener, H. C., Rahlfs, V. W., & Danesch, U. (2004). The first placebo-controlled trial of a special butterbur root extract for the prevention of migraine: Reanalysis of efficacy criteria. *European Neurology, 51*(2), 89–97.

Dodick, D. W., Turkel, C. C., DeGryse, R. E., Aurora, S. K., Silberstein, S. D., Lipton, R. B., et al. (2010). Onabotulinumtoxin A for treatment of chronic migraine: Pooled results from the double-blind, randomized, placebo-controlled phases of the PREEMPT clinical program. *Headache, 50*(6), 921–936.

Edvinsson, L., & Ho, T. W. (2010). CGRP receptor antagonism and migraine. *Neurotherapeutics, 7*(2), 164–175.

Facchinetti, F., Sances, G., Borella, P., Genazzani, A. R., & Nappi, G. (1991). Magnesium prophylaxis of menstrual migraine: Effects on intracellular magnesium. *Headache, 31*(5), 298–301.

Faux, S., & Sheedy, J. (2008). A prospective controlled study in the prevalence of post-traumatic headache following mild traumatic brain injury. *Pain Medicine, 9*(8), 1001–1011.

Feng, F. L., & Schofferman, J. (2003). Chronic neck pain and cervicogenic headaches. *Current Treatment Options in Neurology, 5*(6), 493–498.

Fernandez-De-Las-Penas, C. (2010). *Tension-type and cervicogenic headache.* Boston: Jones & Bartlett.

Fioretti, A., Eibenstein, A., & Fusetti, M. (2011). New trends in tinnitus management. *Open Neurology Journal, 5*, 12–17.

Gall, B., Parkhouse, W., & Goodman, D. (2004). Heart rate variability of recently concussed athletes at rest and exercise. *Medicine and Science in Sports and Exercise, 36*(8), 1269–1274.

Gladstone, J. (2009). From psychoneurosis to ICHD-2: An overview of the state of the art in post-traumatic headache. *Headache, 49*(7), 1097–1111.

Grimshaw, D. N. (2001). Cervicogenic headache: Manual and manipulative therapies. *Current Pain and Headache Reports, 5*(4), 369–375.

Grossmann, M., & Schmidramsl, H. (2000). An extract of *Petasites hybridus* is effective in the prophylaxis of migraine. *International Journal of Clinical Pharmacology and Therapeutics, 38*(9), 430–435.

Hain, T. C., & Yacovino, D. (2005). Pharmacologic treatment of persons with dizziness. *Neurologic Clinics, 23*(3), 831–853.

Heptinstall, S., Groenewegen, W. A., Spangenberg, P., & Loesche, W. (1987). Extracts of feverfew may inhibit platelet behaviour via neutralization of sulphydryl groups. *Journal of Pharmacy and Pharmacology, 39*(6), 459–465.

Heptinstall, S., White, A., Williamson, L., & Mitchell, J. R. (1985). Extracts of feverfew inhibit granule secretion in blood platelets and polymorphonuclear leucocytes. *Lancet, 1*(8437), 1071–1074.

Hershey, A. D., Powers, S. W., Vockell, A. L., Lecates, S. L., Ellinor, P. L., Segers, A., et al. (2007). Coenzyme Q10 deficiency and response to supplementation in pediatric and adolescent migraine. *Headache, 47*(1), 73–80.

Hillier, S. L., & McDonnell, M. N. (2011). *Vestibular rehabilitation for unilateral peripheral vestibular dysfunction* [Review] (Vol. 2).

Ho, T. W., Edvinsson, L., & Goadsby, P. J. (2010). CGRP and its receptors provide new insights into migraine pathophysiology. *Nature Reviews Neurology, 6*(10), 573–582.

Hoskin, K. L., Kaube, H., & Goadsby, P. J. (1996). Sumatriptan can inhibit trigeminal afferents by an exclusively neural mechanism. *Brain: A Journal of Neurology, 119*(Pt. 5), 1419–1428.

IHS. (2004). The international classification of headache disorders—second edition. *Cephalalgia, 24*(Suppl. 1), 9–160.

John, P. J., Sharma, N., Sharma, C. M., & Kankane, A. (2007). Effectiveness of yoga therapy in the treatment of migraine without aura: A randomized controlled trial. *Headache, 47*(5), 654–661.

Jokeit, H., & Reed, V. (2011). Cognitive effects of topiramate in migraine patients aged 12–17 years. *Pediatric Neurology, 44*(5), 396; author reply, 396–397.

Kanjwal, K., Karabin, B., Kanjwal, Y., & Grubb, B. P. (2010). Autonomic dysfunction presenting as postural tachycardia syndrome following traumatic brain injury. *Cardiology Journal, 17*(5), 482–487.

Kirk, C., Nagiub, G., & Abu-Arafeh, I. (2008). Chronic post-traumatic headache after head injury in children and adolescents. *Developmental Medicine and Child Neurology, 50*(6), 422–425.

Kirkwood, M. W., & Kirk, J. W. (2010). The base rate of suboptimal effort in a pediatric mild TBI sample: Performance on the Medical Symptom Validity Test. *The Clinical Neuropsychologist, 24*(5), 860–872.

Kirkwood, M. W., Kirk, J. W., Blaha, R. Z., & Wilson, P. (2010). Noncredible effort during pediatric neuropsychological exam: A case series and literature review. *Child Neuropsychology, 16*(6), 604–618.

Korinthcnberg, R., Schreck, J., Weser, J., & Lehmkuhl, G. (2004). Post-traumatic syndrome after minor head injury cannot be predicted by neurological investigations. *Brain and Development, 26*(2), 113–117.

Kraus, J. F., Fife, D., Cox, P., Ramstein, K., & Conroy, C. (1986). Incidence, severity, and external causes of pediatric brain injury. *American Journal of Diseases of Children, 140*(7), 687–693.

Lane, J. C., & Arciniegas, D. B. (2002). Post-traumatic headache. *Current Treatment Options in Neurology, 4*(1), 89–104.

Langguth, B., Landgrebe, M., Wittmann, M., Kleinjung, T., & Hajak, G. (2010). Persistent tinnitus induced by tricyclic antidepressants. *Journal of Psychopharmacology, 24*(8), 1273–1275.

Lanser, J. B., Jennekens-Schinkel, A., & Peters, A. C. (1988). Headache after closed head injury in children. *Headache, 28*(3), 176–179.

Larson, E. B., & Zollman, F. S. (2010). The effect of sleep medications on cognitive recovery from traumatic brain injury. *Journal of Head Trauma Rehabilitation, 25*(1), 61–67.

Lauwerier, E., Paemeleire, K., Van Damme, S., Goubert, L., & Crombez, G. (2011). Medication use in patients with migraine and medication-overuse headache: The role of problem-solving and attitudes about pain medication. *Pain, 152*(6), 1334–1339.

Lew, H. L., Lin, P. H., Fuh, J. L., Wang, S. J., Clark, D. J., & Walker, W. C. (2006). Characteristics and treatment of headache after traumatic brain injury: A focused review. *American Journal of Physical Medicine and Rehabilitation, 85*(7), 619–627.

Lewis, D., & Paradiso, E. (2007). A double-blind, dose comparison study of topiramate for prophylaxis of basilar-type migraine in children: A pilot study. *Headache, 47*(10), 1409–1417.

Lewis, K. S. (2010). Pediatric headache. *Seminars in Pediatric Neurology, 17*(4), 224–229.

Linde, K., Allais, G., Brinkhaus, B., Manheimer, E., Vickers, A., & White, A. R. (2009). Acupuncture for tension-type headache. *Cochrane Database of Systematic Reviews, 21*(1), 1–45.

Lipton, R. B., Gobel, H., Einhaupl, K. M., Wilks, K., & Mauskop, A. (2004). *Petasites hybridus* root (butterbur) is an effective preventive treatment for migraine. *Neurology*, *63*(12), 2240–2244.

Lipton, R. B., Silberstein, S. D., & Stewart, W. F. (1994). An update on the epidemiology of migraine. *Headache*, *34*(6), 319–328.

Losche, W., Mazurov, A. V., Heptinstall, S., Groenewegen, W. A., Repin, V. S., & Till, U. (1987). An extract of feverfew inhibits interactions of human platelets with collagen substrates. *Thrombosis Research*, *48*(5), 511–518.

Lundin, A., de Boussard, C., Edman, G., & Borg, J. (2006). Symptoms and disability until 3 months after mild TBI. *Brain Injury*, *20*(8), 799–806.

Magis, D., Ambrosini, A., Sandor, P., Jacquy, J., Laloux, P., & Schoenen, J. (2007). A randomized double-blind placebo-controlled trial of thioctic acid in migraine prophylaxis. *Headache*, *47*(1), 52–57.

Maruta, J., Lee, S. W., Jacobs, E. F., & Ghajar, J. (2010a). A unified science of concussion. *Annals of the New York Academy of Sciences*, *1208*, 58–66.

Maruta, J., Suh, M., Niogi, S. N., Mukherjee, P., & Ghajar, J. (2010b). Visual tracking synchronization as a metric for concussion screening. *Journal of Head Trauma Rehabilitation*, *25*(4), 293–305.

Meares, S., Shores, E. A., Batchelor, J., Baguley, I. J., Chapman, J., Gurka, J., et al. (2006). The relationship of psychological and cognitive factors and opioids in the development of the postconcussion syndrome in general trauma patients with mild traumatic brain injury. *Journal of International Neuropsychology Society*, *12*(6), 792–801.

Meienberg, O., & Muri, R. (1992). Nuclear and infranuclear disorders. *Bailliere's Clinical Neurology*, *1*(2), 417–434.

Middleton, K., Krabak, B. J., & Coppel, D. B. (2010). The influence of pediatric autonomic dysfunction on recovery after concussion. *Clinical Journal of Sports Medicine*, *20*(6), 491–492.

Milroy, G., Dorris, L., & McMillan, T. M. (2008). Sleep disturbances following mild traumatic brain injury in childhood. *Journal of Pediatric Psychology*, *33*(3), 242–247.

Nestoriuc, Y., Martin, A., Rief, W., & Andrasik, F. (2008a). Biofeedback treatment for headache disorders: A comprehensive efficacy review. *Applied Psychophysiology and Biofeedback*, *33*(3), 125–140.

Nestoriuc, Y., Rief, W., & Martin, A. (2008b). Meta-analysis of biofeedback for tension-type headache: Efficacy, specificity, and treatment moderators. *Journal of Consulting and Clinical Psychology*, *76*(3), 379–396.

Niemensivu, R., Pyykko, I., Wiener-Vacher, S. R., & Kentala, E. (2006). Vertigo and balance problems in children: An epidemiologic study in Finland. *International Journal of Pediatric Otorhinolaryngology*, *70*(2), 259–265.

Oh, H. J., Kim, J. S., Han, B. I., & Lim, J. G. (2007). Predicting a successful treatment in posterior canal benign paroxysmal positional vertigo. *Neurology*, *68*(15), 1219–1222.

Olesen, J., Diener, H. C., Husstedt, I. W., Goadsby, P. J., Hall, D., Meier, U., et al. (2004). Calcitonin gene-related peptide receptor antagonist BIBN 4096 BS for the acute treatment of migraine. *New England Journal of Medicine*, *350*(11), 1104–1110.

Orff, H. J., Ayalon, L., & Drummond, S. P. (2009). Traumatic brain injury and sleep disturbance: A review of current research. *Journal of Head Trauma Rehabilitation*, *24*(3), 155–165.

Ormos, G. (2003). Cervicogenic headache in children. *Headache*, *43*(6), 693–694.

Pakalnis, A., Gibson, J., & Colvin, A. (2005). Comorbidity of psychiatric and behavioral disorders in pediatric migraine. *Headache*, *45*(5), 590–596.

Peikert, A., Wilimzig, C., & Kohne-Volland, R. (1996). Prophylaxis of migraine with oral magnesium: Results from a prospective, multi-center, placebo-controlled and double-blind randomized study. *Cephalalgia: An International Journal of Headache*, 16(4), 257–263.

Peterson, M. L., Christou, E., & Rosengren, K. S. (2006). Children achieve adult-like sensory integration during stance at 12-years-old. *Gait and Posture*, 23(4), 455–463.

Pfaffenrath, V., Wessely, P., Meyer, C., Isler, H. R., Evers, S., Grotemeyer, K. H., et al. (1996). Magnesium in the prophylaxis of migraine: A double-blind placebo-controlled study. *Cephalalgia: An International Journal of Headache*, 16(6), 436–440.

Podoshin, L., Ben-David, Y., Fradis, M., Malatskey, S., & Hafner, H. (1995). Idiopathic subjective tinnitus treated by amitriptyline hydrochloride/biofeedback. *International Tinnitus Journal*, 1(1), 54–60.

Post, R. E., & Dickerson, L. M. (2010). Dizziness: A diagnostic approach. *American Family Physician*, 82(4), 361–368, 369.

Pothmann, R., & Danesch, U. (2005). Migraine prevention in children and adolescents: Results of an open study with a special butterbur root extract. *Headache*, 45(3), 196–203.

Prakash, S., Mehta, N. C., Dabhi, A. S., Lakhani, O., Khilari, M., & Shah, N. D. (2010). The prevalence of headache may be related with the latitude: A possible role of vitamin D insufficiency? *Journal of Headache and Pain*, 11(4), 301–307.

Prakash, S., & Shah, N. D. (2009). Chronic tension-type headache with vitamin D deficiency: Casual or causal association? *Headache*, 49(8), 1214–1222.

Prisman, E., Ramsden, J. D., Blaser, S., & Papsin, B. (2011). Traumatic perilymphatic fistula with pneumolabyrinth: Diagnosis and management. *Laryngoscope*, 121(4), 856–859.

Pugh, W. J., & Sambo, K. (1988). Prostaglandin synthetase inhibitors in feverfew. *Journal of Pharmacy and Pharmacology*, 40(10), 743–745.

Raj, S. R. (2006). The postural tachycardia syndrome (POTS): Pathophysiology, diagnosis and management. *Indian Pacing and Electrophysiology Journal*, 6(2), 84–99.

Rauschecker, J. P., Leaver, A. M., & Muhlau, M. (2010). Tuning out the noise: Limbic–auditory interactions in tinnitus. *Neuron*, 66(6), 819–826.

Recober, A., Kuburas, A., Zhang, Z., Wemmie, J. A., Anderson, M. G., & Russo, A. F. (2009). Role of calcitonin gene-related peptide in light-aversive behavior: Implications for migraine. *Journal of Neuroscience*, 29(27), 8798–8804.

Register-Mihalik, J. K., Mihalik, J. P., & Guskiewicz, K. M. (2008). Balance deficits after sports-related concussion in individuals reporting posttraumatic headache. *Neurosurgery*, 63(1), 76–80; discussion, 76–80.

Sanchez-Barcelo, E. J., Mediavilla, M. D., & Reiter, R. J. (2011). Clinical uses of melatonin in pediatrics. *International Journal of Pediatrics*, epub article ID 892624.

Sandor, P. S., Di Clemente, L., Coppola, G., Saenger, U., Fumal, A., Magis, D., et al. (2005). Efficacy of coenzyme Q10 in migraine prophylaxis: A randomized controlled trial. *Neurology*, 64(4), 713–715.

Sas, K., Pardutz, A., Toldi, J., & Vecsei, L. (2010). Dementia, stroke and migraine: Some common pathological mechanisms. *Journal of the Neurological Sciences*, 299(1–2), 55–65.

Satz, P., Zaucha, K., McCleary, C., Light, R., Asarnow, R., & Becker, D. (1997). Mild head injury in children and adolescents: A review of studies (1970–1995). *Psychological Bulletin*, 122(2), 107–131.

Schmitz, M., & Jackel, M. (1998). Comparative study for assessing quality of life of patients with exogenous sleep disorders (temporary sleep onset and sleep interruption disorders) treated with a hops–valarian preparation and a benzodiazepine drug. *Wiener Medizinische Wöchenschrift*, 148(13), 291–298.

Schoenen, J., Jacquy, J., & Lenaerts, M. (1998). Effectiveness of high-dose riboflavin in migraine prophylaxis: A randomized controlled trial. *Neurology*, 50(2), 466–470.

Schoenen, J., & Jensen, R. (2006). Differential diagnosis and prognosis of tension-type head-aches. In J. Olesen (Ed.), *The headaches* (3rd ed., pp. 701–706). Philadelphia: Lippincott, Williams & Wilkins.

Schreiber, S., Barkai, G., Gur-Hartman, T., Peles, E., Tov, N., Dolberg, O. T., et al. (2008). Long-lasting sleep patterns of adult patients with minor traumatic brain injury (mTBI) and non-mTBI subjects. *Sleep Medicine, 9*(5), 481–487.

Shields, K. G., & Goadsby, P. J. (2006). Serotonin receptors modulate trigeminovascular responses in ventroposteromedial nucleus of thalamus: A migraine target? *Neurobiology of Disease, 23*(3), 491–501.

Shulman, A., & Strashun, A. M. (2009). Fluid dynamics vascular theory of brain and inner-ear function in traumatic brain injury: A translational hypothesis for diagnosis and treatment. *International Tinnitus Journal, 15*(2), 119–129.

Sjaastad, O., Fredriksen, T. A., & Pfaffenrath, V. (1998a). Cervicogenic headache: Diagnostic criteria. The Cervicogenic Headache International Study Group. *Headache, 38*(6), 442–445.

Sjaastad, O., Salvesen, R., Jansen, J., & Fredriksen, T. A. (1998b). Cervicogenic headache: A critical view on pathogenesis. *Functional Neurology, 13*(1), 71–74.

Solomon, S. (1998). John Graham Senior Clinicians Award Lecture: Posttraumatic migraine. *Headache, 38*(10), 772–778.

Solomon, S. (2009). Post-traumatic headache: Commentary—an overview. *Headache, 49*(7), 1112–1115.

Sprenger, T., & Goadsby, P. J. (2009). Migraine pathogenesis and state of pharmacological treatment options. *BMC Medicine, 7*, 71.

Stiller-Ostrowski, J. L. (2010). Fourth cranial nerve palsy in a collegiate lacrosse player: A case report. *Journal of Athletic Training, 45*(4), 407–410.

Sun-Edelstein, C., & Mauskop, A. (2011). Alternative headache treatments: Nutraceuticals, behavioral and physical treatments. *Headache, 51*(3), 469–483.

Taibi, D. M., Landis, C. A., Petry, H., & Vitiello, M. V. (2007). A systematic review of valerian as a sleep aid: Safe but not effective. *Sleep Medicine Reviews, 11*(3), 209–230.

Taylor, H. G., Dietrich, A., Nuss, K., Wright, M., Rusin, J., Bangert, B., et al. (2010). Post-concussive symptoms in children with mild traumatic brain injury. *Neuropsychology, 24*(2), 148–159.

Thiedke, C. C. (2001). Sleep disorders and sleep problems in childhood. *American Family Physician, 63*(2), 277–284.

Uomoto, J. M., & Esselman, P. C. (1993). Traumatic brain injury and chronic pain: Differential types and rates by head injury severity. *Archives of Physical Medicine and Rehabilitation, 74*(1), 61–64.

Vincent, M. B. (2010). Cervicogenic headache: The neck is a generator: con. *Headache, 50*(4), 706–709.

CHAPTER 16

School-Based Management

John W. Kirk, Beth Slomine, and Jeanne E. Dise-Lewis

M anaging the acute needs of students with a concussion or mild traumatic brain injury (mTBI) can be challenging for school professionals due to limited TBI training, poor communication between medical and school professionals, and lack of formal school reentry protocols for students. Given that the majority of concussions are uncomplicated and mild in nature, most students will recover relatively quickly and not need extensive evaluative or educational services (Cassidy et al., 2004; Kraus, 1995; Langlois, Rutland-Brown, & Wald, 2006). However, even when a child appears physically healthy in the days or weeks after injury, a variety of difficulties can negatively impact school performance, including problems sustaining attention, slowed processing speed, decreased learning of new information, and fatigue. For a minority of students, these types of difficulties may persist beyond the first few weeks. For example, when mTBI is complicated by intracranial findings on neuroimaging (e.g., subdural hematoma), cognitive deficits have been found to persist for months or longer (Levin et al., 2008).

A number of publications provide detailed information about returning students to school after a moderate to severe TBI (Dise-Lewis, Calvery, & Lewis, 2005; Semrud-Clikeman, 2001; Stanford & Dorflinger, 2009; Savage, Depompei, Tyler, & Lash, 2005; Ylvisaker et al., 1995a). These publications focus on providing accommodations and modifications to support the child with new, significant cognitive deficits that are not likely to be short-lived. Among students with more severe TBI, much of the educational and therapeutic focus is on developing systems of care and advocating for services needed to address long-lasting impairments and disability. One challenge in working with children who have sustained an mTBI is that, although subtle difficulties tend to be short-lived for most students, they nonetheless can persist and possibly worsen without proper intervention and support. We believe that a key to successfully managing children with mTBI is to develop a program specific to their short-term academic needs, which will likely be different than those provided for children with moderate to severe TBI. For example, to optimize recovery after mTBI, we believe that students should return to school within a few days to a week, whereas after a moderate to severe injury the transition to school typically needs to occur over a matter of weeks to months.

To date, there has been a handful of guidelines proposed that address when and how to return a student to school following a concussion or mTBI. In this chapter, we present these guidelines and our own five-step model for returning students to school following an mTBI. Before reviewing the available literature, we provide a brief overview of educational supports, including temporary accommodations, a Section 504 Plan, and an individualized education plan (IEP).

OPTIONS FOR EDUCATIONAL ACCOMMODATIONS AND SPECIAL EDUCATION LAW

Most commonly, children with mTBI need only temporary support through informal accommodations and monitoring. Special education law does not mandate that informal accommodations be implemented after mTBI; however, most schools are more than willing to implement a few simple, temporary accommodations at the request of parents or health care professionals. We advocate that temporary supportive accommodations be implemented when a student returns to school following a concussion. Informal accommodations can easily be implemented and do not require the formal review and eligibility determination that are required for a Section 504 Plan or IEP. Therefore, they can be put into place almost immediately, providing the appropriate safety net for the student when he or she most needs it—in the first several days and weeks postconcussion. We believe that putting appropriate documentation in place immediately offers the best chance that a student's postconcussive symptoms will resolve completely within a matter of weeks.

If a child experiences persistent postconcussive difficulties lasting more than several weeks, a Section 504 Plan, which offers a formal mechanism to implement appropriate accommodations in the child's regular education environment, can be utilized. Section 504 of the Rehabilitation Act of 1973 provides protection against discrimination for individuals who have disabilities (Hicks, 1996), and lists accommodations to the regular school program that are intended to help students compensate for physical difficulties that interfere with their ability to learn at a rate commensurate with peers (McIntosh & Decker, 2005). Typically, documentation from a health care provider indicating that the child had a concussion and warrants accommodations is needed to put a 504 Plan in place. Educationally based evaluations are not required to implement a 504 Plan.

In the rare instances when a child with an mTBI requires special education or therapeutic services in school as a result of injury, an IEP is needed. An IEP offers accommodations and modifications to the regular education program and may include remedial instruction and therapeutic services such as speech–language, occupational, and/or physical therapies. Public Law 94-142: Education for All Handicapped Children Act (1975) was the first in the series of federal statutes to mandate that all children have a right to a free and appropriate education and to require that each state develop a plan to ensure that every child who has disabilities receives special education services, as outlined in an IEP (Jacob & Hartshorne, 2003). The Individuals with Disabilities Education Act (IDEA) Amendment of 1997 (Public Law 105-117) ensures that all children with handicapping conditions are identified and served. Mandated by federal law, all children who have an educational disability, including TBI, are entitled to receive free and appropriate educational services, including special education as needed (Education for All Handicapped Children Act, 1975; IDEA, 1990; IDEA Amendment, 1997). The IEP process is more involved and may take much longer to implement than informal accommodations or a 504 Plan. To determine whether a child has an educational disability, a multidisciplinary team is organized that typically includes a special education teacher, regular education teacher, school psychologist, therapists relevant to the services being provided (e.g., speech–language, occupational, or physical therapy), and parents. Evaluations by some or all of these educational professionals are typically required prior to making a determination about eligibility for services. Although the school's multidisciplinary team must determine eligibility for special education services, they often work collaboratively with professionals outside of the school, including psychologists, therapists, and physicians in making that determination.

EXISTING GUIDELINES FOR RETURNING TO SCHOOL

Ylvisaker, Feeney, and Mullins (1995b) were the first to propose a comprehensive protocol for transitioning a student from the hospital to school setting after a pediatric mTBI. The authors note that many children who sustain mTBI will recover quickly and will not likely need any formal accommodations or modifications; however, they highlight that (1) a minority of children experience difficulties lasting from weeks to months, and (2) children who are recovering from concussions benefit from reducing the added stress of full academic demands in the acute period. Their protocol was designed as a "safety net system" to ensure that those children who experience lingering difficulties would not fall behind academically or socially.

The authors provide two separate protocols, one for hospital or medical providers and the other for school personnel. The hospital protocol directs the hospital's discharge planner to provide education regarding recovery (e.g., rarely are there lingering difficulties) and the importance of contacting the school nurse (or other designated school representative) to establish temporary accommodations. Ylvisaker et al. (1995b) recommend that if symptoms persist beyond 4 weeks or if there are "red flags" present, a formal referral should be made to a multidisciplinary team (e.g., pediatric neuropsychologist, special education TBI team) for further evaluation.

The school protocol begins when the school nurse (or other designated representative) receives the information from the medical professional and informs the student's educational team of the injury, prognosis, and potential red flags that would warrant further evaluation and intervention. Although this protocol is specific to the needs of children with mTBI and provides excellent suggestions, the protocol is dependent on medical personnel (e.g., hospital discharge planner) communicating directly with the school. As providers who work in large hospital settings, we believe that placing the responsibility on hospital staff of directly communicating (e.g., via phone contact) with the patient's school could be impractical due to time requirements and is unlikely to occur on a regular basis. In addition, most children with mTBI are never seen in emergency departments (EDs) or are discharged directly from them without hospitalization. Additionally, the recommendations provided by Ylvisaker et al. (1995b) may be most appropriate for children with more complicated mild injuries who are slow to recover and may not be necessary for the majority of children with uncomplicated mTBI who typically recover relatively quickly after injury.

McGrath (2010) recently proposed a five-step model for school-based concussion management for student athletes, with education and assessment provided by a clinical neuropsychologist and the school's athletic trainer. In this model, the athletic trainer is identified as the key professional on the educational team who provides education, support, and communication. McGrath argues that in today's culture of increased concussion awareness and management techniques, schools should be capable of carrying out comprehensive concussion management programs. McGrath's proposed five-step model begins with concussion education provided, ideally, by a neuropsychologist or physician and directed toward athletes, coaches, parents, and school personnel. The second and third steps involve preseason computer-administered neurocognitive testing and postinjury evaluation of neurocognitive functions following a concussion. The fourth step involves tracking postconcussion symptoms during the recovery period, both to determine return-to-play status and to implement appropriate support in the classroom. The goal of this step is to support the recovering student in keeping up with academic demands in a way that does not overstress cognitive functions and potentially exacerbate postconcussion symptoms. The fifth and final step in this model involves consultation between the athletic trainer and the student's physician about returning to physical activity, with the results then integrated into the classroom plan for resumption of full academic demands.

Although McGrath's (2010) return-to-school protocol provides helpful information regarding specific accommodations, it relies on athletic trainers and community-based neuropsychologists to initiate and implement it. Even in today's culture of heightened concussion awareness in sports, many schools do not have specific concussion management programs due to limited funding and resources. Moreover, not all students who sustain an mTBI are athletes who are returning to play and, as such, not all are known to the athletic trainer. Additionally, the supply of neuropsychologists and knowledgeable physicians in the community is not adequate to provide neurocognitive testing for all students who sustain an mTBI, and the ability of serial neurocognitive testing to identify meaningful recovery in all students continues to be debated (Broglio, Ferrara, Macciocchi, Baumgartner, & Elliott, 2007; Kirkwood, Randolph, & Yeates, 2009; Randolph, McCrea, & Barr, 2005). Finally, we believe that the individual who is identified as the lead person in managing the student's educational needs should come from within the school system (e.g., a school nurse or counselor).

In another model, Kirkwood and colleagues (2008) provide a number of strategies to support the transition back to school for children with mTBI. They divided the strategies into three areas: initial transitional support, general school-based support, and specific classroom-based support that involve teachers' taking a greater role in monitoring the children's return. With regard to initial transitional strategies, they recommend that (1) parents or health care providers notify school personnel and educate staff regarding potential consequences of the student's mTBI; (2) the return to school occurs gradually; (3) the student not be expected to complete all missed work; and (4) additional assistance be provided to facilitate completion of schoolwork. In the area of school-based support, school personnel are encouraged to (1) monitor the student closely for at least a few weeks; (2) reduce general school demands (e.g., tests and assignments); and (3) provide organizational assistance, as needed, for demanding assignments or projects. Classroom-based support might include (1) the delay of any standardized exams, (2) additional time on exams, (3) flexible assignment due dates, (4) access to peer or teacher classroom notes, and (5) preferential seating to support attention. Although Kirkwood et al. (2008) provide the basic foundation for appropriate school reentry following concussion, no specific guidelines are offered as to how best to facilitate communication between health care providers and school personnel. As previously mentioned, ideally, health care providers should be available to quickly and efficiently communicate to parents or school personnel (1) the nature of the child's injury, (2) any restrictions on physical activity, (3) accommodations for school participation, (4) expected recovery, and (5) red flags indicative of poor outcome.

THE "COGNITIVE REST" CONTROVERSY

Recently, the idea of cognitive rest and delayed return to school has received some attention in the pediatric concussion literature. For example, in the most recent consensus statement on concussion in sport from the Third International Conference on Concussion in Sport held in Zurich, very specific guidelines were offered to manage an athlete's return to play (McCrory et al., 2009). As part of this consensus statement, a recommendation was included for "physical and cognitive rest" during the "no-activity" rehabilitation stage of the graduated return-to-play protocol. This publication fails to specifically define cognitive rest, but Halstead, Walter, and the Council on Sports Medicine and Fitness (2010) define this as refraining from all activities that involve mental exertion, such as schoolwork, reading for leisure, working on a computer, watching television, and playing video games. They indicate that the child should not return to school "while symptomatic" and recommend a possible temporary leave of absence from school, shortening of the student's day, and/or general reduction in school workload. In actuality, empirical data showing that rest facilitates recovery or reduces risks after mTBI are lacking (for further discussion, see Iverson, Gagnon, & Griesbach, Chapter 14, this volume). Although we agree that rest is likely to be important during the acute period (within the first hours to days postinjury), children with mTBI are apt to benefit most from a return to school as soon as some of their most severe symptoms subside, with accommodations and modifications in place as needed.

Consistent with this view, Kirkwood et al. (2008) recommend a gradual transition back to school after an mTBI, suggesting that too slow of a return to school could potentially protract the child's recovery. For example, a high school student may experience undue stress secondary to falling behind, being away from peers, and disruption of the family's typical routine due to a prolonged school absence. In most cases, a child will be able to return to school within days to, at most, 1 week after injury.

PROPOSED GUIDELINES AND APPROACHES
TO SCHOOL REENTRY FOLLOWING mTBI

Without evidence-based intervention strategies, we believe approaches to school reentry should take into account the research we do have available regarding recovery after pediatric mTBI. Based on the available literature, we propose some basic guidelines, programming, and intervention strategies to help reintegrate the child into school after an uncomplicated mTBI through a five-step protocol. The protocol should be applicable to the majority of children who sustain a concussion, whereas those who sustain a complicated mTBI will likely require a more comprehensive neuropsychological evaluation to assist with formal educational programming. A summary of the steps of the protocol is provided in Table 16.1.

Step 1: Education

The first step to promote successful management of pediatric mTBI involves providing general education to school professionals, students, and their families. Assuring that professionals within the school have a basic appreciation and awareness of mTBI and its potential impact on academics and social performance is essential to any school reentry model. TBI education should focus on identifying acute signs/symptoms, the need for immediate medical attention, the expected recovery trajectory, the potential cognitive and behavioral difficulties that can arise during the days to weeks

TABLE 16.1. Summary of Five-Step Protocol for School Reentry

Schoolwide intervention prior to any injury

Step 1: Educate.
All school professionals, students, and families should be provided with basic education about mTBI to promote appreciation and awareness of the potential impact of mTBI on school functioning.

Child-specific interventions after TBI

Step 2: Communicate.
After a child is injured and evaluated by a medical provider, that professional should provide *documentation* of the TBI and suggested accommodations to the school or to caregivers who can share them with the school.

Step 3: Monitor.
Prior to, or on the first day back to, school, a school professional should be identified as a case manager. The case manager should share injury-related information and suggested accommodations with all of the child's teachers and monitor the child's recovery.

Step 4: Create a safety net.
The case manager should work with the child's teachers to implement temporary accommodations upon return to school to manage common symptoms of mTBI and to develop a plan to address missed work.

Step 5: Refer to health care providers.
For the child who does not recover as expected, the case manager should suggest referral to health care specialists with experience in TBI, who can work with the child's educational team to help guide and refine the educational plan.

postinjury, and specific guidelines for school-based accommodations. Given the limited funding and resources currently available to many public and private schools, much of this education may need to be provided through written and online resources rather than directly by professionals with TBI expertise. Notably, some states have enacted or are proposing concussion legislation that not only provides specific regulations regarding students' return to play sports, but also requires coaches to receive a minimal amount of education about mTBI (see Jake Snakenberg Youth Concussion Act: Colorado Senate Bill 11-040).

In line with the idea of general education, the Centers for Disease Control and Prevention (CDC), through the Children's Health Act of 2000, implemented a national concussion education and awareness initiative. As part of that initiative, the CDC pulled together experts in the field to develop resources for parents, student athletes, health care professionals, and educators. The resources are designed to raise awareness and provide education about concussion, help professionals educate others about concussion, and improve health care providers' and educators' ability to prevent, recognize, and manage concussion in student athletes. More recently, the focus of the resources has broadened beyond sports to include a wide range of etiologies. The materials are available for downloading and ordering at no cost from the CDC's website (*www.cdc.gov/Concussion*).

Several of the CDC resources are useful in considering return-to-school policy following concussion. For instance, the most recently developed toolkit, the *Heads Up to Schools: Know Your Concussion ABCs*, was developed for professionals working with grades K–12 to help them identify and respond to concussions in a range of school settings (Centers for Disease Control and Prevention, 2010). The toolkit contains a fact sheet for educators, counselors, and other school professionals that includes information about common signs and symptoms of concussion, typical course of recovery, problems to look for in the classroom, and common accommodations that may be necessary upon return to school. In addition, the toolkit provides a separate fact sheet for school nurses with more detailed information about the assessment of signs and symptoms, as well as an emphasis on raising awareness and helping educate other professionals within the school system about concussion assessment, management, and prevention. A short fact sheet for parents is also included. The toolkit can be accessed at (*www.cdc.gov/concussion/HeadsUp/schools.html*).

Step 2: Communication

One of the most common pitfalls in implementing appropriate educational services for the child with mTBI is the lack of communication among medical professionals, parents, and educational professionals. The *Heads Up: Brain Injury in Your Practice* toolkit was designed to help physicians prevent concussion as well as to appropriately diagnose and treat children with concussion. The Acute Concussion Evaluation (ACE) tool, an evidenced-based clinical assessment and monitoring measure, developed by Gioia and Collins (2006), is one of several resources included in the kit (see Appendix 6.1). Along with the ACE, the toolkit includes the ACE Care Plan. The school version of the ACE Care Plan includes common recommendations related to managing a student's return to school after a concussion. In addition to general guidelines about return-to-school-related activities, professionals are able to check off specific recommendations on the care plan. Common school recommendations include guidance about when to return to school and whether a full day or partial day is recommended initially, as well as recommendations about rest breaks, extra time, homework load, standardized testing, and requesting a meeting of the educational team. The ACE Care Plan was intended to be completed by the health care provider who assessed the child following injury and provided to the child's family and school to promote a thoughtful return to both physical and mental activities. The toolkit, ACE, and ACE Care Plan can be found at (*www.cdc.gov/concussion/HeadsUp/physicians_tool_kit.html*).

We propose that the medical provider (e.g., pediatrician, ED physician) complete the ACE Care Plan—School Version or a similar document and either fax this directly to the child's school or provide the parent with this documentation to share with the school. Utilizing such a simple yet informative document would likely facilitate communication between medical providers and educational staff, and would not require the medical professional to directly communicate with the school's case manager via telephone or take the additional time to write a specific school note for each patient.

Step 3: Identifying a School Case Manager and Monitoring the Student

Within the school, a case manager should be identified who takes the lead among the child's educational team (e.g., school nurse, counselor, psychologist, special education teacher). Ideally, the case manager would receive initial information regarding the child's injury, expected recovery, and need for accommodations through the ACE Care Plan—School Version or a similar form, provided either by the student's parents or doctor. This type of document would then serve as a starting point to develop a temporary safety net or support system within the school. The case manager should document the student's injury, expected recovery, and individual support plan for reference if concerns arise in the future. The case manager should also convey, either orally or in writing, information regarding the student's injury and specific accommodations to all relevant teachers.

A number of well-controlled studies with children with mTBI due to a variety of etiologies suggests that cognitive deficits are not identifiable within 2–3 months after the injury (Carroll et al., 2004; Satz, 2001, Satz et al., 1997). In contrast, more recent work highlights that postconcussion symptoms may be more pronounced and long-lasting in some children with mTBI, especially those who present acutely with evidence of more severe injury (Yeates et al., 2009). Keeping these basic expectations in mind, if the child is experiencing a change in academic functioning, continues to miss a significant amount of school, has significant behavioral problems either at home or school, or is complaining of unresolved subjective symptoms (e.g., difficulties with concentration, headaches) several weeks after the injury, this information should be shared with the child's family and education and health care team. The case manager should track recovery from a daily to weekly basis through teacher report or monitoring of assignment completion. It is most important that the child is monitored by the case manager to ensure the identification of any difficulties, whether they persist beyond typical recovery periods, or if there appears to be a worsening of symptoms.

Step 4: Providing a Supportive Safety Net

Consistent with previously mentioned school reentry protocols, we believe that establishing at least temporary accommodations upon the child's return to school provides a "safety net" so that the child does not experience undue stress or unrealistic expectations during the acute recovery period (Kirkwood et al., 2008; Ylvisaker et al., 1995). For the majority of students with mTBI, a formal education plan will not be necessary, but temporary accommodations and modifications may be particularly beneficial upon immediate return to the classroom. In Table 16.2, we have provided a list of general accommodations and modifications that would be appropriate as temporary supports or as part of a formal Section 504 Plan.

As previously mentioned, we believe that students should return to school sooner rather than later, because missing a significant amount of school (particularly within high school curriculum) can place undue stress upon the student and could exacerbate headaches, sleep difficulties, and anxiety. During the acute period of recovery, missing a day or two of school, or possibly up to a week, may be reasonable. In addition, in some cases gradual return to school (e.g., participation in half-day classes) is necessary for a brief period of time; however, we have seen the idea of "cognitive rest while symptomatic" be inappropriately applied (e.g., child is forced to take a leave of absence from school for several weeks or months). For the child who is experiencing persistent

---

TABLE 16.2. Potential Accommodations and Modifications in School after mTBI

Develop a transition plan

- Notify school of concussion injury prior to or upon returning to school.
- Develop a plan for a gradual return-to-school day and demands (e.g., child may be allowed to return part-time before building up to a full day schedule as necessary).
- Provide a waiver of any missed assignments/exams or design a plan of assistance to support completion of missing assignments.

Reduce demands, monitor recovery, and provide emotional support

- Provide rest time or breaks during the day (e.g., student is allowed to go to nurse's office when experiencing headaches and then returns to class when feeling better).
- Carefully consider upcoming standardized tests (e.g., college entrance exams) and advise student whether or not to reschedule.
- Excuse student from classes or activities that require rigorous physical activity (e.g., physical education, recess) until cleared by medical personnel.
- Reduce classroom and homework assignments.
- Reschedule exams when student is symptomatic or coordinate and pace exams to no more than one per day.
- Negotiate timing of large assignments so that they do not occur at the same time.
- Assign a counselor to meet with the student at the end of each day at least for the first few days to check in with regarding emotional status (e.g., frustration tolerance, emotional lability), problem-solve, and assure that homework needs are being addressed.

Other common academic accommodations

- Provide preferential seating to reduce exposure to distracting lights or noises, allow for closer teacher monitoring, and facilitate focused attention.
- Allow for tests to be taken in a distraction-free environment.
- Grant additional time for in- and out-of-class exams and assignments.
- Assign a good notetaker in each class whose notes can be photocopied and provided to the student daily.

Note. Based on Kirkwood, Yeates, and Wilson (2006).

headaches that interfere with his or her ability to participate in school beyond 1 week postinjury, we strongly recommend referral to a physician for further evaluation and management. The goal should be to return the student to school as soon as possible, but with appropriate accommodations and modifications implemented.

Step 5: Referral to Health Care Providers as Needed

The majority of children will recover relatively quickly after an mTBI without a Section 504 Plan or formal school-based or neuropsychological evaluation. However, students occasionally require further evaluation and intervention by health care specialists with expertise in TBI to assist with educational programming.

A child who has sustained multiple concussions would benefit from consultation with a concussion expert or specialty clinic to assess for any lingering postconcussion complaints and concerns about future injuries. It is not uncommon for teens who have sustained multiple concussions to continue to participate in competitive high-risk sports (e.g., ice hockey, football, soccer). Often, these athletes will require multiple evaluations to assist with return-to-play decision making. These evaluations could include additional neuroimaging techniques (e.g., magnetic resonance imaging [MRI]), neuropsychological evaluation, and neurological examination. The child who sustains a more severe injury, such as a complicated mTBI or a moderate to severe TBI, should always be referred to medical specialists to assist with rehabilitation and academic interventions. In addition, the child who has a preinjury history of learning disabilities, attention-deficit/hyperactivity disorder (ADHD), or psychiatric concerns may benefit from referral for neuropsychological evaluation, as it can be difficult to discern whether persistent cognitive or behavioral difficulties are lingering postconcussion complaints or due to premorbid problems.

If a child experiences difficulties that seem severe given the nature of the injury, or if it seems that a child's symptoms are either not improving or are worsening over time, the school should also consider involving medical or concussion specialists. For example, if a child who sustains an uncomplicated mTBI continues to experience persistent postconcussion complaints lasting longer than a month, a referral for a neuropsychological evaluation may be warranted. This evaluation can help determine if premorbid psychiatric features or situational stressors are complicating recovery. An essential component of any neuropsychological evaluation of a child who experiences persistent or atypical symptoms related to a poorly resolving concussion should be the formal evaluation of effort and motivation. Kirkwood and Kirk (2010) studied how many children seen for neuropsychological consultation after an mTBI presented with noncredible effort during examination. Among this large sample of 193 patients, 17% of patients provided noncredible effort, yielding invalid neuropsychological data. Why children present with noncredible effort or exaggerate symptoms after a concussion has not been studied much to date, but the reasons are likely multifactorial and complex (Kirkwood, Kirk, Blaha, & Wilson, 2010).

CASE VIGNETTES

To illustrate the utility of these specific school reentry recommendations, we provide three case vignettes. The first case demonstrates what is commonly seen after the majority of concussions, in which the child quickly recovers and does not require a specialty evaluation, whereas the other two cases represent more complex scenarios that typically benefit from the involvement of concussion specialists.

CASE 1: SARA

Sara was 10 years old when she sustained an mTBI while ice skating with her family. She reportedly slipped, fell, and hit her head in the occipital region on the ice. She was not wearing a helmet. The injury was not associated with a loss of consciousness or significant retrograde or anterograde amnesia. Sara experienced the immediate onset of blurry vision, headaches, dizziness, and mental fogginess. Her family took her directly to a local hospital-based urgent care facility. She was diagnosed with a mild concussion and, given her rapidly improving postconcussion symptoms, a computed tomography (CT) of her head was not completed. The physician at the urgent care facility completed the ACE Care Plan—School Version and instructed Sara's parents to share the plan with Sara's elementary school. The concussion occurred on a Thursday, and Sara missed school that Friday secondary to headaches, fatigue, and sensitivity to light/noise. She returned to school on Monday, and her mother brought the ACE form to the school nurse, who was serving as the case manager for Sara. The school nurse shared information about Sara's injury with her teachers and implemented several temporary accommodations, including no test taking, permission to go to the nurse's office if she experienced headaches, no rigorous physical activity at gym/recess, and a reduction of homework assignments. By the end of the week, Sara reported that she was completely asymptomatic, and there was no need for any further academic support or medical follow-up.

This case typifies the expected recovery for the majority of mild concussions in children and adolescents, and demonstrates how, with the right support and services in the acute period, a child will quickly recover. Sara was evaluated in the acute period by a physician at the urgent care facility who appropriately diagnosed and managed the educational needs of the child. The physician was able to quickly complete the ACE Care Plan—School Version, which facilitated communication between the medical and educational teams. The physician also indicated to Sara's family that Sara would likely recover within a matter of 1–2 weeks, but emphasized that within this time period careful observation and support would be needed. The school nurse took the lead in managing Sara's educational support and likely helped to facilitate a quick recovery. Within 10 days, Sara had fully recovered from her concussion and no longer required any medical or academic support.

CASE 2: TOM

Tom was 14 years old when he sustained a TBI while skateboarding at a community skate park. Tom was described as a "straight-A student" who loved to participate in competitive skateboard competitions. He was wearing a helmet when he fell and hit his head on a concrete skate ramp. He had no loss of consciousness, but immediately after his fall, he reported a headache, nausea, vomiting, balance problems, and confusion. Tom's mother immediately took him to the local hospital ED, where he received a CT of the head that revealed a very small, right-frontal subdural hematoma. Tom was kept in the hospital overnight for observation, and repeat neuroimaging did not reveal any worsening of his hematoma. He was discharged the next day and was told to follow up with his pediatrician if his headaches, balance problems, and fatigue did not improve.

Tom sustained his injury 2 weeks before he was to begin his freshman year in high school. Despite displaying significant improvement in many of his postconcussion symptoms, 6 weeks into the school year, Tom was earning C marks across all core academic classes. School personnel were never notified of Tom's injury because it had occurred during the summer, and the teachers did not have any previous experience with Tom's typical academic performance. After repeatedly coming home from school with complaints of persistent headaches and fatigue, Tom's mother followed up with her pediatrician, who eventually referred Tom to a hospital-based concussion clinic, where he was evaluated by a neuropsychologist. The neuropsychologist contacted the school's nurse who was the case manager and implemented recommendations into a Section 504 Plan.

Too often limited communication occurs between medical and school personnel after children and adolescents sustain a TBI. In Tom's case, the lack of communication between medical personnel and educational providers was not unexpected, given that his injury occurred during the summer, when school was not in session. Additionally, Tom's family never followed up with their pediatrician, as instructed by the physicians at the hospital. This is not uncommon. Indeed, Slomine and colleagues (2006) found that as many as 37% of caregivers of children hospitalized for TBI did not follow up with their pediatrician within the first year postinjury. Given the severity of this child's injury (i.e., complicated mTBI), Tom probably should have undergone a formal evaluation to assist with accommodations and modifications for the school. Only after the student demonstrated a clear decline in academic functioning were his difficulties recognized as being associated with the TBI and a referral to appropriate specialists made.

CASE 3: BILL

Bill was 16 years old when he sustained an mTBI while playing in a competitive ice hockey game. He had a history of three previous concussions and was reportedly being recruited by Division I colleges. Bill's injury occurred when he was hit unexpectedly by another player and collided with the wall and ice. He experienced no loss of consciousness but was immediately removed from play because of balance problems, dizziness, confusion, and persistent headache. Bill did not recall sitting on the bench for the remainder of the game, indicating a period of posttraumatic amnesia lasting up to 20 minutes. The following day his parents took him to his pediatrician, who diagnosed him with a concussion and ordered a CT of the head, which was unremarkable. The injury occurred over a weekend, and Bill missed 1 day of school, but returned the following day. The pediatrician provided the school nurse with an educational sheet regarding mTBI and potential lingering symptoms. Based on the documentation from the pediatrician, school personnel excused Bill from his final exams and implemented a number of temporary supports (e.g., extended time to complete assignments, reduced workload, permission to go to nurse's office when experiencing headaches). Approximately 2 weeks later, Bill's symptoms had resolved and he was allowed to take his final exams. Before Bill's pediatrician considered permitting him to return to ice hockey, he required a medical evaluation by a physiatrist and neuropsychological evaluation.

Bill's case demonstrates the appropriate implementation of various educational and medical supports. First, Bill's pediatrician identified that this was his fourth injury and that he needed additional immediate support upon returning to school. Second, the school nurse was identified as the case manager and was able to take the information from the pediatrician and set up temporary accommodations and modifications. Unfortunately, Bill's injury occurred the weekend before finals, but with the temporary support he was able to take his exam 2 weeks later when he was asymptomatic. Finally, the pediatrician realized the seriousness of Bill's multiple concussions and referred him for further medical and neuropsychological evaluation both to address the return to his sport and to potentially identify any lingering cognitive deficits that could interfere with his academic and social functioning.

SUMMARY

Managing the educational needs of the child who sustains an mTBI can be difficult due to limited TBI training among educational professionals, lack of formal school reentry protocols, and poor communication between medical and educational professionals. The majority of children who sustain an mTBI experience a full recovery within a relatively short period of time. However, a minority of children experience persistent postconcussion difficulties lasting weeks to months or longer, including many children who sustain more severe injuries (e.g., complicated mTBI).

We have proposed a five-step school reentry model that integrates many concepts previously recommended in the published literature, as well as many general therapeutic interventions thought to be effective for the child who is recovering from an mTBI. Consistent with Ylvisaker et al. (1995b), we believe that there needs to be communication between the health care and school teams about the child's injury, needs, and expected outcome during the acute recovery period, in order to provide a supportive "safety net." However, we do appreciate that many medical providers do not have time to directly communicate with the school's case manager via telephone or to take additional time to write a specific school note for the patient. Therefore, we propose instead that medical professionals utilize a simple and quick-to-complete document that would likely facilitate the communication between medical providers and educational staff (e.g., ACE Care Plan—School Version in Appendix 16.1).

The scientific literature regarding pediatric mTBI and school reentry is quite sparse, with very few published papers providing clear guidelines or direction for the treatment of children who have sustained a mTBI. As mTBI becomes more publicized by the media, opportunities to provide appropriate education regarding concussion guidelines and management within the educational system will grow. Our hope is that with increased awareness, research, and education, school management of the child who has sustained a concussion will become more standardized and effective, eventually improving outcome.

REFERENCES

Broglio, S. P., Ferrara, M. S., Macciocchi, S. N., Baumgartner, T. A., & Elliott, R. (2007). Test–retest reliability of computerized concussion assessment programs. *Journal of Athletic Training, 42,* 509–514.

Carroll, L. J., Cassidy, J. D., Peloso, P. M., Borg, J., von Holst, H., Holm, L., et al. (2004). Prognosis for mild traumatic brain injury: Results of the WHO Collaborating Centre Task Force on Mild Traumatic Brain Injury. *Journal of Rehabilitation Medicine, 43*(Suppl.), 84–105.

Cassidy, J. D., Carroll, L. J., Peloso, P. M., Borg, J., von Holst, H., Holm, L., et al. (2004). Incidence, risk factors and prevention of mild traumatic brain injury: Results of the WHO Collaborating Centre Task Force on Mild Traumatic Brain Injury. *Journal of Rehabilitation Medicine, 43*(Suppl.), 28–60.

Centers for Disease Control and Prevention. (2010). *Injury prevention and control: Traumatic brain injury.* Retrieved January 8, 2011, from *www.cdc.gov/concussion/HeadsUp/schools.html.*

Dise-Lewis, J. E., Calvery, M. L., & Lewis, H. C. (2005). *Brain STARS.* Wake Forest, IL: Lash & Associates.

Education for all Handicapped Children Act of 1975, Public Law No. 94-142, § 20 U.S.C., 34 C.F.R.

Gioia, G., & Collins, M. (2006). *Heads up: Brain injury in your practice.* Acute Concussion Evaluation (ACE) Care Plan. Retrieved February 6, 2011, from *www.cdc.gov/concussion/HeadsUp/physicians_tool_kit.html.*

Halstead, M. E., Walter, K. D., & the Council on Sports Medicine and Fitness. (2010). Clinical Report: Sport-related concussion in children and adolescents. *Pediatrics, 126*(3), 597–615.

Hicks, P. A. (1996). Section 504 of the Rehabilitation Act. In P. G. Warden & T. K. Fagan (Eds.), *Historical encyclopedia of school psychology* (pp. 353–354). Wesport, CT: Greenwood.

Individuals with Disabilities Act (Public Law No. 101-476), 20 U.S.C. chapter 33. Amended by Public Law No. 105-117 in June 1997. Regulations appear at 34 C.F.R. Part 30.

Individuals with Disabilities Education Act, 1990, Public Law No. 101-476 § 2, 104 Stat. 1103. (1991).

Jacob, S., & Hartshorne, T. S. (2003). *Ethics and law for school psychologists* (4th ed.). Hoboken, NJ: Wiley.

Kirkwood, M. W., & Kirk, J. W. (2010). The base rate of suboptimal effort in a pediatric mild TBI sample: Performance on the Medical Symptom Validity Test. *The Clinical Neuropsychologist, 24*(5), 860–872.

Kirkwood, M. W., Kirk, J. W., Blaha, R. Z., & Wilson, P. (2010). Noncredible effort during pediatric neuropsychological exam: A case series and literature review. *Child Neuropsychology, 16,* 604–618.

Kirkwood, M. W., Randolph, C., & Yeates, K. (2009). Returning pediatric athletes to play after concussion: The evidence of (lack thereof) behind neuropsychological testing. *Acta Paediatrica, 98,* 1409–1411.

Kirkwood, M. W., Yeates, K. O., Taylor, H. G., Randolph, C., McCrea, M., & Anderson, V. A. (2008). Management of pediatric mild traumatic brain injury: A neuropsychological review from injury through recovery. *The Clinical Neuropsychologist, 22,* 769–800.

Kirkwood, M. W., Yeates, K. O., & Wilson, P. E. (2006). Pediatric sport-related concussion: A review of the clinical management of an oft-neglected population. *Pediatrics, 117,* 1359–1371.

Kraus, J. F. (1995). Epidemiological features of brain injury in children: Occurrence, children at risk, causes, and manner of injury, severity, and outcomes. In S. H. M. Broman (Ed.), *Traumatic head injury in children* (pp. 22–39). New York: Oxford University Press.

Langlois, J. A., Rutland-Brown, W., & Wald, M. M. (2006). The epidemiology and impact of traumatic brain injury. *Journal of Head Trauma Rehabilitation, 21*, 375–378.

Levin, H. S., Hanten, G., Roberson, G., Li, X., Ewing-Cobbs, L., Dennis, M., et al. (2008). Prediction of cognitive sequelae based on abnormal computed tomography findings in children following mild traumatic brain injury. *Journal of Neurosurgery: Pediatrics, 1*, 461–470.

McCrory, P., Meeuwisse, W., Johnston, K., Dvorak, J., Aubry, M., Molloy, M., et al. (2009). Consensus statement on concussion in sport: The 3rd International Conference on Concussion in held in Zurich, November 2008. *Journal of Clinical Neuroscience, 16*, 755–763.

McGrath, N. (2010). Supporting the student-athlete's return to the classroom after a sport-related concussion. *Journal of Athletic Training, 45*(5), 492–498.

McIntosh, D. E., & Decker, S. L. (2005). Understanding and evaluating special education, IDEA, ADA, NCLB, and Section 504 in school neuropsychology. In R. C. D'Amato, E. Flecther-Janzen, & C. R. Reynolds (Eds.), *Handbook of school neuropsychology* (pp. 365–382). Hoboken, NJ: Wiley.

Randolph, C., McCrea, M., & Barr, W. B. (2005). Is neuropsychological testing useful in the management of sport-related concussion? *Journal of Athletic Training, 40*, 139–152.

Satz, P. (2001). Mild head injury in children and adolescents. *Current Directions in Psychological Science, 10*, 106–109.

Satz, P., Zaucha, K., McCleary, C., Light, R., Asarnow, R., & Becker, D. (1997). Mild head injury in children and adolescents: A review of studies (1970–1995). *Psychological Bulletin, 122*(2), 107–131.

Savage, R. C., Depompei, R., Tyler, J., & Lash, M. (2005). Paediatric traumatic brain injury: A review of pertinent issues. *Pediatric Rehabilitation, 8*(2), 92–103.

Semrud-Clikeman, M. (2001). *Traumatic brain injury in children and adolescence: Assessment and intervention.* New York: Guilford Press.

Slomine, B. S., McCarthy, M. L., Ding, R., MacKenzie, E., Jaffe, K. M., Aitken, M. E., et al. (2006). Health care utilization and needs after pediatric traumatic brain injury. *Pediatrics, 117*(4), 663–674.

Stanford, L. D., & Dorflinger, J. M. (2009). Pediatric brain injury: Mechanisms and amelioration. In C. R. Reynolds & E. Fletcher-Janzen (Eds.), *Handbook of clinical child neuropsychology* (3rd ed., pp. 169–186). New York: Springer.

Yeates, K. O., Taylor, H. G., Rusin, J., Bangert, B., Dietrich, A., Nuss, K., et al. (2009). Longitudinal trajectories of postconcussive symptoms in children with mild traumatic brain injuries and their relationship to acute clinical status. *Pediatrics, 123*(3), 735–743.

Ylvisaker, M., Feeney, T., Maber-Maxivell, N., Meserve, N., Geary, P., & DeLorenzo, J. (1995a). School reentry following severe traumatic brain injury: Guidelines for educational planning. *Journal of Head Trauma Rehabilitation, 10*, 25–41.

Ylvisaker, M., Feeney, T., & Mullins, K. (1995b). School re-entry following mild traumatic brain injury: A proposed hospital-to-school protocol. *Journal of Head Trauma Rehabilitation, 10*, 42–49.

APPENDIX 16.1. ACE Care Plan—School Version

ACUTE CONCUSSION EVALUATION (ACE)
CARE PLAN

Gerard Gioia, PhD[1] & Micky Collins, PhD[2]
[1]Children's National Medical Center
[2]University of Pittsburgh Medical Center

Patient Name:_____	
DOB: _____ Age:_____	
Date:_____ ID/MR#_____	
Date of Injury:_____	

You have been diagnosed with a concussion (also known as a mild traumatic brain injury). This personal plan is based on your symptoms and is designed to help speed your recovery. Your careful attention to it can also prevent further injury.

Rest is the key. You should not participate in any high risk activities (e.g., sports, physical education (PE), riding a bike, etc.) if you still have any of the symptoms below. It is important to limit activities that require a lot of thinking or concentration (homework, job-related activities), as this can also make your symptoms worse. If you no longer have any symptoms and believe that your concentration and thinking are back to normal, you can slowly and carefully return to your daily activities. Children and teenagers will need help from their parents, teachers, coaches, or athletic trainers to help monitor their recovery and return to activities.

Today the following symptoms are present (circle or check).   _____No reported symptoms

Physical		Thinking	Emotional	Sleep
Headaches	Sensitivity to light	Feeling mentally foggy	Irritability	Drowsiness
Nausea	Sensitivity to noise	Problems concentrating	Sadness	Sleeping more than usual
Fatigue	Numbness/Tingling	Problems remembering	Feeling more emotional	Sleeping less than usual
Visual problems	Vomiting	Feeling more slowed down	Nervousness	Trouble falling asleep
Balance Problems	Dizziness			

RED FLAGS: Call your doctor or go to your emergency department if you suddenly experience any of the following

Headaches that worsen	Look very drowsy, can't be awakened	Can't recognize people or places	Unusual behavior change
Seizures	Repeated vomiting	Increasing confusion	Increasing irritability
Neck pain	Slurred speech	Weakness or numbness in arms or legs	Loss of consciousness

Returning to Daily Activities

1. Get lots of rest. Be sure to get enough sleep at night—no late nights. Keep the same bedtime weekdays and weekends.

2. Take daytime naps or rest breaks when you feel tired or fatigued.

3. **Limit physical activity as well as activities that require a lot of thinking or concentration. These activities can make symptoms worse.**
   • Physical activity includes PE, sports practices, weight-training, running, exercising, heavy lifting, etc.
   • Thinking and concentration activities (e.g., homework, classwork load, job-related activity).

4. Drink lots of fluids and eat carbohydrates or protein to main appropriate blood sugar levels.

5. **As symptoms decrease, you may begin to gradually return to your daily activities. If symptoms worsen or return, lessen your activities, then try again to increase your activities gradually.**

6. During recovery, it is normal to feel frustrated and sad when you do not feel right and you can't be as active as usual.

7. Repeated evaluation of your symptoms is recommended to help guide recovery.

Returning to School

1. If you (or your child) are still having symptoms of concussion you may need extra help to perform school-related activities. As your (or your child's) symptoms decrease during recovery, the extra help or supports can be removed gradually.

2. Inform the teacher(s), school nurse, school psychologist or counselor, and administrator(s) about your (or your child's) injury and symptoms. School personnel should be instructed to watch for:
   • Increased problems paying attention or concentrating
   • Increased problems remembering or learning new information
   • Longer time needed to complete tasks or assignments
   • Greater irritability, less able to cope with stress
   • Symptoms worsen (e.g., headache, tiredness) when doing schoolwork

~Continued on back page~

This form is part of the "Heads Up: Brain Injury in Your Practice" tool kit developed by the Centers for Disease Control and Prevention (CDC).

— SCHOOL VERSION —

Returning to School (Continued)

Until you (or your child) have fully recovered, the following supports are recommended : *(check all that apply)*

__No return to school. Return on (date)_____

__Return to school with following supports. Review on (date)_____

__Shortened day. Recommend ___ hours per day until (date) _____

__Shortened classes (i.e., rest breaks during classes). Maximum class length: _____ minutes.

__Allow extra time to complete coursework/assignments and tests.

__Lessen homework load by _____%. Maximum length of nightly homework: _____ minutes.

__No significant classroom or standardized testing at this time.

__Check for the return of symptoms (use symptom table on front page of this form) when doing activities that require a lot of attention or concentration.

__Take rest breaks during the day as needed.

__Request meeting of 504 or School Management Team to discuss this plan and needed supports.

Returning to Sports

1. **You should NEVER return to play if you still have ANY symptoms** – (Be sure that you do not have any symptoms at rest and while doing any physical activity and/or activities that require a lot of thinking or concentration.)

2. Be sure that the PE teacher, coach, and/or athletic trainer are aware of your injury and symptoms.

3. It is normal to feel frustrated, sad and even angry because you cannot return to sports right away. With any injury, a full recovery will reduce the chances of getting hurt again. It is better to miss one or two games than the whole season.

The following are recommended at the present time:

___ Do not return to PE class at this time

___ Return to PE class

___ Do not return to sports practices/games at this time

___ **Gradual** return to sports practices under the supervision of an appropriate health care provider (e.g., athletic trainer, coach, or physical education teacher).

   • Return to play should occur in gradual steps beginning with aerobic exercise only to increase your heart rate (e.g., stationary cycle); moving to increasing your heart rate with movement (e.g., running); then adding controlled contact if appropriate; and finally return to sports competition.

   • Pay careful attention to your symptoms and your thinking and concentration skills at each stage of activity. Move to the next level of activity only if you do not experience any symptoms at the each level. If your symptoms return, let your health care provider know, return to the first level, and restart the program gradually.

Gradual Return to Play Plan

1. No physical activity

2. Low levels of physical activity (i.e., *symptoms do not come back during or after the activity*). This includes walking, light jogging, light stationary biking, light weightlifting (lower weight, higher reps, no bench, no squat).

3. Moderate levels of physical activity with body/head movement. This includes moderate jogging, brief running, moderate-intensity stationary biking, moderate-intensity weightlifting (reduced time and/or reduced weight from your typical routine).

4. Heavy non-contact physical activity. This includes sprinting/running, high-intensity stationary biking, regular weightlifting routine, non-contact sport-specific drills (in 3 planes of movement).

5. Full contact in controlled practice.

6. Full contact in game play.

*Neuropsychological testing can provide valuable information to assist physicians with treatment planning, such as return to play decisions.

This referral plan is based on today's evaluation:

___ Return to this office. Date/Time_____

___ Refer to: Neurosurgery_____ Neurology_____ Sports Medicine_____ Physiatrist_____ Psychiatrist_____ Other_____
___ Refer for neuropsychological testing
___ Other_____

ACE Care Plan Completed by:_____

PART V

TOPICS OF SPECIAL INTEREST

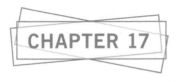

CHAPTER 17

Sport-Related Concussion

Michael W. Kirkwood, Christopher Randolph, Michael McCrea, James P. Kelly, and Keith Owen Yeates

Over the last two decades, sport-related concussion (SRC) has received a great deal of scientific and popular attention. Because the athletic and financial stakes at the university and professional levels are quite high, much of the focus has been on the adult competitive athlete. In the last several years, however, increasing attention has been devoted to young athletes. Multiple scientific reviews on pediatric SRC have now been published (Guskiewicz & Valovich McLeod, 2011; Halstead & Walter, 2010; Kirkwood, Yeates, & Wilson, 2006; Meehan & Bachur, 2009), thousands of media stories about youth concussion have appeared, and, as of February 2012, 31 states in the United States had passed laws aimed at youth SRC. A recent epidemiological study also reported that from 1997 to 2007 hospital emergency department visits for SRC doubled for 8- to 13-year-olds and increased by more than 200% for 14- to 19-year-olds (Bakhos, Lockhart, Myers, & Linakis, 2010). The increased attention to young athletes is understandable given the amount of anxiety and uncertainty often associated with an injury to a child's brain. As nearly all athletic endeavors pose some risk of concussive injury, the sheer number of youth involved in sports provides further justification for ample attention to the topic. In the United States alone, some 40–50 million children participate in organized sports each year (National Council of Youth Sports, 2008; National Federation of Youth Sports Associations, 2010).

DEFINITION AND PATHOPHYSIOLOGY

The term *concussion* or *commotio cerebri* has been used for centuries to imply an alteration in mental status caused by external trauma that may or may not involve a loss of consciousness (Kelly & Rosenberg, 1997; Shaw, 2002). Multiple detailed definitions of mild traumatic brain injury (mTBI) and concussion have been proposed over the years (see Wilde et al., Chapter 1, this volume; McCrea, 2008).

Across age groups, commonalities are apparent in the physical dynamics of SRC, as all injuries primarily involve rotational acceleration and/or deceleration forces that stress or strain the brain tissue, vasculature, and other neural elements. If sufficient enough, such force sets in motion a multilayered pathophysiological response. This complex response, often referred to as the *neurometabolic cascade*, has been documented extensively in animals (see Obenaus et al., Chapter 4, this volume) and can include disruption of the neuronal cell membranes, axonal stretching, unchecked ionic shifts, abrupt neuronal depolarization, widespread release of excitatory neurotransmitters, alteration in glucose metabolism, reduced cerebral blood flow, and overall depletion of brain energy stores. The pathophysiological dysfunction apparent in basic experimental studies is presumed to underlie the neurobehavioral changes seen in individuals soon after a concussion. Although initial electrophysiological and imaging studies have begun to characterize the pathophysiological process after SRC specifically (Davis, Iverson, Guskiewicz, Ptito, & Johnston, 2009), considerable additional work will be required to translate these data and the animal data into evidence-based clinical care guidelines.

TYPICAL CLINICAL OUTCOME

Clinically, the immediate effects of concussion are likely to appear similar in younger and older athletes. Table 17.1 provides many of the most common acute signs and symptoms of SRC. Neurobehavioral outcomes will vary to some extent among individual athletes, likely determined (at least in part) by the initial gradient of injury severity. Nevertheless, methodologically sound studies have begun to converge to paint a picture of what can be considered the "typical" recovery. In the first few days after injury, the effects of SRC can be impressive, with the largest effects usually seen for athlete-reported symptoms and on objective balance and cognitive tests (Broglio & Puetz, 2008). These symptoms and deficits are typically self-limiting and resolve gradually for the majority of teenage and older athletes in the initial days after a single concussion, such that most prospective controlled studies fail to identify significant differences between concussed and control groups after approximately 7–10 days (Bruce & Echemendia, 2003; Echemendia, Putukian, Mackin, Julian, & Shoss, 2001; Macciocchi, Barth, Alves, Rimel, & Jane, 1996; McCrea et al., 2003). Meta-

TABLE 17.1. Common Signs and Symptoms of Sport-Related Concussion

Signs observed by coaching staff	Symptoms reported by athlete
• Appears dazed or stunned	• Can't recall events *after* hit or fall
• Is confused about assignment or position	• Headache or "pressure" in head
• Forgets an instruction	• Nausea or vomiting
• Is unsure of game, score, or opponent	• Balance problems or dizziness
• Moves clumsily	• Double or blurry vision
• Answers questions slowly	• Sensitivity to light
• Loses consciousness (*even briefly*)	• Sensitivity to noise
• Shows mood, behavior, or personality changes	• Feeling sluggish, hazy, foggy, or groggy
• Can't recall events *prior* to hit or fall	• Concentration or memory problems
• Can't recall events *after* hit or fall	• Confusion
	• Does not "feel right" or is "feeling down"

Note. From Centers for Disease Control and Prevention, National Center for Injury Prevention and Control (2009).

analysis of the cognitive studies produces similar results (Belanger & Vanderploeg, 2005).

Many of the most methodologically rigorous SRC studies have involved adult athletes (Comper, Hutchison, Magrys, Mainwaring, & Richards, 2010). For several reasons, recovery for the younger athlete might be different. The compositional and mechanical properties of the head and brain differ between developing and mature organisms. Developmental factors such as brain water content, cerebral blood volume, level of myelination, and skull geometry are known to affect the biomechanics of brain injury and could affect the pathophysiological response to SRC, although exactly how remains largely undetermined (Prins & Hovda, 2003; Thibault & Margulies, 1998). Moreover, in contrast to the historical idea that young age at the time of brain injury has protective benefits, research with patients with more severe TBI indicates that the immature brain is more vulnerable, not more plastic, to diffuse injury (Taylor & Alden, 1997). Most studies demonstrating increased childhood vulnerability, though, have focused on the differential sensitivity of the especially young child (i.e., infants to preschoolers), so their applicability to the older child or teen sustaining an SRC is unclear.

Unfortunately, the current empirical literature leaves a number of questions unanswered with regard to the pediatric athlete's recovery after SRC. First, and most problematic, outcome studies for athletes younger than high school age are virtually nonexistent, so the recovery course for these young athletes cannot yet be characterized with confidence. Second, insufficient data exist to understand if young age itself might serve as an independent risk factor for protracted recovery. Athletes who play collegiate or professional sports, by definition, undergo a selection process. Individuals who are prone to injury or lengthier recoveries are less apt to play competitively after high school, so studies that contrast youth athletes with college or professional athletes are unlikely to be comparing biologically and/or behaviorally equivalent groups. Third, extant pediatric sport-focused studies provide mixed results, with interpretation complicated by a number of methodological shortcomings across studies (e.g., small sample size, lack of matched control groups or collegiate comparison groups, limited test batteries). Several studies do suggest that cognitive recovery may take some days longer for the average high school athlete compared with the average adult athlete (Collins, Lovell, Iverson, Ide, & Maroon, 2006; Field, Collins, Lovell, & Maroon, 2003; Sim, Terryberry-Spohr, & Wilson, 2008). Conversely, other studies suggest that high school athletes return to baseline within time frames similar to those seen in older athletes (Lovell, Collins, Iverson, Johnstone, & Bradley, 2004; McCrea, Kelly, Randolph, Cisler, & Berger, 2002).

To further clarify the average recovery time in high school athletes, data are presented here from one of the largest prospective SRC projects to date, which was led by McCrea, Guskiewicz, and colleagues in the Concussion Research Consortium and has been described elsewhere in detail (Guskiewicz et al., 2003; McCrea, 2008; McCrea et al., 2003). Data were derived from three parallel, multicenter studies involving both high school and college athletes. In the end, more than 16,000 player seasons and 600 concussed athletes were investigated. All players underwent a preseason baseline evaluation. Both injured athletes and matched uninjured control athletes were administered an identical testing protocol at the same retest intervals. Participants were evaluated immediately after injury, at 2–3 hours postinjury, several times within the first week, and at 45 or 90 days.

Data from an initial group of 94 concussed college players and 56 matched controls were presented by McCrea et al. (2003). Figure 17.1 provides a graphic representation of the symptom, cognitive, and balance recovery curves for these athletes, as measured by a Graded Symptom Checklist (GSC), Standardized Assessment of Concussion (SAC), and Balance Error Scoring System (BESS), respectively. Figure 17.1 also presents unpublished data for only the high school athletes (M. A. McCrea, personal communication, June 20, 2011). The high school sample consisted of 81 concussed players and 81 matched controls. As can be seen, the recovery trajectories are virtually identical in both the college and high school athletes. The most severe symptoms, cognitive dysfunction and balance problems, are seen immediately postconcussion, followed by a gradual improvement during the first hours and days after injury. By 5–7 days, group differences are no longer apparent by symptom report for college athletes or on cognitive or balance testing for either group. A small difference between the concussed and control groups is seen at 1 week postinjury for symptoms reported by high school athletes, which is no longer apparent by day 45. As discussed by McCrea (2008), across both high school and college groups, 21% of

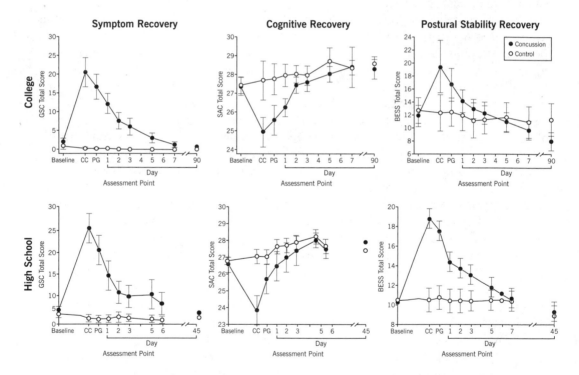

FIGURE 17.1. Symptom, cognitive, and postural stability recovery trajectories for college and high school athletes from the Concussion Research Consortium Project. Higher scores on the Graded Symptom Checklist (GSC) indicate more severe symptoms; lower scores on the Standardized Assessment of Concussion (SAC) indicate poorer cognitive performance; and higher scores on the Balance Error Scoring System (BESS) indicate poorer postural stability. Error bars indicate 95% confidence intervals. CC, time of concussion; PG, postgame/postpractice. On the BESS, multiple imputation was used to estimate means and 95% confidence intervals for control participants for the CC and PG assessments. Top panel (college athletes) from McCrea et al. (2003). Copyright 2003 by American Medical Association. All rights reserved. Reprinted by permission.

athletes reported full symptom recovery within the first day, and 80–90% of injured athletes reported full symptom recovery in less than a week. Fewer than 5% of athletes reported symptoms beyond 1 month postinjury.

ATYPICAL CLINICAL OUTCOMES/RISKS

Although select questions remain with regard to the exact timing of recovery for the average high school and younger athlete, available data suggest that most SRC will result in transient impairment lasting some hours to a few weeks. However, atypical outcomes can occur. In order to modify an unwanted outcome via a prevention or clinical management strategy, these risks and their incidence need to be understood. Randolph (Randolph, 2011; Randolph & Kirkwood, 2009) has recently attempted to quantify the risks of SRC using American football as a model. Four atypical outcomes were identified: (1) prolonged recovery; (2) same-season repeat concussion; (3) permanent brain injury or death, including delayed cerebral swelling or "second-impact syndrome"; and (4) late-life consequences of repeated concussions. Each of these outcomes is reviewed thoroughly in Randolph and Kirkwood (2009) and discussed more briefly here.

Prolonged Recovery

As highlighted above, existing prospective controlled studies indicate that most high school and older athletes appear to return to baseline within 7–10 days after a concussion. These results do not suggest that all individual athletes recover within this time window, as group studies and meta-analyses can mask individual differences (Iverson, 2010). Some percentage of athletes can be expected to display concussion-related problems beyond 1–2 weeks. Prospective controlled studies are the best means to document exactly how large these percentages are. A prospective controlled study in the context of SRC consists of preseason and postconcussion testing for all athletes, as well as a matched nonconcussed control group evaluated under the same conditions at similar time points postinjury. Although noncontrolled studies may be able to provide the number of athletes who display persistent postconcussive problems, they fail to account for the base rate occurrence of common postconcussive symptoms among non-head-injured individuals or account for false positives—that is, the number of nonconcussed athletes who would report "postconcussive" symptoms or would be classified as impaired on objective testing at the time of postinjury measurement.

To date, there have been few attempts in prospective controlled studies to quantify the percentage of athletes who do not return to normal within a well-defined time period. The percentage of high school and older athletes who display lingering problems will probably be fairly small, as these cases have failed to lead to persistent group differences in prospective studies thus far. Ultimately, the precise percentage found to display persistent problems is apt to vary based on, at least to some extent, both methodological factors (e.g., how incomplete recovery is defined, which neurobiological or neurobehavioral domain is examined) and the specific characteristics of the sample under study (e.g., age, severity of injury, previous injury history).

Same-Season Repeat Concussion

Relatively few quality studies have investigated how often same-season repeat concussion occurs in various sports. In American football, the base rate of a single concussion is generally reported to be between 3 and 6% of players per season in prospective studies of high school and older athletes. Repeat concussions occur with about this same frequency (Guskiewicz et al., 2003; Macciocchi, Barth, Littlefield, & Cantu, 2001; McCrea et al., 2009). Because playing time for those athletes who suffered a repeat injury was presumably shortened secondary to injury, the data do suggest at least a modest increase in risk of repeat injury after an initial concussion (Randolph & Kirkwood, 2009). When repeat concussions occur, some data indicate that they are more likely within 10 days of initial injury (Guskiewicz et al., 2003; McCrea et al., 2009). This pattern of reinjury is consistent with findings from the animal and human pathophysiological studies showing that the brain is in a state of increased neurobiological vulnerability within the first days of injury. Interestingly, the risk of reinjury appears more dependent upon time postinjury than whether or not an athlete remains clinically symptomatic (McCrea et al., 2009).

Catastrophic Outcome

To quantify the risk of catastrophic outcome after SRC, Randolph and Kirkwood (2009) analyzed 10 seasons of American football at all levels of play (1997–2006), using data from the National Center for Catastrophic Injury Research (NCCIR) database. During the 10-year period, cerebral injury resulted in 38 deaths and 50 cases of permanent neurological disability. The vast majority of deaths occurred in high school athletes and resulted from an acute subdural hematoma. Based on an annual football participation rate in the U.S. of 1.8 million athletes at all levels of play, one death occurred for every 474,000 player seasons, or at an average rate of 3 to 4 times per year.

In a broader study using the U.S. National Registry of Sudden Death in Young Athletes, Thomas and colleagues (2011) systematically examined sudden death from 1980 to 2009 in U.S. athletes 21 years and younger participating in organized competitive sports. Of the 1,827 total deaths recorded over the 30-year period, 62% were attributable to cardiovascular events (38 per year on average) and 14% resulted from bodily trauma (9 per year on average). Head, neck, and/or spine-related injury accounted for 89% of all trauma-related deaths. American football was by far the most frequent cause of the trauma-related fatalities, accounting for 57% of all cases. Track and field accounted for the next most deaths (10%), followed by baseball (7%), boxing (5%), and soccer (4%).

Diffuse or malignant cerebral edema is a well-documented phenomenon after minor head injury, with numerous reported cases in the pediatric neurosurgical literature (see Davis, Chapter 6, this volume). Typically, the child or teen suffers a blow to the head, which is followed by a period of lucidity, which is in turn followed by rapid neurological deterioration. The pathology or pathologies responsible for the edema have not yet been determined definitively, although this phenomenon appears linked at least in certain cases to a calcium channel gene mutation apparent in familial hemiplegic migraine (Kors et al., 2001; Stam et al., 2009).

"Second-impact syndrome" (SIS), as commonly described, involves diffuse cerebral swelling resulting from a second blow to the head while an athlete is still symptomatic from a previous concussion. This second blow to the head is said to trigger vascular congestion, diffuse edema, increased intracranial pressure, brain herniation, and ultimately severe neurological injury or death. Whether or not two closely spaced blows to the head trigger cerebral edema is controversial. In the only identified systematic review of SIS, McCrory and Berkovic (1998) found just 17 cases of diffuse cerebral edema after SRC in the world literature (all males ranging in age from 16 to 24 years old and all appearing in the United States). Using the authors' classification system, none was considered a definite case of SIS. Only 5 of the 17 cases were considered "probable" SIS; three of these were boxers, one a football player, and one an ice hockey player. Given the rarity of the phenomenon and the lack of back-to-back concussions in most cases, the authors questioned the existence of SIS as a distinct syndrome. In the review by Randolph and Kirkwood (2009), only a single death was attributed to diffuse cerebral swelling at all levels of American football across the analyzed 10-year period, which translated to a risk of 1 event for every 18 million player seasons. In a study by McCrory, Berkovic, and Cordner (2000), all Australian football-related deaths in the State of Victoria were reviewed from 1968 to 1999. In the 32-year time frame, nine deaths were attributed to neurotrauma; three deaths involved diffuse cerebral swelling associated with intracranial bleeding; no cases of SIS were identified.

In sum, catastrophic outcomes from cerebral trauma can and do happen in a variety of sports, and young athletes are at higher risk for these outcomes than adults. Most cases result from acute intracranial bleeding from a single blow to the head, not from isolated edema from two closely spaced concussions. Regardless, the fact that death or severe neurological impairment occurs after head injury in sports needs to be appreciated by all athletes, parents, athletic staff, school staff, and health care personnel, especially those involved in sports such as football that involve repeated high-velocity force to the head and neck. At the same time, given the many psychosocial and health benefits of athletic participation, it may be worth noting that these catastrophic outcomes are extremely rare. Without minimizing the devastation or singular tragedy associated with any catastrophic outcome, the risk at the individual level is low. In the face of tens of millions of U.S. youth participating in organized athletics, pediatric deaths resulting from sport-related cerebral trauma occur somewhere around 6 times per year on average, in a largely unpredictable fashion. In the United States, these injuries account for fewer deaths per year in those 1 to 21 years old than motor vehicles (8,973), homicide (4,088), suicide (2,481), stroke (246), meningitis (67), sport-related cardiovascular events (38), and lightning (10) (cardiovascular data from Thomas et al., 2011; all other data 1999–2009 average from National Center for Injury Prevention and Control, 2011).

Potential for Late-life Consequences of Repeated Concussions or Repetitive Head Trauma

Based largely on anecdotal data and single autopsy reports from professional athletes, a great deal of recent media coverage has highlighted the potential for sport-related head trauma to lead to later cognitive decline, psychiatric problems, and neurological deficits. One means by which these undesirable outcomes may occur is a distinct neuropathological process such as that reported in chronic traumatic encephalopathy (CTE). Although well-specified clinical and pathological diagnostic criteria still do not exist, CTE is thought to occur in a small subset of individuals who have been exposed to repeated head trauma. CTE is reported to be associated clinically with memory, personality, and motor disturbance; pathologically with atrophy in multiple brain regions; and microscopically with extensive tau-based neurofibrillary tangles (McKee et al., 2009).

Environmental factors are well known to affect the clinical expression of late-life neurodegenerative disorders, presumably through their effect on cerebral or cognitive "reserve" (Randolph & Kirkwood, 2009). Factors that are thought to bolster reserve, such as increased years of education, are associated with the delayed onset of dementia, whereas factors that are assumed to diminish reserve, such as moderate–severe TBI earlier in life, may predispose an individual to the expression of dementia. Multiple concussions or multiple subconcussive blows could theoretically serve to diminish reserve in a similar fashion. Preliminary studies with boxers and American football players seem to provide support for this idea (Guskiewicz et al., 2005; Jordan et al., 1997). Whether these effects are attributable to CTE, a more generic pathological process, or some combination of the two is not yet known.

Some media and scientific reports seem to suggest simply that concussions cause late-life neurodegeneration; however, the vast majority of individuals who sustain concussions do not go on to develop significant neuropathology, so many other factors undoubtedly play a role (e.g., genetic vulnerability, age, history of steroid and other substance abuse). Moreover, multiple published case studies with pathologically reported CTE actually do not have a history of any known concussion (McCrory, 2011). As speculated by Randolph and Kirkwood (2009), this raises the possibility that the concussion itself might be a *sign* of underlying diminished reserve, rather than the cause of it. In other words, concussions per se might not be as damaging to the brain as the repeated exposure to significant high-impact forces experienced in certain sports. Recent biomechanical studies in American football and ice hockey have demonstrated that the cumulative force to the head to which the average teen and adult athlete is exposed each season is substantial (see Mihalik, Chapter 3, this volume). The idea that concussions may represent a sign of diminished reserve is perhaps supported by data that the risk of concussion continues to increase with each observed concussion, such that a player with a history of one concussion has an increased risk of further concussion, and this risk of future concussion increases with each additional concussion (Randolph & Kirkwood, 2009).

To summarize, current data indicate that long-term neurological problems after repeated head injury are possible, with or without a history of concussion, and that this occurs most often in sports involving exposure to years of high-impact forces to the head (e.g., boxing, American football). Which, if any, pediatric athletes are at risk for developing long-term neuropathology is entirely unknown at present, as is the amount of distinct or cumulative trauma necessary to produce such pathology. Thus, for the pediatric practitioner, raising the possibility that a young athlete is at risk for CTE, dementia, or neurodegeneration because of a history of concussion should be done very judiciously, if at all, given the amount of anxiety such a statement is apt to cause. To more fully understand the relationship between sport-related head trauma and later pathology, scientific studies clearly need to move beyond anecdotal case reports to include prospective, longitudinal, population-based, blinded neuropathological studies of concussed and nonconcussed athletes participating in high-impact sports.

CLINICAL MANAGEMENT

To date, over 20 different published expert guidelines geared toward managing SRC have appeared in the scientific literature. The set of recommendations from the 3rd International Conference on Concussion in Sport is probably one of the most well known at this point (McCrory et al., 2009). Many clinically oriented literature reviews, several books, and numerous journal issues have also been devoted entirely to the topic. All of these publications can help direct the clinical care of the young concussed athlete. However, none of the management guidelines can yet be considered evidence-based, so the need for sound judgment from a clinician familiar with the natural clinical history and risks of SRC cannot be overstated. Some of the most important sport-specific pediatric clinical management issues are reviewed below. Given the many non-sport-related demands young athletes face, broad-based management after any pediatric concussion is necessary to ensure that medical, cognitive, emotional, social, school, and family issues are all addressed adequately (Kirkwood et al., 2008).

Preparticipation Assessment and Prevention

Prior to participation in organized sports, medical examination is frequently mandated and certainly advisable to rule out any condition that might preclude participation (Wingfield, Matheson, & Meeuwisse, 2004). One aspect of any preparticipation contact should be a thorough TBI history that delineates the number of prior concussions, timing and severity of each, and duration and intensity of the resulting symptoms. A structured concussion assessment is important when taking the history, as simply asking more generally about previous concussions is apt to lead to underreporting (Labotz, Martin, Kimura, Hetzler, & Nichols, 2005). McCrory (2004) offers a convenient clinical baseline assessment form to facilitate the documentation of this information.

Another central goal of any preseason contact should be concussion prevention. Several recent articles review the available empirical evidence for sport-based prevention strategies (Benson, Hamilton, Meeuwisse, McCrory, & Dvorak, 2009; Navarro, 2011). Using cause-of-injury data, other authors have offered recommendations to prevent catastrophic outcomes in particular (Cantu & Mueller, 2009; Zemper, 2010). These include new rules or strict enforcement of current rules (e.g., mandating that all baseball players wear helmets while batting, even during practice; ensuring that all rules with regard to checking in ice hockey are strictly enforced), proper use and maintenance of equipment (e.g., in cheerleading, using proper floor mats during stunts; in youth soccer, keeping goals anchored and supervised), and player education (e.g., teaching tackling and blocking with the head up in American football; teaching how to safely "bail out" during pole vault).

An additional essential ingredient of any preparticipation contact is providing education to athletes and parents so that concussions are quickly and accurately recognized. Many athletes still do not report concussive injuries, likely because they either lack awareness of concussion or do not want to be withheld from competition (Cusimano, 2009; McCrea, Hammeke, Olsen, Leo, & Guskiewicz, 2004). In this context, education should be provided about the signs and symptoms of concussion, as well as the fact that concussions are types of brain injuries and need to be taken quite seriously. Many resources are available to assist in the provision of such education, including those provided by the Centers for Disease Control and Prevention (*www.cdc.gov/concussion*).

Evaluation

Given the rare but serious pathology that can be associated with sport-related blows to the head, acute evaluation of any athlete after a head injury must be focused on the prompt identification and initial management of medical emergencies (see Grubenhoff & Provance, Chapter 10, this volume). After emergencies have been ruled out, attention can be turned to tools that can assist in diagnosing concussion, characterizing severity, and tracking recovery. A multidimensional approach is recommended for all concussion assessment protocols. Ideally, this approach includes a physical examination, survey of postconcussion symptoms, performance-based measures of acute mental status and postural stability, and careful consideration of individual host factors (athlete's history of prior concussion, other neurological conditions, current medications, family history, etc.). As mentioned previously, the domains that have been shown to be the most sensitive to concussion are postconcussion symptoms, balance, and cognition. Multiple tools are available to assess each of these domains in children, many of which are reviewed in detail in other chapters of the current volume (see Part III).

In the athletic setting specifically, a commonly used instrument is the Sport Concussion Assessment Tool–2 (SCAT2), which was developed at the Zurich Concussion in Sport conference (McCrory et al., 2009) and is built around a multidimensional approach to concussion assessment. The psychometric properties of the entire instrument are largely unexplored. Nonetheless, the popularity of the SCAT2 is growing, likely because it is freely available (*www.sportconcussions.com/html/SCAT2.pdf*), allows for a standardized method to evaluate the most important domains in concussion assessment, and is comprised largely of more specific tools that have been well validated in TBI populations (e.g., Glasgow Coma Scale, SAC, BESS). Of note, the SCAT2 was not designed specifically for young athletes, so care is needed when using the instrument with children, as they are apt to perform differently than older teens and adults (Schneider, Emery, Kang, Schneider, & Meeuwisse, 2010).

The instruments used to detect the neurocognitive effects of concussion, in particular, can be divided into two broad categories: (1) brief screening tools designed for use on the sideline or in the acute health care setting and (2) lengthier cognitive test batteries designed to be interpreted by neuropsychologists. Brief screening tools such as the SAC have good sensitivity to concussion in the first hours to days after injury (McCrea et al., 2002) and are widely considered a key component of any diagnostic or postacute evaluation. More controversy surrounds the value of lengthier neuropsychological assessment in the "baseline" model for return-to-play purposes. Baseline testing calls for preinjury neurocognitive testing lasting approximately 20–30 minutes, followed by postinjury comparison testing for athletes who sustain concussions during the season. The baseline battery originally consisted of paper-and-pencil instruments. Over the last decade, computerized tests have grown in popularity, in part because they have a number of practical advantages over paper-and-pencil measures (e.g., ease of administration and data storage). Even so, existing computerized measures seem to be no more, or less, sensitive than paper-and-pencil measures (Belanger & Vanderploeg, 2005; Broglio & Puetz, 2008).

Whether paper-and-pencil or computerized measures are used, evaluation within a baseline model is appealing because of its potential to provide objective information about an athlete's recovery from a concussive injury. However, as we have discussed elsewhere, a number of questions about baseline testing exist, including whether it has adequate methodological/statistical support and demonstrated real-life utility to justify the financial costs, time, and energy needed for its implementation (Kirkwood, Randolph, & Yeates, 2009; Randolph, 2011; Randolph, McCrea, & Barr, 2005).

Simply showing that cognitive effects can be detected soon after injury is insufficient to justify baseline testing, because athletes also commonly report postconcussive symptoms during this same period, and expert guidelines do not recommend a return to competition until athletes themselves endorse the absence of symptoms. To establish the incremental validity of neuropsychological testing for return-to-play decision making, cognitive deficits need to be detected *after* self-reported symptoms resolve, which has not yet been shown consistently in prospective controlled studies. The baseline testing model involves evaluating concussed athletes on at least two different occasions, so the stability of the tests over time is also in need of close scrutiny. In pediatric populations, the baseline paradigm has been questioned because youth are rapidly developing, so test results obtained at baseline may no longer be a valid comparison once a concussion occurs (Guskiewicz & Valovich McLeod, 2011). More generally, several studies suggest that the stability of existing paper-and-pencil and computerized tests is below the standards needed to make reliable return-to-play decisions (Barr, 2003; Broglio, Ferrara, Macciocchi, Baumgartner, & Elliott, 2007; Randolph, 2011; Randolph et al., 2005; Schatz, 2010). Regardless of the psychometric merit of the tests, the utility of baseline testing in the end rests upon evidence that the results improve real-life outcomes. At present, no identified empirical data are available to demonstrate that such testing actually improves a clinical outcome or reduces any known risk associated with concussive injury (Randolph & Kirkwood, 2009).

Despite the current limitations of neuropsychological testing within the baseline model, experts agree that such assessment has a role in evaluating and managing certain athletes postinjury. Because most pediatric athletes are expected to meet the demands of school soon after injury, neuropsychological evaluation can be beneficial in identifying cognitive and/or psychosocial problems that might interfere with educational performance. When recovery is not progressing in a typical fashion (i.e., symptom clearance within 1 to 2 weeks), neuropsychological assessment can also provide valuable information to guide treatment. Given expertise in child development, brain injury, and psychology, pediatric neuropsychologists are well positioned to disentangle the many factors that can contribute to persistent symptoms, including injury-related pathology, developmental learning and attentional issues, emotional reactions to injury or more general psychosocial issues, and family and school factors. Objective testing can also help to identify individuals who may exert noncredible effort on formal testing or may exaggerate symptoms, which likely happens in a sizable minority of pediatric patients who present with persistent symptoms following concussion (Kirkwood & Kirk, 2010).

When to Return to Play

Most experts agree that returning an athlete to play following concussion should be approached with due caution. The most publicized reason given for this caution is probably "second impact syndrome," although given the questionable etiology and rarity of this phenomenon, stronger arguments can be made for other rationales. For example, after a concussion, a temporal window of vulnerability likely exists during which cerebral performance is disturbed. As mentioned, this idea has support from both animal and human studies, pertaining especially in the first 1–2 weeks after injury (Barkhoudarian, Hovda, & Giza, 2011; Guskeiwicz et al., 2003; McCrea et al., 2009). The risk for cumulative damage after sustaining multiple concussions or multiple subconcussive blows is another commonly stated reason for caution when making the return-to-play decision. This idea also has some empirical support (Bruce & Echemendia, 2004; Collins et al., 2002; Guskiewicz et al., 2003; Iverson, Gaetz, Lovell, & Collins, 2004), although other studies have not found much evidence for cumulative effects (Belanger, Spiegel, & Vanderploeg, 2010; Broglio, Eckner, Surma, & Kutcher, 2011; Bruce & Echemendia, 2009). In the pediatric athlete specifically, the fact that we do not yet have a clear understanding of how repeated brain insult could change neurobiological or neurobehavioral development over the short or long run should provide sufficient reason for caution in and of itself. In comparison to adult competitive athletes, the risk–benefit analysis for most youth will differ considerably and should be weighted much more heavily on the potential for functional disruption and future loss than on any immediate gain from returning to competition.

Regardless of the underlying rationale, some commonalities around when to allow a return to play have emerged in recent years. Most experts now agree that youth athletes should always be removed from the day's competition after a concussion. Consensus opinion also suggests that all concussed athletes should undergo a thorough clinical examination soon after injury and be monitored serially in the subsequent days. Until athletes no longer display evidence of concussion-related problems, the common recommendation is that they should be restricted from activities in which they would be at increased risk for sustaining another concussion. Put simply, most experts would agree that the earliest an athlete should return to play is when (1) no concussion-related symptoms or functional disruption is apparent at rest or during exertion; (2) neurological examination is normal; and (3) neuroimaging is unremarkable, when conducted.

We agree with these guidelines in principle and believe that they are particularly sensible in the initial days to weeks after injury. At the same time, the recommendations should probably not be followed rigidly, as minimal to no data suggest that managing athletes in this manner actually improves outcomes. This fact was illustrated by a recent study by McCrea et al. (2009), who analyzed data from the multisite Concussion Research Consortium project. As one of the only core recommendations across all concussion management guidelines is that no athlete should return to play while symptomatic, the researchers grouped the concussed athletes ($n =$ 635) by whether or not a symptom-free waiting period was required by team/medical officials before a return to competition. They then examined clinical outcomes for the two groups, comparing symptom duration, cognitive functioning, postural stability, and likelihood of repeat injury. Contrary to expectations, 40% of the sample was allowed to return to play without a symptom-free waiting period and these individuals had recovery characteristics that were no different from the other athletes. In fact, the players who observed a symptom-free waiting period actually displayed an increased risk for sustaining a repeat concussion. We do not believe that this study should be used to endorse returning athletes to play while symptomatic; however, it does highlight the role that empirical data can play in challenging some commonly accepted ideas about which factors are important in reducing risk after SRC.

For those youth who display longer-term problems, whether to allow a return to relatively high-risk sports and other physical activities is a complicated decision. On the one hand, most experts recommend a restriction when persistent difficulties are apparent. On the other, no identified empirical data indicate that athletes with persistent difficulties are actually at increased risk for a negative outcome if they return to play. Moreover, the further in the past from injury, the less likely that injury-related pathology is the exclusive explanation for functional problems, as multifactorial etiological explanations tend to predominate weeks to months after injury. Activity restriction itself can also have adverse effects on lifestyle, mood, and identity (Bloom, Horton, McCrory, & Johnston, 2004; Dunn, Trivedi, & O'Neal, 2001).

We certainly support a conservative approach when making return-to-play decisions for young athletes, all the more so for those athletes with neuroimaging findings, a history of repeated concussions, or evidence of either a lowered threshold for sustaining concussive injury or cumulative effects from the experienced injuries. In the end, though, the return-to-play decision is unlikely to be driven successfully by a one-size-fits-all algorithm and should be grounded in a thoughtful and individualized cost–benefit analysis that weighs the largely unknown risks of multiple insults to an actively developing brain with the many psychosocial and other benefits of allowing a return to play.

How to Return to Play

As seen in Table 17.2, the International Concussion in Sport group has offered a detailed graduated protocol for how to return athletes to play after a concussion (McCrory et al., 2009). Once an athlete is judged free of all symptoms at rest, he or she is encouraged to progress through a series of steps, with the athlete needing to remain symptom-free without medication before proceeding to the next step. Each step is recommended to take 24 hours, so approximately 1 week is needed after the athlete is asymptomatic before a return to play. If symptoms recur while in one of the stages, the recommendation is for the athlete to drop down to the previous level and try to progress again after a 24-hour period.

Returning an athlete to play in a graduated fashion is intuitively appealing and sensible to us, though, again, recommendations here are not evidence-based, so strict

TABLE 17.2. Graduated Return-to-Play Protocol Recommended in the Zurich Consensus Statement on Concussion in Sport

Rehabilitation stage	Functional exercise at each stage of rehabilitation	Objective of each stage
1. No activity	Complete physical and cognitive rest	Recovery
2. Light aerobic exercise	Walking, swimming, or stationary cycling keeping intensity < 70% MPHR. No resistance retraining.	Increase HR
3. Sport-specific exercise	Skating drills in ice hockey, running drills in soccer. No head-impact activities.	Add movement
4. Noncontact training drills	Progression to more complex training drills (e.g., passing drills in football and ice hockey). May start progressive resistance training).	Exercise, coordination, cognitive load
5. Full-contact practice	Following medical clearance, participate in normal training activities	Restore confidence, assessment of functional skills by coaching staff
6. Return to play	Normal game play	

Note. HR, heart rate; MPHR, maximum predicted heart rate. From McCrory et al. (2009). Copyright 2009 by Elsevier Limited. Reprinted with permission.

adherence to this type of protocol is not yet warranted. The group's recommendation for "no activity" and "complete physical and cognitive rest" until asymptomatic also deserves careful consideration. Taken literally, the idea of *complete rest until asymptomatic* is not only impractical but conceptually impossible (how does one engage in "no" physical or cognitive activity?). Clinically, we have seen this recommendation used as the basis to tell athletes that they are to "do absolutely nothing" for not just hours or a few days but for many weeks after injury, despite the athlete's desire to return to school, homework, reading, socializing, aerobic activities, etc. Unsurprisingly, such a recommendation in these situations has often had iatrogenic effects, leading to increased lethargy, fatigue, apathy, and feelings of helplessness and hopelessness.

A designated period of reduced activity and rest soon after concussion may be beneficial and is grounded in experimental work suggesting that injured rodents who exercise too soon after injury may have more protracted recoveries (see the work of Griesbach, summarized in Chapter 14, this volume). However, total bed rest for more than a short period of time is unlikely to be effective, and intensive rest is probably only sensible for some postinjury hours to days (Allen, Glasziou, & Del Mar, 1999; Asher, 1947; de Kruijk, Leffers, Meerhoff, Rutten, & Twijnstra, 2002; Relander, Troupp, & Af Bjorkesten, 1972). The idea that the rest needs to be "complete" and to encompass "all" activities should also probably be tempered and reframed as a reduction in rigorous or overly stimulating activities, especially those that worsen symptomatology.

At some point within the first few weeks of injury, transitioning athletes back to their usual activities (in which they are unlikely to sustain a repeat concussion) is apt to be helpful, even if they remain symptomatic. Too slow of a return to activities such as school could actually protract recovery by causing undue stress secondary to feelings of falling behind, being away from friends, and disrupting the child's and family's normal routine (Kirkwood et al., 2008). An overemphasis on extensive rest or other non-evidence-based management strategies may also have iatrogenic effects, given that recovery expectations, anxiety, and the misattribution of unwanted but common symptomatology (e.g., forgetfulness, fatigue) to head injury are well known to affect the perception and reporting of persistent problems following mTBI (Ferguson, Mittenberg, Barone, & Schneider, 1999; Gunstad & Suhr, 2001). Finally, data from animal studies and limited data from high school athletes suggest that reengaging in activities in the days to initial weeks after injury is likely to have no effect or a beneficial one (Griesbach, Hovda, Gomez-Pinilla, & Sutton, 2008; Majerske et al., 2008; McCrea et al., 2009). An "active" rehabilitation approach is also likely to be more helpful than an exclusively rest-based approach for those athletes who display persistent symptoms (see Iverson et al., Chapter 14, this volume).

Ultimately, how to transition an athlete back to play after a concussion has a straightforward goal: to return the athlete to his or her usual activities as soon as possible without worsening symptomatology or increasing the risk of a negative outcome. Gradually reintegrating athletes back to play is prudent in most cases, although until additional empirical data are available to direct this process, decisions about the progression of activities should be predicated on a heavy dose of clinical judgment that accounts for the likely etiology, type, and severity of symptoms, severity of initial injury, time since injury, the athlete's feelings about returning to activities, and the individual circumstances involved in each case.

The Special Case of Permanent Disqualification

When clinicians should recommend seasonal or lifetime retirement to an athlete is another area especially devoid of empirical data. Several authors have, however, offered points to consider (Cantu, 2003; McCrory, 2001; Sedney, Orphanos, & Bailes, 2011). Disqualification has not been addressed specifically with reference to the pediatric athlete, although a conservative approach is almost certainly appropriate in most cases, and both parents and youth should be actively engaged in the decision-making process.

As highlighted above, general contraindications to return to play soon after injury include ongoing symptoms, abnormalities on neurological examination, or neuroimaging findings. Clear evidence of impairment on balance or cognitive testing may indicate ongoing problems as well and thus could support a recommendation for retirement. Other potential reasons to consider disqualification include evidence of an increasingly prolonged recovery course after successive injuries and concussions or lasting symptoms incurred by less force. Even without evidence of cumulative injury or ongoing symptoms, many experts recommend disqualification for athletes who sustain multiple concussions in one season, a recommendation without clear scientific validation but one with intuitive appeal when dealing with the developing brain of a young athlete. Table 17.3 summarizes some of the questions that we use clinically to help determine whether to recommend disqualification for a given athlete. If seasonal or permanent disqualification is deliberated but ultimately deemed inappropriate, consideration could still be given to recommending other options that would lessen the young athlete's risk of concussion, including changing sports, positions, or style of participation (e.g., changing from football to baseball, from quarterback to punter, from aggressive to more cautious skiing).

TABLE 17.3. Questions to Consider When Deliberating Permanent Disqualification for an Athlete

1. Are concussions occurring closer together in time?
2. Are concussions occurring as a result of a lesser blow or impact (e.g., the impact that caused the most recent concussion would not have caused an injury 3 years ago)?
3. Is the rate of recovery slower after each concussion?
4. Is there incomplete recovery after a concussion (e.g., only getting back to 80% of typical functioning)?
5. Is there a persisting decline in academic, cognitive, social, emotional, or other personal function after a concussion?

CONCLUSION

The sport-related concussion story has been unfolding with impressive rapidity in recent years, driven by a remarkable amount of work by researchers around the globe. Although the recovery trajectory for the preteen athlete requires further specification, current data suggest that most young athletes will achieve a favorable outcome, characterized by complete recovery over a period of days to several weeks after a single, uncomplicated SRC. Clinically, optimal care and resource expenditure should be informed by, and yoked to, a clear understanding of this natural clinical history, including the possible atypical outcomes reviewed here. At this point, many guidelines and recommendations exist that can be used to inform the management of the young concussed athlete. However, none can yet be considered evidence-based, so inflexible adherence to any particular approach is unwarranted. Clinical management broadly, and return to play decisions specifically, should continue to be characterized by increased conservatism for the young athlete and rest upon an individualized cost–benefit analysis conducted by providers who carefully weigh the many benefits of youth sports participation with the largely unknown risks associated with repeated concussive or subconcussive blows to an actively developing brain.

REFERENCES

Allen, C., Glasziou, P., & Del Mar, C. (1999). Bed rest: a potentially harmful treatment needing more careful evaluation. *Lancet, 354*, 1229–1233

Asher, R. A. (1947). The dangers of going to bed. *British Medical Journal, 2*, 967–968.

Bakhos, L. L., Lockhart, G. R., Myers, R., & Linakis, J. G. (2010). Emergency department visits for concussion in young child athletes. *Pediatrics, 126*, e550–e556.

Barkhoudarian, G., Hovda, D. A., & Giza, C. C. (2011). The molecular pathophysiology of concussive brain injury. *Clinics in Sports Medicine, 30*, 33–48.

Barr, W. B. (2003). Neuropsychological testing of high school athletes: Preliminary norms and test–retest indices. *Archives of Clinical Neuropsychology, 18*, 91–101.

Belanger, H. G., Spiegel, E., & Vanderploeg, R. D. (2010). Neuropsychological performance following a history of multiple self-reported concussions: A meta-analysis. *Journal of the International Neuropsychological Society, 16*, 262–267.

Belanger, H. G., & Vanderploeg, R. D. (2005). The neuropsychological impact of sports-related concussion: A meta-analysis. *Journal of the International Neuropsychological Society, 11*, 345–357.

Benson, B. W., Hamilton, G. M., Meeuwisse, W. H., McCrory, P., & Dvorak, J. (2009). Is protective equipment useful in preventing concussion?: A systematic review of the literature. *British Journal of Sports Medicine, 43*(Suppl. 1), 56–67.

Bloom, G. A., Horton, A. S., McCrory, P., & Johnston, K. M. (2004). Sport psychology and concussion: New impacts to explore. *British Journal of Sports Medicine, 38,* 519–521.

Broglio, S. P., Eckner, J. T., Surma, T., & Kutcher, J. S. (2011). Post-concussion cognitive declines and symptomatology are not related to concussion biomechanics in high school football players. *Journal of Neurotrauma, 28,* 2061–2068.

Broglio, S. P., Ferrara, M. S., Macciocchi, S. N., Baumgartner, T. A., & Elliott, R. (2007). Test–retest reliability of computerized concussion assessment programs. *Journal of Athletic Training, 42,* 509–514.

Broglio, S. P., & Puetz, T. W. (2008). The effect of sport concussion on neurocognitive function, self-report symptoms and postural control: A meta-analysis. *Sports Medicine, 38,* 53–67.

Bruce, J. M., & Echemendia, R. J. (2003). Delayed-onset deficits in verbal encoding strategies among patients with mild traumatic brain injury. *Neuropsychology, 17,* 622–629.

Bruce, J. M., & Echemendia, R. J. (2004). Concussion history predicts self-reported symptoms before and following a concussive event. *Neurology, 63,* 1516–1518.

Bruce, J. M, & Echemendia, R. J. (2009). History of multiple self-reported concussions is not associated with reduced cognitive abilities. *Neurosurgery, 64,* 100–106.

Cantu, R. C. (2003). Recurrent athletic head injury: Risks and when to retire. *Clinics in Sports Medicine, 22,* 593–603.

Cantu, R. C., & Mueller, F. O. (2009). The prevention of catastrophic head and spine injuries in high school and college sports. *British Journal of Sports Medicine, 43,* 981–986.

Centers for Disease Control and Prevention. (2009). *How can I recognize a concussion?* Retrieved from *www.cdc.gov/concussion/sports/recognize.html.*

Collins, M. W., Lovell, M. R., Iverson, G. L., Cantu, R. C., Maroon, J. C., & Field, M. (2002). Cumulative effects of concussion in high school athletes. *Neurosurgery, 51,* 1175–1179.

Collins, M. W., Lovell, M. R., Iverson, G. L., Ide, T., & Maroon, J. (2006). Examining concussion rates and return to play in high school football players wearing newer helmet technology: A three-year prospective cohort study. *Neurosurgery, 58,* 275–286.

Comper, P., Hutchison, M., Magrys, S., Mainwaring, L., & Richards, D. (2010). Evaluating the methodological quality of sports neuropsychology concussion research: A systematic review. *Brain Injury, 24,* 1257–1271.

Cusimano, M. D. (2009). Canadian minor hockey participants' knowledge about concussion. *Canadian Journal of Neurological Sciences, 36,* 315–320.

Davis, G. A., Iverson, G. L., Guskiewicz, K. M., Ptito, A., & Johnston, K. M. (2009). Contributions of neuroimaging, balance testing, electrophysiology and blood markers to the assessment of sport-related concussion. *British Journal of Sports Medicine, 43*(Suppl. 1), i36–i45.

de Kruijk, J. R., Leffers, P., Meerhoff, S., Rutten, J., & Twijnstra, A. (2002). Effectiveness of bed rest after mild traumatic brain injury: A randomised trial of no versus six days of bed rest. *Journal of Neurology, Neurosurgery, and Psychiatry, 73,* 167–172.

Dunn, A. L., Trivedi, M. H., & O'Neal, H. A. (2001). Physical activity dose–response effects on outcomes of depression and anxiety. *Medicine and Science in Sports and Exercise, 33*(Suppl. 6), S587–S597.

Echemendia, R. J., Putukian, M., Mackin, R. S., Julian, L., & Shoss N. (2001). Neuropsychological test performance prior to and following sports-related mild traumatic brain injury. *Clinical Journal of Sport Medicine, 11,* 23–31.

Ferguson, R. J., Mittenberg, W., Barone, D. F., & Schneider, B. (1999). Postconcussion syndrome following sports-related head injury: Expectation as etiology. *Neuropsychology, 13,* 582–589.

Field, M., Collins, M. W., Lovell, M. R., & Maroon, J. (2003). Does age play a role in recovery from sports-related concussion?: A comparison of high school and collegiate athletes. *Journal of Pediatrics, 142,* 546–553.

Griesbach, G. S., Hovda, D. A., Gomez-Pinilla, F., & Sutton, R. L. (2008). Voluntary exercise or amphetamine treatment, but not the combination, increases hippocampal brain-derived neurotrophic factor and synapsin I following cortical contusion injury in rats. *Neuroscience, 23,* 530–540.

Gunstad, J., & Suhr, J. A. (2001). "Expectation as etiology" versus "the good old days": Postconcussion syndrome symptom reporting in athletes, headache sufferers, and depressed individuals. *Journal of the International Neuropsychological Society, 7,* 323–333.

Guskiewicz, K. M., Marshall, S. W., Bailes, J., McCrea, M., Cantu, R. C., Randolph, C., et al. (2005). Association between recurrent concussion and late-life cognitive impairment in retired professional football players. *Neurosurgery, 57,* 719–726.

Guskiewicz, K. M., McCrea, M., Marshall, S. W., Cantu, R. C., Randolph, C., Barr, W., et al. (2003). Cumulative effects associated with recurrent concussion in collegiate football players: The NCAA Concussion Study. *Journal of the American Medical Association, 290,* 2549–2555.

Guskiewicz, K. M., & Valovich McLeod, T. C. (2011). Pediatric sports-related concussion. *PM & R, 3,* 353–364.

Halstead, M. E., & Walter, K. D. (2010). American Academy of Pediatrics: Clinical report—sport-related concussion in children and adolescents. *Pediatrics, 126,* 597–615.

Iverson, G. L. (2010). Mild traumatic brain injury meta-analyses can obscure individual differences. *Brain Injury, 24,* 1246–1255.

Iverson, G. L., Gaetz, M., Lovell, M. R., & Collins, M. W. (2004). Cumulative effects of concussion in amateur athletes. *Brain Injury, 18,* 433–443.

Jordan, B. D., Relkin, N. R., Ravdin, L. D., Jacobs, A. R., Bennett, A., & Gandy, S. (1997). Apolipoprotein E epsilon4 associated with chronic traumatic brain injury in boxing. *Journal of the American Medical Association, 278,* 136–140.

Kelly, J. P., & Rosenberg, J. H. (1997). Diagnosis and management of concussion in sports. *Neurology, 48,* 575–580.

Kirkwood, M. W., & Kirk, J. W. (2010). The base rate of suboptimal effort in a pediatric mild TBI sample: Performance on the Medical Symptom Validity Test. *The Clinical Neuropsychologist, 24,* 860–872.

Kirkwood, M. W., Randolph, C., & Yeates, K. O. (2009). Returning pediatric athletes to play after concussion: The evidence (or lack thereof) behind baseline neuropsychological testing. *Acta Paediatrica, 98,* 1409–1411.

Kirkwood, M. W., Yeates, K. O., Taylor, H. G., Randolph, C., McCrea, M., & Anderson, V. A. (2008). Management of pediatric mild traumatic brain injury: A neuropsychological review from injury through recovery. *The Clinical Neuropsychologist, 22,* 769–800.

Kirkwood, M. W., Yeates, K. O., & Wilson, P. E. (2006). Pediatric sport-related concussion: A review of the clinical management of an oft-neglected population. *Pediatrics, 117,* 1359–1371.

Kors, E. E., Terwindt, G. M., Vermeulen, F. L., Fitzsimons, R. B., Jardine, P. E., Heywood, P., et al. (2001). Delayed cerebral edema and fatal coma after minor head trauma: Role of the CACNA1A calcium channel subunit gene and relationship with familial hemiplegic migraine. *Annals of Neurology, 49,* 753–760.

Labotz, M., Martin, M. R., Kimura, I. F., Hetzler, R. K., & Nichols, A. W. (2005). A comparison of a preparticipation evaluation history form and a symptom-based concussion survey in the identification of previous head injury in collegiate athletes. *Clinical Journal of Sport Medicine, 15,* 73–78.

Lovell, M. R., Collins, M. W., Iverson, G. L., Johnston, K. M., & Bradley, J. P. (2004). Grade 1 or "ding" concussions in high school athletes. *American Journal of Sports Medicine, 32,* 47–54.

Macciocchi, S. N., Barth, J. T., Alves, W., Rimel, R. W., & Jane, J. A. (1996). Neuropsychological functioning and recovery after mild head injury in collegiate athletes. *Neurosurgery, 39,* 510–514.

Macciocchi, S. N., Barth, J. T., Littlefield, L. M., & Cantu, R. (2001). Multiple concussions and neuropsychological functioning in collegiate football players. *Journal of Athletic Training, 36,* 303–306.

Majerske, C. W., Mihalik, J. P., Ren, D., Collins, M. W., Reddy, C. C., Lovell, M. R., et al. (2008). Concussion in sports: Postconcussive activity levels, symptoms, and neurocognitive performance. *Journal of Athletic Training, 43,* 265–274.

McCrea, M. A. (2008). *Mild traumatic brain injury and postconcussion syndrome.* Oxford, UK: Oxford University Press.

McCrea, M. A., Guskiewicz, K. M., Marshall, S. W., Barr, W., Randolph, C., Cantu, R. C., et al. (2003). Acute effects and recovery time following concussion in collegiate football players: The NCAA Concussion Study. *Journal of the American Medical Association, 290,* 2556–2563.

McCrea, M. A., Guskiewicz, K. M., Randolph, C., Barr, W. B., Hammeke, T. A., Marshall, S. W., et al. (2009). Effects of a symptom-free waiting period on clinical outcome and risk of reinjury after sport-related concussion. *Neurosurgery, 65,* 876–882.

McCrea, M. A., Hammeke, T., Olsen, G., Leo, P., & Guskiewicz, K. (2004). Unreported concussion in high school football players: Implications for prevention. *Clinical Journal of Sport Medicine, 14,* 13–17.

McCrea, M. A., Kelly, J. P., Randolph, C., Cisler, R., & Berger, L. (2002). Immediate neurocognitive effects of concussion. *Neurosurgery, 50,* 1032–1040.

McCrory, P. R. (2001). When to retire after concussion? *British Journal of Sports Medicine, 35,* 380–382.

McCrory, P. R. (2004). Preparticipation assessment for head injury. *Clinical Journal of Sport Medicine, 14,* 139–144.

McCrory, P. R. (2011). Sports concussion and the risk of chronic neurological impairment. *Clinical Journal of Sport Medicine, 21,* 6–12.

McCrory, P. R., & Berkovic, S. F. (1998). Second impact syndrome. *Neurology, 50,* 677–683.

McCrory, P. R., Berkovic, S. F., & Cordner, S. M. (2000). Deaths due to brain injury among footballers in Victoria, 1968–1999. *Medical Journal of Australia, 172,* 217–219.

McCrory, P. R., Meeuwisse, W., Johnston, K., Dvorak, J., Aubry, M., Molloy, M., et al. (2009). Consensus statement on concussion in sport: The 3rd International Conference on Concussion in Sport held in Zurich, November 2008. *Journal of Clinical Neuroscience, 16,* 755–763.

McKee, A. C., Cantu, R. C., Nowinski, C. J., Hedley-Whyte, E. T., Gavett, B. E., Budson, A. E., et al. (2009). Chronic traumatic encephalopathy in athletes: Progressive tauopathy after repetitive head injury. *Journal of Neuropathology and Experimental Neurology, 68,* 709–735.

Meehan, W. P., & Bachur, R. G. (2009). Sport-related concussion. *Pediatrics, 123,* 114–123.

National Center for Injury Prevention and Control. (2011). *WISQARS leading causes of death reports, 1999–2009* [Data file]. Retrieved from *http://webappa.cdc.gov/sasweb/ncipc/leadcaus10.html.*

National Council of Youth Sports. (2008). *Market research report NCYS membership survey—2008 edition.* Retrieved from *www.ncys.org/pdfs/2008/2008-ncys-market-research-report.pdf.*

National Federation of Youth Sports Associations. (2010). *2009–2010 high school athletics participation survey results.* Retrieved from *www.nfhs.org/content.aspx?id=3282.*

Navarro, R. R. (2011). Protective equipment and the prevention of concussion: What is the evidence? *Current Sports Medicine Reports, 10,* 27–31.

Prins, M. L., & Hovda, D. A. (2003). Developing experimental models to address traumatic brain injury in children. *Journal of Neurotrauma, 20,* 123–137.

Randolph, C. (2011). Baseline neuropsychological testing in managing sport-related concussion: Does it modify risk? *Current Sports Medicine Reports, 10,* 21–26.

Randolph, C., & Kirkwood, M. W. (2009). What are the real risks of sport-related concussion, and are they modifiable? *Journal of the International Neuropsychological Society, 15,* 512–520.

Randolph, C., McCrea, M., & Barr, W. B. (2005). Is neuropsychological testing useful in the management of sport-related concussion? *Journal of Athletic Training, 40,* 139–152.

Relander, M., Troupp, H., & Af Bjorkesten, G. (1972). Controlled trial of treatment for cerebral concussion. *British Medical Journal, 4,* 777–779.

Schatz, P. (2010). Long-term test–retest reliability of baseline cognitive assessments using ImPACT. *American Journal of Sports Medicine, 38,* 47–53.

Schneider, K. J., Emery, C. A., Kang, J., Schneider, G. M., & Meeuwisse, W. H. (2010). Examining Sport Concussion Assessment Tool ratings for male and female youth hockey players with and without a history of concussion. *British Journal of Sports Medicine, 44,* 1112–1117.

Sedney, C. L., Orphanos, J., & Bailes, J. E. (2011). When to consider retiring an athlete after sports-related concussion. *Clinics in Sports Medicine, 30,* 189–200.

Shaw, N. A. (2002). The neurophysiology of concussion. *Progress in Neurobiology, 67,* 281–344.

Sim, A., Terryberry-Spohr, L., & Wilson, K. R. (2008). Prolonged recovery of memory functioning after mild traumatic brain injury in adolescent athletes. *Journal of Neurosurgery, 108,* 511–516.

Stam, A. H., Luijckx, G. J., Poll-Thé, B. T., Ginjaar, I. B., Frants, R. R., Haan, J., et al. (2009). Early seizures and cerebral edema after trivial head trauma associated with the CACNA1A S218L mutation. *Journal of Neurology, Neurosurgery, and Psychiatry, 80,* 1125–1129.

Taylor, H. G., & Alden, J. (1997). Age-related differences in outcomes following childhood brain insults: An introduction and overview. *Journal of the International Neuropsychological Society, 3,* 555–567.

Thibault, K. L., & Margulies, S. S. (1998). Age-dependent material properties of the porcine cerebrum: Effect on pediatric inertial head injury criteria. *Journal of Biomechanics, 31,* 1119–1126.

Thomas, M., Haas, T. S., Doerer, J. J., Hodges, J. S., Aicher, B. O., Garberich, R. F., et al. (2011). Epidemiology of sudden death in young, competitive athletes due to blunt trauma. *Pediatrics, 128,* 1–8.

Wingfield, K., Matheson, G. O., & Meeuwisse, W. H. (2004). Preparticipation evaluation: An evidence-based review. *Clinical Journal of Sport Medicine, 14,* 109–122.

Zemper, E. D. (2010). Catastrophic injuries among young athletes. *British Journal of Sports Medicine, 44,* 13–20.

CHAPTER 18

Injury in Preschool-Age Children

Audrey McKinlay

T raumatic brain injury (TBI) occurs frequently during childhood, with children under 5 years old (preschool) being one of the most vulnerable groups. In the preschool-age group, over 90% of the TBI events will be classified as mild (mTBI). Despite the frequency of preschool mTBI, there is limited information regarding the outcomes of these injuries, and the information that is available conflicts as to whether or not the injury results in deficits. These conflicting findings may be due to the methodological difficulties that hamper research in this area. Preschool mTBI, in particular, presents unique problems that need to be considered when conducting or evaluating research. This chapter provides an overview of the research and issues particularly pertinent to preschool mTBI.

EPIDEMIOLOGY

The preschool period represents a time of rapid development in terms of motor coordination and body awareness (see Figure 18.1). It is not surprising, therefore, that during this period a high rate of accidental injuries occurs, including mTBI. The most common source of injury for this age group is falls (Langley, Dodge, & Silva, 1979; Langley & Silva, 1979; McKinlay et al., 2008). Reported incidence rates for children vary widely from around 100–300 per 100,000 per year (Cassidy et al., 2004; Hawley, Ward, Long, Owen, & Magnay, 2003; Peloso, von Holst, & Borg, 2004) up to 1,850 per 100,000 per year (McKinlay et al., 2008). Rates depend in part on how TBI is defined (e.g., International Classification of Diseases [ICD] code, Abbreviated Injury Scale, Glasgow Coma Scale) and the inclusion criteria used. Most studies have used hospital admission or discharge data, which may seriously underestimate the incidence of these injuries. Information from cohort studies show that a high percentage of young children are seen in a variety of emergency settings and discharged

Skill	Brain maturation age bands		
	Years 1 & 2	**Years 3 & 4**	**Years 5 & 6**
Motor	Gross motor skills develop; holding head, sitting, standing, walking. Basic fine motor skills developing; able to pick up small objects, scribble with crayons, and stack blocks.	Developing coordination and strength. Running, jumping, climbing, balancing on one foot, able to walk up stairs and ride a tricycle.	Able to hop, skip, and jump, throw and catch a ball, and climb the stairs competently. Capable of tying their own shoes and buttoning their clothes.
Behavior/ Emotion	Children become aware of the emotions of others—anger, affection, pleasure. They experience anxiety and begin to develop self-soothing skills.	Able to engage in make-believe and pretend. Developing the ability to work through emotional conflicts.	Able to interact with others and regulate behavior to conform with their surroundings (e.g., formal schooling).
Social	Aware of their surroundings, seen as increased fear of strangers and distress when their parents leave the room. Toward the end of this stage they begin to explore their environment independently when in familiar surroundings.	Increasing awareness of other people's emotions, reacting to pleasure, affection, and anger. Increasing use of imitative play. Using games of pretend with other children. Developing theory of mind.	Developing the ability to cooperate and share with others. Able to develop independent friendships.
Language	Progress from babbling to speaking single words and putting two words together. Able to follow directions and understand the words for familiar objects. By the time they are 2 years of age they can say between 30 and 50 words.	By this time, most children are fully understandable in their production of speech. Sentences increase in length and complexity, able to use pronouns (*I*, *me*, *you*, *we*, etc.).	Increasingly able to understand and apply more complex concepts such as *why*, *under*, and *over*. Vocabularies typically contain between 1,000 and 5,000 words.

Relative level of brain maturation occurring over each age band (Peterson, 1989).

FIGURE 18.1. Skill development and relative level of brain maturation from birth to age 6 years.

home (McKinlay et al., 2008). Other factors may also result in an underestimation of mTBI during this period. For example, very young children may have difficulty expressing symptoms, and further, young children require a parent or guardian to understand the nature of the injury and to present them to a hospital for treatment.

Sex

In general, when all injury types and levels of severity are considered, males are more at risk of injury than females (McKinlay et al., 2008; Rivara, 1984). This difference begins to appear during the preschool years and remains even when corrected for level of exposure to risky activities (Rivara, 1984). The increased rate for males is thought to be related, at least in part, to socialization, with males being encouraged to engage in higher-risk activities (Rivara, 1984). However, sex differences in terms of incidence are much less marked during the preschool period than during any other in the lifespan (McKinlay et al., 2008). This similarity in rates of male and female mTBI may be related to the fact that preschool children are generally under the direct supervision of an adult for the majority of their waking hours. In contrast, school-age children are often unsupervised for periods of time, providing more opportunity for sex differences in higher-risk activities to become apparent.

OUTCOMES

Few studies have exclusively examined outcomes for children who have experienced mTBI in the preschool-age group. (In the current literature review, studies focused on children in the 0- to 7-year age range are considered.) The vast majority of current research focuses on outcomes for school-age children or preschoolers with mTBI combined with children who have experienced moderate TBI (Ewing-Cobbs et al., 1997; Goldstrohm & Arffa, 2005; Marsh & Whitehead, 2005). Because of this lack of focused research, very little is known about the clinical recovery curves and outcomes of mTBI in very young children.

Behavioral Outcomes

Behavioral problems appear to be the most consistent finding following mTBI in preschool children (see Table 18.1), and there is evidence that these problems may continue for some time postinjury. For example, McKinlay, Grace, Horwood, and Fergusson (2010) reported longitudinal outcomes of mTBI for a birth cohort born in 1977, which included information on child and family characteristics from 1,265 children. This study demonstrated that, compared to controls, children with an mTBI prior to age 10, whose injury required overnight observation in a hospital, received significantly poorer mother and teacher assessments of attention and conduct ratings averaged over the age range of 10–13 years. Increased behavioral problems were more prevalent if injuries occurred prior to age 5. These findings remained substantially unchanged after accounting for child and family factors. This study also examined academic outcomes, but found no evidence of deficits in this area. Children who had experienced an mTBI prior to age 5 were followed up at ages 14–16 years. At that time, six psychiatric outcomes were examined: attention-deficit/hyperactivity disorder (ADHD), conduct disorder, mood disorder, substance abuse, alcohol abuse, and anxiety. Again, the groups were divided according to mTBI severity (inpatient hospitalization and outpatient care). Relative to other children in the cohort who did not experience a TBI, preschool injury requiring hospitalization was associated with significantly more cases with symptoms of ADHD (odds ratio 4.2), conduct disorder (odds ratio 6.2), and substance abuse (odds ratio 3.6). After accounting for child and family factors, these findings remained substantially unchanged.

However, although behavioral deficits are a common finding following preschool mTBI (see Table 18.1), they are not unequivocal. For example, Wetherington, Hooper, Keenan, Nocera, and Runyan (2010) reported no evidence of behavior problems following preschool mTBI. In this study, 31 children, who were injured prior

TABLE 18.1. mTBI Outcomes for Children under 7 Years of Age Ordered by Publication Date

Study	Definition	N	Age at injury	Control group	Follow-up	Skills assessed	Outcome
Wrightson et al. (1995)	4–6 hours ED monitoring; not hospitalized	79	2.5–4.5 y.o.	Other injury group	1, 6, and 12 mths. and 6.5 yrs.	Behavior and cognition	Deficits in visual closure; more likely to need help with reading when 6.5 y.o.
Anderson et al. (2000)	GCS on admission 13–15; no evidence of mass lesion	19	2–7 y.o.	Noninjured children	3, 6, and 18 mths.	Memory	Memory problems
McKinlay et al. (2002)	Medical diagnosis of concussion; GCS 14–15	22	0–5 y.o.	Outpatient and noninjured children	2–13 yrs.	Behavior and cognition	Behavior problems
Anderson et al. (2004)	GCS on admission 13–15; no evidence of mass lesion	14	2–7 y.o.	Noninjured children	12 and 30 mths.	Intellectual, language, and memory	No deficits
Anderson, Catroppa, Morse, Haritou, & Rosenfeld (2005)	GCS on admission 13–15; no evidence of mass lesion	10	2–7 y.o.	Noninjured children	30 mths.	Attention, processing speed, reaction time	Deficits in some aspects of attention
Anderson et al. (2006)	GCS on admission 13–15; no evidence of mass lesion	14	2–7 y.o.	Noninjured children	12 and 30 mths.	Intellectual, memory, behavior, and educational	Behavior problems
Catroppa et al. (2007)	GCS on admission 13–15; no evidence of mass lesion	12	2–7 y.o.	Noninjured children	5 yrs.	Intellectual and attention	Sustain attention and processing speed deficits

Study	Inclusion criteria	N	Age	Comparison group	Follow-up	Domain assessed	Outcome
Nadebaum et al. (2007)	GCS on admission 13–15; no evidence of mass lesion	12	1–7 y.o.	Noninjured children	5 yrs.	Executive functions: cognitive flexibility, information processing, behavior	No deficits
McKinlay, Grace, Horwood, Fergusson, & MacFarlane (2009)	Medical diagnosis of concussion; GCS 14–15	21	0–5 y.o.	Outpatient and noninjured children	9–16 yrs.	Psychiatric outcomes, based on DSM-IV	Increased rates of ADHD, CD/ODD, and substance abuse
Anderson et al. (2009)	GCS 13–15; no evidence of mass lesion	12	Mean 4.3 y.o.	Noninjured children	5 yrs.	Cognition	Initial effect on cognition; recovered over time
Gerrard-Morris et al. (2009)	GCS 13–15 with neuroimaging abnormalities	43	3–6 y.o.	Other injury group	6, 12, and 18 mths.	Cognition	Cognitive deficits
Keenan, Hooper, Wetherington, Nocera, & Runyan (2007)	GCS 13–15	29	All < 2 y.o.	Noninjured children	2 yrs.	Cognition, behavior, visual reception, fine motor, expressive and receptive language	Below normal on composite score for cognitive skills
McKinlay, Grace, Horwood, & Fergusson (2010)	Medical diagnosis of concussion; GCS 14–15	22	0–5 y.o.	Outpatient and noninjured children	2–13 yrs.	Behavior	Behavior problems
Wetherington, Hooper, Keenan, Nocera, & Runyan (2010)	GCS 13–15	31	All < 2 y.o.	Noninjured children	1–2 yrs. (when 3 y.o.)	Behavior and developmental functioning	No deficits

Note. ED, emergency department; y.o., years of age; mths., months; yrs., years; GCS, Glasgow Coma Scale; ADHD, attention-deficit/hyperactivity disorder; CD, conduct disorder; ODD, oppositional defiant disorder.

to 2 years of age, were assessed at age 3 years, using the Child Behavior Checklist. These authors reported no behavioral difference for children with mTBI compared to the noninjured controls. One possible explanation for the conflicting findings here may be the differences in the follow-up period, with behavioral outcomes in the latter study being assessed while the children were still in the preschool period, prior to behavioral control being fully developed.

A major area of controversy has surrounded the issue of whether any behavioral problems found following mTBI reflect the outcomes of the injury or preexisting problems. This issue is particularly problematic with the assessment of preschool children for whom there is often no objective preinjury data. However, considerable attention has been given to this issue by Anderson and colleagues, who have reported comparable child and family preinjury functioning for children both with and without mTBI (Anderson & Catroppa, 2005; Anderson et al., 2006; Anderson, Catroppa, Morse, Haritou, & Rosenfeld, 2009; Anderson, Morse, Catroppa, Haritou, & Rosenfeld, 2004).

Cognitive Outcomes

Unlike behavioral outcomes, a less consistent picture appears when considering cognitive outcomes. Although some researchers have found evidence of deficits, others have not (see Table 18.1 for an overview). There is little evidence that global intellectual functioning is compromised following early mTBI (Anderson et al., 1997, 2004, 2006; Catroppa, Anderson, Morse, Haritou, & Rosenfeld, 2007; McKinlay, Dalrymple-Alford, Horwood, & Fergusson, 2002). However, skills that are in the process of developing at the time of injury appear to be more vulnerable. For example, Wrightson, McGinn, and Gronwall (1995) examined outcomes for children (N = 76) who experienced an mTBI between the ages of 2.5 and 4.5 years. Outcomes were assessed at 6 and 12 months postinjury and again when the children reached 6.5 years. Compared to controls, children who had experienced an mTBI showed no differences immediately following injury. However, assessment at 6 months and 1 year postinjury showed evidence of deficits in visual closure, and by 6.5 years, children with mTBI were more likely to require assistance with reading. This finding was related to visual closure scores obtained at 1 year postinjury. Anderson and colleagues have assessed outcomes for preschoolers at 6, 12, 30, and 60 months post mTBI, and found evidence of deficits in attention and processing speed, both acutely and long term (Anderson et al., 2004; Catroppa et al., 2007; Nadebaum, Anderson, & Catroppa, 2007). However, this research group did not find statistically consistent deficits for children with mTBI in the areas of language, memory, or executive function, although a trend for increased problems was frequently evident (Anderson, Catroppa, Rosenfeld, Haritou, & Morse, 2000; Anderson et al., 2004).

METHODOLOGICAL ISSUES

Overview

In contrast to the literature on school-age children, the majority of studies on preschool outcomes of mTBI have occurred over the last 10 years. Therefore, many of the methodological problems that historically plagued the research for older children

(Satz, 2001; Satz, Zaucha, McCleary, & Light, 1997) are not evident in the preschool studies. For example, across the extant studies in this area, a reasonably consistent definition has been used to categorize mTBI. These studies have used standardized methods of assessment, appropriate control groups, and longitudinal follow-up. However, there are other methodological limitations within the literature on preschool mTBI that make it difficult to come to any firm conclusions regarding the outcomes of these injuries. For example, many of the studies in this area use very small sample sizes. Given the variability of functioning that would be expected for this age group and the relatively small effect sizes that might be expected after mTBI, it is surprising that many of the studies still reported either negative outcomes or trends toward a more negative outcome for preschool children following mTBI. Further, the assessment of pre- and postinjury functioning, length of longitudinal follow-up, and the appropriate skills assessed raises questions as to whether the full extent of any problems following preschool mTBI have been fully elucidated.

Assessment of Preinjury Behavior

One of the most difficult aspects in evaluating the outcomes of preschool mTBI is the assessment of preinjury behavior, the accuracy of which is vital to determine the true effect of the injury on postinjury behavior (Dennis, Yeates, Taylor, & Fletcher, 2007). In the case of school-age children, there is often access to objective information regarding their level of preinjury functioning (both in terms of formal assessment and teacher report). In contrast, preinjury information is frequently absent for younger children. This lacuna is particularly pertinent given the large percentage of preschool children who are injured prior to the development of language (i.e., those under 2 years old; Kraus, Fife, & Conroy, 1987; Kraus, Rock, & Hemyari, 1990; McKinlay et al., 2008). Because of this, the vast majority of research to date has relied on parental reporting of preinjury functioning. Reliance on parent report is problematic for a number of reasons. First, parents are often approached for a report within a short time frame following the injury and may be under considerable stress if their child was hospitalized, even if only for a brief period. Second, parents may tend to minimize any problems to reduce their own anxiety regarding the possibility that the injury may have ongoing effects. Further, parents may minimize problems if they believe that they were in some way responsible for the injury. Furthermore, when a longer period of time elapses between the injury event and assessment, parents may begin to evaluate their child's preinjury functioning based on postinjury functioning (Chess, Thomas, & Birch, 1966; Robbins, 1963).

Postinjury Functioning

Unlike any other age group, preschool children are in a process of rapid physical, social, behavioral, and neurocognitive development (see Figure 18.1). Whereas assessment of adults and older children has often focused on loss of already consolidated skills, assessment of outcomes following preschool mTBI requires careful consideration of the developmental period during which the injury occurred.

In this regard, it is not surprising that the research on mTBI in preschoolers has found little evidence for deficits in global IQ. The common standardized tests used to measure this skill set are relatively gross. Although outcomes may be fairly stable in older school-age children, there can be considerable variability in what is considered normal for younger children, with marked changes over time as new skills develop and consolidate (Moffit, Caspi, Harkness, & Silva, 1993). It is interesting to note that when more fine-grained analysis of skills that could be considered to be at a "critical stage of development," such as behavioral control, attentional control, speed of processing, or language, are assessed, a more consistent pattern of deficits appears (Anderson & Catroppa, 2005; McKinlay et al., 2002).

Longitudinal Follow-Up

Children from 0 to 7 years of age cannot be considered a homogeneous group. As outlined in Figure 18.1, the skill set of a 2-year-old is considerably different from that of a 7-year-old. Moreover, a follow-up of even 5 years for a child injured under the age of 2 years cannot be considered comparable to a similar length of follow-up of a child who is injured at age 7. As Dennis et al. (2007) point out, multiple age-related factors impact outcomes, including age at injury, time since injury, and age at time of evaluation. These age-based factors are particularly relevant for very young children for whom recovery from injury occurs during a period of rapid physical and cognitive development. Yet, there are few studies that have specifically examined mTBI outcomes more than 5 years postinjury, long before the developmental process is complete. A notable exception to this is the research findings reported by Hessen and colleagues (Hessen, Nestvold, & Anderson, 2007; Hessen, Nestvold, & Sundet, 2006). For this research a cohort of children who had experienced a minor head injury was recruited between 1974 and 1975 and invited to take part in a 23-year follow-up ($N = 45$; mean age at injury 8.9 years). Results indicated that increased neuropsychological deficits were evident for this group. Nevertheless, given the lack of truly longitudinal follow-up after early mTBI, it is reasonable to suggest that the eventual consequences of these injuries remain unclear.

BRAIN MATURATION

As depicted in Figure 18.2, the human brain is in the most active period of development during the preschool years. A recent study used high-resolution magnetic resonance images to more accurately quantify the maturation of the brain in individuals ages 3 months to 30 years (87 females and 71 males; Groeschel, Vollmer, King, & Connelly, 2010). This study reported that total gray matter peaked during childhood, whereas white matter increased into adulthood. Gender-specific development of white and gray matter volumes was also found. These periods of brain maturation have also been found to correspond with growth spurts in other areas of neurocognitive development (Thatcher, 1992; Toga, Thompson, & Sowell, 2006).

It has been suggested that the marked neuronal maturation evident in the immature brain will result in greater plasticity, protecting it from adverse outcomes of TBI regardless of severity or site of lesion. Although it is clearly evident that the immature brain exhibits a high level of plasticity, compared to the mature brain, the suggestion that this plasticity will provide unlimited protection requires some consideration.

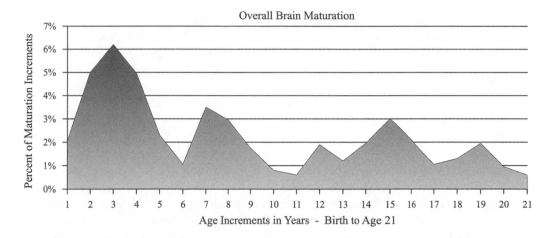

FIGURE 18.2. Incremental brain maturation. From Savage (2010). Copyright 2010 by Lash & Associates Publishing/Training Inc. *www.lapublishing.com*. Reprinted by permission.

Early versus Later Injury

Brain plasticity has been defined in terms of structural components (i.e., structural connectivity and brain volume) and is assessed in terms of neurobehavioral outcomes (Dennis et al., 2007). Much of the earlier research on child TBI assumed an advantage for the immature brain due to greater plasticity. The enhanced plasticity in the immature brain, compared to the mature brain, has been referred to as the *Kennard principle* (Kennard, 1940). Research from both animal and human studies have supported remarkable plasticity in the immature brain, and examples of this are seen in the literature regarding hemispherectomies in cases of epilepsy, in which early surgeries have been associated with more positive outcomes (Dunkley et al., 2010). However, this apparent plasticity is not common to all areas of function. Others have argued for an early vulnerability model that suggests that the immature brain is more vulnerable because early skills, on which later functioning relies, may be interrupted or may fail to develop fully (Hebb, 1942; Jacobs, Harvey, & Anderson, 2007).

There is increasing evidence that for emerging skills, an early vulnerability model may be more accurate than models assuming protection from early plasticity (Anderson & Moore, 1995; Ewing-Cobbs et al., 1997; McKinlay, Grace, Horwood, Fergusson, & MacFarlane, 2009). As Dennis et al. (2007) point out in their review on factors related to brain plasticity in children, normal cognitive development may, in fact, require greater neural reserves than the maintenance of developed skills. Few studies have directly examined the possibility of greater plasticity following childhood brain impairment. A study conducted by Anderson et al. (2010) examined executive function performance for groups of children who had experienced early focal brain insult during six different periods: (1) congenital, (2) perinatal, (3) infancy, (4) preschool, (5) middle childhood, and (6) late childhood. They found that children who experienced brain impairment prior to age 3 were more likely to show global and severe deficits in executive function compared to older children, who tended to perform closer to the normal range. These authors noted that skills emerging at the time of insult were particularly vulnerable, in keeping with the concept of "critical stages" of development. Dennis and colleagues (2007) reported that selective attention was more impaired with young, compared to older, children in the context of congenital and acquired brain injury in children. In a study that focused on early mTBI, McKinlay and colleagues (2002) reported evidence of increased behavior problems for children injured prior to age 5, whereas few deficits were evident in those injured between ages 5 and 10 years. Further, increased neuropsychological deficits were reported for those injured prior to age 15 in the study by Hessen and colleagues (2006, 2007), whereas no significant deficits were found for individuals with mTBI after age 15 years.

Unlike adults and older school-age children, preschoolers have very few established skills. Therefore, although the initial deficits associated with the injury may appear minimal, deficits may appear later in life as expected skills fail to emerge. For example, early TBI may interrupt the development of basic skills such as visual closure, which in turn could lead to later problems with learning to read (Wrightson et al., 1995). Further, particular areas of the brain (e.g., the prefrontal cortex) are not fully developed until early adulthood, and deficits in functions associated with injury in this area (e.g., planning and inhibitory control; Samango-Sprouse, 1999) may not become evident for sometime following the injury. The length of time that the prefrontal cortex takes to fully mature is particularly relevant in terms of outcomes after TBI, as it is also the area of the brain most likely to be injured due to its proximity to the bony protrusions of the orbitofrontal and anterior temporal regions (Kraus & Levin, 2001).

CONCLUSIONS

mTBI is a common event during the preschool years. Assessing outcomes for children who experience injury during these early years is a complex process and requires consideration of methodological issues, brain maturation, and stages of developmental change. Assessment of outcomes must be focused on the developmental stage of the child because emerging skills are considered to be most vulnerable. Further, because recovery occurs in conjunction with rapid maturation and skill development, assessing the outcomes of these injuries requires a considerable period of follow-up to evaluate whether any deficits in skill development are evident, and whether age-appropriate skills emerge over time. Currently, there is little information regarding the impact of mTBI in very early childhood on adolescent or adult functioning, resulting in uncertainty about the eventual outcomes of these injuries. However, those studies that do exist suggest that deficits may continue long after the injury is forgotten, especially for those children who display evidence of more severe initial injury.

REFERENCES

Anderson, V., & Catroppa, C. (2005). Recovery of executive skills following paediatric traumatic brain injury (TBI): A 2 year follow-up. *Brain Injury, 19*(6), 459–470.

Anderson, V., Catroppa, C., Dudgeon, P., Morse, S., Haritou, F., & Rosenfeld, J. (2006). Understanding predictors of functional recovery and outcome 30 months following early childhood head injury. *Neuropsychology, 20*(1), 42–57.

Anderson, V., Catroppa, C., Morse, S., Haritou, F., & Rosenfeld, J. (2005). Attentional and processing skills following traumatic brain injury in early childhood. *Brain Injury*, *19*(9), 699–710.

Anderson, V., Catroppa, C., Morse, S., Haritou, F., & Rosenfeld, J. (2009). Intellectual outcome from preschool traumatic brain injury: A 5 year prospective, longitudinal study. *Pediatrics*, *124*, e164–e171.

Anderson, V., Catroppa, C., Rosenfeld, J., Haritou, F., & Morse, S. (2000). Recovery of memory function following traumatic brain injury in pre-school children. *Brain Injury*, *14*(8), 679–692.

Anderson, V., & Moore, C. (1995). Age at injury as a predictor of outcome following pediatric head injury: A longitudinal perspective. *Child Neuropsychology*, *1*(3), 187–202.

Anderson, V., Morse, S., Catroppa, C., Haritou, F., & Rosenfeld, J. (2004). Thirty month outcome from early childhood head injury: A prospective analysis of neurobehavioural recovery. *Brain*, *127*(12), 2608–2620.

Anderson, V., Morse, S., Klug, G., Catroppa, C., Haritou, F., Rosenfeld, J., et al. (1997). Predicting recovery from head injury in young children: A prospective analysis. *Journal of the International Neuropsychological Society*, *3*(6), 568–580.

Anderson, V., Spencer-Smith, M., Coleman, L., Anderson, P., Williams, J., Greenham, M., et al. (2010). Children's executive functions: Are they poorer after very early brain insult. *Neuropsychologia*, *48*, 2041–2050.

Cassidy, J. D., Carroll, L. J., Peloso, P. M., Borg, J., von Holst, H., Holm, L., et al. (2004). Incidence, risk factors and prevention of mild traumatic brain injury: Results of the WHO Collaborating Centre Task Force on Mild Traumatic Brain Injury. *Journal of Rehabilitation Medicine*, *43*, 28–60.

Catroppa, C., Anderson, V., Morse, S., Haritou, F., & Rosenfeld, J. (2007). Children's attentional skills 5 years post-TBI. *Journal of Pediatric Psychology*, *32*(3), 354–369.

Chess, S., Thomas, A., & Birch, H. G. (1966). Distortions in developmental reporting made by parents of behaviorally disturbed children. *Journal of the American Academy of Child Psychiatry*, *5*(2), 226–234.

Dennis, M., Yeates, K. O., Taylor, H. G., & Fletcher, J. M. (2007). *Brain reserve capacity, cognitive reserve capacity, and age-based functional plasticity after congenital and acquired brain injury in children*. Philadelphia: Taylor & Francis.

Dunkley, C., Kung, J., Scott, R. C., Nicolaides, P., Neville, B., Aylett, S. E., et al. (2010). Epilepsy surgery in children under 3 years. *Epilepsy Research*, *93*(2–3), 96–106.

Ewing-Cobbs, L., Fletcher, J. M., Levin, H. S., Francis, D. J., Davidson, K., & Miner, M. E. (1997). Longitudinal neuropsychological outcome in infants and preschoolers with traumatic brain injury. *Journal of the International Neuropsychological Society*, *3*(6), 581–591.

Gerrard-Morris, A., Taylor, H. G., Yeates, K. O., Walz, N. C., Stancin, T., Minich, N., et al. (2009). Cognitive development after traumatic brain injury in young children. *Journal of the International Neuropsychological Society*, *16*, 157–168.

Goldstrohm, S. L., & Arffa, S. (2005). Preschool children with mild to moderate traumatic brain injury: An exploration of immediate and post-acute morbidity. *Archives of Clinical Neuropsychology*, *20*(6), 675–695.

Groeschel, S., Vollmer, B., King, M. D., & Connelly, A. (2010). Developmental changes in cerebral grey and white matter volume from infancy to adulthood. *International Journal of Developmental Neuroscience*, *28*, 481–489.

Hawley, C. A., Ward, A. B., Long, J., Owen, D. W., & Magnay, A. R. (2003). Prevalence of traumatic brain injury amongst children admitted to hospital in one health district: A population-based study. *Injury*, *34*, 256–260.

Hebb, D. O. (1942). The effect of early and late brain injury upon test scores, and the nature of adult intelligence. *Proceedings of the American Philosophical Society, 85,* 275–292.

Hessen, E., Nestvold, K., & Anderson, V. (2007). Neuropsychological function 23 years after mild traumatic brain injury: A comparison of outcome after paediatric and adult head injuries. *Brain Injury, 21*(9), 963–979.

Hessen, E., Nestvold, K., & Sundet, K. (2006). Neuropsychological function in a group of patients 25 years after sustaining minor head injuries as children and adolescents. *Scandinavian Journal of Psychology, 47*(4), 245–251.

Jacobs, R., Harvey, A. S., & Anderson, V. (2007). Executive function following focal frontal lobe lesions: Impact of timing of lesion on outcome. *Cortex, 43*(6), 792–805.

Keenan, H. T., Hooper, S. R., Wetherington, C. E., Nocera, M., & Runyan, D. K. (2007). Neurodevelopmental consequences of early traumatic brain injury in 3-year-old children. *Pediatrics, 119*(3), e616–e623.

Kennard, M. A. (1940). Relation of age to motor impairment in man and subhuman primates. *Archives of Neurology and Psychiatry, 43,* 377–397.

Kraus, J. F., Fife, D., & Conroy, C. (1987). Pediatric brain injuries: The nature, clinical course, and early outcomes in a defined United States' population. *Pediatrics, 79,* 501–507.

Kraus, J. F., Rock, A., & Hemyari, P. (1990). Brain injuries among infants, children, adolescents, and young adults. *American Journal of Diseases of Children, 144,* 684–691.

Kraus, M. F., & Levin, H. S. (2001). The frontal lobes and traumatic brain injury. In S. P. Salloway, P. F. Malloy, & J. D. Duffy (Eds.), *The frontal lobes and neuropsychiatric illness* (pp. 199–213). Washington, DC: American Psychiatric Association.

Langley, J., Dodge, J., & Silva, P. A. (1979). Accidents in the first five years of life: A report from the Dunedin Multidisciplinary Child Development Study. *Australian Paediatric Journal, 15*(4), 255–259.

Langley, J., & Silva, P. A. (1979). *Falls: The most common accident experienced by New Zealand children—a report to the Accident Compensation Commission.* Dunedin Multidisciplinary Child Development Study, New Zealand.

Marsh, N. V., & Whitehead, G. (2005). Skull fracture during infancy: A five-year follow-up. *Journal of Clinical and Experimental Neuropsychology, 27*(3), 352–366.

McKinlay, A., Dalrymple-Alford, J. C., Horwood, L. J., & Fergusson, D. M. (2002). Long term psychosocial outcomes after mild head injury in early childhood. *Journal of Neurology, Neurosurgery, and Psychiatry, 73*(3), 281–288.

McKinlay, A., Grace, R., Horwood, L. J., & Fergusson, D. (2010). Long-term behavioural outcomes of pre-school mild traumatic brain injury. *Child: Care, Health and Development, 36*(1), 22–30.

McKinlay, A., Grace, R. C., Horwood, L. J., Fergusson, D. M., & MacFarlane, M. R. (2009). Adolescent psychiatric symptoms following preschool childhood mild traumatic brain injury: Evidence from a birth cohort. *Journal of Head Trauma Rehabilitation, 24*(3), 221–227.

McKinlay, A., Grace, R. C., Horwood, L. J., Fergusson, D. M., Ridder, E. M., & MacFarlane, M. R. (2008). Prevalence of traumatic brain injury among children, adolescents, and young adults: Prospective evidence from a birth cohort. *Brain Injury, 22*(2), 175–181.

Moffit, T., Caspi, A., Harkness, A., & Silva, P. A. (1993). The natural history of change in intellectual performance: Who changes? How much? Is it meaningful? *Journal of Child Psychology and Psychiatry, 34*(4), 455–506.

Nadebaum, C., Anderson, V., & Catroppa, C. (2007). Executive function outcomes following traumatic brain injury in young children: A five year follow-up. *Developmental Neuropsychology, 32*(2), 703–728.

Peloso, P. M., von Holst, H., & Borg, J. (2004). Mild traumatic brain injuries presenting to Swedish hospitals. *Journal of Rehabilitation Medicine,* (Suppl. 43), 22–27.

Peterson, C. (1989). *Looking forward through the lifespan: Developmental psychology* (2nd ed.). New York: Prentice Hall.

Rivara, F. (Ed.). (1984). *Epidemiology of childhood injuries*. New York: Wiley-Interscience.

Robbins, L. C. (1963). The accuracy of parental recall of aspects of child development and of child rearing practices. *Journal of Abnormal and Social Psychology, 66*(3), 261–270.

Samango-Sprouse, C. (Ed.). (1999). *Frontal lobe development in childhood*. New York: Guilford Press.

Satz, P. (2001). Mild head injury in children and adolescents. *Current Directions in Psychological Science, 10,* 106–109.

Satz, P., Zaucha, K., McCleary, C., & Light, R. (1997). Mild head injury in children and adolescents: A review of studies (1970–1995). *Psychological Bulletin, 122*(2), 107–131.

Savage, R. (2010). *Brain development in children and adolescents*. Youngsville, NC: Lash & Associates Publishing/Training Inc.

Thatcher, R. (1992). Cyclic cortical reorganization during early childhood. *Brain and Cognition, 20,* 24–50.

Toga, A. W., Thompson, P. M., & Sowell, E. R. (2006). Mapping brain maturation. *Trends in Neurosciences, 29,* 148–159.

Wetherington, C. E., Hooper, S. R., Keenan, H. T., Nocera, M., & Runyan, D. (2010). Parent ratings of behavioural functioning after traumatic brain injury in very young children. *Journal of Pediatric Psychology, 35*(6), 662–671.

Wrightson, P., McGinn, V., & Gronwall, D. (1995). Mild head injury in pre-school children: Evidence that it can be associated with a persisting cognitive defect. *Journal of Neurology, Neurosurgery, and Psychiatry, 59,* 375–380.

CHAPTER 19

Forensic Considerations

Jacobus Donders

Pediatric neuropsychologists usually see children with mild traumatic brain injury (mTBI) as part of their regular clinical practice. This chapter, however, deals with those cases that are the subject of litigation. Typically, the matter of dispute is whether the child has any neurobehavioral sequelae of an alleged mTBI. Another common and related question pertains to the degree to which any currently known behavioral or cognitive deficits can be attributed to mTBI. This chapter reviews some of the variables that need to be considered routinely in the context of forensic neuropsychological evaluations of children with mTBI. There are also other legal and administrative matters for which input from pediatric neuropsychologists may be sought, such as adjustment issues after child abuse or eligibility for special education services, but these fall outside the scope of this chapter and have been discussed elsewhere (Donders, 2012). The term *forensic* is used here specifically as pertaining to a civil medicolegal context and is not intended to apply to cases involving child custody or criminal responsibility.

There is general consensus in the literature that uncomplicated mTBI in children is most often not associated with long-term neurobehavioral sequelae (Babikian & Asarnow, 2009; Kirkwood et al., 2008). However, even when standard neuropsychological tests suggest good recovery, there appears to be a small subgroup of children who are at increased risk for more persistent parent- or self-reported subjective symptomatology. This appears to be the case primarily in children whose otherwise "mild" injury, as reflected in the absence of any prolonged coma or posttraumatic amnesia, is complicated by acute intracranial lesions on neuroimaging (Taylor et al., 2010; Yeates et al., 2009). In this chapter, the term *mTBI* is used to refer to children whose mild injury was uncomplicated, with duration of coma < 30 minutes, duration of posttraumatic amnesia < 24 hours, and negative findings on neuroimaging.

This chapter first reviews some basic aspects of legal procedures and contingencies that the pediatric neuropsychologist needs to consider before embarking on a forensic evaluation. Next, issues that are pertinent to the content of the evaluation as well as the interpretive process are discussed, including psychometrics as well as child and family history. Finally, some general guidelines are provided with regard to documentation and sworn testimony.

BASIC LEGAL ISSUES

The forensic arena is distinctly different from regular clinical practice. Some of these differences are summarized in Table 19.1. During clinical evaluations, the child's parent or guardian is the client, and the pediatric neuropsychologist may become a treating doctor or a patient advocate. In contrast, in a forensic evaluation, the client is the referring agent, typically an attorney working for the "other side" or an insurance company. Furthermore, whereas the clinical practitioner is likely used to the collegial and caring atmosphere of a health care environment, the forensic arena is, by design, adversarial in nature. This does not mean that the pediatric neuropsychologist needs to sell his or her soul to one of the parties in the case, or even try to "win" the case for one side. In fact, if anything, he or she should make every attempt at personal neutrality and scientific objectivity within his or her boundaries of expertise, and that neutrality and objectivity should be communicated to the referring agent prior to accepting the referral. Several authors have provided practical suggestions

TABLE 19.1. Differences between Clinical and Forensic Practice

Neuropsychologist variable	Clinical practice	Forensic practice
Typical referral agent	Physician or other health care provider	Attorney or insurance case manager
Professional role	Treating doctor, patient advocate	Objective/independent expert
Relationship with other professionals	Collegial	Adversarial
Who is the client?	Patient and/or family	Referring agent
Confidentiality	Maintained unless under extreme conditions (e.g., suspicion of child abuse)	Privilege has been waived; "private" information becomes a matter of public record
Audience for the report	Treating professionals	Attorneys, judges, and juries
Level of certainty required	Common confidence intervals (e.g., 90%)	More likely than not (> 50%)
Handling of raw data	Maintain test security	Must often be made available
HIPAA rules	Applicable	Superseded by discovery rules
Feedback to, or follow-up with, patient	Routine	Typically not allowed
Witness during deposition or trial	Fact witness	Expert witness

for neuropsychologists to self-screen for potential bias during the forensic evaluation process (Sweet & Moulthrop, 1999; Van Gorp & McMullen, 1997).

A complete review of all the legal terms, rules of evidence, and procedural issues that may arise in the context of a forensic neuropsychological evaluation is beyond the scope of this chapter. The reader is referred to Greiffenstein (2008) and Sweet, Ecklund-Johnson, and Malina (2008) for details in this regard. However, a few issues that arise commonly merit discussion. The first of these is that, at all times, the pediatric neuropsychologist should aspire to the highest ethical, professional, and scientific standards, consistent with the ethics code of the American Psychological Association (APA; 2002) but with the understanding that the law may have different standards and that law will ultimately trump the preferences of a professional guild. For example, when faced with a subpoena for the raw data to be sent to the opposing attorney, the neuropsychologist may express a preference to send those data directly to another neuropsychologist, citing issues of test security and the like. However, except in cases where state law prohibits such direct disclosure or when the neuropsychologist can clearly demonstrate the likelihood of substantial harm to the child, a judge may ultimately order direct release of the raw data anyway. In that case, the neuropsychologist had best comply, unless he or she wants to risk being held in contempt of court and face the legal consequences. More detailed guidelines for dealing with such circumstances have been described by Attix and colleagues (2007).

Another big difference in standards pertains to the degree of certainty that is required for an opinion. Pediatric neuropsychologists who conduct research have historically been enamored with the $p < .05$ criterion, sometimes with a Bonferroni correction that results in a more conservative threshold, and even in regular clinical evaluations, they often use 90% confidence intervals (e.g., around obtained standard scores). It is important to realize that the basic evidentiary standard in civil personal injury cases is whether something is "more likely than not," or whether the "preponderance of the evidence" supports a specific position. Essentially, that translates into anything that is ≥ 51% likely. The standard is different if the neuropsychologist gets asked about a "reasonable degree of scientific/neuropsychological certainty." In such instances, one can assume a 90% certainty level (Kagehiro, 1990). It is typically a good idea for pediatric neuropsychologists to qualify their professional opinions with reference to a degree of certainty or a degree to which the phenomenon deviates from expected patterns. For example, if two tests have 95% specificities based on various independent empirical studies, then "positive" findings on both tests in the same child with mTBI would typically be expected less than 1% of the time ($0.05 \times 0.05 = .0025$). Phrasing this in the report or during testimony as something that would most likely occur in less than 3 out of every 1,000 patients places the information in a context that is intelligible to those who are not experts in psychometrics.

The most common roles that pediatric neuropsychologists are likely to play in a case of civil litigation pertaining to alleged sequelae of mTBI are those of a fact witness or an expert witness (Greiffenstein & Cohen, 2005). If the neuropsychologist has been a treating doctor, then he or she will most likely be called as a fact witness, whereas an expert witness is retained by an attorney to provide an independent opinion about the child's neuropsychological status without entering into a doctor–patient relationship. Although a fact witness can technically speak directly only to the actual findings in this particular client, an expert witness has more leeway to offer professional opinions that include attribution of causality and discussion of the consensus in the literature. In reality, these lines are often blurred, and neuropsychologists are typically treated as experts by most magistrates and judges. However, it is very important to avoid dual relationships, as stated in standard 3.05(a) of the APA ethics code (2002). Therefore, a pediatric neuropsychologist who has at one time evaluated a child with mTBI at the request of a primary care physician (i.e., a regular clinical referral, resulting in a doctor–patient relationship) should definitely not later accept a referral from the attorney who represents the parents of the child in a personal injury lawsuit, for an "expert" evaluation.

It is crucial for pediatric neuropsychologists to (1) accept only forensic referrals that are actually within their boundaries of professional competence, and (2) be reasonably familiar with judicial and administrative rules affecting their forensic work, as documented in standards 2.01(a) and 2.01(f) of the APA ethics code (2002). Therefore, a person with little or no training in TBI, and who almost exclusively sees children with learning disability in his or her private practice, should most likely decline a request for an independent medicolegal evaluation of a child with mTBI. At the same time, a pediatric neuropsychologist with considerable experience in the evaluation of the entire range of TBI severities should, after agreeing to an expert role, make sure he or she understands how the local legal system works.

At the time of the initial contact with the referring attorney or other agent, the pediatric neuropsychologist needs to ascertain that he or she can conduct an unbiased and objective examination, with access to relevant records as well as the child with mTBI. Fees and/or retainers for services should also be made explicit at that time. Sometimes the neuropsychologist will simply be asked to do a records review, which is permissible as long as he or she documents the limits this places on his or her ability to actually make diagnostic impressions, consistent with standards 9.01(b) and 9.01(c) of the APA ethics code (2002). More often, though, the request is for an actual neuropsychological evaluation. Details of that process are discussed below.

A particular challenge that is unique to forensic evaluations is that the pediatric neuropsychologist may receive a request from the opposing attorney for the presence of a third-party observer during the evaluation. Magistrates and judges may have considerable leeway in the degree to which they allow such a presence, but this varies considerably from state to state, so familiarity with local jurisdictions is needed. With that reservation in mind, it is highly advisable for the pediatric neuropsychologist to object to the presence of third-party observers during the actual psychometric assessment process, because of the deviation from standardized procedures and the likely confounding impact on the behavior of the examinee. Several professional organizations, including the National Academy of Neuropsychology (2000) and the American Academy of Clinical Neuropsychology (2001), have issued position papers to this effect. However, it is typically more persuasive to also cite, in a notarized affidavit, some empirical literature that documents the perils and negative influences associated with third-party observers (e.g., Constantinou, Ashendorf, & McCaffrey, 2005; Lynch, 2005). Most often, attorneys are agreeable to limiting the presence of a third person to the interview, with no subsequent direct observation or electronic recordings during the actual test administration; however, this is not universal. Howe and McCaffrey (2010) provide further suggestions about how to deal with third-party observer requests.

Following the evaluation, the neuropsychologist is typically expected to prepare a report, although the retaining attorney may sometimes request that this be deferred until he or she and the neuropsychologist have verbally discussed the findings. When a report is prepared, the neuropsychologist can send this only to his or her client (i.e., the agent who retained the neuropsychologist) and cannot share it routinely with the child's parents in the absence of a valid subpoena or court order. The report should be evidence-based and explain in professional yet intelligible language if the child has any current neuropsychological deficits and to what degree those are related to mTBI or other factors.

At some point after completion of the evaluation, the pediatric neuropsychologist is likely to be asked to provide some kind of sworn testimony about the case. This testimony can be in the form of a deposition, where only attorneys from both sides of the case plus a court recorder are present, or an actual court room appearance during trial in front of a judge and/or jury. Some depositions are videotaped for later presentation at trial in lieu of live testimony. It is far more common for neuropsychologists to give deposition than live trial testimony because a lot of mTBI cases get settled out of court. It should be noted that the entire file of the pediatric neuropsychologist on the case in question is "discoverable" as part of the deposition or trial process; i.e., the opposing attorney has the right to inspect the complete file.

With both deposition and trial testimony, there are direct examination and cross-examination phases. The former occurs by the retaining attorney and serves to establish the pediatric neuropsychologist's qualifications and to elicit definitive statements about the degree to which the child has any neuropsychological sequelae of mTBI. The cross-examination is performed by the opposing attorney and is designed to demonstrate either weaknesses in the doctor's expertise or impartiality or to challenge his or her conclusions. During this entire process, it is important for the pediatric neuropsychologist to understand that he or she is primarily there to assist the trier of fact (i.e., a jury or judge), and that tough or challenging questions by attorneys are part of their trade and are most often not to be taken personally. The best testimony comes from pediatric neuropsychologists who (1) are thoroughly prepared, with recent review of their own case file as well as awareness of the current state of the art of the literature on pediatric mTBI; (2) are capable of prompt and active answering in a way that is responsive to the question while also addressing ambiguities or possible misperceptions; (3) maintain a calm and professional composure without being completely devoid of emotion; and (4) are familiar with common courtroom strategies or gambits (see section on "Practical Suggestions" below).

NEUROPSYCHOLOGICAL ASSESSMENT

A forensic neuropsychological evaluation of a child with mTBI needs to start off with a clear question: What is the purpose of the evaluation? Sometimes an insurance company may want a delineation of the degree to which a child's reported current neurobehavioral problems are due to mTBI as opposed to a known premorbid history of learning disability or family psychiatric history. In other instances, an attorney may be looking for some kind of statement with regard to the child's future ability to drive a car or hold a competitive job. Obtaining from the referring agent a specific set of questions for the evaluation will allow the neuropsychologist to understand what issues will be brought to the trier of fact. This knowledge may facilitate inclusion in the report of specific language that speaks to those issues in a way that nonpsychologists can understand. This does not mean that the neuropsychologist has to limit him- or herself to the insurance company's or the attorney's issues, or that he or she should feel forced to answer questions that are outside his or her area of expertise. For example, even if the referral questions are all about cognition, that does not allow the neuropsychologist to simply ignore emotional–behavioral functioning. Pediatric neuropsychologists should also be clear about their boundaries of expertise—for example, that they cannot comment with scientific certainty on the healing time of a femur fracture. In addition, they should be careful not to make substantive predictions about likely adult outcomes without explaining the associated margin of error and the limited degree of empirical foundation for such long-term estimates.

Once the reason for referral is clear, and once all the contingencies regarding fees and other professional relationships are mutually understood, the neuropsychologist should request from the referring agent any and all relevant medical and academic records. It may be helpful to define *relevant*. For example, in the case of mTBI, it would be typical to review the day-of-injury emergency room report and any neuroimaging findings, but the neuropsychologist may not need to read all the records about the ingrown toenail that the child had 3 years previously. In contrast, premorbid medical and academic records pertaining to treatment for any kind of emotional or learning disorder should routinely be reviewed. Exclusive reliance on postinjury neuropsychological test scores is grossly insufficient in cases with prior psychiatric or special education histories (Donders & Strom, 2000; Farmer et al., 2002). More recent research has also demonstrated that standardized postinjury parental ratings of the daily functioning of children with mTBI who had a premorbid history of attention-deficit/hyperactivity disorder (ADHD) or psychiatric treatment were essentially indistinguishable from the corresponding parental ratings of children with severe TBI who did not have any such premorbid histories (Donders, DenBraber, & Vos, 2010). *Bottom line*: A pediatric forensic neuropsychological evaluation needs to include a thorough review of academic as well as relevant medical records. If the child has already undergone a prior evaluation with a different neuropsychologist, it is standard of care to request the associated report as well as the raw data.

When the child is brought in for the evaluation, it is incumbent on the neuropsychologist to obtain informed consent from the parent or guardian, as well as assent from the child, in a language that they can understand, consistent with standard 3.10(a–d) of the APA ethics code (2002). Sample consent forms are available from the website of the National Academy of Neuropsychology (*www.nanonline.org*). The specific contingencies of the medicolegal context that make the evaluation different from a normal doctor–patient relationship should be made very clear. This includes explanation of the limits of confidentiality as well as clarification of who the client is, and that the neuropsychologist can typically not initiate new treatment or even discuss the test results.

Although neuropsychologists are often known for pouring on the tests, it is typically much more advisable to start the forensic evaluation of the child with mTBI with a thorough history. This should address the child's prenatal environment, early development, subsequent psychosocial adjustment, any prior medical events, educational experiences, and recent stressors that the child or family may have experienced that could confound the current presentation. Family socioeconomic status, genetic as well as social history, and coping style should also be explored. All of this is important because there is research to suggest that the relative risk for suboptimal outcome after mTBI is increased in children with premorbid complications such as special education history or family dysfunction (Ponsford et al., 1999). If permissible under the arrangement of the evaluation (and this needs to be determined a priori with the referring agent), obtaining collateral information through standardized rating scales that can be completed by school teachers can also be very helpful.

It is not unusual for the pediatric neuropsychologists to face barriers when performing his or her "usual" intake during a forensic evaluation. For example, a plaintiff's attorney may object to the inquiry about any kind of family medical history when the examination is performed by an expert who was retained by the defense. Families may consequently decline to answer such questions, or a judge may even order such inquiry off limits. Under such circumstances it is important for the neuropsychologist to (1) respect any boundaries imposed by a judge, (2) clearly note these restrictions in the report, and (3) explain in the same report how those restrictions limit the scope of the conclusions that can be made on the basis of an essentially incomplete evaluation.

There is no single test or battery that can be considered required or to be superior to all others for the neuropsychological evaluation of children with mTBI. That being said, it is advisable to assure that the evaluation is sufficiently comprehensive and that the chosen measures have established reliability and validity in the assessment of pediatric TBI. For example, it would be easy to defend the choice of the California Verbal Learning Test—Children's version (CVLT-C; Delis, Kramer, Kaplan, & Ober, 1994), given that this instrument has been standardized and norm-referenced not only nationally but also extensively researched with regard to its construct and criterion validity in children with TBI (Donders & Nesbit-Greene, 2004; Miller & Donders, 2003; Mottram & Donders, 2005). However, such information is not available for all pediatric neuropsychological tests, and it would also not do to limit the evaluation or the interpretation to only one instrument. In general, it is advisable to make sure that the assessment includes instruments that (1) capture the domains that are most likely to be affected by mTBI (see Bodin & Shay, Chapter 13, this volume), and that (2) are commonly accepted in the scientific and clinical community (Greiffenstein & Cohen, 2005). Formal tabletop tests should also be supplemented with standardized rating scales of daily functioning because of concerns about the ecological validity of exclusively laboratory-based assessments (Silver, 2000) and also because subjectively distressing or concerning symptoms may be reported by parents, even when cognitive test scores are fairly unremarkable, particularly in cases of mTBI (Gioia, Isquith, Schneider, & Vaughan, 2009).

There is now sufficient evidence to suggest that inclusion of objective measures of symptom validity should be an integral part of forensic neuropsychological evaluations of children with mTBI. Kirkwood and Kirk (2010) recently found that a sizable minority (17%) of a 3-year series of consecutive clinically referred children with complicated and uncomplicated mTBI failed actuarial effort criteria. That translates into one out of every six examinees. The vast majority of these cases did not involve litigation or other external incentives, which suggests that they simply were not putting forth good effort—for reasons that were not always clearly evident. Failure to take such test-taking behavior into account is prone to lead to diagnostic errors. It has been established that several symptom validity tests that were originally developed for use with adults can easily be passed by children with serious neurological compromise. For example, the Test of Memory Malingering (TOMM; Tombaugh, 1996) and the Medical Symptom Validity Test (MSVT; Green, 2004) are both associated with a ≥ 95% specificity in children with various neurological disorders (Carone, 2008) and specifically those with TBI (Donders, 2005). Therefore, application of those instruments in pediatric samples is justified by the empirical literature. Failure of actuarial validity criteria on the TOMM or MSVT in school-age children with mTBI is strongly suggestive of invalid test results. That does not necessarily mean that the child was malingering, but it does mean that something else, other than cerebral compromise, was confounding his or her performance.

As was suggested previously, inclusion of standardized rating scales that can be completed by parents can be a helpful component of the diagnostic process. However, particularly in a forensic context, it is advisable to choose instruments that have checks and balances built in for possible overly negative or inconsistent reporting by parents. For example, during a recent study of parental ratings on the Behavioral Rating Inventory of Executive Function (Gioia, Isquith, Guy, & Kenworthy, 2000) in a 4-year consecutive series of clinically referred children with TBI, almost 8% of the profiles had to be eliminated because of invalid responding (Donders et al., 2010).

During the evaluation, it is important to record behavioral observations. These can range from descriptions of how the child reacted to test failure to documentation of spontaneous comments that the child made about peer and family dynamics. Behaviors that may affect success on tests, such as apparent or subjectively reported pain or sleep, should be accounted for. At a minimum, the neuropsychologist should be able to comment on the child's general appearance, affect, speech, and whether the child's general sensory and motor abilities appeared sufficient for the purposes of the assessment. It should be realized that observations are just that: documentation of potentially relevant information, but not necessarily proof of a specific interpretation. For example, poor grooming might be due to a host of factors, ranging from socioeconomic family stress to parental neglect to teenage rebelliousness. It is the task of the pediatric neuropsychologist to objectively integrate observations with quantifiable data and historical records.

INTERPRETIVE ISSUES

Various issues need to be carefully considered when interpreting data from a forensic pediatric neuropsychological evaluation. Assuming that there is objective evidence that the data can be considered valid, and that relevant premorbid history and behavioral observations during assessment have been duly considered, the neuropsychologist must keep a number of important principles in mind.

Base Rates

One important consideration is that of base rates. Symptoms that are common shortly after mTBI, such as irritability or headaches, are not specific to this condition and actually occur with considerable frequency in the general population (Nacajauskaite,

Endziniene, Jureniene, & Schrader, 2006). Therefore, reverse reasoning on the basis of subjective symptoms is not scientifically sound. This consideration is likely to become increasingly important with longer time spans between the occurrence of the mTBI and the neuropsychological evaluation. For example, it may be tempting to attribute a depressive disorder in an adolescent to an mTBI that occurred 3 years previously, just because that happens to be the only "positive" medical history finding. However, to do so would ignore the fact that, at any time, approximately 1 out of every 10 children and adolescents will have a psychiatric disorder that causes sufficient distress or social impairment to warrant treatment, and that about 1 in every 3 will have at least one brief period of psychiatric impairment during childhood, most often in the absence of any head trauma (Costello, Mustillo, Erkanli, Keeler, & Angold, 2003; Ford, Goodman, & Meltzer, 2003).

Base rates also need to be considered when determining whether a "statistically significant" discrepancy between two test scores, or even the presence of a single "impaired" score, has any clinical significance, let alone a causal relationship to the mTBI. If the neuropsychologist just administers more and more tests, it is just about inevitable that at least a few of the obtained scores or discrepancies are going to appear abnormal. In fact, it has been demonstrated that the majority of presumably normal children will have at least one or two scores in the "impaired" range on a test with multiple variables (Brooks, Iverson, Sherman, & Holdnack, 2009a). The same applies when patterns of performance are considered. For example, a profile of Verbal Comprehension < Perceptual Reasoning by 13 points is statistically significant at any age level in the standardization sample of the Wechsler Intelligence Scale for Children—Fourth Edition (WISC-IV; Wechsler, 2003) but a discrepancy of that magnitude or greater also has a base rate of 18% in that same standardization sample. This base rate indicates that such a pattern is not uncommon in neurologically healthy children and therefore not necessarily indicative of acquired pathology in a child with mTBI. This point is not to suggest that the pediatric neuropsychologist should just ignore norms or any aberrant scores. However, it does mean that caution is needed with the overinterpretation of isolated poor scores or performance discrepancies, and that the data need to be interpreted, whenever possible, in the context of known base rates in the general population as well as the rest of the neuropsychological evaluation. In the context of the above-described WISC-IV profile, the case for a deficit related to mTBI could be made more convincingly if the child's premorbid school records demonstrated above-average performance in language subjects and if the current neuropsychological evaluation yielded quantitative evidence for selective fine motor impairment on the right side of the body.

Premorbid Status

Another important psychometric issue is the estimation of a child's premorbid status. As was stated above, review of prior academic records needs to be performed routinely, but in most cases that present for forensic pediatric neuropsychological assessment, there will be no prior IQ or neuropsychological test scores. Methods have therefore been developed to estimate premorbid intelligence in children on the basis of demographic and postinjury WISC-IV variables (e.g., Schoenberg, Lange, Brickell, & Saklofske, 2007; Schoenberg, Lange, Saklofske, Suarez, & Brickell, 2008). These actuarial algorithms do not include WISC-IV subtests such as Coding or Symbol

Search, which is important because those are the very ones with the most sensitivity to severity of TBI (Donders & Janke, 2008). Instead, they include subtests of "crystallized" skills that are relatively more robust to the effect of TBI (e.g., Information) and therefore more appropriate to include in estimates of premorbid functioning. However, it still needs to be realized that such algorithms yield estimates that are associated with standard errors of estimation of about two-thirds of a standard deviation (*SD*), yielding 90% confidence intervals that are typically ± one *SD*. It is important for the pediatric neuropsychologist to appreciate this wide margin of error, in order to avoid drawing inaccurate conclusions about the premorbid level of functioning of a child with mTBI.

Measurement Error

Measurement error also needs to be considered carefully in case of repeat assessments. It is common in a forensic context for a child with mTBI to have undergone at least one prior neuropsychological evaluation. Readministering the same test can be problematic if the prior exposure really alters the basic nature of the test and is therefore associated with large practice effects. For example, an adolescent who was exposed to the Wisconsin Card Sorting Test within the past 6–12 months is very likely to do much better during a second administration because of the prior experience with what was originally a more ambiguous problem-solving task (Basso, Bornstein, & Lang, 1999). Furthermore, no neuropsychological test has perfect reliability, and even neurologically healthy children may demonstrate considerable variability in performance on tests that, on face value, may not appear to be as prone to practice effects (Zabel, von Thomsen, Cole, Martin, & Mahone, 2009). This does not mean that such tests can never be readministered, but the pediatric neuropsychologist should do so with caution, not repeating every single task while also including some "new" measures in order to get a broader and more accurate impression of the child's current status. Several methods, including reliable change and regression approaches, have been described in the literature to evaluate whether change in pediatric psychometric test performance over time is statistically reliable and clinically meaningful (for a review, see Brooks, Strauss, Sherman, Iverson, & Slick, 2009b).

Psychosocial Stressors

A final issue that is crucial to consider during the interpretive process is the influence of psychosocial stressors, occurring either at the time of the original mTBI or that may have affected the child within a relatively close time window, before and/or after the injury. Children can be affected by a host of family stressors, ranging from parental unemployment to sibling terminal illness. However, in the context of mTBI, one confounding factor that often comes up in forensic neuropsychological evaluations is posttraumatic stress disorder (PTSD). Children with mTBI can develop symptoms of PTSD because they may have witnessed a vehicle coming toward them at high speed just before impact, or family members being injured or killed. Research has shown that PTSD is common in children after motor vehicle accidents but that the presence or absence of mTBI has little influence on the presence or degree of PTSD symptomatology (Mather, Tate, & Hannan, 2003). At the same time, subjective symptoms of mTBI and PTSD are known to be correlated but not redundant with each other in children (Hajek et al., 2010). Since pediatric PTSD is, in and by itself, often associated with impairments of attention, memory, and/or executive functioning (Beers & De Bellis, 2002; Moradi, Doost, Taghavi, Yule, & Dalgleish, 1999), the forensic neuropsychologist must be extra careful in the diagnostic process when evaluating children in whom the differential of mTBI and PTSD is an issue.

PRACTICAL SUGGESTIONS

Brodsky (1991, 1999, 2004) has written a series of very practical books about testifying during depositions or trials, and they are recommended reading for any pediatric neuropsychologist venturing into the forensic arena. Other reasonable and pragmatic recommendations for this purpose are provided by Greiffenstein and Kaufmann (2012) and by Tsushima and Anderson (1996). This section draws heavily from their collective wisdom, as well as from my personal experience with medicolegal cases of mTBI. The following should not be misconstrued as either legal advice or as foolproof instruction for how to be invincible in the forensic arena. These guidelines are simply offered as practical suggestions for consideration. In addition, in a chapter like this, it is not possible to cover every possible deposition or courtroom strategy or dilemma, so only the most common ones that often arise in the context of civil litigation regarding pediatric mTBI are discussed.

The first rule of thumb is to keep any written documentation as objective as possible. If a child with mTBI was found to be violating validity criteria on the TOMM, it is ill advised to simply call the child a malingerer or to berate his or her assumed dishonesty. Instead, the pediatric neuropsychologist should objectively document the nature and implications of this finding in factual terms that are devoid of emotional overtones. For example:

> "On a forced-choice picture recognition task where the chances of getting the answers right were equal to the flip of a coin, John answered correctly only 30% of the time, which is statistically significantly worse than chance. That means that a person who had just turned his or her back to the table, never saw the pictures, and just randomly guessed at the answers would likely have done better than John did on this visual test."

A related maxim is to remain professional, both in writing and during sworn testimony, about any difference in opinion with another neuropsychologist. Often, the opposing side in a lawsuit will enter into evidence an evaluation by the child's treating doctor or by a third, independent expert, who may very well have come to a different diagnostic conclusion. It is advisable to maintain the high road in these kinds of situations and to avoid derisive comments or guild squabbles (e.g., about differences in board certification) that are likely to be perceived as childish or nitpicky by juries. For example, the pediatric neuropsychologist may be asked if he or she would not agree that a treating doctor who has seen the child multiple times would be in a better position to make an accurate diagnosis than a "hired gun who has only once done a very limited evaluation of this child." Rather than touting the superiority of his or her own training, or dismissing the other neuropsychologist as an enmeshed quack who cannot tell a cucumber from a frontal lobe, the pediatric neuropsychologist should correct any latent misconceptions and restate the basis for his or her professional opinion. For example:

> "With the understanding that I base my opinions simply on the facts in evidence, and distinctly not because anybody offered me money for them, I respectfully disagree with the premise that just because Dr. Smith has seen John more than once makes her a better judge of his current test performance. For example, if one doctor looks at an X-ray of a bone, he or she should be able to see the same fracture, regardless of whether he or she knew the child from before. It is the same with the interpretation of John's performance during the very comprehensive assessment that I performed."

Often, the pediatric neuropsychologist will be asked whether he or she is familiar with the work of Dr. X and whether he or she would consider it to be "authoritative." Simply saying "yes" to that question will likely be used as an implication that the witness will defer to specific opinions that are stated in that particularly referenced work, sometimes presented out of context. Instead, the pediatric neuropsychologist can acknowledge the presence and level of importance of the work, while still making it clear that it is not the word of God. An effective answer may be:

> "I am well aware of Dr. X's book and I have even found it helpful in some cases, just like I rely on hundreds of other writings to stay informed about the field of traumatic brain injury, but that does not mean that I necessarily agree with everything Dr. X has written. If you want me to comment on any particular part of his book, I would be happy to do so if you just give me a minute to read that section again."

Another common scenario is that the pediatric neuropsychologist is asked whether it isn't "possible" that this particular child might be an outlier who deviates from the norm of what would often be expected after mTBI, and if that is indeed possible, does that not actually demonstrate the severity of his or her impairment? It is important to avoid coming across as dismissive or too authoritarian. However, at the same time, simply acknowledging that something is "possible," without further qualification, is likely to be perceived or misconstrued as supporting a position that may be in conflict with the witness' actual opinion. The following are examples of this dilemma, and some ways to deal with them.

Q: Isn't it possible, doctor, to have severe brain damage even though there was no loss of consciousness?

A: It is indeed possible to experience some brain injury without it resulting in coma, but this would be very unusual if there was also no memory loss for the event and especially when neuroimaging was also normal. This particular child was able to remember all the circumstances surrounding her fall, and she had an unremarkable CT scan in the emergency room, and again 1 month later. That would make it extremely unlikely that she sustained the kind of severe brain damage that you referred to.

Q: But, Doctor, you evaluated this child within less than 1 year after her injury. Isn't it possible that she might have much more serious problems when she gets older, like 5 or 10 years from now?

A: I cannot rule it out with 100% certainty, but I would consider it highly unlikely.

Q: But it is possible, correct?

A: Possible but extremely unlikely.

Sometimes, attorneys will insist on phrasing issues in extreme terms or insist on a "yes" versus "no" answer. If the matter is too complex or delicate for such purposes, the pediatric neuropsychologist should attempt to preface his or her answer with a dependent clause, in a way that shows responsiveness to the original question while leaving room to subsequently elaborate with a strong statement that more accurately reflects his or her expert opinion. Words such as *although* and *whereas* are often effective in this regard. If the attorney interrupts and insists on a dichotomous answer, the pediatric neuropsychologist should calmly state that he or she is not comfortable with this and has a need to explain matters. If the attorney still persists, the pediatric neuropsychologist has the option, during a deposition, of refusing to answer or, during a trial, to turn to the judge.

Q: Doctor, please answer me with "yes" or "no" to the following questions. Is it your testimony that my client sustained an uncomplicated mild traumatic brain injury in the motor vehicle accident of November 27, 2010?

A: Yes.

Q: And is it your testimony that the vast majority of children with uncomplicated mild traumatic brain injury do not have problems for more than a few weeks or months?

A: Yes.

Q: But do you agree that there are *some* children with uncomplicated mild traumatic brain injury who continue to have problems for much longer, even years after injury?

A: Although there is a tiny minority . . .

Q: "Yes" or "no," Doctor!

A: I cannot answer that with a simple "yes" or "no," and would like to explain why.

Q: I am asking the questions here, they are very simple questions, and I am instructing you to answer "yes" or "no."

A: [deposition variant] In that case I am going to decline to answer and suggest that we get a ruling from the judge upon this before we proceed any further.

A: [trial variant] Your Honor, if it pleases the court, I would really like to qualify my answer with a very brief explanation because I am concerned that otherwise, it could be misleading or confusing to the jury. I will be careful not to take too much of the court's valuable time.

A: [after permission has been granted by the judge] Although the research shows that there is a very small percentage of children with uncomplicated mild traumatic brain injury who continue to have longer-term problems, this research also shows that those children typically have a lot of other things going against them, like a severe learning disability before the accident, or coming from an environment that is not very healthy. In this particular case, the unfortunate facts are that the police had been called to the home several times, both before and after the accident, because of neighbors' concerns about domestic violence. In my professional opinion, that has a lot more to do with the fact that this child continues to have adjustment problems than his uncomplicated mild traumatic brain injury does.

When the deposition or trial testimony has concluded, the pediatric neuropsychologist should leave the proceedings in a dignified manner. Shaking hands, not only with the retaining attorney but also with the opposing attorney, would show professional courtesy at the end of a deposition. In a court room, after having been excused, the pediatric neuropsychologist may simply say "Thank you, your Honor," briefly nod to the jury, and then walk out without further interaction with the attorneys from either side. In order to maintain one's own level of professional distance and scientific objectivity, it is also highly advisable not to try to find out later who "won" or how much money the plaintiff got. However, particularly for those who are novices to the legal arena, it may be helpful to have the deposition or court testimony observed by a senior colleague and to receive feedback on one's verbal and nonverbal demeanor during the proceedings, at some later point.

CONCLUSION

Pediatric neuropsychologists can make important contributions to the accurate evaluation of mTBI in a forensic context, as long as they adhere to an ethical and scientifically defensible approach, without personalized investment in the outcome of the legal proceedings. It is important to be aware of not only the current state of the literature on pediatric mTBI but also of basic legal contingencies and proceedings as well as of psychometric and interpretive pitfalls. Particular care must be taken to present information in a way that is intelligible to members of a jury, who are typically a cross-section of the local population. The pediatric neuropsychologist who offers reliable and evidence-based services to the legal system serves not only his or her own profession but also supports the principle of justice and protects the public.

REFERENCES

American Academy of Clinical Neuropsychology. (2001). Policy statement on the presence of third party observers in neuropsychological assessment. *The Clinical Neuropsychologist, 15,* 433–439.

American Psychological Association. (2002). Ethical principles of psychologists and code of conduct. *American Psychologist, 57,* 1060–1073.

Attix, D. K., Donders, J., Johnson-Greene, D., Grote, C. L., Harris, J. G., & Bauer, R. M.

(2007). Disclosure of neuropsychological test data: Official position of Division 40 (Clinical Neuropsychology) of the American Psychological Association, Association of Postdoctoral Programs in Clinical Neuropsychology, and American Academy of Clinical Neuropsychology. *The Clinical Neuropsychologist, 21,* 232–238.

Babikian, T., & Asarnow, R. (2009). Neurocognitive outcomes and recovery after pediatric TBI: Meta-analytic review of the literature. *Neuropsychology, 23,* 283–296.

Basso, M. R., Bornstein, R. A., & Lang, J. M. (1999). Practice effects on commonly used measures of executive function across twelve months. *Clinical Neuropsychologist, 13,* 283–292.

Beers, S. R., & De Bellis, M. D. (2002). Neuropsychological function in children with maltreatment-related posttraumatic stress disorder. *American Journal of Psychiatry, 159,* 483–486.

Brodsky, S. L. (1991). *Testifying in court: Guidelines and maxims for the expert witness.* Washington, DC: American Psychological Association.

Brodsky, S. L. (1999). *The expert witness: More maxims and guidelines for testifying in court.* Washington, DC: American Psychological Association.

Brodsky, S. L. (2004). *Coping with cross-examination and other pathways to effective testimony.* Washington, DC: American Psychological Association.

Brooks, B. L., Iverson, G., Sherman, E., & Holdnack, J. (2009a). Healthy children and adolescents obtain some low scores across a battery of memory tests. *Journal of the International Neuropsychological Society, 15,* 613–617.

Brooks, B. L., Strauss, E., Sherman, E. M. S., Iverson, G. L., & Slick, D. J. (2009b). Developments in neuropsychological assessment: Refining psychometric and clinical interpretive methods. *Canadian Psychology, 50,* 196–209.

Carone, D. A. (2008). Children with moderate/severe brain damage/dysfunction outperform adults with mild-to-no brain damage on the Medical Symptom Validity Test. *Brain Injury, 22,* 960–971.

Constantinou, M., Ashendorf, L., & McCaffrey, R. J. (2005). Effects of a third-party observer during neuropsychological assessment: When the observer is a video camera. *Journal of Forensic Neuropsychology, 4,* 39–48.

Costello, E. J., Mustillo, S., Erkanli, A., Keeler, G., & Angold, A. (2003). Prevalence and development of psychiatric disorders in childhood and adolescence. *Archives of General Psychiatry, 60,* 837–844.

Delis, D. C., Kramer, J. H., Kaplan, E., & Ober, B. A. (1994). *California Verbal Learning Test—Children's Version.* Austin, TX: Psychological Corporation.

Donders, J. (2005). Performance on the Test of Memory Malingering in a mixed pediatric sample. *Child Neuropsychology, 11,* 221–227.

Donders, J. (2012). Forensic aspects of pediatric traumatic brain injury. In G. Larrabee (Ed.), *Forensic neuropsychology: A scientific approach* (2nd ed., pp. 211–230). New York: Oxford University Press.

Donders, J., DenBraber, D., & Vos, L. (2010). Construct and criterion validity of the Behavior Rating Inventory of Executive Function (BRIEF) in children referred for neuropsychological assessment after pediatric traumatic brain injury. *Journal of Neuropsychology, 4,* 197–209.

Donders, J., & Janke, K. (2008). Criterion validity of the Wechsler Intelligence Scale for Children—Fourth Edition after pediatric traumatic brain injury. *Journal of the International Neuropsychological Society, 14,* 651–655.

Donders, J., & Nesbit-Greene, K. (2004). Predictors of neuropsychological test performance after pediatric traumatic brain injury. *Assessment, 11,* 275–284.

Donders, J., & Strom, D. (2000). Neurobehavioral recovery after pediatric head trauma: Injury, pre-injury, and post-injury issues. *Journal of Head Trauma Rehabilitation, 15,* 792–803.

Farmer, J. E., Kanne, S. M., Haut, J. S., Williams, J., Johnstone, B., & Kirk, K. (2002). Memory functioning following traumatic brain injury in children with premorbid learning problems. *Developmental Neuropsychology, 22,* 455–469.

Ford, T., Goodman, R., & Meltzer, H. (2003). The British child and adolescent mental health survey 1999: The prevalence of DSM-IV disorders. *Journal of the American Academy of Child and Adolescent Psychiatry, 42,* 1203–1211.

Gioia, G. A., Isquith, P. K., Guy, S. C., & Kenworthy, L. (2000). *Behavior Rating Inventory of Executive Function.* Odessa, FL: Psychological Assessment Resources.

Gioia, G. A., Isquith, P. K., Schneider, J. C., & Vaughan, C. G. (2009). New approaches to assessment and monitoring of concussion in children. *Topics in Language Disorders, 29,* 266–281.

Green, P. (2004). *Green's Medical Symptom Validity Test.* Edmonton, AB: Author.

Greiffenstein, M. F. (2008). Basics of forensic neuropsychology. In J. E. Morgan & J. H. Ricker (Eds.), *Textbook of clinical neuropsychology* (pp. 905–941). New York: Taylor & Francis.

Greiffenstein, M. F., & Cohen, L. (2005). Neuropsychology and the law: Principles of productive attorney–neuropsychologist relations. In G. L. Larrabee (Ed.), *Forensic neuropsychology: A scientific approach* (pp. 29–91). New York: Oxford University Press.

Greiffenstein, M. F., & Kaufmann, P. M. (2012). Neuropsychology and the law: Principles of productive attorney-neuropsychologist relations. In G. L. Larrabee (Ed.), *Forensic neuropsychology: A scientific approach* (2nd ed., pp. 23–69). New York: Oxford University Press.

Hajek, C. A., Yeates, K. O., Taylor, H. G., Bangert, B., Dietrich, A., Nuss, K. E., et al. (2010). Relationships among post-concussive symptoms and symptoms of PTSD in children following mild traumatic brain injury. *Brain Injury, 24,* 100–109.

Howe, L. L. S., & McCaffrey, R. J. (2010). Third-party observation during neuropsychological evaluation: An update on the literature, practical advice for practitioners, and future directions. *The Clinical Neuropsychologist, 24,* 518–537.

Kagehiro, D. (1990). Defining the standard of proof in jury instructions. *Psychological Science, 1,* 194–200.

Kirkwood, M. W., & Kirk, J. W. (2010). The base rate of suboptimal effort in a pediatric mild TBI sample: Performance on the Medical Symptom Validity Test. *The Clinical Neuropsychologist, 24,* 860–872.

Kirkwood, M. W., Yeates, K. O., Taylor, H. G., Randolph, C., McCrea, M., & Anderson, V. A. (2008). Management of pediatric mild traumatic brain injury: A neuropsychological review from injury through recovery. *The Clinical Neuropsychologist, 22,* 769–800.

Lynch, J. K. (2005). Effects of a third-party observer on neuropsychological test performance following closed head injury. *Journal of Forensic Neuropsychology, 4,* 17–25.

Mather, F. J., Tate, R. L., & Hannan, T. J. (2003). Post-traumatic stress disorder in children following road traffic accidents: A comparison of those with and without mild traumatic brain injury. *Brain Injury, 17,* 1077–1087.

Miller, L. J., & Donders, J. (2003). Prediction of educational outcome after pediatric traumatic brain injury. *Rehabilitation Psychology, 48,* 237–241.

Moradi, A. R., Doost, H. T. N., Taghavi, M. R., Yule, W., & Dalgleish, T. (1999). Everyday memory deficits in children and adolescents with PTSD: Performance on the Rivermead Behavioral Memory Test. *Journal of Child Psychology and Psychiatry, 40,* 357–361.

Mottram, L., & Donders, J. (2005). Construct validity of the California Verbal Learning Test—Children's Version (CVLT-C) after pediatric traumatic brain injury. *Psychological Assessment, 17,* 212–217.

Nacajauskaite, O., Endziniene, J., Jureniene, K., & Schrader, H. (2006). The validity of post-concussion syndrome in children: A controlled historical cohort study. *Brain and Development, 28,* 507–514.

National Academy of Neuropsychology. (2000). Presence of third-party observers during neuropsychological testing: Official statement of the National Academy of Neuropsychology. *Archives of Clinical Neuropsychology, 15,* 379–380.

Ponsford, J., Wilmott, C., Rothwell, A., Cameron, P., Ayton, G., Nelms, R., et al. (1999). Cognitive and behavioral outcome following mild traumatic brain injury in children. *Journal of Head Trauma Rehabilitation, 14,* 360–372.

Schoenberg, M. R., Lange, R. T., Brickell, T. A., & Saklofske, D. H. (2007). Estimating premorbid general cognitive functioning for children and adolescents using the American Wechsler Intelligence Scale for Children—Fourth Edition: Demographic and current performance approaches. *Journal of Child Neurology, 22,* 379–388.

Schoenberg, M. R., Lange, R. T., Saklofske, D. H., Suarez, M., & Brickell, T. A. (2008). Validation of the child premorbid intelligence estimate method to predict premorbid Wechsler Intelligence Scale for Children—Fourth Edition Full Scale IQ among children with brain injury. *Psychological Assessment, 20,* 377–384.

Silver, C. H. (2000). Ecological validity of neuropsychological assessment in childhood traumatic brain injury. *Journal of Head Trauma Rehabilitation, 15,* 973–988.

Sweet, J. J., Ecklund-Johnson, E., & Malina, A. (2008). Forensic neuropsychology: An overview of issues and directions. In J. E. Morgan & J. H. Ricker (Eds.), *Textbook of clinical neuropsychology* (pp. 869–890). New York: Taylor & Francis.

Sweet, J. J., & Moulthrop, M. A. (1999). Self-examination questions as a means of identifying bias in adversarial assessments. *Journal of Forensic Neuropsychology, 1,* 73–88.

Taylor, H. G., Dietrich, A., Nuss, K., Wright, M., Rusin, J., Bangert, B., et al. (2010). Postconcussive symptoms in children with mild traumatic brain injury. *Neuropsychology, 24,* 148–159.

Tombaugh, T. N. (1996). *Test of Memory Malingering.* Toronto, ON: Multi-Health Systems.

Tsushima, W. T., & Anderson, R. M. (1996). *Mastering expert testimony: A courtroom handbook for mental health professionals.* Mahwah, NJ: Erlbaum.

Van Gorp, W. G., & McMullen, W. J. (1997). Potential sources of bias in forensic neuropsychological evaluations. *The Clinical Neuropsychologist, 11,* 180–187.

Wechsler, D. (2003). *Wechsler Intelligence Scale for Children—Fourth Edition.* San Antonio, TX: Harcourt.

Yeates, K. O., Taylor, H. G., Rusin, J., Bangert, B., Dietrich, A. Nusss, K., et al. (2009). Longitudinal trajectories of post-concussive symptoms in children with mild traumatic brain injuries and their relationship to acute clinical status. *Pediatrics, 123,* 735–743.

Zabel, T. A., von Thomsen, C., Cole, C., Martin, R., & Mahone, M. (2009). Reliability concerns in the repeated computerized assessment of attention in children. *The Clinical Neuropsychologist, 23,* 1213–1231.

Index

Page numbers followed by t or f indicate tables and figures.